HANDBOOK OF NEUROPSYCHOLOGY, 2nd Edition

VOLUME 8, PART I

CHILD NEUROPSYCHOLOGY

# HANDBOOK OF NEUROPSYCHOLOGY, 2nd Edition

*Series Editors*

## FRANÇOIS BOLLER

INSERM, Unité 324, Centre Paul Broca, 75014 Paris, France

*and*

## JORDAN GRAFMAN

National Institute of Neurological Disorders and Stroke, National Institutes of Health, Bethesda, MD 20892, USA

Volume 8, Part I

# CHILD NEUROPSYCHOLOGY, PART I

*Editors*

## SID J. SEGALOWITZ

Department of Psychology, Brock University, 500 Glenridge Avenue, St. Catharines, ON L2S 3A1, Canada

*and*

## ISABELLE RAPIN

Department of Neurology, Albert Einstein College of Medicine, K 807, Bronx, NY 10461, USA

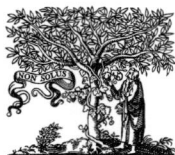

ELSEVIER

Amsterdam – Boston – London – New York – Oxford – Paris
San Diego – San Francisco – Singapore – Sydney – Tokyo
2002

ELSEVIER SCIENCE B.V.
Sara Burgerhartstraat 25
P.O. Box 211, 1000 AE Amsterdam, The Netherlands

First edition 1993
Second edition, first printing 2002

Library of Congress Cataloging in Publication Data
A catalog record from the Library of Congress has been applied for.

British Library Cataloguing in Publication Data
A catalogue record from the British Library has been applied for.

ISBN series 0 444 50376 5 (HB)
ISBN series 0 444 50377 3 (PB)
ISBN this edition (hardbound) 0 444 50364 1
ISBN this edition (paperback) 0 444 50373 0

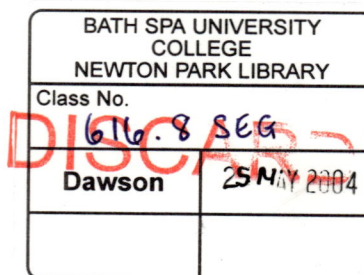

♾ The paper used in this publication meets the requirements of ANSI/NISO Z39.48-1992 (Permanence of Paper).
Printed in The Netherlands

# Preface

We are pleased to present the eighth volume of the second edition of the Handbook of Neuropsychology. As already demonstrated by the first edition and by the first seven volumes of the second edition of the Handbook, neuropsychology is a field of science that has undergone extraordinary growth and changes in recent years. Planning for the first edition of the Handbook started over sixteen years ago and even though the more recent volumes of the first edition were designed to reflect some of the changes that have taken place in the field of neuropsychology, we have decided, with the encouragement of the Publisher, that it would be worthwhile to prepare a new edition. As the series co-editors, we intend to ensure that the new edition of the Handbook of Neuropsychology remains the principal reference source in the field, continuing to provide comprehensive and current coverage of both experimental and clinical aspects of neuropsychology. To this end, we have asked the authoritative chapter authors to produce new in-depth reviews that go beyond a summary of their results and point of view. Each chapter is up-to-date, covering the latest developments in methodology and theory. Discussion of 'bedside' evaluations, laboratory techniques, as well as extensive discussions of theoretical models are all to be found in the Handbook. The Handbook also presents the latest findings and methodologies of functional neuroimaging techniques such as PET, fMRI, and transcranial magnetic stimulation (TMS).

We are confident that the Handbook will continue to be an essential reference source for clinicians such as neuropsychologists, neurologists, psychiatrists, and psychologists, as well as for all scientists engaged in research in the cognitive neurosciences. This second all-new edition is designed to update chapters covering research domains where considerable developments have occurred. In addition, there has been an in-depth reorganization of content areas that have spawned new approaches since the first edition. All the chapters included in this new edition will provide the most recent data and references for further studies and research.

The first volume included an Introduction section that focused on practical and theoretical issues of general interest. Two chapters covered, in a novel and comprehensive fashion, clinical evaluation and neuropsychological assessment, with an emphasis not so much on the description of tests, but on their rationale. One of the features of Neuropsychology in recent years has been the spectacular comeback of single case studies and that is why the chapter on statistical approaches compared statistical procedures appropriate for groups to those of single cases. Hemispheric specialization remains an important topic, which was examined in the introduction under two different points of view. One chapter summarized the contribution to neuropsychology provided by the commissurotomy ('split brain') model, while another chapter reviewed experimental assessments of hemispheric specialization in normal individuals. An introduction to current neuroimaging techniques used language disorders as an illustration.

Neurophysiological techniques were reviewed with an emphasis on evoked potentials (ERPs). Several chapters dealt with the application of theoretical models to neuropsychology including a discussion of the lesion method and of computer modeling.

In the first volume, the Introduction was followed by the Section on Attention edited by Giacomo Rizzolatti. It included four chapters. Two of them concerned selective attention.

The first was essentially devoted to visuospatial attentional phenomena, while the focus of the second was on the temporal aspects of attention. The phenomenon of failure to orient, neglect and neglect related phenomena was dealt with in the third chapter. This chapter included a large section devoted to the anatomical localization of lesions producing neglect in humans. Finally, the last chapter reviewed the anatomy and the neurophysiological properties of the circuits whose lesion produces neglect deficits in primates. In that chapter, the various theories of neglect were reviewed and their validity discussed from a neurophysiological perspective.

The second volume of the Handbook was a special 'in memoriam' volume. It was dedicated to the memory of Laird Cermak who, despite his grave illness, vigorously and resolutely took on the task of preparing a new section on memory and its disorders. The volume included chapters on animal models and neuropsychological assessment. Memory was discussed from the anatomical and clinical viewpoints, and memory disorders resulting from specific diseases such as herpes simplex encephalitis and Alzheimer's disease were considered in detail. The section further provided a cognitive neuropsychological analysis of various forms of memory, including explicit memory, remote memory and semantic memory. Chapters on confabulation and on functional amnesia were also included. We were all deeply saddened by the news of Laird's untimely death. We are very much indebted to Mieke Verfaellie for supervising the final stages of the preparation of this volume for the revised handbook.

The third volume, edited by Rita Sloan Berndt, covered traditional approaches to, as well as new techniques for, investigating language disorders by leading researchers in the field of language and aphasia research. The volume is divided into four parts. The first part, entitled the study of aphasia, includes a chapter on historical developments, a discussion of the relationship between neuroanatomy and language, one on sign language, one on cross-lingual studies and a review of aphasia in bilinguals and polyglots. The second section ('understanding the symptoms of aphasia') discussed and analyzed the symptoms of aphasia and related disorders including reading and writing. The next section went further into related disorders with chapters that discuss the relationship between language and memory and attention as well as disorders of skilled movements, of body representation and of number processing. The volume concluded with a review of emerging methods for the study of language and aphasia including neuroimaging, ERP, TMS and studies of 'split brain' subjects.

Volume 4, edited by Marlene Behrmann, covered disorders of visual behavior. The volume began with a chapter reviewing the neurophysiology of spatial vision with special emphasis on single unit recordings in non-human primates. The next three chapters reviewed the recent work on recognition deficits for faces (prosopagnosia), objects (visual object agnosia) and words (peripheral dyslexias). Disorders of spatial representation, of color processing and of mental imagery, were presented next including a detailed discussion of the neuropsychological behavior as well as the underlying neural substrate of these disorders. Additional chapters dealt with Balint's syndrome, with blindsight and with visuospatial or constructional disorders. Finally, the relationship between eye movements and brain damage has been described in detail.

The fifth volume, edited by Guido Gainotti, covered emotional behavior and its disorders. It included introductory chapters dealing with basic theoretical and anatomical issues in the neuropsychological study of emotions. A central part of this volume addressed the problem of hemispheric asymmetries in emotional representation and a final group of chapters examined the neural mechanisms of the stress response and reviewed the main emotional disorders. In the introductory chapters, an effort was made to present both neurobiologically oriented and cognitively oriented theories of emotion. Both the detailed anatomo-clinical and theoretical aspects of the anatomical substrates of emotions were covered in depth. In the central part of the volume, the claims for right hemisphere dominance for emotions and emotional communication were contrasted with those assuming a different hemispheric specialization for positive versus negative emotions and with models assuming asymmetric cortico-limbic control of human emotion. Finally, in the last chapters of the volume, individual differences in the hemispheric control of the stress response were discussed and the neural mechanisms of affective/emotional disturbances were approached with neuropsychological methods and with functional neuroimaging techniques.

The sixth volume of the Handbook, edited by François Boller and Stefano Cappa, was devoted to topics related to Aging and Dementia. The volume began with two chapters dealing with age-related cognitive and neurobiological alterations in animals, including a detailed review of data obtained with transgenic and knockout mouse technology. The next chapter reviewed the cognitive changes associated with normal aging. The gamut of symptoms that occur in Alzheimer's disease (AD) were then described and analyzed. They include effects on attention, language, memory, non-verbal functions with emphasis on spatial abilities, olfaction and the motor system. The discussion of dementia syndromes was presented in two sections. The first concerned AD, discussed from the points of view of epidemiology, neuropathology and neurochemistry, concluding with a review of current and future treatments. The other section dealt with non-AD dementias including fronto-temporal and Lewy body dementias and specific conditions such as Parkinson's and Huntington's disease, as well as HIV infection. The volume included a review of brain imaging and cerebral metabolism findings in aging and dementia. The final chapters reviewed the relations between culture and dementia and the special syndrome of severe dementia.

Volume 7 comprises a completely revamped section on the Frontal Lobes edited by Jordan Grafman. A chapter on the neural architecture/anatomy of the prefrontal cortex leads off this volume. Animal research has contributed greatly to our understanding of the special capability of the frontal lobes to respond to a variety of input from 'lower order' sensory and posterior association cortex and this and other observations are reported in this volume. Functions dependent on the frontal lobes emerge late in ontogeny and appear to decline early in normal aging. These findings are reviewed and their implications for neuropsychology discussed. Over the last 15 years, the functioning of the frontal lobes has become associated with the term working memory. In this volume the concept of working memory is discussed in relationship to both functional neuroimaging and patient studies. Gross distinctions in the functioning of the prefrontal cortex have divided it topographically into dorsolateral and ventromedial sectors. This volume offers chapters highlighting the role of each sector from both neuroimaging and lesion perspectives. Many of the views of the prefrontal cortex characterize it as involved in 'processing'. A chapter in this volume takes a slightly different perspective and attempts to characterize the nature of knowledge representation within the frontal lobes. Many theories of the frontal lobes suggest that they are concerned with maintaining information across time. A chapter reviews the role of the frontal lobes in temporal processing. Since the frontal lobes are affected by many neuropsychiatric disorders, a chapter in this volume places their dysfunction in the context of the parallel fronto-subcortical networks and suggests that each network, when damaged, contributes specific symptoms to the patient's clinical presentation. Finally, computational modeling has taken center-stage in cognitive neuroscience and its usefulness in testing different theoretical stances about the role of the frontal lobes in information processing is presented in a concluding chapter.

The Child Neuropsychology Section consists of Volume 8, Parts I and II, edited by Sid Segalowitz and Isabelle Rapin. They rest on the fact that the impact of acquired and degenerative disorders in childhood is strongly colored by the immaturity of the brain, so that what is said in other volumes of the Handbook rarely applies directly to children. The first part considers theoretical perspectives in bridging developmental neuroscience with child psychology, with the role of neuroscience furthering our understanding of the child's mental development, and a separate chapter outlines the importance of plasticity in this growth. Chapters also cover methodological issues arising from epidemiological perspectives and from psychometric concepts and issues. Methods for measuring biological brain function and structure and their particular application to child neuropsychological disorders are covered next, including ERP, PET, SPECT, MRI and fMRI technologies. Included here is a chapter devoted to childhood seizure disorders. Next follow separate chapters on neuropsychological assessment in infancy, in the preschool child, and in school-aged children. Following this are presentations on the development of motor control, including handedness, and somatosensory perception. The second part begins with chapters on visual development and on development in visually impaired children, followed by chapters on cognitive development in deaf children and on central auditory functions and their evaluation. This is followed by chapters on early language development and its neural correlates, developmental language disorders, and on acquired aphasia in childhood. Two chapters on dyslexia and another on dyscalculia follow. Next are presented a chapter on disorders of memory with a special focus on temporal lobe disease and autism, one on attention disorders, and one on executive functions in normal and abnormal development. Following this are chapters on the development of emotional regulation and on mechanisms and influences on addiction in children and adolescents. Final chapters include one on eating disorders, and another focussing on autism spectrum disorders.

The final volume on Rehabilitation, edited by Jordan Grafman and Ian Robertson, contains topics not specifically covered in the previous edition of the Handbook. In particular, we were so impressed by the advances and current direction of studies on neuroplasticity and rehabilitation that we thought the time was right to include these topics in the new edition of the Handbook of Neuropsychology. Neuroplasticity is among the most exciting areas of research in cognitive neuroscience. In this volume, there are chapters on animal models of neuroplasticity, cortical map changes with practice and following brain damage, cross-modal reassignment of function, auditory system reassignment following learning and brain damage, the effects of amputation on phantom limb and pain perceptions, the effects of age on plasticity, the ability of the non-damaged hemisphere to take over functions of the damaged hemisphere, and the effects of cognitive skill learning on neural organization and function. A section describing how basic science findings can be translated into practical rehabilitation of patients follows. Rehabilitation programs for neglect, language, executive functions, and motor skills are described. The use of functional neuroimaging to provide a neural window on cognitive plasticity is discussed. The last section of the Handbook has traditionally been reserved for a discussion of the state-of-the-art of new technologies. Here we provide updates on MRI, fMRI, PET, transcranial magnetic stimulation, and other technologies that have burst upon the cognitive neuroscience scene in the last ten years.

As can be seen, there are important changes between the first edition and the present one in terms of organization and content. Other changes include timing, presentation and availability. The eleven volumes of the first edition appeared over a span of ten years because in most cases, volumes were written and edited consecutively.

In the second edition, several volumes have been concurrently planned and we estimate that the entire series will appear over a span of approximately two years. The first edition consisted of hardbound volumes that were followed by paperback volumes after an interval ranging from two to three years. In the current edition, the paperback edition appears at the same time as the hardbound one and its price will make it more easily available to students and fellows.

Besides the printed second edition of the Handbook of Neuropsychology that you have in your hands, there are already plans for a web-based version. This will make it easier to adapt the Handbook to changes that will undoubtedly occur in the near future. For example, neuroimaging techniques are rapidly developing, opening new in-roads into the mapping of brain and behavior relationships. The rising interest in the aging population is also very likely to increase even further, as new advances will occur concerning the early detection of cognitive impairment and the maintenance of cognitive functions into old age. The same advances will undoubtedly also occur for the developing brain.

Many people have contributed to the successful preparation of the Handbook. We again wish to emphasize our appreciation for the commitment of the Volume Editors who have spent long hours in the planning stage and in the actual compiling of the various sections. Throughout the development and production of the Series, the editorial staff of Neurology and Neuroscience of Elsevier Science B.V. in Amsterdam has provided invaluable assistance.

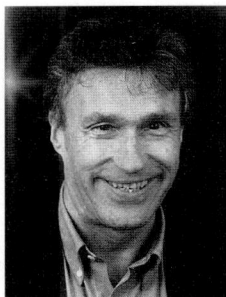

François Boller          Jordan Grafman

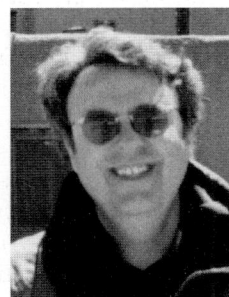

# List of Contributors

**Beers, N.B.**  Department of Pediatrics, Harvard Medical School, Boston, MA 02115, USA

**Bellinger, D.C.**  Department of Neurology, Children's Hospital, CA-503, 300 Longwood Avenue, Boston, MA 02115-5747, USA

**Casey, J.E.**  Department of Psychology, University of Windsor, Windsor, ON N9B 3P4, Canada

**Chugani, D.C.**  Departments of Pediatrics and Radiology, PET Center, Children's Hospital of Michigan, Wayne State University School of Medicine, 3901 Beaubien Blvd., Detroit, MI 48201, USA

**Chugani, H.T.**  Departments of Pediatrics, Radiology, and Neurology, Children's Hospital of Michigan, Wayne State University School of Medicine, Detroit, MI 48201, USA

**Corbetta, D.**  Department of Health and Kinesiology, and Department of Psychological Sciences, Purdue University, Lambert Fieldhouse, 800 West Stadium Avenue, West Lafayette, IN 47907-2046, USA

**Deuel, R.K.**  Department of Neurology, Saint Louis University Health Sciences, 3635 Vista at Grand Blvd., P.O. Box 15250, St. Louis, MO 63110-0250, USA

**Dunn, M.**  Department of Neurology, Rose F. Kennedy Center, Albert Einstein College of Medicine, 1300 Morris Park Avenue, Bronx, NY 10461, USA

**Fein, D.**  Department of Psychology, University of Connecticut, 406 Babbidge Road, U-1020, Storrs, CT 06269-1020, USA

**Filipek, P.A.**  Department of Neurology, University of California, Irvine, College of Medicine, UC Irvine Medical Center, Route 81-4482, 101 City Drive South, Orange, CA 92868-3298, USA

**Fletcher, J.M.**  Department of Pediatrics, University of Texas Health Science Center-Houston, Houston, TX, USA

**Francis, D.J.**  Department of Psychology, University of Houston, Houston, TX, USA

**Gangestad, S.W.**  Department of Psychology, Logan Hall, University of New Mexico, Albuquerque, NM 87131-1161, USA

**Harel, B.**  Department of Psychology, University of Connecticut, 406 Babbidge Road, U-1020, Storrs, CT 06269-1020, USA

| | |
|---|---|
| **Hiscock, M.** | Department of Psychology, University of Houston, Houston, TX, USA |
| **Juranek, J.** | Department of Pediatrics (Division of Child Neurology), University of California, Irvine, College of Medicine, UC Irvine Medical Center, Route 81-4482, 101 City Drive South, Orange, CA 92868-3298, USA |
| **Luck, D.Z.** | Mattis and Luck Center for Neuropsychological Services, LLP, 34 South Broadway, Suite 100, White Plains, New York, 10601, USA |
| **Masur, D.M.** | Department of Neurology and Comprehensive Epilepsy Management Center, Montefiore Medical Center, and Albert Einstein College of Medicine, Bainbridge Avenue and 210th Street, Bronx, NY 10467, USA |
| **Mattis, S.** | Mattis and Luck Center for Neuropsychological Services, LLP, 34 South Broadway, Suite 100, White Plains, New York, 10601, USA |
| **Molfese, V.** | Center for Research in Early Childhood Education, College of Education and Human Development, University of Louisville, Louisville, KY 40292, USA |
| **Morris, R.D.** | Department of Psychology, Georgia State University, University Plaza, Atlanta, GA 30303, USA |
| **Nass, R.** | Department of Neurology, New York University Medical Center, 400 E 34th Street, New York, NY 10016, USA |
| **O'Shea, A.G.** | Department of Psychology, University of Connecticut, 406 Babbidge Road, U-1020, Storrs, CT 06269-1020, USA |
| **Price, B.** | Center for Research in Early Childhood Education, College of Education and Human Development, University of Louisville, Louisville, KY 40292, USA |
| **Rapin, I.** | Department of Neurology, Albert Einstein College of Medicine, K 807, 1410 Pelham Parkway South, Bronx, NY 10461, USA |
| **Rappaport, L.A.** | Department of Medicine, Children's Hospital and Harvard Medical School, 300 Longwood Avenue, Boston, MA 02115-5747, USA |
| **Rourke, B.P.** | Department of Psychology, University of Windsor, Windsor, ON N9B 3P4, Canada and Yale University, New Haven, CT, USA |
| **Segalowitz, S.J.** | Department of Psychology, Brock University, 500 Glenridge Avenue, St. Catharines, ON L2S 3A1, Canada |
| **Shinnar, S.** | Departments of Neurology and Pediatrics, and Comprehensive Epilepsy Management Center, Montefiore Medical Center, and Albert Einstein College of Medicine, Bainbridge Avenue and 210th Street, Bronx, NY 10467, USA |
| **Steinschneider, M.** | Departments of Neurology and Neuroscience, Rose F. Kennedy Center, Rm. 322, Albert Einstein College of Medicine, 1300 Morris Park Avenue, Bronx, NY 10461, USA |

**Stowe, M.T.**    Department of Neurology and Comprehensive Epilepsy Management Center, Montefiore Medical Center, and Albert Einstein College of Medicine, Bainbridge Avenue and 210th Street, Bronx, NY 10467, USA

**Thelen, E.**    Department of Psychology, Indiana University, 1101 E 10th Street, Bloomington, IN 47405, USA

**Thoma, R.J.**    Department of Psychiatry, Albuquerque Veterans Administration Medical Center, Albuquerque, NM, USA

**Weiler, M.D.**    Department of Psychiatry, Children's Hospital and Harvard Medical School, Boston, MA 02115-5747, USA

**Yeo, R.A.**    Department of Psychology, Logan Hall, University of New Mexico, Albuquerque, NM 87131-1161, USA

# Contents

Contents

CHAPTER 1

# On the nature and scope of child neuropsychology

Isabelle Rapin [a,*] and Sidney J. Segalowitz [b]

[a] *Department of Neurology, Albert Einstein College of Medicine, K807, 1410 Pelham Parkway South, Bronx, NY 10461, USA*
[b] *Department of Psychology, Brock University, 500 Glenridge Avenue, St. Catharines, ON L2S 3A1, Canada*

From its start, neuropsychology has been interdisciplinary, addressing normal and pathological development of brain function and behavior. Consideration of childhood disorders involves embryologists, geneticists, developmental psychologists, pediatricians, child neurologists and neurosurgeons, child psychiatrists, pediatric speech and language pathologists and psycholinguists, and now child neuropsychologists. The questions they ask of young children differ greatly from those asked of adults and require quite different instruments and test strategies.

Child neuropsychology is no more adult neuropsychology than developmental psychology is adult psychology. Much of the excitement in child neuropsychology stems from the belief (and hope) that unraveling some of the basic processes that govern brain growth and maturation will help illuminate psycholinguistic development, emotional regulation, and such associated issues as peer socialization, attachment, identification processes, and models of cognitive memory. In order to truly understand the relationship between brain and behavior, we must come to grips with the developmental aspects of the relationship, which means that developmental neuropsychology is relevant to all of neuropsychology.

Developmental neuropsychology thus encompasses more than pediatric behavioral neurology, the clinical importance of which remains one of its central concerns. Our mandate was to cover both the clinical and the experimental aspects of child neuropsychology, a large enterprise limited somewhat by the newness of the field, so that many critical questions had to remain unanswered.

## Etiological differences between behavioral syndromes of children and adults

Most of the major pathologies responsible for neuropsychological disorders in children differ from those of adults. Even similar acquired pathologies such as trauma, neoplasms, diffuse ischemia, and infarctions may have quite different impacts on the immature brain than at maturity. Adult neuropsychology has depended upon two major sources of information: the impact of documented focal and diffuse acquired brain lesions on behavior, and the results of experimental lesions in animals. In the past decade, a third source has come on line, functional imaging of the active, living brain. Experiments on immature animals have yielded important data for pediatric neuropsychology, but only some of the information from adult pathologies can be transferred to children. Strokes and penetrating wounds produce particularly informative focal lesions in adults because they produce permanent, stable anatomical deficits whose location and extent are assessable with current imaging techniques. This type of lesion is less common in children in whom congenital malformations, pre- and peri-natal insults — notably prematurity, intraventricular hemorrhage and ischemia/anoxia — and the consequences of bacterial meningitis and other encephalopathies predom-

_____
* Corresponding author. E-mail: rapin@aecom.yu.edu

inate. A major portion of the neuropsychological disorders of early life is not associated with brain insults nor with lesions detectable with current clinical neuroimaging technology. This is true of most cases of mental deficiency, autism, dysphasia, attention deficit, and so-called learning disabilities in which genetics, not 'damage', plays a major role in their causation.

In the past two decades, newer neuroimaging technologies like magnetic resonance imaging (MRI) morphometry, functional MRI, positron emission tomography (PET), single photon emission computed tomography (SPECT), event-related potentials (ERPs), and magnetoencephalography (MEG) are increasingly being used clinically in children and adolescents with known or suspected brain lesions and diseases, and they are increasingly being applied to elucidate the neural basis of developmental disorders. These technologies have started to delineate the distributed networks implicated in complex tasks like language comprehension and production, reading, attention, and even emotion. The great challenge, of course, is to determine whether brain activation patterns associated with clinical disorders are simply reflecting the disordered thinking or form the basis for the disorder in the first place.

Genetics plays a more important etiologic role in pediatric than adult neuropsychology. Chromosome abnormalities and single gene defects associated with major malformations, systemic diseases, or obviously progressive brain degenerations can have profound effects on brain development. The etiologic role of as yet largely undefined genetic disorders in the learning disabilities and, indeed, the role of genetic programs for the development of various brain systems, neuromodulators, and neurotransmitters are topics at the forefront of current research in developmental neuroscience and neuropsychology.

The past decade has also seen cross-fertilization between clinical genetics and molecular biology. Twin studies that show a high level of concordance for a developmental disorder in monozygotic twins and significant but much lower concordance in dizygotic twins and siblings have provided strong evidence for a genetic role for complex abilities. Gene linkage studies applied to families with multiple affected individuals indicate linkage of dyslexia to loci on chromosome 15 in some families and to chro-

mosome 6 in others, and linkage of dysphasia to chromosome 7 in one large family. With respect to autism, it is now clear that single gene defects are infrequent causes, and that differing combinations of interacting genes contribute to within and between family variability. For example, family histories of children with autism suggest that in some families there is a broader phenotype that encompasses such related disorders as developmental language disability, obsessive–compulsive disorder, bipolar disease, and even Tourette's syndrome. Similarly, tuberous sclerosis, which has a dramatically varied phenotype, can arise from either of two separate genes on chromosomes 9 and 16. Besides poly- and multigenic etiologies, there are other causes for phenotypic variability. Molecular studies have revealed that any given gene can harbor multiple mutations, some more frequent than others. Some single nucleotide substitutions are inconsequential harmless polymorphisms, in contrast to others, and to other genetic alterations such as the expansion of trinucleotide repeats or the truncation of the gene that result in the assembly of a defective protein or preclude its assembly altogether. Some complex syndromes may be caused by chromosomal microdeletions which affect a variable number of adjacent genes, depending on the size of the deletion. In some cases phenotypes vary depending on whether genes are of maternal or paternal origin. A frequent consequence of this molecular variability is that particular gene defects may give rise to quite dissimilar phenotypes.

Genes are responsible for the assembly of proteins, some of which are enzymes for the synthesis or degradation of molecules, others of which define structural components of cells such as subcellular organelles or the ion channels required for intercellular and intracellular trafficking of ions and molecules. Alterations in enzymes and structural proteins may have profound consequences for brain development, cellular well being and function, and intercellular communication. But elucidating these molecular mechanisms does not provide adequate explanations for behavioral phenotypes such as dyslexia or mental retardation. Assembly of the complex networks that sustain such acquired skills depends equally on the orchestration of multiple genes that come into play at various times in development, and on the effects of the individual's life experience that shapes these networks. Progress in functional imaging and electrophysiology shows that plasticity in brain structure and function is much more extensive than previously appreciated and that, as had long been suspected, postnatal experience and specific training play major roles in molding the brain.

## Behavioral versus biological classification

When investigators from different fields pool their efforts to address common research questions or provide services to overlapping populations, communication may become a significant problem. Each discipline develops its own jargon. Each may use the same words as another discipline but attach a somewhat different meaning to them. Each discipline uses its own tools, classifications, and perspectives and may be blind to aspects of the problem that fall beyond its expertise. An example in point is the major classification problems that plague the behaviorally defined developmental disorders whose biological characteristics are only starting to be defined or remain ill-defined or unknown.

Classification at the descriptive or behavioral level, even when internally valid, is not isomorphic with biological classification, there being two distinct biologic levels: *pathophysiology* (the identification of dysfunctional brain systems, their location, the nature of their pathologies, what neurotransmitter or neuromodulator may be in inadequate supply, etc.), and *etiology* (the genetic or acquired biologic conditions responsible for the occurrence of disorders). It is legitimate to make inferences from a behavioral syndrome to the pathophysiology and localization of the underlying brain dysfunction, not to its etiology. For example, a quite specific behavioral syndrome, Broca's aphasia which reflects a reasonably well-defined brain lesion, can have any of several etiologies, e.g., trauma, neoplasm, stroke. Classification among disorders must respect the level of classification: it is not enough to ask whether a child is autistic, or has epileptic aphasia, or fragile-X syndrome. A child with fragile-X may or may not have an attention disorder, may or may not have a learning disability, may or may not be mentally deficient, may or may not be autistic, may or may not

have seizures. The child may legitimately be diagnosed as having one, more than one, or all of these conditions. Autism, mental deficiency, and attention deficit are behaviorally defined disorders, epilepsy is defined at the pathophysiologic level, fragile-X syndrome at the biologic level. It is productive to look for specific biologic clusters among autistic, or dyslexic, or specifically language impaired, or epileptic children, but defining the biologic etiology or pathophysiology of a child's behaviorally defined disorder in no way substitutes for behavioral diagnosis.

Present classifications of the developmental disorders are descriptive and are largely based on numerical (continuous) criteria, i.e. test scores, supplemented to some degree by clinical observation which relies more strongly on pathognomonic (categorical) signs. Validation of behavioral classifications depends largely on follow-up. Not so biological classification, which is usually categorical and can be validated by external tests. A person does or does not have AIDS, does or does not have increased intracranial pressure, does or does not have a mass on MRI or evidence of an infection on examination of the cerebrospinal fluid. While biological classification (including medical diagnosis) does at times depend on numerically continuous data, for example head circumference to diagnose microcephaly or the amount of immunoglobulin in the spinal fluid to support a diagnosis of multiple sclerosis, much of the time biological classification has access to categorical confirmatory diagnostic criteria such as neuroimaging, chromosome analysis, the demonstration of an abnormal metabolite in body fluids, or of epileptiform activity in the EEG.

In comparison, most neuropsychological deficits in children are defined quantitatively by the amount of deviation from more or less well-established age-dependent norms for questionnaires, observation schedules, or tests. How much deviance is required to diagnose mental deficiency, or dysphasia, or motor clumsiness is statistical and depends on the goals of the classification, rather than on the categorical criteria that define biological diagnoses. What is statistically significant may not be medically significant, and vice versa.

## Bridging the clinical gap

Definitions of normal and pathologic behaviors rest on psychologic constructs such as cognition, affect, memory, motivation, attention, perception, etc. Detailed analysis of pathologic behaviors often provides critical data upon which to base cognitive hypotheses, and cognitive psychology suggests hypotheses regarding brain organization but does not provide direct biological data. Neuropsychology attempts to bridge the gap between these social/cognitive psychological constructs and neuroscience. There are classic syndromes common to adults and children with acquired brain lesions that provide strong data on the localization and, in some cases, on the cause of the underlying brain pathology. Hybrid classifications in child neuropsychology, for example the attribution of a particular childhood learning disability to the right or the left hemisphere, or to the white matter without neuroimaging, neurophysiological, or neuropathological corroborative evidence, is at most a hypothesis which may or may not be warranted, even if some of the symptoms are similar to those of adults with right or left focal lesions. Because of the organizational plasticity of the immature brain, it is hazardous in children to predict behavioral symptoms from the nature and localization of a known lesion, and even more hazardous to predict the pathophysiology, localization, and etiology of a brain dysfunction from a developmental behavioral syndrome.

These principles are less likely to be ignored in adult neuropsychology than in child neuropsychology where there are very few data on underlying brain pathology and function, especially in the very young child, and where there are more stringent limitations on ethically acceptable tools for investigation in view of the non-life-threatening types of disorders and long life expectancy of most of the children. This situation is exacerbated by the well developed (some may say 'overdeveloped') theoretical formulations of psychological development.

Finally, child neuropsychology offers greater potential than adult neuropsychology for altering outcome by early diagnosis and the provision of effective habilitation and education. However, in order to devise maximally effective remediations, there is a need to elucidate the mechanisms underlying altered behaviors, while in turn, response to effective remediation sheds light on brain organization and maturation. These complementary dialectical processes make child neuropsychology especially exciting.

## Bridging the experimental gap

The purely clinical questions of assessment are, of course, what has driven the field for many years. However, the multiplicity of chances to follow interesting cases has once again taught those of us from the developmental psychology laboratory that the brain, like the genotype, places constraints on development; it does not determine it. By focusing on how the growth of the CNS structures the growth of psychological characteristics, we will advance some of the basic goals of developmental psychology: the explication of universal laws of development and the sources of individual differences.

Developmental psychology as a discipline has fed developmental neuropsychology, until recently without reciprocation. Given that the child can do some task, the job for developmental neuropsychology was simply to ask: what is the brain organization for that function and is it the same as that in adults? We now are seeing developmental neuropsychology returning the favor, since we are able to bring some principles of brain growth to bear on the developmental questions. Various examples include virtually all the core areas of developmental psychology. Consider the following issues. The development of emotional regulation in early and middle childhood: is it due solely to the acquisition of cognitive and linguistic mechanisms or also due to the growth of frontal lobe regulatory control over limbic systems? Development of memory and learning skills: what is the role of cognitive constructivism (whether Piagetian or a learning theory framework) versus the increase in information processing speed due to physiological maturation? Indeed, what is the nature of constructivism? Language development: what role, if any, does normal hemispheric specialization play in easing or stressing the task of learning a first language? Even when these issues have been well explored, we will still have to deal with the fundamental but more complex question of synergy: how do experience and learning affect the brain growth that in turn affects experience and learning?

**Bringing together the clinical and the experimental**

Longitudinal studies of the neuropsychological development of normal and non-normal children have the potential to shed light on the consequences of early choices that shape the development of adult abilities and talents. Early detection of differences among children may help uncover the roots of some adult personality traits and pathologies such as substance abuse, antisocial behavior, manic/depressive illness, schizophrenia, and others. Differences in the potential for recovery from acquired brain lesions in adults and children at different ages illuminate the trajectory of plasticity in the reorganization of the brain following an injury. Studies in children have shown that certain abilities are more stable in their functional localization than others, since children suffer behavioral deficits similar to those of adults following lesions in similar locations and since recovery may be incomplete, while lesions in other locations do not cause permanent deficits. Limitations in functional plasticity provide evidence for determined organization of some but not other behaviors in the brain.

At any age, some recovery is attributable to the reversible changes that follow an acute lesion. Further recovery may be a function of the complexities of the many tasks whose accomplishment depends upon the contributions of multiple, widely distributed and therefore spared, brain systems. These systems provide flexibility in task performance and resiliency in the face of focal damage. Skills in the process of acquisition may call upon undamaged circuits unavailable in the more mature, more committed brain, which may be one of the bases for greater plasticity of the immature brain. The seizure of uncommitted (which is not the same as non-specialized) circuits may render them unavailable to the acquisition of other skills. For example, children who sustain large enough lesions of their left perisylvian cortex to push the development of language to the right hemisphere may have deficits in visuospatial skills that, presumably, have been 'crowded out' by the establishment of language on the right, although this is still a highly controversial notion.

**Scope of the section**

The goal of these volumes devoted to child neuropsychology is to discuss the relationship between normal brain development and some of its pathologies. We begin by covering some of the issues that bridge development neuroscience to child psychology, and the nature of cortical specialization and plasticity, and the similarities and differences between developmental and acquired neuropsychological syndromes. A chapter on the epidemiology of the developmental disorders of brain function cautions that there are many naive assumptions about the prevalence and causes of childhood developmental disorders, and warns of the pitfalls of extrapolating from single or few cases to children in general.

The next few chapters review current neurobiological methodologies applicable to the investigation of brain structure and function in children, including electrophysiology (especially ERPs), neuroimaging (MRI) and metabolic imaging (PET, SPECT, and fMRI). A major disorder of activation is, of course, epilepsy, which is much more prevalent and more likely to have a genetic etiology in children than adults, and complicates many types of brain dysfunction. The chapter on epilepsy attempts to dispel some of the many misconceptions about the behavioral and neurologic consequences of this disorder in childhood. We next turn to neuropsychologic assessment of infants, toddlers, and school-age/adolescent children, discussed separately since the test strategies and measures differ so widely across ages. Each of the authors has provided a list of tests appropriate to the age group they are considering. Child neuropsychologists need to address the urgent need for instruments that span development, and for better definition of the psychological functions of interest across ages so as to enable longitudinal assessment. Despite the considerable advances in the field, conceptual difficulties in the measurement of change remain. We close the first part of this section with several chapters on the development and disorder of movement, complementing the primarily cognitive focus of child neuropsychological assessment.

In the second part, we cover the developmental neuropsychology of vision and hearing, together with the implications of their dysfunction, drawing attention to the cognitive and affective consequences of these sensory deprivations and the pitfalls in testing these children. These conditions also illustrate the drastic reorganization of brain anatomy and function resulting from peripheral sensory deficits, changes which are starting to be explored.

Both developmental and acquired language disorders are strongly anchored by the structure of language and the phases of its development. The academic disorders of written language and calculation and their remediation raise a fundamental question in neuropsychology and child neuropsychology: what are the cognitive information processing deficits responsible for incompetent acquisition of these learned skills? The need to consider motivational and social factors as well as neuropsychologic ones is stressed, especially for remediation. While neuroscientists and neuropsychologists are intrigued by investigations of the neurologic bases of these disorders, the present lack of evidence make these largely irrelevant as far as classification and remediation are concerned.

While the neuropsychology of memory and attention at one time seemed fairly straightforward, developments in the last decade emphasize their complexities in a developmental framework. These are reflected in the progress made in describing executive function disturbance in clinical disorders. The field is starting to focus also on the complexities of disorders of affect and drives, systems also increasingly implicating frontal lobe circuits. In addition, these disorders raise strongly the question of the relationship of environmental factors to serious behavioral disorders. Substance abuse, one of the burning issues of our time, has its roots in childhood and adolescence. Understanding substance abuse rests on progress in psychopharmacology, and the elucidation of neurotransmitters and reward systems of the brain.

Autism is indeed a pervasive developmental disorder of brain function. Its prevalence has been underestimated in the past and is only now receiving the concentrated multidisciplinary attention afforded the adult dementias, for example. Its clinical prevalence and centrality to developmental neuropsychology is underscored in this section by the variety of contexts in which it is discussed, being independently chosen as a focus for the discussion of memory and executive functions, as well as a specific clinical disorder. Research in autism may pay rich dividends in terms of understanding tics and stereotypies, compulsions, anxiety, disorders of attention and affect, sociability, and higher order cognition. It is a life-long disorder which neurologists and neuropsychologists concerned with adults need to recognize, especially in its less flagrant forms. The fact that early intensive individual education is able to alter its symptomatology provides a model for remediation of other developmental disorders. Its differentiation from the psychoses and character disorders of adolescents and young adults, especially schizophrenia, deserves further study.

In this second edition of the Handbook, we have only two chapters that are essentially unchanged from the first edition, one dealing with methodological issues which still are of concern in research today, and the other covering somatosensory disorders, where there has been unfortunately little new work in the last decade. All other chapters present either entirely new or heavily revised material, an exceptionally arduous task for some fields where the research advances have been prolific.

There has been an exponential growth in the advances in the research base for child neuropsychology over the last decade, to the point where neuropsychology can be seen as a contributing factor to every aspect of child development. This increase in the knowledge base has fed on and nourished this cross-disciplinary collaboration, leading to a welcomed integration of behavioral and neurobiological perspectives on the growth of the child.

*Handbook of Neuropsychology*, 2nd Edition, Vol. 8, Part I
S.J. Segalowitz and I. Rapin (Eds)

CHAPTER 2

# The neuropsychology of normal development: developmental neuroscience and a new constructivism

Sidney J. Segalowitz [a,*] and Merrill Hiscock [b]

*[a] Department of Psychology, Brock University, St. Catharines, ON L2S 3A1, Canada*
*[b] University of Houston, Houston, TX, USA*

## Introduction

Developmental psychologists during much of the late 20th century viewed the growing influence of neuroscience with some concern because of the widely held assumption that biological influences necessarily lead to a philosophy of predeterminism, with political and social implications considered unacceptable (Segalowitz and Rose-Krasnor, 1992). After all, developmentalists have been charting the influence of varied experience on behavioural outcome for some time with considerable success, while not denying that biological sources of variance also exist. For much of the past 20 years, however, there have been several attempts to grow beyond an uneasy mutual acknowledgment with the argument that there must be some ways to bridge the gap (Crnie and Pennington, 1987; Dawson and Fischer, 1994; Segalowitz and Hiscock, 1992). During the last 10 years especially, the gap has truly begun to be bridged with the development and growing availability of new brain imaging technologies that allow in vivo measurements of brain structure and function. Most importantly, developmental neuroscience has been discovering the biological bases for this bridge, and the result is a startling support for a constructivist developmental psychology. Because of this fundamental meeting of minds, developmental psychology

is embracing the new developmental neuroscience with much less scepticism. In addition, a neuropsychology of normal development has complemented clinical child neuropsychology.

The traditional reasons for developmentalists disregarding biological growth as useful may now partly be history, but it is nonetheless instructive to acknowledge them: (1) the physiological bases of mind can only reflect changes at a molecular level and changes at that level do not carry much explanatory power at the molar level, which is of primary concern to developmental psychologists; (2) we do not know enough about brain physiology and certainly not enough about brain maturation to be able to map brain growth onto behavioural development in a systematic or reliable way; and (3) the variables that affect the most interesting aspects of development (i.e., mental developments that are distinctly human) are assumed to be either primarily environmental in nature, or to interact with environmental factors so strongly that the context in which these mental developments occur should be the prime focus of study.

These are powerful arguments against the integration for which this Section of the Handbook strives, but we think that developmental neuropsychologists are now in a position to respond to them. We will do so by discussing realms in which traditional assumptions in developmental psychology are starting to break down, ways in which neuropsychological discoveries in the near future may well lead to ex-

---

* Corresponding author. E-mail: ssegalow@spartan.ac.brocku.ca

citing new developmental insights, and instances in which developmental neuroscience now provides the material basis for some of the constructs central to developmental psychology. We will state our conclusions at the start so that the reader may preview the thrust of our argument. We will conclude (1) that the child is born without a tabula rasa, but neither is he or she born with a preprogramming for the growth of mind; (2) that developmental psychology will find that the neuropsychological perspective furthers its own ends, i.e., neuropsychological data can reflect traditional developmental constructs in contexts where behavioural measures are inadequate or impossible and even solve some persistent problems in developmental psychology; and most importantly (3) that this integration provides the best concrete arguments for a new view on the primary approach to psychological development — constructivism: the idea that mental growth is self-constructed by the child.

The primary difficulty in the integration has been the task of reconciling two major developments in the field of neuroscience itself: (1) the growing evidence that much of our genome is devoted to growth and regulation of the central nervous system, and (2) that the brain also shows phenomenal plasticity with its structural outcome being heavily influenced by its own experience. While developmental neuroscientists have known for a long time that growth involves a highly dynamic interaction between genetic heritage and environmental experiences, pulling these together in concrete terms of brain maturation is still a major challenge. However, a tremendous amount of progress has been made on this issue, and we will outline some of it in broad strokes in this chapter. In fact, we now see learning and plasticity as reflecting different sides of similar phenomena, and that separating these notions has become increasingly difficult and unnecessary (see Nass, 2002, this volume; and Stiles, 2000). For example, extremely high heritability has been reported for several brain structures, including language regions and frontal cortices (Thompson et al., 2001). Although heritability values from twin studies are now known to not necessarily reflect only genetic factors (Segalowitz, 1999; Sokol, Moore, Rose et al., 1995), it is clear that biological factors are heavily involved in determining the gross morphology of the brain. On the other hand, it is now well documented that the fine structure of the brain is heavily influenced by experience and by traumatic insult, and that this period of plasticity is not restricted to the early period after birth (Cameron and McKay, 1999; Kaas, 2000; Muhlnickel, Elbert, Taub and Flor, 1998; Rosenzweig and Bennett, 1996; Schoups, Vogels, Qian and Orban, 2001; Stiles, 2000). We will argue that the new constructivism requires that both these aspects be true, i.e., not only is experience influenced by maturation but maturation is also influenced by experience, and a key mechanism is the individual's personal influence over some aspects of this process.

Our model of constructivism is based on a developmental neuroscience that rejects the Cartesian distinction between mind and body that plagued developmental psychology for most of the 20th century. While rejection of such a dualist position is standard practice in psychology today, we should acknowledge that a variant of this position has a long heritage in behaviourism and is manifested even today in cognitive psychology. The discoveries of the latter 19th century concerning the genetic basis for heredity were even used to reinforce this distinction: the body's design was seen to be fixed by the genotype, whereas the mind was seen as shaped by experience, dividing behaviour into instincts and acquired traits. Ironically, the debate between extreme hereditarians and radical behaviourists only exacerbated the dichotomy, when the real solution lay in removing it (Gottlieb, 1976; McGraw, 1946).

## General relationships: brain growth and behaviour change

Describing the relationship between brain development and behavioural development, even in the most general terms, is a difficult undertaking. The multidimensional character of growth in both spheres is an obvious challenge. We must specify which aspects of neural development are related to which facets of behavioural development. For example, we must explore what the behavioural implications are of neuronal proliferation and migration, of glial proliferation and migration, of synaptic attrition and axonal myelination. We must detail the neural underpinnings of attention, language, or memory. Once the dimensions of interest are identified, we must choose the relevant points on the temporal dimension. Again, this is not an easy choice. Nature not only fails to guarantee that a behavioural characteristic will emerge simultaneously with its neural substrate, but nature fails even to guarantee a fixed lag time. We can infer this temporal variability from observations that prenatal neuropathology in the human manifests itself in behavioural abnormality anywhere from soon after birth to several years later (Towbin, 1978).

Even if associated neural and behavioural changes were to occur simultaneously, the investigator is often handicapped by an inability to measure the two dimensions simultaneously. The most detailed knowledge about neural development pertains to prenatal development, during which time behaviour is relatively sparse and difficult to measure. Conversely, during early and middle childhood, when the behavioural repertoire is rich and when developmental advances are readily documented, the corresponding physiological changes are almost entirely covert, although advances during the last decade in brain imaging technology are rectifying this (see Juranek and Filipek, 2002, this volume, and Chugani and Chugani, 2002, this volume).

An additional problem of neurobehavioural correlation in development is that neither brain development nor behavioural development is linear over time. The concept of developmental stages is as familiar to neurobiologists (e.g., Cowan, 1979, 1990) as it is to developmental psychologists (e.g., Kagan, 1980). Furthermore, the relation between neural change and behavioural change is probably nonlinear as well. A critical level of neural growth, differentiation, and organization is necessary before a given behaviour begins to emerge. Below that threshold, the behaviour will be absent irrespective of developmental changes in the neural substrate. Once the threshold is crossed, behavioural change will be related to neural change. There can be an upper threshold as well, though, where skilled behaviour comes to rely on processes that are quite different from those involved in learning. For example, frontal lobe activation reduces with automatization of an activity (Jueptner, Stefan, Frith et al., 1997), or fully fluent reading may not correlate with the same left hemisphere structures as does not-so-fluent reading (Segalowitz, Wagner and Menna, 1992). Thus, once

some further developmental threshold is crossed, behavioural change may be more related to the acquisition of some new strategies, and these new strategies may no longer be linearly related to the original neural change in question.

*Brain growth and mental development*

Brain maturation in the child consists of (mostly) prenatal neural production, the proliferation of many more connections (synapses) than will be normally present at maturity, and of changes in biochemical systems. For example, an early estimate put the number of neurons per cubic millimetre of tissue at birth as 100,000 dropping to 20,000 by one year after birth, although some argue that this is an artifact of expanding cortex making the density reduce (Shankle, Landing, Rafii et al., 1998). More importantly, the number of synapses grows simultaneously from a few thousand per neuron at birth to 10 to 15 times this at the age of 1 year (Huttenlocher, 1979; Quartz and Sejnowski, 1997).

The neurons and connections that survive, at least within sensory parts of the nervous system, are largely determined by the stimulation to which the organism is exposed during a 'critical' or 'sensitive' period (Mitchell and Timney, 1984; Movshon and Van Sluyters, 1981). This is dramatically demonstrated in the expansion of auditory or visual functions into the cortex normally reserved for the other modality in blind (Leclerc, Saint-Amour, Lavoie et al., 2000; Weeks, Horwitz, Aziz-Sultan et al., 2000) or deaf (Finney, Fine and Dobkins, 2001) individuals. As described by Greenough, Black and Wallace (1987), ". . . many species seem to have evolved such that the genes need only to roughly outline the pattern of neural connectivity in a sensory system, leaving the more specific details to be determined through the organism's interactions with its environment" (p. 543). Thus, the role of the genome is critical in specifying this sequence of growth and the general structure — no amount of special experience will turn a sheep brain into a human brain or vice versa — but this is not the same as saying that the genome rigidly determines the outcome (Wahlsten, 2002; Wahlsten and Gottlieb, 1997). Although the genome is set at fertilization, the pattern of gene activation through life may well be influenced by the hormonal environment, metabolic and nutritional factors, by the activation of neural systems, and these in turn are affected by social and physical stress. Once the basic structures are set, the fine tuning is influenced by a variety of factors. The growth pattern of the brain is by no means fixed at birth, and its growth represents a dynamic interplay with its environment. The extent of this interplay is sometimes astonishing, for what at first seem to be fixed species-specific characteristics turn out to be dependent on experience (see Moore, 1992, for an elegant illustration of sex-specific mating behaviour in mice, and Post and Weiss, 1997, for a model of molecular neurobiological alterations affecting behaviour). This is positive directive development and is more than just the result of harmful factors, which of course also exist, e.g., cocaine administered during embryogenesis of the cortex alters dendritic growth in the anterior cingulate, a region closely associated with executive functions of the frontal lobes (Stanwood, Washington and Levitt, 2001).

Most of what we know of the environmental sculpting concerns specific sensory and motor experiences and their representation in the cortex. This sculpting may be an efficient way of fine-tuning sensory and motor systems that develop early and remain relatively fixed throughout subsequent development. Such a process may, however, impose too many constraints on the development of other systems (Greenough et al., 1987). For instance, systems that subserve learning throughout the lifespan would have to remain modifiable long beyond the 'critical periods' for sensory and motor development. Moreover, lack of early exposure to a particular category of information, e.g., a foreign language, does not preclude subsequent learning of that information (even though the information may be more difficult to learn at a more advanced age, and the capability to acquire perfect pronunciation and use of grammar may be reduced, e.g., Kim, Relkin, Lee and Hirsch, 1997; Werker and Tees, 1984).

Greenough et al. (1987) suggest that the storage of different kinds of information depends on different neural mechanisms. These authors use the term 'experience-expectant information storage' to refer to the process of incorporating information that is "ubiquitous and has been so throughout much of the evolutionary history of the species" (p. 540).

It is this category of storage that is traditionally associated with critical periods. Thus the organism expects (in an evolutionary sense) certain events to occur, and to occur within a specific context and time-frame, because these events or experiences occurred with enough regularity during its evolution that the organism's growth plan could rely on them. Experience-expectant circuits have a strong disposition to develop in a certain way but require triggering or enabling events. These circuits may have relatively limited sensitive periods for their activation. For example, the visual system develops a highly consistent structure when mammals are presented with the natural world made up of lines and shapes in various orientations, with movement in all possible directions. When the environment presents these highly reliable experiences, the visual system progresses quickly and solidifies after relatively little exposure (Mower, Christen and Caplan, 1983). If we artificially restrict the input (e.g., limiting vision to vertical stripes), the resulting system does not develop the normal structures and some bizarre but permanent alterations ensue (e.g., being blind to horizontally oriented objects) (Blakemore, 1991; Chapman, Godecke and Bonhoeffer, 1999; Daw, 1995; Hirsch, 1985). A similar experience-expectant situation appears to exist in the auditory system (Ponton, Moore and Eggermont, 1999). The baby's brain also seems to expect linguistic input within the first year or two, and such experience sets off a pattern of growth that forms a firm basis for later development, along with diminishing ability to alter (hence, the diminishing ability to acquire a second language). This approach is consistent with a purely maturationist approach. Greenough et al. (1987) also outlined another type — 'experience-dependent' circuits — that are more guided by the specifics of the environment, and to which we will return later.

*Evidence for a maturationist position*

The best example for a maturational approach to understanding the child's cognitive development is that of the frontal lobe, whose associated cognitive functions are central to child development. Goldman-Rakic and her colleagues (Goldman, 1971, 1974; Goldman and Alexander, 1977; Goldman, Rosvold and Mishkin, 1970) showed that monkeys' ability to perform a particular task depends on different brain structures at different stages of development. What appears to be plasticity may be the consequence of an irrelevant lesion, i.e., a lesion within a brain structure that has not yet become necessary for performing a particular task. With further development, which normally would have made the structure essential for the behaviour in question, the irrelevant lesion becomes relevant and deficits are observed. This pattern was obtained in monkeys given dorsolateral prefrontal lesions at the age of 50 days. When lesioned monkeys were tested for delayed response performance at the age of 1 year, they performed as well as unoperated controls. If, however, testing was delayed until the animals were 2 years old, at least some of the early-lesioned monkeys showed a striking impairment. It seems that they 'grew into' their lesion. Subsequent work utilizing reversible cryogenic depression of the dorsolateral cortex again implied that this region does not contribute to delayed-response performance during the first 16 postnatal months, and that its contribution remains rather minor until the age of 3 years (Goldman and Alexander, 1977).

Parallel findings were reported for monkeys' performance on an object discrimination reversal task following early lesions to the orbital prefrontal cortex. Again the functional sparing observed at an early age of testing was followed by impairment at a later age of testing. The main difference between the dorsolateral and orbital findings was that the deficits began appearing at an earlier age following orbital lesions (Goldman, 1974).

Goldman (1974) concluded that the consequences of early brain damage depend not only on the maturational status of the damaged structure, but also on the maturational status of alternative substrates for the functions affected by the lesion. An early cortical lesion will have no measurable effect on behaviour if testing takes places before the damaged region would have become functional and if alternative structures, particularly subcortical structures, have developed normally. Under such circumstances, "functions will appear to have been compensated when, in fact, they had not been lost" (Goldman, 1974, p. 168).

Do these findings of Goldman-Rakic and her colleagues imply that any plasticity observed in the immature brain is merely an artifact of premature testing? Apparently not, because monkeys le-sioned in infancy ultimately are able to perform at least some delayed-response tasks that adult-lesioned monkeys cannot accomplish (Goldman-Rakic, Isseroff, Schwartz et al., 1983). The outcome may be even better for animals with prenatal lesions (Goldman and Galkin, 1978). Goldman-Rakic et al. (1983) attribute this advantage of early-operated animals to reorganization in neural systems left intact following the cortical lesion. With respect to delayed-response tasks, the caudate nucleus and the mediodorsal nucleus of the thalamus are probable alternative substrates. Lesions to these subcortical structures cause impaired delayed-response performance in both immature and adult monkeys (Alexander, Witt and Goldman-Rakic, 1980; Battig, Mishkin and Rosvold, 1960; Goldman, 1974; Goldman and Rosvold, 1972; Isseroff, Galkin, Rosvold and Goldman-Rakic, 1982; Schulman, 1964).

When the various findings concerning the development of delayed-response performance in monkeys are assembled, a fairly coherent picture emerges. Early lesions to the dorsolateral prefrontal cortex have no immediate effects on delayed-response performance because the capability to perform this task depends on subcortical structures in the immature animal. With further maturation of the prefrontal cortex, the dorsolateral cortex becomes the primary neural substrate for delayed-response performance. Removal of the dorsolateral cortex now will cause impaired performance on the delayed-response task. At the same time, the delayed effects of early lesions now have become apparent. The enigmatic part of this picture, as acknowledged by Goldman-Rakic et al. (1983), is the failure of subcortical structures to subserve delayed-response performance in the adult monkey following cortical damage. The maturational change being proposed is not a complete elimination of subcortical contributions to delayed-response performance, but rather an enlargement of the substrate to include the dorsolateral prefrontal cortex, which acquires primary control over the behaviour. If the involvement of the mediodorsal thalamic and caudate nuclei in delayed-response performance persists into adulthood, then why can these subcortical structures not compensate for loss of the dorsolateral cortex in the adult? Goldman-Rakic et al. (1983) propose two possible explanations. As one possibility, they suggest that the early organization of the subcortical substrate, which is capable of controlling delayed-response behaviour in the immature animal, is a transitory organization that is modified after the prefrontal cortex develops. Alternatively, Goldman-Rakic et al. suggest that cortical lesions in adult animals, but not infants, permanently affect the functioning of subcortical structures by depriving them of essential cortical inputs.

*Relevance to human infants*

The delayed-response task demands that behaviour be guided by stored information that changes from one trial to the next (Goldman-Rakic, 1987b). The task thus engages a kind of memory that is often referred to as representational (Fuster, 1985; Goldman-Rakic, 1987a; Passingham, 1985) or working (Baddeley, 1981; Olton, 1983) memory. Goldman-Rakic (1987b) emphasized the distinction between representational memory and associative learning, in which the same stimulus–response association is maintained and reinforced across trials. Although both kinds of memory may be dependent on the hippocampus in rodents (cf., Morris, Garrud, Rawlins and O'Keefe, 1982; Olton and Papas, 1979), primate studies indicate a "sharp dissociation in the neural mechanisms that mediate representational and associative guidance of behaviour, respectively, and implicates prefrontal cortex primarily in the former" (Goldman-Rakic, 1987b, pp. 602–603), whereas the latter rely on posterior and limbic structures.

The concept of representational memory can serve as a nexus between studies of delayed-response performance in primates and studies of humans (as well as between studies of rodents and other species). A more specific link between primate studies and studies of human cognitive development arises from the similarity between the primate delayed-response task and the Piagetian A-not-B Stage IV object permanence task (Goldman-Rakic, 1987b). As pointed out by Goldman-Rakic, both tasks entail hiding a reward in one of two locations as the subject watches and then allowing the subject to choose the correct location after a delay of a few seconds. Recognizing that there are some procedural differences between the two tasks — primarily in the way in which the location of the reward is varied across trials — Diamond and Goldman-Rakic (1989) showed that dorsolateral

prefrontal damage in adult monkeys impairs performance on the Piagetian object permanence task just as it impairs performance on the delayed-response task. Conversely, human infants show the same developmental pattern on the delayed-response task as on the A-not-B task (Diamond and Doar, 1989).

When the A-not-B performance of lesioned monkeys is compared with that of normal human infants, it is obvious that they make similar errors, i.e., when the reward is hidden in the location opposite to the location that was rewarded on the previous trial, subjects tend to respond to the previously rewarded location rather than the current location (Diamond, 1985, 1990; Diamond and Goldman-Rakic, 1989). This kind of error — the A-not-B error — may indicate that responding is guided by associative learning rather than representational memory: "When the A-not-B error occurs, the conditioned habit to return to the location where the infant was previously rewarded (A) appears to override the 'intention' to reach to B, based on the memory of where the toy was just hidden" (Diamond, 1985, p. 880).

If A-not-B errors are ascribed to competition between representational and associative memory on trials when the rewarded location is reversed, then the number of such errors should increase as the retention interval (the delay between hiding and retrieving) increases. Longer delays place a greater demand on representational memory, thus increasing the likelihood of an incorrect response based on 'conditioned habit'. Accordingly, longer delays yield A-not-B errors in older children who would tend not to make errors with short retention intervals (Diamond, 1985; Gratch and Landers, 1971). In comparing human infants and adult rhesus monkeys, Diamond and Goldman-Rakic (1989) found that adult monkeys with bilateral dorsolateral prefrontal lesions performed similarly to human infants at 7.5–9 months of age. Both groups committed A-not-B errors at delays of 2–5 s and showed only chance performance at delays of 10 s. In contrast, unoperated control animals, as well as monkeys with bilateral parietal lesions, performed successfully at delays up to 10 s. The performance of the unoperated and parietal animals was comparable to that of 12-month-old human infants.

The role of the dorsolateral prefrontal cortex is not limited to delayed-response (or A-not-B) performance. Diamond and Goldman-Rakic (1985) found that adult monkeys with bilateral lesions to the dorsolateral prefrontal cortex were also impaired in their ability to retrieve objects from an open transparent box when successful retrieval required indirect reaching, i.e. reaching for the object via a route other than the direct line of sight. Monkeys with dorsolateral lesions again performed comparably to human infants in the age range of 7.5–9 months, and intact animals and animals with parietal lesions performed comparably to 12-month-old children.

Since Diamond and Goldman-Rakic's (1985) object retrieval task does not require the subject to remember the locus of the object, failure to perform this task successfully cannot be attributed to a defect of representational memory. Conversely, since the delayed-response and A-not-B tasks do not require indirect reaching, failure to perform these tasks cannot be ascribed to an inability to reach around barriers. Is there a common defect underlying the parallel results for the two categories of tasks? Can the effect of dorsolateral lesions on both kinds of performance be explained in terms of a single mechanism? Goldman-Rakic (1987a) suggested that the prefrontal cortex utilizes stored information to control behaviour while inhibiting response tendencies based on external, situational variables. In Goldman-Rakic's (1987b) words, "the prefrontal cortex may be necessary to override the tendency to behave strictly on the basis of reinforcement or on the basis of stimulation present at the moment of response" (p. 604). According to Diamond (1991), the role of the dorsolateral prefrontal cortex can be specified in greater detail. The dorsolateral cortex not only involves inhibitory control of prepotent response tendencies but also the integration of information over time or space. Diamond argues that the A-not-B task requires the subject to relate a cue and a response which are separated in time, and that the object retrieval task requires the subject to relate two objects — the reward and the box opening — which are separated in space. Unless a task requires temporal or spatial integration as well as the inhibition of a competing response, performance will not be disrupted by dorsolateral lesions.

Diamond has extended this work by studying infants and young children under treatment for phenylketonuria (PKU). This condition demonstrates the contribution of dopamine to cognitive abilities associated with the dorsolateral prefrontal cortex. Children with PKU, despite being treated continuously from an early age, have reduced dopaminergic innervation of the prefrontal region and show selective impairment of the skills that are thought to be dependent on that region (Diamond, 1998, 2001; Diamond, Prevor, Callender and Druin, 1997).

This linkage between the dorsolateral cortex and delayed responding is also demonstrated in the growth of healthy infants whose performance on the delayed-response (A-not-B) task increases from 7 months to 12 months. They also show an age-related increase in EEG power from the frontal region, while those infants who do not improve do not have an EEG power increase (Bell and Fox, 1992).

*Implications*

The studies of Goldman-Rakic and her associates have contributed to developmental neuropsychology in a number of ways. The developmental approach to examining lesion effects in nonhuman primates offers a framework for disentangling the confound between developmental changes in plasticity and developmental changes in functional localization that has so bedevilled clinical studies. Recovery of function following early damage may be better understood if the maturational status of the damaged structure, as well as the status of alternative substrates, is considered. For instance, the primate data provide empirical support for the conclusion that cognitive deficits with apparent onset in middle childhood reflect the delayed effects of early lesions to slow-maturing cortical structures (Kinsbourne, 1973).

In addition to adding a new dimension to clinical neuropsychological studies, Goldman-Rakic's work illustrates how different topics of neuropsychological enquiry — topics that are often examined in relative isolation — must be linked together if a complete understanding is to be attained. The studies of early lesions in monkeys show clearly that the development of prefrontal cortical functioning cannot be understood in isolation. The high degree of anatomical connectivity between prefrontal cortex and subcortical structures, as well as the developmental progression from subcortical to cortical control over behaviour, justifies the incorporation of subcortical as well as cortical functions into a single, complex functional system. Moreover, one of the subcortical structures implicated in delayed-response performance, the mediodorsal nucleus of the thalamus (MD), which is often damaged in patients with Korsakoff's syndrome, is thought to contribute to the learning of new information (cf., Markowitsch, 1988; Squire, Amaral, Zola-Morgan et al., 1989). The common involvement of MD in delayed-response performance and learning provides a potential anatomical link between systems for acquiring and storing new information and for using that information to guide behaviour. Such a link would be consistent with the hypothesized role of recently acquired representational memory in delayed-response performance. Finally, the work of Diamond and Goldman-Rakic illustrates the power of a research strategy that conjoins developmental neuropsychology with developmental psychology and primate neurobiology. The strategy entails investigating normal development in the human infant, normal development in the nonhuman primate infant, and lesion effects in the adult primate. Using lesion studies to establish the anatomical basis of a function at maturity, and normative studies to specify the temporal relationship between human and nonhuman development, investigators can determine the age at which a particular substrate becomes functional in both the human and nonhuman primate. Not all human skills can be studied in this manner. Nonetheless, this research strategy has already proven to be a particularly effective means of gaining information about the brain basis of cognitive development in the infant.

This paradigm presents us with a good example of the developmental neuropsychologist's response to the first and second objections raised earlier. For example, the classic Piagetian explanation for the emergence of the object concept, that is, the development of a stable representation of an object in the world (Piaget, 1952), is that through the sensorimotor period of infancy the child engages the world in a series of sensorimotor operations that culminate in the cognitive structures necessary for emergence of the object concept. Since Piaget observed behaviour while performing interesting, but minor, modifications of the environment to see what the child would do, the descriptions he developed can only be seen as models of what the child would do in certain circumstances, such as the infant's efforts to retrieve an object that was out of sight or in a new place. Why should we ascribe the emergence of the object concept to the sensorimotor practice the child has experienced, as opposed to the maturation of a brain structure suitably connected to put together the present with memories of the past? Perhaps practice plays a relatively minor role in this developmental stage, primarily reflecting the growth in cognitive structures rather than leading the growth. On the other hand, it is hard to see the simple growth of a brain structure as sufficient cause to develop cognitive structures, since they must be embedded within contexts. Both aspects may be necessary but each in themselves is insufficient to account for the intellectual development of the child.

In summary, developmental psychologists can heed the simple reminder by Nadel and Zola-Morgan (1984): "If the machinery is not there, the system will not function" (p. 158). On the other hand, possessing too much machinery too early in development might impede learning (Elman, Bates, Johnson et al., 1996; Newport, 1990). Using neural networks to model selected aspects of language learning, Elman (1993) found that learning occurred only when restrictions of working memory were imposed on the network. This somewhat counterintuitive finding can be understood readily if one assumes that one brain system may process input before presenting it to another brain system. Limited processing capacity of the first system, due to its immaturity, may constitute a form of selective filtering that is adaptive and perhaps essential for the functioning of an immature second system.

## Maturation modulated by experience

### The concept of 'constructivism'

After dismissing the notions of pure maturation and of pure learning as inadequate explanations for anything but the simplest of psychological behaviours, much of contemporary developmental psychology has found comfort in the notion of 'constructivism' (Piaget, 1970). While compatible with a neuropsychological approach in many ways, there are some basic points of contrast on which we would like to focus. Constructivism is the idea that one can bootstrap one's way to cognitive maturity. It is interesting to note that while Piaget originally suggested that maturation alone would account for cognitive changes (Piaget, 1930), he never elaborated on specific mechanisms and would appear to have abandoned this task. The underlying notion in constructivism is that simple cognitive constructs, such as the sensorimotor actions applied to an object in the world by a child, combine in such a way as to evolve a mental representation of the object. Similarly, representations can combine to produce relationships, and relationships can combine to produce logical concepts. Along the way, there are adaptations that the environment requires of the child ('accommodation') and generalizations that the child makes to the world of new objects and events ('assimilation'). All this is prompted by an inherent desire of the system to resolve conflicts in the mental structure of ideas, i.e., to turn the mental representation of the world into an organized whole. Of course, there are limits to how well the child (or adult) can organize these constructs and adapt them to the world. However, the notion that the organism is capable of building complex mental structures from simple ones without being driven by biological maturation is basic to the cognitive constructivist approach to development. Although clearly there must be synaptic changes associated with new learning, this is not the same as suggesting that maturational change prompts the growth of new cognitive systems.

In contrast to this purely constructivist argument, for which brain maturation is not a needed component, the developmental neuropsychologist focuses on the following sort of questions. What happens when sensorimotor actions on the environment, which are proposed to be the primary basis for cognitive development, are so severely restricted from birth due to paralysis that they could not reasonably form the basis for the development of cognitive structures? Jordan (1972) documents such a case that cannot fit the constructivist's rubric (Segalowitz, 1979). Similarly, one may ask why it is that children develop certain cognitive skills at certain times. The traditional developmentalist's explanation for this is that bootstrapping cognitive structures (or, for the behaviourist, learning behavioural response contingencies) takes a certain amount of time, although this is a somewhat nonempirical position. The neuropsychological response is that the brain

structures required for the child to develop fluency in the cognitive operations only mature at certain ages. For example, histological and metabolic evidence suggests that sensory and motor areas mature earlier (Barkovich, Kjos, Jackson and Norman, 1988; Chugani and Phelps, 1986) than areas associated with visual memory, spatial skills and language processes (Scheibel, 1990), while areas involving tertiary association functions such as the prefrontal lobe mature later still, such areas enabling the child to integrate information over time and space (Fuster, 1989). Being able to integrate information over time and space is essential for monitoring oneself and the environment (Schacter, 1987), as well as for inhibiting responses and planning complex behaviours (Fuster, 1989; Goldman-Rakic, 1987b).

The purely constructivist doctrine requires a logical sequence in conceptual development: certain basic concepts must emerge before the complex cognitive structures dependent on them. For example, one should not be able to place oneself within a perceptual context (Piaget's perceptual egocentrism task) without having developed certain cognitive skills (integration across frames of concrete reference). Yet we know from the long history of research on concept formation that this neat pattern is not the way cognitive skills emerge. Rather, there are simple familiar contexts in which the supposedly advanced concept emerges first, contexts in which the subject is not too distracted and the materials are not too novel (Donaldson, 1978; Gelman, 1978). In other words, there are some contexts in which integration of information over time and space is easier than others. For example, children find a variety of logically demanding tasks are easier when the props are familiar dolls and toys than when they are unfamiliar, yet simple, novel objects. That is, the restraining factor is not only the theoretical complexity of the to-be-learned construct, but also the contextual complexities associated with it. This is compatible with the notion that brain maturation places constraints on the ontogeny of cognition through its effect on the amount of new information that can be easily processed and integrated.

The idea of brain maturation constraining behaviour is complicated by the notion discussed above that early experience influences the physiological maturation of the brain. Such a mutual constraint system has yet to be articulated within the context of human development, and one of the complexities to deal with is the differentiation of thought into various levels, such as metacognitive–late maturing versus simple perceptual–early maturing systems (Stuss, 1992). We should expect for logical reasons alone that the latest maturing and most functionally complex areas should be the most influenced by prior experience since there is more opportunity for such an influence. Such a view would be compatible with the notion that rearing style during the child's infancy has an influence on the later cognitive metacontrol processes usually associated with prefrontal lobe systems (White, 1975). However, so far there have been virtually no animal studies that have shown that this prefrontal area is as easily affected by early experience as are the primary sensory areas. The one exception we know of showed that cognitive stimulation in infancy increased the glucose metabolism over the long term in the dorsolateral prefrontal cortex of simians (Raleigh, McGuire, Melega et al., 1996). The lack of more studies such as this one may stem from the fact that the advanced functions associated with the primate prefrontal lobe are not as evident in the rodents and cats which are usually used in this kind of research. In fact, it is not clear how one could specify appropriately enriched experiences for cats, rats and mice.

To recapitulate, the new maturational constructivist model requires several factors to hold: (1) maturational changes must be influenced by experience; (2) the length of time of this influence must be adequately prolonged in order to allow it to affect his or her own development over the long term; and (3) the individual must be able to influence his or her own development by means of choices of behaviour, especially by means of conscious choices. We review the evidence for each of these postulates.

*Effects of stress on brain growth*

One of the main influences on a child's psychological development is the primary caregiver through social and emotional interactions. Social interaction and affective arousal alter catecholamine levels, and engage the sympathetic nervous system. The role of the caregiver for the developing young child is to regulate these, by reducing overarousal, soothing negative affect, and increasing attentional engagement to objects in the environment, including other people. Presumably during the early period of considerable neural growth, plasticity and vulnerability, these systems can reach a more healthy or less healthy outcome. Reducing anxiety from an unacceptable level, or alternatively increasing excitement and arousal to an acceptable level, is a major responsibility. A lack of involvement or insensitive intrusiveness, such as happens sometimes with depressed mothers, can presumably alter the neural response in the child (Dawson, Frey, Self et al., 1999). Without appropriate external stimulation and modulation, it is not clear how well a child can develop affective self-regulation. We do not know whether the affective system requires a relatively small amount of stable and healthy attachment to facilitate adequate emotional self-regulation or whether its healthy development cannot tolerate large amounts of instability. However, the literature on emotional resiliency suggests that some children are capable of benefiting from amazingly small pockets of stability and emotional guidance in an otherwise neglectful context (Werner, 2000).

On the other hand, heightened levels of chronic stress can have deleterious effects on the central nervous system. The stress response involves altered activation of the hypothalamic–pituitary–adrenocortical (HPA) system, resulting in increased levels of the catecholamine neurotransmitters dopamine and noradrenaline, and subsequently of ACTH and cortisol. While normal, everyday challenges may be beneficial for the development of the HPA system, there are also deleterious effects of chronic heightened stress. Such stress can be brought about by either neglect or abuse, with the result of either dampened HPA responsiveness or inappropriately heightened stress response, depending on a variety of complex factors (for summaries of these complexities, see Glaser, 2000, and Gunnar, 1998). Inappropriately high levels of dopamine and noradrenaline are associated with dysfunction of the prefrontal cortex, a region acutely involved in emotional self-regulation (Arnsten, 1999; Schore, 1994). Of course, individual infants will differ in the amount of stress response shown, and their caregivers will vary in their proficiency in soothing. In this way, individual differences naturally arise not only from congenital variations in central nervous system structure, but also from the experiences during infancy, and such effects have been demonstrated in primates experiencing prenatal stress (Schneider, Clarke, Kraemer et al., 1998).

Another implication of high levels of stress during infancy is the effect of cortisol on various aspects of nervous system function. High levels of cortisol have documented effects on the immune response, and more importantly for the discussion here, on the growth of the hippocampus (Sapolsky, 1996). High levels of cortisol (whether achieved through chronic stressors or through medication) lead to atrophy of hippocampal connections, although this is reversible if the levels are reduced. Survivors of severe childhood abuse have been reported to show reduced hippocampal size, and this is associated with diagnosis of post-traumatic stress disorder (PTSD) (Bremner, Randall, Vermetten et al., 1997). Interestingly, the reduced hippocampal size may be a response that only appears later in adulthood (De Bellis, Keshavan, Clark et al., 1999), and therefore may be linked to the normal generation of new cells in that region, which in these cases would be reduced.

Perry and colleagues have also demonstrated that children with post-traumatic stress disorder have overactive sympathetic nervous system responses (Perry, Pollard, Blakley et al., 1995; Perry, Southwick, Yehuda and Giller, 1994), including raised heart rate which has been linked to lowered vagal tone and inhibited social communication (Porges, 1995). Of even more concern is the report that boys who experienced severe neglect (with or without abuse) before the age of 3 years also had lowered plasma levels of dopamine beta hydroxylase, which was correlated with reduced valuation of authority and rules of conscience (Galvin, Stilwell, Shekhar et al., 1997). The authors suggest that this represents a reduced development of the behavioural inhibition system, which is associated with the prefrontal cortex. Similarly, such children show signs of hypervigilance and hyperactivity, with heightened readiness to respond to perceived threats (Perry et al., 1995), traits that may be symptomatic of a reduced efficiency of the behavioural inhibition system (Koenen, Driver, Oscar-Berman et al., 2001). Similarly, in a series of maltreated children and adolescents, brain size correlated positively with age of onset of the abuse and negatively with its duration, while tissue loss (ventricular size) correlated with intrusive thoughts, hyperarousal and dissociation (De Bellis et al., 1999).

*Exuberant growth and sensitivity to experience*

The notion that there is major brain maturation in early childhood accords well, of course, with what we know of changes in the child's functional capacity. In early infancy, there is considerable reorganization of primitive reflexes and this is reflected in the maturation of the electroencephalogram and to the increases in cortical glucose metabolism during this period (Chugani, 1994, 1996). Such increases in visual and sensory cortex correspond to improvements in visual and sensory integrative functions during the second and third month after birth (Bronson, 1974). This pattern of exuberant growth of neuronal processes followed by subsequent elimination of these excess connections (known as 'pruning') extends over much of the period of dramatic cognitive growth in infancy, childhood and adolescence (Chugani, 1996). The advantage of such an extended dynamic growth period is increased sensitivity to the environmental factors that may shape the development, i.e., the child is sensitive to experience allowing for structural changes in the brain to reflect influences of the experience even into complex thought processes. This may be the major hallmark of human development, and may separate us from other mammals.

Because experience fine-tunes brain structure through pruning, the pruning itself is a marker of important advances in information processing. For example, primary auditory and visual sensory cortex reach maximal thickness with subsequent thinning during the middle of the first year after birth, and the electrocortical evoked potential matures in parallel with this change, at first rising in amplitude dramatically and then reducing to a reduced amplitude by the end of the first year (Vaughan and Kurtzberg, 1992). Failure to prune back connections in brain regions associated with conceptual and motor control appropriately may be a source of a variety of developmental disabilities, such as ADHD (Andersen and Teicher, 2000), schizophrenia (Hoffman and Dobscha, 1989), and disabilities associated with fragile-X syndrome (Irwin, Galvez and Greenough, 2000). There are also sex differences in the growth and pruning processes that may account for gender differences in some syndromes (Andersen and Teicher, 2000; De Bellis, Keshavan, Beers et al., 2001).

An important feature of the model of exuberant growth followed by experience-influenced pruning is that each individual develops uniquely. The sculpting of the neural connections can be influenced by many factors. For example, Panksepp (1998) has speculated that early rough-and-tumble play influences the maturation of frontal lobe systems that are responsible for impulse control, and cultural changes limiting such early play behaviour is at the root of the increase in rates of ADHD. He shows in animals that rough-and-tumble play can serve as a mediator and therapy for impulse control (Panksepp, Burgdorf and Gordon, 2002). Whether these effects are due to dendritic pruning or changes in biochemical responses is not yet known, but either would support a model of experience altering some fundamental parameters of child development.

*The long period of maturation*

As was mentioned earlier, the process responsible for learning, including that which takes place later in life, is referred to by Greenough et al. (1987) as "experience-dependent information storage". The mechanism of experience-dependent circuits differs from that of experience-expectant in important ways. The maturational period of the human brain is certainly long enough to permit some aspects of brain function to be guided by experience rather than being driven by a prespecified program. The evidence for a very long period of maturation has been growing rapidly (De Bellis et al., 2001; Giedd, Blementhall, Jeffries et al., 1999; Jernigan, Trauner, Hesselink and Tallal, 1991; Paus, Zijdenbos, Worsley et al., 1999; Sowell and Jernigan, 1998; Sowell, Thompson, Holmes et al., 1999; Sowell, Thompson, Tessner and Toga, 2001; Van Bogaert, Wikler, Damhaut et al., 1998). One mechanism is the prolific production of neuronal connections during the early years that leads to a 'surfeit' that has been documented as thicker cortical tissue (Greenough et al., 1987) and the early over-production of synapses relative to those in the adult (Huttenlocher, 1979;

Huttenlocher and Dabholkar, 1997). This exuberant growth is what makes some elimination feasible and perhaps necessary, and we presume that the lost material represents less efficient or unused aspects of the networks (although there really is no way to prove this at present). This pruning process represents a tremendous opportunity for change that, at least in principle, could be coordinated by specific experiences. The discovery of such initial excess and subsequent elimination of neurons and dendritic material was first made in animals, and the pattern seemed to progress on such a well-defined schedule that it was referred to as 'apoptosis' or 'programmed cell death' (Cowan, Fawcett, O'Leary and Stanfield, 1984; Frost, 1990; Gordon, 1995). However, one of the special qualities of human development is a lengthening of this maturational period, which suggests that any such 'programming' is not well specified beforehand. This longer period is one of plasticity, when the nervous system can organize itself according to its needs. It may extend well into the second decade after birth (Chugani, 1996), and maturational changes indeed occur throughout life (Bartzokis, Beckson, Lu et al., 2001). This period also can be characterized as an especially long period of vulnerability, since the outcome could be for the worse as well as for the better (e.g., White, Coppola and Fitzpatrick, 2001). The question for the developmentalist is how the normal period of childhood presents a set of specific challenges to make best use of this vulnerable period.

In contrast to the experience-expectant networks associated with critical periods, the experience-dependent networks do not have a predisposed pattern for fulfilment and can be influenced by specific experiences throughout life. This characterizes most normal learning (admittedly some learning skills diminish with age, but others improve up to a point), and is supported by the notion of life-long growth of neurons in the hippocampus associated with experience (Gross, 2001; Shors, Miesegaes, Beylin et al., 2001). This experience would not produce specific new neurons (it is unclear how this could possibly happen), but rather may increase the chances of survival of neurons that are created.

While specialists in child development might like to categorize some aspects of growth as representing experience-expectant or experience-dependent networks, there is no biological reason to assume that the two types are entirely separable, and therefore no reason to separate maturation from learning.

### Late maturation of the frontal lobe

Whereas there is some controversy concerning the extent to which the prefrontal cortex structurally matures later than other cortex, there seems to be consensus, as discussed earlier, that this region matures later than others in some functional manner (Goldman-Rakic, Bourgeois and Rakic, 1997; Huttenlocher and Dabholkar, 1997). Indeed, the controversy over whether frontal cortex increases in synaptic density later than other regions of the neocortex may come down to differences in the maturation rate of tissue in humans versus great apes.

In humans, this late frontal maturation applies to infancy and early childhood (Greenough et al., 1987; Kolb and Fantie, 1997) and continues into adolescence and young adulthood (Chugani, 1996; Giedd et al., 1999; Kostovic, Petanjek, Delalle and Judas, 1992; Sowell et al., 1999, 2001; Stuss, 1992). For example, cerebral blood flow as measured by positron emission tomography (PET) is a reasonable reflection of synaptic activity. It rises to adult levels by about 1 year, with the frontal region lagging slightly behind the posterior regions. However, cerebral blood flow continues to rise to almost double the normal adult level and then begins a dramatic reduction at about 8 years through the second decade after birth. Similarly, there is a thinning of the cortex (as shown on MRI) during adolescence (Jernigan and Tallal, 1990; Jernigan et al., 1991), especially in the dorsal (upper) frontal and parietal regions (Sowell et al., 1999), presumably due to the pruning process. Dopamine receptors, found in much of the cortex but especially in frontal lobe tissue, have also been shown (in rats) to dramatically diminish in number through adolescence (Andersen, Thompson, Rutstein et al., 2000). Thus, it appears that there are greater than adult levels of connections, cerebral metabolism, and cortical thickness throughout adolescence. Synapse elimination during this period would be a reasonable mechanism for the dramatic increase in a wide variety of skills, with a gradual reduction in plasticity for most functions (Chugani, 1996). However, while it is healthy to have selective pruning, it is better to have this based on more cortex to begin with (De Bellis et al., 2001).

### Behavioural inhibition, self-regulation, and plasticity

The prefrontal cortex and its connecting networks are critically involved in some of the functions that reflect maturation later in childhood and adolescence. As described earlier, Goldman-Rakic showed that the animals had grown into the deficit, a 'sleeper effect' concept than can be readily understood in terms of brain growth. This is counterintuitive to traditional views of child development where we assume that the brain will show plasticity in development, i.e., that early losses are more easily compensated for. This assumption of plasticity is pervasive in psychology and in our society. Sameroff and his colleagues articulated this notion as a 'self-righting' processes, or 'movement towards health' and espoused a continuity model in which early events were explicitly not seen as having later effects unless some way of linking them over time could be specified (Sameroff and Chandler, 1975; Sameroff and Fiese, 2000). In their examples, children with early neglect or abuse are at risk later because the interactional repertoire first developed is counterproductive and is maintained as the world reacts to them as a negative influence, and they again react counterproductively, thereby continuing the cycle. The plasticity principle rests on the usually reasonable notion of the adaptive quality of growth. If the organism's growth is halted in one direction, then it will grow in some other direction. Growth implies taking advantage of new opportunities, and that this adaptability will lead to positive outcomes if the negative pressure is released, i.e., there will be self-righting. However, the hidden assumption is also that all the necessary tools will be available for that growth. Goldman-Rakic's work shows that this assumption is not always warranted.

Since Goldman-Rakic's studies on monkeys, much work has been done with children who have been victims of frontal lobe damage with a variety of etiologies. There are many fascinating case studies in this literature (Ackerly, 1986; Eslinger, Biddle and Grattan, 1997; Grattan and Eslinger, 1992; Marlowe, 1992; Williams and Mateer, 1992). One well-documented case was of a woman who at the age of 7 years had surgery on her left frontal lobe to correct a congenital venous malformation. Even though she certainly showed some subsequent learning problems in school, her real psychological difficulties started at the age of 12, when puberty brought on its usual new agenda of social temptations, concerns and responsibilities. However, her mechanism for self-regulation and planning was awry. The difficulties she encountered appeared long after one would have expected recovery, and were considerably greater than the intervening psychological profile would have predicted (Grattan and Eslinger, 1992).

Another example involves two teenage boys, guilty of sociopathic delinquent behaviour, who were each reported to have acquired frontal lobe damage through a closed head injury at the ages of 4 and 6 years (Vargha-Khadem, Cowan and Mishkin, 2000). Not only did they fail to show neural plasticity and recovery of function, their behaviour deteriorated considerably. Without knowledge of the earlier brain injuries, we might be tempted to blame their unacceptable behaviour solely on poor parenting or their peer group. But their problem was an inherent difficulty in self-monitoring and utilization of feedback that may only seriously affect behaviour long after the lesion occurred. Two similar extreme cases were documented of young adults showing reasonable intelligence levels but high risk-taking and gross deficiencies in planning, empathy, and emotional self-regulation (Anderson, Bechara, Damasio et al., 1999). They had suffered serious frontal damage in infancy (in one case in a motor vehicle accident, and the other due to surgery to remove a tumour) but both seemed to show immediate good recovery. Both came from families that were stable, highly supportive and well-educated. Yet by adolescence, both children had become unmanageable. These case studies reflect the more general association between antisocial personality disorder and loss of tissue in the prefrontal cortex (Devinsky, Morrell and Vogt, 1995; Raine, Lencz, Bihrle et al., 2000).

### The constant rewiring of functions

There is a highly dynamic competition among cortical neurons for functional connectivity. The representation of the motor and sensory functions in cortical tissue is not fixed. There is always a dynamic struggle going on for the use of neurons and this is illustrated by the way in which connections alter with experience. For example, continued exercise of a specific finger will increase the representation of that finger in the motor and sensory cortex by 'stealing' territory from the representation for neighbouring fingers, not by increasing motor representation overall. Presumably the finger with the increased experience also shows improvement in skilled actions, but whether that improvement is due to its representation by an increased number of neurons or due to some other function (such as the pruning of connections from those neurons) is not known. A violinist has more fine motor exercise with the fingers of the left hand than the right, and also has a greater cortical representation for those fingers. The left thumb does not experience the exercise and does not have increased representation, and the extent of this asymmetry is related to the number of years playing (Elbert, Pantev, Wienbruch et al., 1995). The competition for neural sites is also shown in the finger denervation studies on primates (where the nerve connecting the incoming peripheral sensory input is cut). These studies have shown that the sensory representation of the fingers with intact nerve connections take over the newly disconnected cortical tissue very quickly, indicating that there were already connections available but that these were silent until the competition was removed (for a review, see Kaas, 2000). However, it is not clear that simply by virtue of having a larger representation do the fingers gain in skill. There is some evidence to suggest that the opposite can be true in the visual modality.

### Visual skill development

Maurer and Lewis (2001) report that children with monocular cataracts at birth have reduced vision in the occluded eye even when the cataract is removed in early infancy. This presumably is because a reduced expanse of visual cortex is being driven by the deprived eye. As was shown many years ago, a healthy nondeprived eye takes over many of the cells in the visual cortex that otherwise would be driven by the other eye (Wiesel and Hubel, 1963, 1965). If the number of neurons being driven by the eye is all that mattered, then the nondeprived eye would have better than normal acuity, since it now governs more cells than it would normally. However, the opposite result is found; the nondeprived eye shows less acuity than it normally would have, although clearly more than the deprived eye (Maurer and Lewis, 2001). Thus, although cortical plasticity may be intricately involved in the physiological changes associated with experience, the development of new neural connections is not necessarily synonymous with higher levels of ability.

Visual development also illustrates another important principle in development, that of sleeper effects mentioned earlier. The primary visual cortex of kittens that are raised with distorted or degraded vision show evidence of having altered cell specialization in primary visual cortex. Astigmatism does the same in humans (Freeman and Thibos, 1973). The case of the children with congenital cataracts mentioned above allows us to examine the critical or sensitive period for early visual development in humans. When children have bilateral cataracts removed, they quickly show improvement in their visual acuity since their visual input is now clear, but it is essentially at the level of a newborn, i.e., visual acuity does not mature beyond neonatal levels (about 1/40 that of adults) without visual input. However, they subsequently improve in acuity until 4 years, although they do not completely catch up with peers; however, at 4 years they start to fall further behind again. Thus, while peers continue to improve until they reach adult levels at 6 or 7 years (Ellemberg, Lewis, Liu and Maurer, 1999), those with early deprivation asymptote at 4 years (Maurer and Lewis, 2001). They also remain behind their peers in form perception and visual spatial processing (Goldberg, Maurer, Lewis and Brent, 2001). These effects are thought to occur because the early deprivation hampers proper later development at the primary visual (striate) cortex, with the initial early improvement occurring because of remaining plasticity in this area and perhaps by increased skills in the visual system outside the striate cortex. While some primary visual and such extra-striate regions may be adequate for the continued advancement of visual acuity during the early years, a healthy striate cortex is really needed for full development, and children with early binocular degradation are at serious risk only in later stages (Maurer and Lewis, 2001).

## Top-down control

Since the 1960s, there have been many studies illustrating the now classic finding that activity is a necessity for the healthy development of the cortex, and that activity causes the cortical mantle to grow. There are many excellent reviews of this literature available (e.g., Diamond, 1988; Greenough, 1975; Rosenzweig and Bennett, 1996; Sur and Leamey, 2001), the main point of which is that mental and physical activity are major factors in the healthy robust growth of cortical tissue, and affect the connectivity of the cortex (Elbert et al., 1995). Gottlieb's (1976) insightful summary of some animal embryological work gave psychologists a new awareness that the experience of function is critical for the development of physical structures. Only recently, however, has the technology of developmental neuroscience started to examine the mechanisms involved in activity-dependent growth (Thoenen, 1995).

The firing of neurons is a critical feature in their own growth, and accounts for the maintenance of synapses that might otherwise be withdrawn, or might even stimulate the growth of new synapses (Quartz and Sejnowski, 1997). For children to be directing their own mental growth, it would have to be shown that simply attending to one experience over others increases the neuronal activity in the brain region responsible for that experience (Singer, 1982). We now have such evidence. Putting these together, we can now conclude that children's mental engagement furthers healthy maturation of the specific function in which the child is engaged. Anyone working with children knows that at a functional level children spontaneously engage in challenging activities, and that this is probably a requirement for healthy mental growth. Indeed, Held and Hein (1963) showed many years ago that perceptual experience must be active to be an effective vehicle for learning. What is the nature of the newer evidence?

### Attending increases neuronal firing selectively
Much of the work on attention-directing with humans involves visual stimuli for the simple reason that we know a great deal about the neural pathways for vision and manipulating visuospatial attention. For example, cueing people to attend to one region of the visual field over another changes the activation

of the visual cortex selectively and this is reflected in the scalp EEG. EEG alpha activity (a sign of reduced focal activation in the cortex) increases over visual cortex corresponding to the to-be-ignored visual field even though the stimulus has not been presented yet (Worden, Foxe, Wang and Simpson, 2000). Similarly, when subjects are presented with a visual display containing both moving and stationary dots, the visual-movement region of the cortex (V5) either increases in activation or decreases depending on which set of dots are attended (see also Hopfinger, Buonocore and Mangun, 2000; Macaluso, Frith and Driver, 2000; O'Craven, Rosen, Kwong et al., 1997). Similarly, somatosensory cortex increases activation when a vibratory stimulus is attended to (Meyer, Ferguson, Zatorre et al., 1995). In this sense, practice makes perfect in that increased activation of a particular primary function fine-tunes the cortex at the most fundamental level, not just at the level of strategic planning. This was shown in the visual modality: practising visual orientation identification improves coding in primary visual cortex even in adult brains (Schoups et al., 2001).

This alteration in the cortex may be mediated through the reward system: when a sound is followed by stimulation of dopamine neurons in the ventral tegmental area, a region activated by unexpected rewards and by novel stimuli, the cortical representation of that sound is increased, while the representation of nearby sound frequencies is reduced (Bao, Chan and Merzenich, 2001). We are also starting to understand some of the details of this increased activation. Steinmetz, Roy, Fitzgerald et al. (2000) showed that attention synchronizes the neural firing (in somatosensory cortex) in monkeys, and the more challenging the task, the greater is the increase in synchronized firing. When we have developed the technology to measure such neuronal coordination at the cellular level noninvasively, we will be able to see whether children with attentional difficulties have problems with this particular mechanism, and whether this mechanism is one that requires maturation of the cortex or simply experience. Thus, circuits keep changing physically by growing connections, and the functioning of the brain alters the degree to which regions become activated, thereby feeding back on the growth pattern. With this neuronal growth model in mind, it is not surprising that early

propensities lead to later talents. The system is built to take advantage of what experience has to offer to develop expertise in the world as it presents itself.

## Conclusions

Developmental psychology and developmental neuroscience are finding mutual interests in the constructivist–maturational model, finding that they have more in common than was at all realized even just a decade ago. Developmental neuroscience is now in a position to resolve some of the controversies that seemed unresolvable in developmental psychology (see Segalowitz and Hiscock, 1992, for more examples of these). More importantly, developmental neuroscience presents concrete evidence for a modified model of constructivist development, a modification that integrates many aspects of developmental psychology in a way that was not being as readily accepted earlier. This rapprochement between the two developmental fields will no doubt continue at the current fast pace with the development and increased availability of brain imaging technologies that we are now seeing.

## Acknowledgements

Portions of this chapter appear in SJ Segalowitz and LA Schmidt: Developmental psychology and the neurosciences. In J Valsiner and K Connolly (Eds), Handbook of Developmental Psychology. London: Sage.

## References

Ackerly SS: A case of paranatal bilateral frontal lobe defect observed for thirty years. In Warren JM, K Ackert (Eds), The Frontal Granular Cortex and Behavior. New York, NY: McGraw-Hill, pp. 192–218, 1986.

Alexander GE, Witt E, Goldman-Rakic PS: Neuronal activity in the prefrontal cortex, caudate nucleus and mediodorsal thalamic nucleus during delayed response performance of immature and adult rhesus monkeys. Neuroscience Abstracts: 6; 86, 1980.

Andersen SL, Teicher MH: Sex differences in dopamine receptors and their relevance to ADHD. Neuroscience and Biobehavioral Reviews: 24; 137–141, 2000.

Andersen SL, Thompson AT, Rutstein M, Hostetter JC, Teicher MH: Dopamine receptor pruning in prefrontal cortex during the periadolescent period in rats. Synapse: 37; 167–169, 2000.

Anderson SW, Bechara A, Damasio H, Tranel D, Damasio AR: Impairment of social and moral behavior related to early damage in human prefrontal cortex. Nature Neuroscience: 2; 1032–1037, 1999.

Arnsten AFT: Development of the cerebral cortex: XIV. Stress impairs prefrontal cortical function. Journal of the American Academy of Child and Adolescent Psychiatry: 38; 220–222, 1999.

Baddeley AD: The concept of working memory: A view of its current state and probable future development. Cognition: 10; 17–23, 1981.

Bao S, Chan VT, Merzenich MM: Cortical remodelling induced by activity of ventral tegmental dopamine neurons. Nature: 412; 79–83, 2001.

Barkovich AJ, Kjos BO, Jackson DE Jr, Norman D. Normal maturation of the neonatal and infant brain: MR imaging at 1.5 T. Radiology: 166; 173–80, 1988.

Bartzokis G, Beckson M, Lu PH, Nuechterlein KH, Edwards N, Mintz J: Age-related changes in frontal and temporal lobe volumes in men. Archives of General Psychiatry: 58; 461–465, 2001.

Battig K, Mishkin M, Rosvold HE: Comparison of the effects of frontal and caudate lesions on delayed response and alternation in monkeys. Journal of Comparative and Physiological Psychology: 53; 400–404, 1960.

Bell MA, Fox NA: The relations between frontal brain electrical activity and cognitive development during infancy. Child Development: 63; 1142–1163, 1992.

Blakemore C: Sensitive and vulnerable periods in the development of the visual system. Ciba Foundation Symposium: 156; 129–147, 1991.

Bremner JD, Randall P, Vermetten E, Staib L, Bronen RA, Mazure C, Capelli S, McCarthy G, Innis RB, Charney DS: Magnetic resonance imaging-based measurement of hippocampal volume in posttraumatic stress disorder related to childhood physical and sexual abuse: A preliminary report. Biological Psychiatry: 41; 23–32, 1997.

Bronson G: The postnatal growth of visual capacity. Child Development: 45; 873–890, 1974.

Cameron HA, McKay RDG: Restoring production of hippocampal neurons in old age. Nature Neuroscience: 2; 894–897, 1999.

Chapman B, Godecke I, Bonhoeffer T: Development of orientation preference in the mammalian visual cortex. Journal of Neurobiology: 41; 18–24, 1999.

Chugani HT: Development of regional brain glucose metabolism in relation to behavior and plasticity. In Dawson G, Fischer KW (Eds), Human Behavior and the Developing Brain. New York, NY: Guilford, pp. 153–175, 1994.

Chugani HT: Neuroimaging of developmental nonlinearity and developmental pathologies. In Thatcher TW, Lyon GR, Rumsey J, Krasnegor N (Eds), Developmental Neuroimaging. San Diego, CA: Academic Press, pp. 187–195, 1996.

Chugani DC, Chugani HT: Positron emission tomography (PET) and single photon emission computed tomography (SPECT) in developmental disorders. In Segalowitz SJ, Rapin I (Eds), Child Neuropsychology, Handbook of Neuropsychology, 2nd Edition, vol. 8, part I. Amsterdam: Elsevier, pp. 195–215, 2002.

Chugani HT, Phelps M: Maturational changes in cerebral function in infants determined by [18]FDG Positron Emission tomography. Science: 231; 840–843, 1986.

Cowan WM: Selection and control of neurogenesis. In Schmitt FO, Worden F (Eds), The Neurosciences: Fourth Study Program. Cambridge, MA: MIT Press, 1979.

Cowan WM: The development of the brain. In Llinas RR (Ed.), The Workings of the Brain: Development, Memory, and Perception. New York, NY: Freeman, pp. 39–57, 1990.

Cowan WM, Fawcett JW, O'Leary DDM, Stanfield BB: Regressive events in neurogenesis. Science: 225; 1258–1265, 1984.

Crnie LS, Pennington BF: Special Section: Developmental psychology and the neurosciences: Building a bridge. Child Development: 58; 533–717, 1987.

Daw N: Visual Development. New York, NY: Plenum, 1995.

Dawson G, Fischer KW (Eds): Human Behavior and the Developing Brain. New York, NY: Guilford, 1994.

Dawson G, Frey K, Self J, Panagiotides H, Hessl D, Yamada E, Rinaldi J: Frontal brain electrical activity in infants of depressed and nondepressed mothers: Relation to variations in infant behavior. Development and Psychopathology: 11; 589–605, 1999.

De Bellis MD, Keshavan MS, Beers SR, Hall J, Frustaci K, Masalehdan A, Noll J, Boring AM: Sex differences in brain maturation during childhood and adolescence. Cerebral Cortex: 11; 552–557, 2001.

De Bellis MD, Keshavan MS, Clark DB, Casey BJ, Giedd JN, Boring AM, Frustaci K, Ryan ND: Developmental traumatology Part II: Brain development. Biological Psychiatry: 45; 1271–1284, 1999.

Devinsky O, Morrell MJ, Vogt BA: Contributions of anterior cingulate cortex to behaviour. Brain: 118; 279–306, 1995.

Diamond A: Development of the ability to use recall to guide action, as indicated by infants' performance on A-not-B. Child Development: 56; 868–883, 1985.

Diamond MC: Enriching Heredity: The Impact of the Environment on the Anatomy of the Brain. New York, NY: The Free Press, 1988.

Diamond A: The development and neural bases of memory functions as indexed by the AB and delayed response tasks in human infants and infant monkeys. Annals of the New York Academy of Sciences: 608; 267–317, 1990.

Diamond A: Neuropsychological insights into the meaning of object concept development. In Carey S, Gelman R (Eds), The Epigenesis of Mind: Essays on Biology and Cognition. Hillsdale, NJ: Erlbaum, pp. 67–110, 1991.

Diamond A: Evidence for the importance of dopamine for prefrontal cortex functions early in life. In Roberts AC, Robbins TW, Weiskrantz L (Eds), The Prefrontal Cortex: Executive and Cognitive Functions. New York, NY: Oxford University Press, pp. 144–164, 1998.

Diamond A: A model system for studying the role of dopamine int the prefrontal cortex during early development in humans: Early and continuously treated phenylketonuria. In Nelson CA, Luciana M (Eds), Handbook of Developmental Cognitive Neuroscience. Cambridge, MA: MIT Press, pp. 433–472, 2001.

Diamond A, Doar B: The performance of human infants on a measure of frontal cortex function, the delayed response task. Developmental Psychobiology: 22; 271–294, 1989.

Diamond A, Goldman-Rakic PS: Comparison of human infants and rhesus monkeys on Piaget's AB task: Evidence for dependence on dorsolateral prefrontal cortex. Experimental Brain Research: 74; 24–40, 1989.

Diamond A, Prevor MB, Callender G, Druin DP: Prefrontal cortex cognitive deficits in children treated early and continuously for PKU. Monographs of the Society for Research in Child Development; 62: 1–205, 1997.

Diamond E, Goldman-Rakic P. Evidence for involvement of prefrontal cortex in cognitive changes during the first year of life: Comparison of performance of human infants and rhesus monkeys on a detour task with transparent barrier. Neuroscience Abstracts: 11; 832, 1985.

Donaldson M: Children's Minds. New York, NY: Norton, 1978.

Elbert T, Pantev C, Wienbruch C, Rockstroh B, Taub E: Increased cortical representation of the fingers of the left hand in string players. Science: 270; 305–307, 1995.

Ellemberg D, Lewis TL, Liu CH, Maurer D: The development of spatial and temporal vision during childhood. Vision Research: 39; 2325–2333, 1999.

Elman JL: Learning and development in neural networks: The importance of starting small. Cognition; 48: 71–99, 1993.

Elman JL, Bates EA, Johnson MH, Karmiloff-Smith A, Parisi D, Plunkett K: Rethinking Innateness: A Connectionist Perspective on Development. Cambridge, MA: MIT Press, 1996.

Eslinger PJ, Biddle KR, Grattan LM: Cognitive and social development in children with prefrontal cortex lesions. In Krasnegor NA, Lyon GR, Goldman-Rakic P (Eds), Development of the Prefrontal Cortex. Baltimore, MD: Paul H. Brookes, pp. 295–335, 1997.

Finney EM, Fine I, Dobkins KR: Visual stimuli activate auditory cortex in the deaf. Nature Neuroscience: 4; 1171–1173, 2001.

Freeman RD, Thibos LN: Electrophysiological evidence that abnormal early visual experience can modify the human brain. Science: 180; 876–878, 1973.

Frost DO: Sensory processing by novel, experimentally induced cross-modal circuits. Annals of the New York Academy of Sciences: 608; 92–112, 1990.

Fuster JM: The prefrontal cortex and temporal integration. In Jones EG, Peters A (Eds), Cerebral Cortex. New York, NY: Plenum, pp. 151–157, 1985.

Fuster JM: The Prefrontal Cortex: Anatomy, Physiology, and Neuropsychology of the Frontal Lobe (2nd edn.). New York, NY: Raven Press, 1989.

Galvin MR, Stilwell BM, Shekhar A, Kopta SM, Goldbarb SM: Maltreatment, conscience functioning and dopamine beta hydroxylase in emotionally disturbed boys. Child Abuse and Neglect: 21; 83–92, 1997.

Gelman R: Cognitive development. In Rosenzweig MR, Porter LW (Eds), Annual Review of Psychology, Vol. 29. Palo Alto, CA: Annual Reviews, 1978.

Giedd JN, Blementhall J, Jeffries NO, Castellanos FX, Liu H, Zijdenbos A, Paus T, Evans AC, Rapoport JL: Brain development during childhood and adolescence: a longitudinal MRI study. Nature Neuroscience: 2; 861–863, 1999.

Glaser D: Child abuse and neglect and the brain: A review. Journal of Child Psychology and Psychiatry: 41; 97–116, 2000.

Goldberg MC, Maurer D, Lewis TL, Brent HP: The influence of binocular visual deprivation on the development of visual–spatial attention. Developmental Neuropsychology: 19; 55–83, 2001.

Goldman PS: Functional development of the prefrontal cortex in early life and the problem of neuronal plasticity. Experimental Neurology: 32; 366–387, 1971.

Goldman PS: An alternative to developmental plasticity: heterology of CNS structures in infants and adults. In Stein DG, Rosen JJ, Butters N (Eds), Plasticity and Recovery of Function in the Nervous System. New York, NY: Academic Press, pp. 149–174, 1974.

Goldman PS, Alexander GE: Maturation of prefrontal cortex in the monkey revealed by local reversible cryogenic depression. Nature: 267; 613–615, 1977.

Goldman PS, Galkin TW: Prenatal removal of frontal association cortex in the fetal rhesus monkey: Anatomical and function consequence in postnatal life. Brain Research: 152; 451–485, 1978.

Goldman PS, Rosvold HE: The effects of selective caudate lesions in infant and juvenile rhesus monkeys. Brain Research: 43; 53–66, 1972.

Goldman PS, Rosvold HE, Mishkin M: Selective sparing of function following prefrontal lobectomy in infant monkeys. Experimental Neurology: 29; 221–226, 1970.

Goldman-Rakic PS: Circuitry of the prefrontal cortex and the regulation of behavior by representational knowledge. In Plum F, Mountcastle V (Eds), Handbook of Physiology: Vol. 5. Bethesda, MD: American Physiological Society, pp. 373–417, 1987a.

Goldman-Rakic PS: Development of cortical circuitry and cognitive function. Child Development: 58; 601–622, 1987b.

Goldman-Rakic PS, Bourgeois J-P, Rakic P: Synaptic substrate of cognitive development. In Krasnegor NA, Lyon GR, Goldman-Rakic P (Eds), Development of the Prefrontal Cortex. Baltimore, MD: Paul H. Brookes, pp. 27–47, 1997.

Goldman-Rakic PS, Isseroff A, Schwartz ML, Bugbee NM: The neurobiology of cognitive development. In Mussen PH (Ed.), Handbook of Child Psychology (4th edn.): Vol. 2. Infancy and Developmental Psychobiology (Vol. Eds MM Haith and JJ Campos). New York, NY: Wiley, pp. 281–344, 1983.

Gordon N: Apoptosis (programmed cell death) and other reasons for elimination of neurons and axons. Brain Development: 17; 73–77, 1995.

Gottlieb G: Conceptions of prenatal development: behavioral embryology. Psychology Review: 83; 215–234, 1976.

Gratch G, Landers W: Stage IV of Piaget's theory of infants' object concepts: a longitudinal study. Child Development: 42; 359–372, 1971.

Grattan LM, Eslinger PJ: Long-term psychological consequences of childhood frontal lobe lesion in patient DT. Brain and Cognition: 20; 185–195, 1992.

Greenough WT: Experiential modification of the developing brain. American Scientist: 63; 37–46, 1975.

Greenough WT, Black JE, Wallace CS: Experience and brain development. Child Development: 58; 539–559, 1987.

Gross CG: Neurogenesis in the adult brain: death of a dogma. Nature Reviews Neuroscience: 1; 67–72, 2001.

Gunnar MR: Quality of early care and buffering of neuroendocrine stress reactions: Potential effects on the developing human brain. Preventive Medicine: 27; 208–211, 1998.

Held R, Hein A: Movement-produced stimulation in the development of visually guided behavior. Journal of Comparative and Physiological Psychology: 56; 872–876, 1963.

Hirsch HV: The role of visual experience in the development of cat striate cortex. Cell Molecular Neurobiology: 5; 103–121, 1985.

Hoffman RE, Dobscha SK: Cortical pruning and the development of schizophrenia: a computer model. Schizophrenia Bulletin: 15; 477–490, 1989.

Hopfinger JB, Buonocore MH, Mangun GR: The neural mechanisms of top-down attentional control. Nature Neuroscience: 3; 284–291, 2000.

Huttenlocher PR: Synaptic density in human frontal cortexdevelopmental changes and effects of aging. Brain Research: 163; 195–205, 1979.

Huttenlocher PR, Dabholkar AS: Developmental anatomy of prefrontal cortex. In Krasnegor NA, Lyon GR, Goldman-Rakic PS (Eds), Development of the Prefrontal Cortex. Baltimore, MD: Brookes, pp. 69–83, 1997.

Irwin SA, Galvez R, Greenough WT: Dendritic spine structural anomalies in fragile-X mental retardation syndrome. Cerebral Cortex: 10; 1038–1034, 2000.

Isseroff A, Galkin T, Rosvold HE, Goldman-Rakic PS: Spatial memory impairments following damage to the mediodorsal nucleus of the thalamus in rhesus monkeys. Brain Research: 232; 97–113, 1982.

Jernigan TL, Tallal P: Late childhood changes in brain morphology observable with MRI. Developmental Medicine and Child Neurology: 32; 379–385, 1990.

Jernigan TL, Trauner DA, Hesselink JR, Tallal PA: Maturation of human cerebrum observed in vivo during adolescence. Brain: 114; 2037–2049, 1991.

Jordan N: Is there an Achilles' heal in Piaget's theorizing? Human Development: 15; 379–382, 1972.

Jueptner M, Stefan K, Frith CD, Brooks DJ, Fackowiak RSJ, Passingham RE: Anatomy of motor learning, I. Frontal cortex and attention to action. Journal of Neurophysiology: 77; 1313–1324, 1997.

Juranek J, Fikipek PA: Neuroimaging in the developmental disorders. In Segalowitz SJ, Rapin I (Eds), Child Neuropsychology, Handbook of Neuropsychology, 2nd Edition, vol. 8, part I. Amsterdam: Elsevier, pp. 175–194, 2002.

Kaas JH: The reorganization of sensory and motor maps after injury in adult mammals. In Gazzaniga MS (Ed), The New Cognitive Neurosciences. Cambridge, MA: MIT Press, pp. 223–236, 2000.

Kagan J: Perspectives on continuity. In Brim OG Jr, Kagan i (Eds), Constancy and Change in Human Development. Cambridge, MA: Harvard University Press, 1980.

Kim KH, Relkin NR, Lee KM, Hirsch J: Distinct cortical areas associated with native and second languages. Nature: 388; 171–174, 1997.

Kinsbourne M: School problems. Pediatrics: 52; 697–710, 1973.

Koenen KC, Driver KL, Oscar-Berman M, Wolfe J, Folsom S, Huang MT, Schlesinger L: Measures of prefrontal system dysfunction in posttraumatic stress disorder. Brain and Cognition: 45; 64–78, 2001.

Kolb B, Fantie B: Development of the child's brain and behavior. In Reynolds CR, Fletcher-Janzen E (Eds), Handbook of Clinical Child Neuropsychology. New York, NY: Plenum, pp. 17–41, 1997.

Kostovic I, Petanjek Z, Delalle I, Judas M: Developmental reorganization of the human association cortex during perinatal and postnatal life. In Kostovic I, Knezevic S, Wisniewski HM, Spilich GJ (Eds), Neurodevelopment, Aging and Cognition. Boston, MA: Birkhauser, pp. 3–17, 1992.

Leclerc C, Saint-Amouir D, Lavoie ME, Lassonde M, Lepore F: Brain functional reorganization in early blind humans revealed by auditory event-related potentials. NeuroReport: 11; 545–550, 2000.

Macaluso E, Frith CD, Driver J: Modulation of human visual cortex by crossmodal spatial attention. Science: 289; 1206–1208, 2000.

Markowitsch HJ: Diencephalic amnesia: a reorientation towards tracts. Brain Research Review: 13; 351–370, 1988.

Marlowe WB: The impact of a right prefrontal lesion on the developing brain. Brain and Cognition: 20; 205–213, 1992.

Maurer D, Lewis TL: Visual acuity: The role of visual input in inducing postnatal change. Clinical Neuroscience Research: (in press); 2001.

McGraw MB: Maturation of behavior. In Carmichael L (Ed), Manual of Child Psychology. New York, NY: Wiley, pp. 332–369, 1946.

Meyer E, Ferguson SSG, Zatorre RJ, Alivisatos B, Marrett S, Evans AC, Hakim AM: Attention modulates somatosensory cerebral blood flow response to vibrotactile stimulation as measured by positron emission tomography. Annals of Neurology: 29; 440–443, 1995.

Mitchell DE, Timney B: Postnatal development of function in the mammalian nervous system. In Brookhart JM, Mountcastle VR (Eds), Handbook of Physiology, Sec. 1. The Nervous System: Vol. 3. Bethesda, MD: American Physiological Society, pp. 507–555, 1984.

Moore C: The role of maternal stimulation in the development of sexual behavior and its neural basis. Annals of the New York Academy of Sciences: 622; 160–177, 1992.

Morris RGM, Garrud P, Rawlins JNP, O'Keefe J: Place navigation impaired in rats with hippocampal lesions. Nature: 297; 681–683, 1982.

Movshon JA, Van Sluyters RC: Visual neuronal development. Annual Review of Psychology: 32; 477–522, 1981.

Mower G, Christen W, Caplan C: Very brief visual experience

eliminates plasticity in the cat visual cortex. Science: 221; 178–180, 1983.

Muhlnickel W, Elbert T, Taub E, Flor H: Reorganization of auditory cortex in tinnitus. Proceedings of the National Academy of Sciences USA: 95; 10340–10343, 1998.

Nadel L, Zola-Morgan S: Infantile amnesia: a neurobiological perspective. In Moscovitch M (Ed.), Infant Memory: Its Relation to Normal and Pathological Memory in Humans and Other Animals. New York, NY: Plenum, pp. 145–172, 1984.

Nass R: Plasticity: mechanisms, extents and limits. In Segalowitz SJ, Rapin I (Eds), Child Neuropsychology, Handbook of Neuropsychology, 2nd Edition, vol. 8, part I. Amsterdam: Elsevier, pp. 29–68, 2002.

Newport EL: Maturational constraints on language learning. Cognitive Science: 14; 11–28, 1990.

O'Craven KM, Rosen BR, Kwong KK, Triesman A, Savoy RL: Voluntary attention modulates fMRI activity in human MT-MST. Neuron: 18; 591–598, 1997.

Olton DS: Memory functions and the hippocampus. In Siefert W (Ed), Neurobiology of the Hippocampus. New York, NY: Academic Press, pp. 335–373, 1983.

Olton DS, Papas BC: Spatial memory and hippocampal function. Neuropsychologia: 17; 669–682, 1979.

Panksepp J: Attention deficit hyperactivity disorders, psychostimulants and intolerance of childhood playfulness: A tragedy in the making? Current Directions in Psychological Science; 7; 91–98, 1998.

Panksepp J, Burgdorf J, Gordon N: Modeling ADHD-type arousal with unilateral frontal cortex damage in rats and beneficial effects of play therapy. Brain and Cognition: 2002, in press.

Passingham RE: Memory of monkeys (*Macaca mulatto*) with lesions in prefrontal cortex. Behavioral Neuroscience: 99; 3–21, 1985.

Paus T, Zijdenbos A, Worsley K, Collins DL, Blumenthal J, Giedd JN, Rapoport JL, Evans AC: Structural maturation of neural pathways in children and adolescents: In vivo study. Science: 283; 1908–1911, 1999.

Perry BD, Pollard RA, Blakley TL, Baker WL, Vigilante D: Childhood trauma, the neurobiology of adaptation, and 'use-dependent' development of the brain: How 'states' become 'traits'. Infant Mental Health Journal: 16; 271–289, 1995.

Perry BD, Southwick SM, Yehuda R, Giller EL: Adrenergic receptor regulation in posttraumatic stress disorder. In Giller EL (Eds), Biological Assessment and Treatment of Posttraumatic Stress Disorder. Washington, DC: American Psychiatric Press, pp. 87–114, 1994.

Piaget J: The Child's Conception of Physical Causality. London: Routledge and Kegan Paul, 1930.

Piaget J: The Origins of Intelligence in Children. New York, NY: Norton, 1952.

Piaget J: Genetic Epistemology. New York, NY: Columbia University Press, 1970.

Ponton CW, Moore JK, Eggermont JJ: Prolonged deafness limits auditory system developmental plasticity: evidence from an evoked potentials study in children with cochlear implants. Scandinavian Audiology: 28; 13–22, 1999.

Porges SW: Orienting in a defensive world: Mammalian modifications of our evolutionary heritage: A polyvagal theory. Psychophysiology: 32; 301–318, 1995.

Post RM, Weiss SRB: Emergent properties of neural systems: How focal molecular neurobiological alterations can affect behavior. Development and Psychopathology: 9; 907–929, 1997.

Quartz S, Sejnowski TJ: The neural basis of cognitive development: A constructivist manifesto. Behavioral and Brain Sciences: 20; 537–596, 1997.

Raine A, Lencz T, Bihrle S, LaCasse L, Colletti P: Reduced prefrontal gray matter volume and reduced autonomic activity in antisocial personality disorder. Archives of General Psychiatry: 57; 119–127, 2000.

Raleigh M, McGuire M, Melega W, Cherry S, Huang S-C, Phelps M: Neural mechanisms supporting successful social decisions in simians. In Damasio AR, Damasio H, Christen Y (Eds), Neurobiology of Decision-Making. Berlin: Springer, pp. 63–82, 1996.

Rosenzweig MR, Bennett EL: Psychobiology of plasticity: Effects of training and experience on brain and behavior. Behavioral and Brain Research: 78; 57–65, 1996.

Sameroff AJ, Chandler MJ: Reproductive risk and the continuum of caretaking casualty. In Horwitz FD, Hetherington M, Scarr-Salapatek S (Eds), Review of Child Developmental Research. Chicago, IL: University of Chicago Press, pp. 187–244, 1975.

Sameroff AJ, Fiese BH: Transactional regulation: The developmental ecology of early intervention. In Shonkoff JP, Meisels SJ (Eds), Handbook of Early Childhood Intervention. Cambridge: Cambridge University Press, pp. 135–159, 2000.

Sapolsky RM: Why stress is bad for your brain. Science: 273; 749–750, 1996.

Schacter DL: Memory, amnesia, and frontal lobe dysfunction. Psychobiology: 15; 21–36, 1987.

Scheibel AB: Dendritic correlates of higher cognitive function. In Scheibel AB, Wechsler AF (Eds), Neurobiology of Higher Cognitive Function. New York, NY: Guilford, pp. 239–270, 1990.

Schneider ML, Clarke S, Kraemer GW, Roughton EC, Lubach GR, Rimm-Kaufman S, Schmidt D, Ebert M: Prenatal stress alters brain biogenic amine levels in primates. Development and Psychopathology: 10; 427–440, 1998.

Schore AN: Affect Regulation and the Origin of the Self. Hillsdale, NJ: Erlbaum, 1994.

Schoups A, Vogels R, Qian N, Orban G: Practising orientation identification improves orientation coding in V1 neurons. Nature: 412; 549–553, 2001.

Schulman HS: Impaired delayed response from thalamic lesions. Archives of Neurology: 11; 477–499, 1964.

Segalowitz SJ: Piaget's Achilles' heel: a safe soft spot? Human Development: 23; 137–140, 1979.

Segalowitz SJ: Why twin studies don't really tell us much about human heritability. Behavioral and Brain Sciences: 22; 904–905, 1999.

Segalowitz SJ, Hiscock M: The emergence of a neuropsychology of normal development: Rapprochement between neuroscience and developmental psychology. In Rapin I, Segalowitz SJ (Eds), Child Neuropsychology (in F. Boller and J. Grafman (series editors), Handbook of Neuropsychology). Amsterdam: Elsevier, pp. 45–71, 1992.

Segalowitz SJ, Rose-Krasnor L: The construct of brain maturation in theories of child development. Brain and Cognition: 20; 1–7, 1992.

Segalowitz SJ, Wagner WJ, Menna R: Lateral versus frontal ERP predictors of reading skill. Brain and Cognition: 20; 85–103, 1992.

Shankle WR, Landing BH, Rafii MS, Schiano A, Chen JM, Hara J. Evidence for a Postnatal Doubling of Neuron Number in the Developing Human Cerebral Cortex Between 15 Months and 6 years. Journal of Theoretical Biology: 191; 115–140, 1998.

Shors TJ, Miesegaes G, Beylin A, Zhao M, Rydel T, Gould E: Neurogenesis in the adult is involved in the formation of trace memories. Nature: 410; 372–376, 2001.

Singer W: The role of attention in developmental plasticity. Human Neurobiology: 1; 41–43, 1982.

Sokol DK, Moore CA, Rose RJ, Williams CJ, Reed T, Christian JC: Intra-pair differences in personality and cognitive ability among young monozygotic twins distanced by chorion type. Behavior Genetics: 25; 457–466, 1995.

Sowell ER, Jernigan TL: Further MRI evidence of late brain maturation: limbic volume increases and changing asymmetries during childhood and adolescence. Developmental Neuropsychology: 14; 599–617, 1998.

Sowell ER, Thompson PM, Holmes CJ, Jernigan TL, Toga AW: In vivo evidence for post-adolescent brain maturation in frontal and striatal regions. Nature Neuroscience: 2; 859–861, 1999.

Sowell ER, Thompson PM, Tessner KD, Toga AW: Mapping continued brain growth and gray matter density reduction in dorsal frontal cortex: Inverse relationships during postadolescent brain maturation. The Journal of Neuroscience: 21; 8819–8829, 2001.

Squire LR, Amaral DG, Zola-Morgan S, Kritchevsky M, Press G: Description of brain injury in the amnesia patient N.A. based on magnetic resonance imaging. Experimental Neurology: 105; 23–35, 1989.

Stanwood GD, Washington RA, Levitt P: Identification of a sensitive period of prenatal cocaine exposure that alters the development of the anterior cingulate cortex. Cerebral Cortex: 11; 430–440, 2001.

Steinmetz PN, Roy A, Fitzgerald PJ, Hsiao SS, Johnson KO, Niebur E: Attention modulates synchronized neuronal firing in primate somatosensory cortex. Nature: 404; 187–190, 2000.

Stiles J: Neural plasticity and cognitive development. Developmental Neuropsychology: 18; 237–272, 2000.

Stuss DT: Biological and psychological development of executive functions. Brain and Cognition: 20; 8–23, 1992.

Sur M, Leamey C: Development and plasticity of cortical areas and networks. Nature Neuroscience Reviews: 2; 251–262, 2001.

Thoenen H: Neurotrophins and neuronal plasticity. Science: 270; 593–598, 1995.

Thompson PM, Cannon TD, Narr KL, Van Erp T, Poutanen V-

P, Huttunen M, Lönnqvist J, Standertskjöld-Nordenstam C-G, Kaprio J, Khaledy M, Dail R, Zoumala CI, Toga AW: Genetic influences on brain structure. Nature Neuroscience: 4; 1253–1258, 2001.

Towbin A: Cerebral dysfunctions related to perinatal organic damage. Journal of Abnormal Psychology: 87; 617–635, 1978.

Van Bogaert P, Wikler JD, Damhaut P, Szliwowski HB, Goldmant S: Regional changes in glucose metabolism during brain development from the age of 6 years. Neuroimage: 9; 62–68, 1998.

Vargha-Khadem F, Cowan J, Mishkin M: Sociopathic behaviour after early damage to prefrontal cortex. Society for Neurosciences, 2000.

Vaughan HG, Kurtzberg D: Electrophysiologic indices of human brain maturation and cognitive development. In Gunnar MR, CA Nelson (Eds), Developmental Behavioral Neuroscience. Hillsdale, NJ: Erlbaum, pp. 1–36, 1992.

Wahlsten D: Genetics and the development of brain and behavior. In Valsiner J, Connolly K (Eds), Handbook of Developmental Psychology. London: Sage, in press.

Wahlsten D, Gottlieb G: The invalid separation of effects of nature and nurture: Lessons from animal experimentation. In Sternberg RJ, Grigorenko EL (Eds), Intelligence, Heredity, and Environment. New York, NY: Cambridge University Press, pp. 163–192, 1997.

Weeks R, Horwitz B, Aziz-Sultan A, Tian B, Wessinger CM, Cohen LG, Hallett M, Rauschecker JP: A positron emission tomographic study of auditory localization in the congenitally blind. Journal of Neuroscience: 20; 2664–2672, 2000.

Werker JF, Tees RC: Cross-language speech perception: Evidence for perceptual reorganization during the first year of life. Infant Behavior and Development: 7; 49–63, 1984.

Werner EE: Protective factors and individual resilience. In Shonkoff JP, Meisels SJ (Eds), Handbook of Early Childhood Intervention. Cambridge: Cambridge University Press, pp. 115–132, 2000.

White B: The First Three Years of Life. Englewood Cliffs, NJ: Prentice-Hall, 1975.

White LE, Coppola DM, Fitzpatrick D: The contribution of sensory experience to the maturation of orientation selectivity in ferret visual cortex. Nature: 411; 1049–1052, 2001.

Wiesel TN, Hubel DH: Single-cell responses in striate cortex of kittens deprived of vision in one eye. Journal of Neurophysiology: 26; 1002–1017, 1963.

Wiesel TN, Hubel DH: Comparison of the effects of unilateral and bilateral eye closure on cortical unit responses in kittens. Journal of Neurophysiology: 28; 1029–1040, 1965.

Williams D, Mateer CA: Developmental impact of frontal lobe injury in middle childhood. Brain and Cognition: 20; 196–204, 1992.

Worden MS, Foxe JJ, Wang N, Simpson GV: Anticipatory biasing of visuospatial attention indexed by retinotopically specific alpha-band electroenephalography increases over occipital cortex. The Journal of Neuroscience: 20; RC63, 2000.

*Handbook of Neuropsychology*, 2nd Edition, Vol. 8, Part I
S.J. Segalowitz and I. Rapin (Eds)

CHAPTER 3

# Plasticity: mechanisms, extent and limits

Ruth Nass [*]

*Department of Neurology, New York University Medical Center, 400 E 34th Street, New York, NY 10016, USA*

## Introduction

Plasticity can be defined as the brain's capacity to change. All of normal development and learning represent forms of plasticity. Most studies of plasticity, however, assess the brain's response to injury (Bach-y-Rita, 1990). In this chapter, which addresses both the upper and lower limits of plasticity in the immature nervous system, the most frequently referred to models will be those of early focal brain injury and of early sensory deprivation (e.g., deafness). Mechanisms underlying plasticity, factors that affect it, and features in specific skill systems will be discussed.

## Mechanisms of plasticity

### *Normal development: synaptogenesis and myelination*

Synaptogenesis (Nitkin, 2000) (including formation of synaptic connections, growth of axons and dendrites and increased efficacy of synaptic interactions) and myelination are the major events of early central nervous system development (Nelson and Luciana, 2001). Synaptogenesis and resultant synaptic density reach an apex in late infancy and then decline significantly during childhood. Both the addition and elimination of synapses are crucial to learning. Synaptic development and elimination occur at different rates in different cortical regions and have clinical correlates. For example, synaptogenesis in

the angular gyrus and Broca's area occur at similar rates in the right and left hemispheres (Huttenlocher, 1994), but ultimate synaptic density is greater in the left perisylvian language region (Scheibel, Conrad, Perdue et al., 1990), suggesting that there are different patterns of elimination in the two hemispheres. Beginning as early as at the age of 9 years synaptic density and extent of dendritic arborization in Wernicke's area is greater in females than males (Jacobs, Schall and Scheibel, 1993), consistent with the gender difference for some verbal skills. Myelination is a more prolonged process than synaptogenesis, and continues into adolescence and beyond. Clinical correlates include improved performance on both cognitive (e.g., some language tasks) and sensorimotor learning tasks (e.g., crossed tactile localization) that depend on the corpus callosum, the largest and latest structure to myelinate (Jeeves, 1992).

Experience alters brain development by modifying existing neural circuitry and by creating novel circuitry. (During initial brain development all circuitry is, by definition, novel.) In animal models the effects of experience vary both qualitatively and quantitatively with even minor variations in age. For example, 'enriched' experiences during the immediate postnatal period have no measurable effect on dendritic length, but lead to a decrease in spine density. Enriched experiences during the juvenile and adolescent period produce increases in dendritic length, but decreases in spine density. Similar experiences later in life increase both dendritic length and spine density. All these scenarios have behavioral sequela in adulthood (Kolb and Gibb, 2001). Human data are limited, but education has been shown to

---

[*] E-mail: ruth.nass@nyu.edu

affect dendritic arborization. The cortical neurons of people with a university education have more dendritic arbors than those of people with a high-school education who, in turn, have more than those without a high-school education (Taylor and Alden, 1997). Dendritic complexity is greater in the motor cortex of people whose occupations involve more dexterity (Scheibel, 1990). Of course, neural complexity could be the cause of success rather than its result.

The age-dependent changes in the cortex and the differential sensitivity of the brain to experience during development factor into plasticity. The developing brain may amplify relatively minor differences in experience and the environment. How different experiences at different times in development interact and to what extent the absence of a particular experience can be compensated for later in life are areas of active investigation.

The immature brain's ability to change (plasticity) is critical for learning and development. But these early critical periods are also vulnerable periods. Rapidly changing structures are more sensitive to injury/environmental stresses, e.g., anoxia, trauma, malnutrition, sensory deprivation. The same metabolic insult often has a less detrimental effect in the mature nervous system than in the immature nervous system. The enhanced plasticity of the immature nervous system contrasts with its greater vulnerability to injury. The extent of recovery after injury reflects a balance between these two factors.

*Regeneration*

Regeneration does not generally occur in either the mature or immature central nervous system. Fetal neural stem cell transplants have been used to bypass the relative inability of the central nervous system to regenerate. However, the success of transplants requires that developmental cues be preserved. For example, the radial glial cell scaffolding necessary for long-distance migration of cortical neurons is no longer present in the adult cortex. Transplanted neurons may not migrate or differentiate appropriately in the adult brain. Furthermore, doing so may not be sufficient to restore function. Neurons operate via precise, long-distance connections; reestablishing such connections is not trivial (Rakic, 1998). Nonetheless, the possibility of therapeutic neuron re-

placement in both the immature and mature nervous system is fast becoming a reality (Studer, 2001).

Embryonic progenitor cells in the adult human hippocampus (Eriksson, Perfilieva and Björk-Eriksson et al., 1998) and ventricular temporal horn have recently been shown to have the capability to generate new neurons. In animal models the hippocampus, 'old' archicortex, continues to gain neurons during adulthood, while neurogenesis of the phylogenetically 'new' neocortex is completed by or around the time of birth. Neurogenesis in the adult human brain would theoretically be more likely to occur in the dentate gyrus, a region involved in memory formation, rather than in the neocortex, where long-term memories are stored. The decline in neuronal turnover in cortex may have evolved to promote the retention of long-term memory in species dependent on learned behavior. However, although preservation of neurons during the lifespan may enhance memory storage, the decline in the capacity for neurogenesis is detrimental when lost neurons need replacement in neurodegenerative disorders, e.g., brain injury or aging (Rakic, 1998).

*Diaschisis and release from diaschisis*

The term diaschisis refers to a functional impairment at an anatomically connected site, remote from the area of injury. Diaschisis results from a loss of afferent input to the remote site. Release from diaschisis was one of the earliest mechanisms proposed to explain recovery from injury and as such is a form of plasticity. To the extent that injuries to the immature nervous system are generally subject to longer follow-up than injuries to the adult nervous system, release from diaschisis may be in part an artifact of length of follow-up. Indeed, longitudinal studies in adults indicate that the presence or absence of crossed cerebellar diaschisis relates to the time since injury, i.e., diaschisis disappears over time (Di Piero, Chollet, Dolan et al., 1990).

Different patterns of diaschisis are described after early versus late injury. Crossed cerebellar diaschisis (common after strokes in adults) has been ascribed to a functional disconnection between the cerebral cortex and the contralateral cerebellar hemisphere. Dynamic imaging reveals cerebellar hypometabolism. Crossed cerebellar hypometabolism is less common in children (Niimura, Chugani, Muzik et al., 1999). Furthermore, diaschisis patterns appear to be age-dependent even during infancy. In one series (Shamoto and Chugani, 1997) crossed cerebellar hypometabolism was present in 22 children; symmetric cerebellar metabolism was found in 16 children. The presence of crossed cerebellar hypometabolism was typically associated (75% of cases) with a postnatal injury, while symmetric cerebellar metabolism was seen only in patients whose injury occurred prior to 4 weeks of age. Recovery from crossed cerebellar diaschisis occurred only in those whose injury occurred before the age of 10 years. In view of the cerebellum's role in cognition, particularly language (Leiner, Leiner and Dow, 1991), age-dependent patterns of and recovery from diaschisis could underlie some of the differences in cognitive recovery related to age.

Factors in addition to age affect diaschisis. Cerebellar metabolism is state-dependent during the chronic phase after injury; it is symmetrical at rest and asymmetrical during a motor task (Di Piero et al., 1990). (The greater difficulty in performing dynamic studies in the young child could artefactually bias our view of the role of maturational status in diaschisis.) Cerebellar diaschisis is a dynamic process and this fact may partially explain the lack of obvious clinical correlates.

*Crowding*

Teuber (1974) proposed his theory of crowding to explain his seemingly paradoxical clinical finding that Verbal IQ was higher than Performance IQ in children with early left hemisphere lesions (Nass, Peterson and Koch, 1989; Woods and Teuber, 1973). He speculated that this form of plasticity reflected competition for the intact neural space with priority to and resultant sparing of Verbal IQ and language at the expense of ordinarily right hemisphere mediated functions — Performance IQ and spatial skills.

Data from patients with documented right hemisphere language are consistent with the occurrence of crowding. In an exemplary case study an adult with a history of a congenital left hemisphere injury developed an aphasia after a right hemisphere stroke in adulthood, presumably because language was mediated by the right hemisphere. In addition,

some deficits typical of acquired right hemisphere lesions were absent (e.g., neglect), consistent with the view that these functions had been crowded out when reorganization occurred after the early injury (Guerreiro, Castro-Caldas and Martins, 1995). In another case study Ogden (1988) assessed two patients with early left hemisphere injury followed by hemispherectomy in the late teens. After 16- to 28-year recovery periods IQ scores revealed intact language and verbal memory abilities. This finding suggests that crowding can affect some and not other right hemisphere functions. Some functions normally mediated by the right hemisphere were impaired (e.g., nonverbal memory, complex visuospatial skills and extra-personal orientation ability), while other right hemisphere functions were intact (e.g., simple visuospatial perception and orientation, emotional expression, and face recognition). Several group studies have shown that when early left hemisphere damage is associated with right hemisphere language representation (reflecting a shift of language from the damaged left to the intact right hemisphere) performance is reduced on non-language tasks (Helmstaedter, Pohl and Elger, 1995; Lansdell, 1969; Strauss, Satz and Wada, 1990).

Most discussions of crowding are based on the effects of early left hemisphere lesions. The capacity for recovery after early right hemisphere injury may be less extensive (see also the discussions of maturational gradients and computational biases below). Asymmetric crowding/crowdability is one possible explanation. Verbal sparing (VIQ is greater than PIQ) occurs after early left lesions, but there is no right hemisphere counterpart (PIQ is not greater than VIQ). In general, the left hemisphere does not take over, or at least take over to the same degree, functions ordinarily mediated by the right hemisphere; therefore left hemisphere functions are not affected. The left hemisphere appears to be less crowdable (be it because of differing degrees of innate specialization, differing maturation rate and/or differing computational biases (see below). Contrary to this, Sandson, Manoach, Price et al. (1994) report a patient in whom a right hemisphere lesion produced a non-verbal learning disability associated with left hemisphere language dysfunction The more consistent finding that deficits are relatively fixed after early right hemisphere injury (see below and Stiles,

2001 for review) supports the theory of asymmetrical crowding (and/or earlier specialization of the left hemisphere or stronger computational biases, see below). In Cohen, Holmes, Campbell et al. (1990) patient verbal memory skills were not affected, despite the shift of non-verbal memory skills from right to left after early right hemisphere injury. Asymmetric crowding is also documented in some behavioral dichotic listening studies (Nass, Sadler and Sidtis, 1992). Paralleling verbal sparing, consonant vowel perception remains intact whereas complex-pitch discrimination, the province of the right hemisphere, is relatively impaired after early left hemisphere injury, putatively because shifting left hemisphere skills encroach upon the neural space for this right hemisphere function. By contrast, after early right hemisphere injury complex-pitch discrimination remains there/does not shift leftward, and is therefore relatively impaired because of right hemisphere damage (Fig. 1). Consonant vowel perception, on the other hand, dominated by the left hemisphere, is unaffected because there is no encroachment by ordinarily right hemisphere functions into its neural space. Nonetheless, despite the lack or relative lack of transfer of function after early right hemisphere injury to an intact left hemisphere, complex-pitch discrimination is less impaired overall after early than late injury to either hemisphere because the immature right hemisphere is still more plastic than the mature right hemisphere, and thus more capable, relatively speaking of intrahemispheric and/or interhemispheric recovery.

Age affects performance in a manner consistent with asymmetric crowding. In the congenital left lesion group performance on the dichotic listening complex-pitch discrimination task, the test for which the intact right hemisphere is normally specialized, declines with age. As language develops (presumably mediated by the right hemisphere) the increasingly complex linguistic demands result in decreasing capacity for complex-pitch discrimination, because of decreasing capacity in appropriate, functional neural space. By contrast, in the congenital right lesion group, age correlates strongly with left ear performance on the complex-pitch discrimination task and somewhat less strongly with overall accuracy. Continuing recovery of this right hemisphere function within the right hemisphere may be

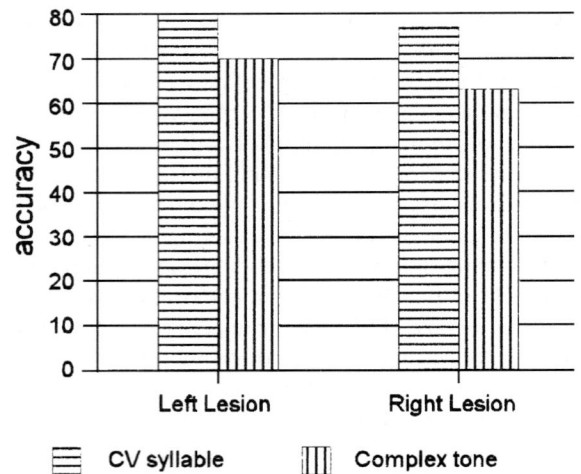

Fig. 1. Dichotic listening results support the theory of asymmetric crowding. Paralleling verbal sparing, consonant vowel perception remains intact whereas complex-pitch discrimination, the province of the right hemisphere, is relatively impaired after early left hemisphere injury, putatively because shifting left hemisphere skills encroach upon the neural space for this right hemisphere function. By contrast, after early right hemisphere injury complex-pitch discrimination remains there/does not shift leftward, and is therefore relatively impaired because of right hemisphere damage. Consonant vowel perception, on the other hand, dominated by the left hemisphere, is unaffected because there is no encroachment by ordinarily right hemisphere functions into its neural space. From Nass et al., 1992.

occurring over time. The absence of any correlation between speech and complex-pitch discrimination suggests that crowding is not a factor in right hemisphere recovery.

Overall, the evidence for crowding suggests that right hemisphere plasticity is affected by the extent and timing of the left hemisphere injury, as well as by the complexity and phylogenetic status of the function requiring restitution (e.g., specific language skill, verbal cognition, verbal memory). Regardless of the decline in right hemisphere functions after early left hemisphere injury, the very fact that the right hemisphere can mediate language with only subtle resulting difficulties highlights the extent of plasticity. Crowding may be asymmetric, i.e., less pronounced after right than left hemisphere lesions. Other related factors including innate specialization, ontogenetic/emergent specialization, hemispheric computational biases, type of hemispheric organization (diffuse versus focal (Kornhuber, Bechinger, Jung et al., 1985), and differing hemispheric maturation rates (a putative mechanism for asymmetric crowding) are discussed in more detail in other sections of this chapter.

*Reorganization*

Reorganization allows for sparing (pre-acquisition injury) and/or recovery (post-acquisition injury) of a skill ordinarily mediated by the region damaged. Both intra- and inter-hemispheric reorganization occurs. Reorganization, generally with transfer and sparing of function to the intact hemisphere, is more pronounced for language than for somatosensory or motor functions (Muller, Chugani, Muzik et al., 1998a; Muller, Rothermel, Behen et al., 1998b) (Fig. 2).

Within the cognitive domain, memory may be spared more than language after early injury, possibly because of its more primitive phylogenetic status. For example, Sass, Silberfein, Platis et al. (1995) found that the right hemisphere of right hemisphere speech dominant epileptic adults mediated both language and verbal memory (measured by the Buschke Selective Reminding Task and the Wechsler Memory Scale Logical Memory subtest). Verbal memory was less compromised than language. Right hemisphere language dominant epileptic adults with left temporal lobe seizures had less verbal memory loss than left hemisphere language dominant patients with left temporal lobe seizures. Language skills did not differ (Rausch, Boone and Ary, 1991).

Factors modifying extent of reorganization include: specific cognitive skill, age at the time of injury, time since injury, size, location and type of lesion, integrity of brain areas surrounding and contralateral to the lesion, presence, severity and duration of epilepsy, effect and extent of innate specialization, maturational status of the brain region injured, and hemispheric computational biases. Specific examples are presented in detail in the sections on language, sensory and motor skills.

Vertical plasticity (in contrast to traditional inter-hemispheric reorganization which is horizontal) (Shewmon, Holmes and Byrne, 1999) occurs when cortical functions are taken over by subcortical structures in settings where the appropriate cortex is absent. Conscious functions like distinguishing familiar from unfamiliar people (e.g., recognizing mother), affective responses and preferences in the hydranencephalic child or visual orientation in patients with complete destruction of occipital cortex (blindsight, Tapp, 1997) are examples of vertical plasticity.

*Redundancy*

Redundancy can take several forms. Equipotentiality of the hemispheres for a particular cognitive function is one form of redundant brain. While equipotentiality was considered the explanation for 'complete' recovery of language after early left hemisphere injury (Lenneberg, 1965), equipotentiality no longer seems tenable in the face of documented incomplete recovery (albeit requiring subtle linguistic measures to demonstrate) and increasing data supporting innate specialization or at least ontogenetic/emergent specialization (Bates, 1999; Vargha-Khadem, Isaacs, Watkins et al., 2000). 'Extra' neural space is another form of redundancy, although again the increasing evidence for early specialization in many modalities means that even though redundant, the function cannot be performed to quite the same degree or in the same way. The possibility of redundant neural space is supported by the occurrence of clinically silent injuries, although it is always possible that the 'correct' tests were not used to define the deficit.

*Compensation*

Compensation is a form of plasticity in which the cognitive strategies used to perform a task differ from the strategies which would have obtained were the damaged area still mediating the skill in question. The differing computational biases of the two hemispheres — left focal/analytic, right global/gestalt — affect the extent of possible compensation. Specific examples are discussed in the sections on language, sensory and motor skills.

**General cognitive factors affecting plasticity**

*The interaction between innate/emergent hemispheric specialization and plasticity*

Innate/emergent hemispheric specialization (see for reviews: Best, 1985; Hellige, 2001; Molfese and

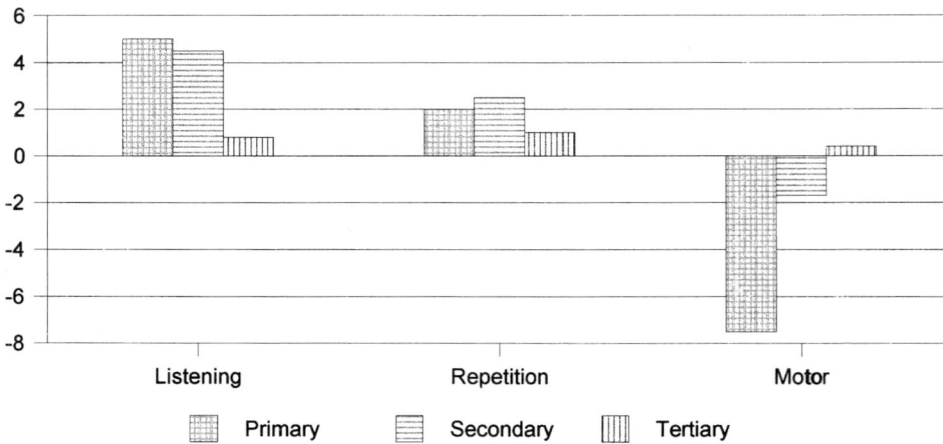

Fig. 2. Relative reorganization of language, motor, and somatosensory functions after early focal injury. Language undergoes considerably more reorganization than motor and somatosensory functions. Positive changes in cerebral blood flow represent shifts in function to the intact hemisphere. Negative changes represent persistent functions in the damaged hemisphere. Modified from Muller et al., 1998a,b.

Segalowitz, 1988) and plasticity are in essence competing phenomena: the greater the specialization, the more limited plasticity. In practical terms innate/emergent hemispheric specialization means that one hemisphere is better equipped (e.g., anatomically, biochemically) to mediate a particular cognitive function. Plasticity allows for the other/non-dominant hemisphere or other parts of the damaged hemisphere to mediate the particular cognitive function at issue. Outcome reflects extent of specialization versus degree of available plasticity. How well we can determine the relative contribution of these two factors depends at least in part on the status of the cognitive function at the time of injury (Fig. 3). When the cognitive function in question is already in effect, an acute and apparent deficit occurs after a unilateral hemispheric insult (e.g., acquired aphasia). Recovery of function after injury reflects both degree of hemispheric dominance at the age of injury and relative central nervous system plasticity at different ages. When the cognitive function in question is already lateralized to one or the other hemisphere, but has not yet been expressed developmentally, no apparent deficit occurs immediately after a unilateral hemispheric insult. The degree of plasticity available here is more difficult to determine and is probably best reflected by the relative normalcy of the development and ultimate capacity for the function (see language section) in question,

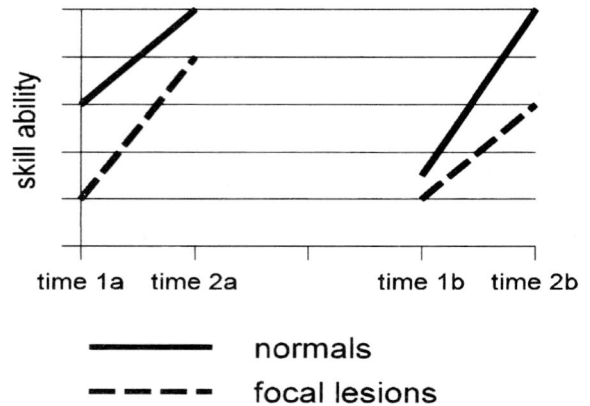

Fig. 3. Pre- and post-skill acquisition effects. Hypothetical developmental changes in established (time 1a to time 2a) versus to be acquired (time 1b to time 2b) skills in children with focal lesions (broken line) and in normal children (solid line). The injury affects an established skill, hence the lesion group performs less well than normals. Over time, however, recovery takes place in the focal lesion group and the skill performance levels start to converge. The effect of the focal injury on a skill yet to be established cannot be ascertained. Over time, the children with lesion show inferior performance compared with normal children. From Taylor and Alden, 1997, with permission.

as well as the status of other skills (trade offs for recovery, see crowding). But, the greater the degree of innate specialization, the more any resulting deficit could reflect specialization, rather than reflect the extent of plasticity or lack thereof. Thus, innate specialization is one factor that defines the limits of plasticity.

Recently, several investigators (Bates, 1999; Vargha-Khadem et al., 2000) have proposed, based on the findings for language in the early focal lesion population, an alternative view to that of innate specialization counterbalanced by plasticity as the determinant of outcome. The emergent view, constrained plasticity, or ontogenetic specialization as this view has been dubbed assumes that hemispheric specialization has an anatomic basis that is genetically determined and under normal circumstances expresses itself very early in life. Its functional expression is determined during development by the interaction between environmentally evoked neural activity and the form of neuroplasticity that extends until puberty. Early brain damage may counteract the genetic disposition by affecting and modifying the neural activity/plasticity interaction.

*The interaction between hemispheric computational biases and plasticity*

Like specialization, hemispheric computational biases and plasticity are competing phenomena: the more discrepant the hemisphere's cognitive styles, the less latitude for the intact hemisphere to take over adequately/optimally. Assuming a computational bias for detail (left hemisphere) and for integration (right hemisphere), recovery and reorganization/plasticity are limited by the degree to which the intact hemisphere can mediate a specific cognitive function utilizing a different cognitive style than the one that best suits it. For example, Bates, Thal, Aram et al. (1997) suggest that the developmental language deficits seen after early left and right hemisphere focal lesions reflect the effects of computational biases at various stages in the process of language acquisition. Learning words/vocabulary for the first time may depend more on the integration of multimodal sources, while learning grammar depends on detail analysis. Hence, those with right hemisphere lesions lag during initial receptive language learning, especially word meaning, and those with left (especially temporal) lesions lag during the development of early grammatical expression. By the age of 5 years, however, both groups have caught up and have nearly normal language (Reilly, Bates

and Marchman, 1998). In this instance plasticity ultimately takes precedence over computational biases.

The particulars of hemispheric computational bias may explain at least in part the differences in plasticity for language and manipulospatial functions. Unlike manipulospatial functions, language can be mediated by a wide variety of strategies. Bates (1999) described language as a parasite that can work off any sort of hardware. The limiting effects of computational biases on plasticity is epitomized by the performance of children with congenital focal lesions on a task requiring the reproduction by copy and from memory of a series of hierarchical letter and form stimuli (Fig. 4) (Stiles, 2001). The patterns of deficit are consistent with those reported for adults with comparable injury. The children with left lesions have difficulty reproducing pattern detail; they draw the global level of the hierarchical pattern, but fail to produce the local level of the form. The children with right lesions perform somewhat better on the task, but they too show evidence of processing difficulty. Two strategies were evident. In one a large pattern composed of smaller parts was produced. However, the local level form was produced at both pattern levels, suggesting difficulty in remembering global level information. In another, a verbal memory strategy ("The large letter-Y made up of small letter Bs") was adopted. However, retaining the visuospatial code for the letter form was difficult as evidenced by the fact that both upper and lower case letters appear at the local level of the reproductions (T–t; B–b). Because of the specific features of this task (requiring both analytic (left hemisphere) and gestalt (right hemisphere) contributions to different degrees) those with left lesions actually had more difficulty, despite the visuospatial nature of the task (Stiles, Stern, Trauner et al., 1996). With respect to the issue of plasticity, it is notable that neither lesion group improved with age, i.e., plasticity was limited by computational bias constraints.

*The interaction between plasticity and cognitive skills: general and specific*

In general, plasticity decreases with age for specific cognitive skills. Recovery is better after early than late injury, i.e., language recovery is better after an injury in childhood than after an injury in adult-

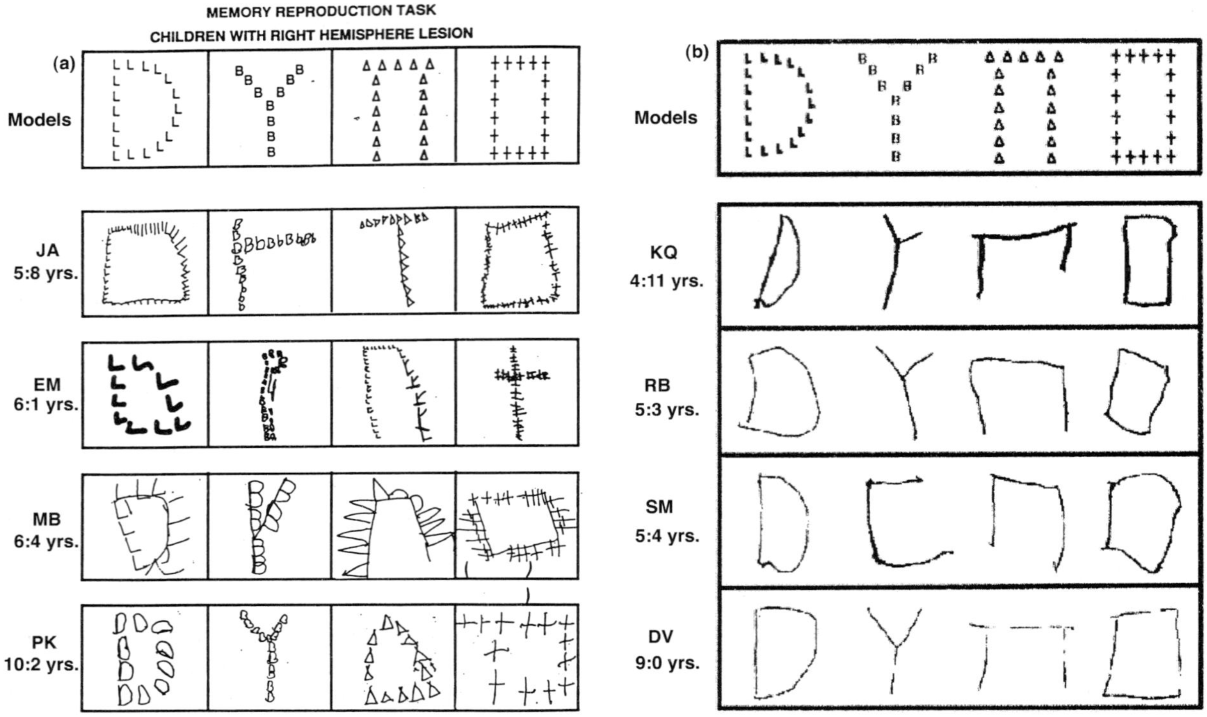

Fig. 4. Effects of early focal lesions on global and local functioning. (a) Memory reproduction of hierarchical letters and form stimuli by children with right hemisphere lesions. These children tend to ignore the gestalt element of the stimuli. (b) Memory reproduction of hierarchical letters and form stimuli by children with left hemisphere lesions. These children tend to ignore the detailed elements of the stimuli. From Nass and Stiles, 1996.

hood. However, despite the general principle that the immature nervous system is more plastic than the mature nervous system, early injury impedes general cognitive development more than late injury impairs already acquired skills. In other words a cognitive system that has already acquired knowledge appears to be more resilient than a system that lacks knowledge (Dennis, 1989) and/or is in the process of very actively acquiring it. The high metabolic rate documented during the first two years (Chugani and Phelps, 1986; Yamada, Sadato, Konishi et al., 2000) could be the physiologic basis of this increased vulnerability (see below). Furthermore, after early injury 'recovered' abilities may decline over time. With age the increasing demands on a compromised cognitive system may tax its capacities. Plasticity has limits even in the immature nervous system. These limits may differ for left and right hemisphere.

Skoyles (1997) theorizes that cognitive evolution (and by extrapolation cognitive recovery) reflects the combined potential of neural plasticity (neural networks in the brain underlying cognition available to process and develop new skills) and prefrontal working memory refashioning old neural networks to do newly evolved novel tasks. While the immature nervous system has a greater capacity to develop new neural networks, the mature nervous system has preformed neural networks to refashion. General versus specific cognitive skills may be relatively more or less dependent on these two different mechanisms of recovery. Two clinical examples discussed below highlight this dichotomy.

*Plasticity and general cognitive ability: intelligence*
Intelligence is less specifically (absence of a consistent left and right hemisphere dichotomy for Verbal versus Performance IQ), but more severely affected by focal injury in childhood than in adulthood. However, despite congenital unilateral lesions, intelligence measured at school age is within the normal

range (Nass et al., 1989), but compromised compared with siblings (Woods and Teuber, 1973). Some studies document a lower IQ in those with congenital right hemisphere lesions, while others do not (see Vargha-Khadem et al., 2000, for review). IQ in the early focal lesion population probably declines over time, despite static brain pathology (Banich, Levine, Kim et al., 1990; Cohen, Huttenlocher, Banich et al., 1987; Levine, Huttenlocher, Banich et al., 1987). Interestingly, the decline in Verbal IQ appears to be particularly prominent in the right focal lesion group (Aram and Eisele, 1994a) (see below for further discussion of the right hemisphere role in language acquisition). There may a continuum of vulnerability from the pre-perinatal period through adolescence. Some studies document lower IQ after pre-perinatal injury than after focal lesions incurred later in childhood (toddler and elementary school years) (see below for further discussion of age at injury).

*Plasticity and specific cognitive ability:*
*visuoperceptual and manipulospatial skills*
Adults with right hemisphere lesions evidence constructional apraxia, difficulty with drawing and manipulating objects in space, more frequently, in different ways and to a more severe degree than those with left hemisphere lesions. Cognitive profiles typical of the right brain damaged adult have been demonstrated in children after early focal lesions and with focal seizure disorders. The deficits are much less severe, however. Stiles and colleagues (Nass and Stiles, 1996; Stiles, 2001) have demonstrated through longitudinal studies a deficit pattern in the early focal lesion population, wherein those with left hemisphere lesions show a delay in the development of a specific spatial skill, but recover over time. By contrast, those with right hemisphere lesions show both delayed and atypical acquisition, yet with apparent recovery. However, when both process and product are evaluated, the process underlying the product is abnormal. Hence the recovery is really a pseudorecovery. When task complexity increases the atypical nature of the process underlying the product becomes apparent, and new delays and atypical patterns of processing emerge. Unlike the effects of early focal lesions on language, increasing age does not appear to mute the degree of deficit. Indeed, after congenital injury, the right hemisphere appears more

wedded to mediating manipulospatial functions than the left to mediating language. In that sense plasticity is more limited after early right hemisphere injury than early left injury. Recovery is nevertheless better than in the adult regardless of lesion side.

Between ages of 1 and 3 years children with right focal lesions evidence a deficit in spatial manipulative classification skills. They fail to build toy arrays with 'next to' constructions at the appropriate age. They create atypical spatial arrays, for example, trying to do the impossible — stack pyramids, rather than place them next to one another. At preschool age the children with early focal brain injury played as actively with the blocks as normal children, but the spatial grouping constructions they produced differed systematically. Children with right hemisphere injury had difficulty organizing objects into coherent spatial groupings, while children with left hemisphere injury had difficulty with local relations within the spatial arrays. The spatial integrative deficits observed in the children with right hemisphere injury persisted, while those of the left lesion children resolved. When the children with right hemisphere lesions began to produce spatial constructions using complex grouping procedures, those constructions were heaps or disordered clusters. When children with left hemisphere injury began to use complex procedures, they generated the same kinds of constructions as normal children, e.g., arches and enclosures (Stiles et al., 1996; Stiles and Nass, 1991; Stiles-Davis, Sugarman and Nass, 1985).

Both lesion groups have difficulty with representational drawing during preschool and early elementary school. The persons and houses drawn by 5-year-old children with left lesions are delayed, while those drawn by children with right lesions are unusual (Stiles-Davis, Janowski, Engel et al., 1988). Over time, however, both groups develop the graphic formula required to draw standard constructions. However, when the system is taxed, for example, by asking for an impossible house, the right lesion children's ability to perform the task breaks down. Unlike children with left lesions and normals, the children with right hemisphere lesions are unable to utilize their graphic formula to produce an impossible version. Answers like "it's impossible because it's invisible or it's too small" are only given by children in the right lesion group. Unlike normal children, the right lesion children tend to merely substitute other graphic formulas from their limited repertoire (Stiles, Trauner, Engel et al., 1997) (Fig. 5).

Longitudinal examination of the copy and immediate memory version of the Rey Osterrieth Complex Figure of 6 to 13 year olds initially revealed similar deficit patterns in the two lesion groups (Akshoomoff, Feroleto, Doyle et al., 2002; Stiles, 2001). Both groups approached the copy task using an immature piecemeal strategy and both lesion groups improved over time. The failure to find group differences on the copy task could reflect the underlying task demands that place equal emphasis on the segmentation and integration processes and thus equally disrupt task performance. The memory task did distinguish between the two lesion groups. Almost none of those with early right hemisphere lesions were able to make use of the central rectangle in the memory version, while many of those with left lesions used it, albeit inefficiently. The failure of the right lesion group to access the gestalt of the Rey Osterrieth Complex Figure interfered with the development of a mature procedural approach to the task.

## Plasticity: the maturational gradient

In this section the cases for right to left and left to right maturational gradients will be presented. The maturation gradient issue relates to plasticity because it affects its extent. The earlier maturing/more mature and therefore less plastic hemisphere is less capable than the later maturing and therefore more plastic hemisphere of taking on or taking over additional functions after early injury.

### The case for a right–left gradient

The right–left maturational gradient position trades on the theory of 'right hemisphere conservatism' (Geschwind and Galaburda, 1987). According to this theory the right hemisphere matures first because it dominates the functions necessary for survival, i.e., visuospatial functions (required to analyze extrapersonal space and orient the body within space), emotion (a preamble to and a necessary part of communication with others), and attention (required to shift focus among external stimuli to enhance survival). Geschwind and Galaburda (1987) suggest that brain damage is more likely to affect the hemisphere that is more immature rather than the more mature, and that these crucial survival functions are therefore less likely to become impaired if they develop early and quickly. Hellige (2001) has proposed that the more established/mature hemisphere has priority in dealing with classes of input for which dominance is not already established. For example, in utero various non-language sounds are experienced by the fetus, e.g., heartbeat, digestive sounds. The more advanced right hemisphere learns more from these noises than does the less advanced left hemisphere. These very early experiences provide the foundation for right hemisphere dominance for a variety of non-language sounds. Later in fetal development when the left hemisphere has reached a critical point in development, the brain is presented, as a result of changes in the acoustic transmission properties of the uterus as its expands, with additional 'noises' including mother's voice. In a sense the right hemisphere's early dominance for non-language sounds actually enhances/contributes to the left hemisphere's availability/dominance for language sounds. Hellige (2001) further speculates that if the right hemisphere is more mature/advanced at birth, it will be more responsive to incoming visual stimuli. However, the range of visual stimuli that the newborn can process is limited to relatively low spatial frequencies. The right hemisphere dominance granted by advanced maturation for processing these relatively degraded visual stimuli could contribute to the right hemisphere's ultimate global processing style. In addition, Hellige speculates that

Fig. 5. Impossible house. (a) Possible and impossible houses by a child with a congenital left hemisphere lesion. Note the marked change in the child's production of the impossible figure. (b) Possible and impossible houses by a child with a congenital right hemisphere lesion. Note the minor changes in the child's production of the impossible house. (c) Examples of possible and impossible houses by two children with right hemisphere lesions using a formula substitution strategy which is not seen in normal controls. This probably reflects the inability of the right lesion patient to access a normal graphic formula. From Nass and Stiles, 1996.

**(a)**

POSSIBLE AND IMPOSSIBLE DRAWINGS BY A CHILD WITH LEFT-HEMISPHERE INJURY

HOUSE (9 yrs, 10 mos)      IMPOSSIBLE HOUSE (9 yrs, 10 mos)

**(b)**

POSSIBLE AND IMPOSSIBLE DRAWINGS BY A CHILD WITH RIGHT-HEMISPHERE INJURY

HOUSE (10 yrs, 8 mos)      IMPOSSIBLE HOUSE (10 yrs, 8 mos)

**(c)**

POSSIBLE AND IMPOSSIBLE DRAWINGS BY CHILDREN WITH RIGHT-HEMISPHERE INJURY

**a**

HOUSE (9 yrs, 7 mos)      IMPOSSIBLE HOUSE (9 yrs, 7 mos)      AIRPLANE (9 yrs, 7 mos)

**b**

HOUSE (5 yrs, 10 mos)      IMPOSSIBLE HOUSE (5 yrs, 10 mos)      FLOWER (5 yrs, 10 mos) the putatively later maturing left hemisphere could be biased toward processing local information, both because the right maintains precedence for the low-frequency spatial input and because, by the time of the left hemisphere's involvement in visual processing, it is more advanced/mature and thus better able to process high-frequency stimuli (Turkewitz, 1988). Mancini, De Schonen, Deruelle and Massoulier (1994) have proposed an innate neural network for face perception dominated by the right hemisphere, but Hellige (2001) suggests that it is more parsimonious to draw a parallel with visual perception in general, since face perception depends on low spatial frequency processing, the presumed province of the right hemisphere.

A number of clinical studies support the right–left maturational gradient position. In keeping with 'right hemisphere conservatism', congenital left hemisphere strokes are considerably more common than right sided ones and post-seizure brain damage occurs more frequently on the left (Chiron, Jambaque, Nabbout et al., 1997). More focal febrile seizures emanate from the left hemisphere in the first 2 years, which suggests, considering the association of febrile seizures with immaturity of brain, later left hemisphere maturation as attested to by the timing of its greater vulnerability (Taylor and Ounsted, 1971). To the extent that innate/early specialization is synonymous with early maturation, studies showing innate/early right hemisphere dominance support the right–left gradient argument. However, few studies compare the timing of right versus left hemisphere specialization on parallel tasks, which is the critical factor. In one behavioral dichotic listening study (based on a non-nutritive sucking habituation paradigm) (Best, 1988), right hemisphere specialization appeared to precede left, inasmuch as the right hemisphere advantage for musical stimuli appeared in younger infants than the left for speech. Helmstaedter, Kurthen and Gleibner et al. (1997a), Helmstaedter, Kurthen, Linke et al. (1994), and Helmstaedter, Kurthen, Linke et al. (1997b) report a higher than normal frequency of bilateral language in patients with right hemisphere pathology. In addition, they present data supporting transfer of language from right to left in a time window generally considered to exceed the usual limits of cerebral plasticity. These investigators speculate that this un-usual pattern is a reflection of the left hemisphere's innate specialization for language, making the right–left language shift more natural and long lasting than the left–right switch. Although not intended to address the maturational gradient issue, prolongation of the critical period after right hemisphere injury is consistent with a right–left gradient.

Anatomically, the right inferior frontal region and the cortical markings surrounding the right sylvian fissure develop earlier (as discussed in Geschwind and Galaburda, 1987). Microscopically, mature folds surrounding the sylvian fissure, as well as higher-order dendritic connections, appear earlier on the right (Chi, Dooling and Gilles, 1977; Simonds and Scheibel, 1989). At the biochemical level choline acetyltransferase levels are higher in the right than left temporal region at term (Amaducci, Sorbi and Albanese, 1981). Assessing longitudinal EEG changes, Thatcher (1994) and Thatcher, Walker and Giudice (1987) found that the right hemisphere is more functionally advanced than the left, particularly with respect to frontal pole activity. Functional imaging (SPECT scanning) demonstrates that blood flow in the right hemisphere predominates between 1 and 3 years, particularly in the posterior associative regions. Around 3 years of age the asymmetry clearly shifts leftward (Chiron et al., 1997).

*The case for a left–right gradient*
On the other hand Corballis and Morgan (1978) postulated, based on an extrapolation from phylogenetic evidence, that the maturational gradient goes from left to right. Asymmetrical crowding (see above) is a strong clinical argument for a left–right gradient pattern. Applying the left–right maturational gradient model to the theory of crowding, the earlier maturing, and therefore less plastic, left hemisphere is less capable/less crowdable than the later maturing and therefore more plastic right hemisphere of taking on additional functions after early injury, i.e., of being crowded. The generally better overall compensation after left than right hemisphere injury is also consistent with a left–right gradient. In the context of a maturational gradient the left hemisphere is equivalent to the mature nervous system and the right to the immature nervous system. Both case and group studies in focal lesion and hemispherectomy patients demonstrate this left

hemisphere advantage. Smith (1981) found higher IQ, better language, and better spatial skills in a left hemispherectomy patient as compared to a right hemispherectomy patient. In group studies the IQ of those with early left lesions is generally better (Nass et al., 1989). Hemispherectomy studies indicate greater compensation by right hemisphere after left hemispherectomy than the reverse (Burkland and Smith, 1977; Smith, 1981). The comparatively more prolonged recovery/reorganization period after early left hemisphere injury with right hemisphere functions progressively crowded out could also trade on a left–right maturational gradient. For example, Smith and Sugar (1975) described a patient with a congenital right hemiplegia who underwent hemispherectomy at 5 years. At the age of 26, the patient had a Verbal IQ of 126, a Performance IQ of 102, and normal scores on a standard language battery; documented improvement of Verbal IQ had occurred over many years.

Innate specialization of the left hemisphere for linguistic processing is consistent with a left–right maturational gradient, but as noted above is not a direct argument for it unless the study compares the two hemispheres. St. James-Roberts (1981), analyzing all reported left and right hemispherectomy cases (tested mainly as adults), found a main effect of age at lesion on intelligence only for right hemispherectomy patients. Left infantile hemiplegics had higher Performance IQ scores; those with later acquired left hemiplegia had higher Verbal IQ scores. These results, assuming that comparable hemispheric damage occurs with congenital and acquired lesions, suggest that right hemisphere specialization, at least for some cognitive abilities, develops with time, i.e., later than left hemisphere specialization. Some U-shaped normal developmental curves (see below) suggest initial left hemisphere dominance consistent with the view that it is the earlier maturing hemisphere.

The anatomical substrate for language, the planum temporale, is larger on the left in most adults (Geschwind and Galaburda, 1987). This asymmetry is already present in the fetus, and persists in the neonate and child. Assessing longitudinal EEG changes, Thatcher (1994) and Thatcher et al. (1987) found that some left sided activity (frontal, occipital and frontal–temporal regions) developed earlier than in homologous regions on the right.

*Mixed maturational gradients*

The hemispheres may develop at different rates from region to region (Chugani, 1994), leaving room for differing maturational gradients depending on both the function at issue and its intrahemispheric location. For example, Mancini et al. (1994) evaluated three children with early left or right focal lesions in various intrahemispheric locations on a variety of face recognition tasks: famous faces, emotional expression, identity, sex, divided visual field presentation of unfamiliar faces. All subjects showed different patterns of strength and weaknesses, suggesting that various skills involved in facial processing developed independently in time and space. As noted above Thatcher's (Thatcher, 1994; Thatcher et al., 1987) EEG activity studies suggest different maturational gradients for different brain regions. Chiron, Raynaud, Maziere et al. (1992) demonstrate that the time needed to reach adult metabolic levels differ for various cortical regions.

U-shaped developmental curves are reported for a number of cognitive skills (Kagan, 1991). What appears to be a modest peripubertal deterioration may reflect shifting dominance. Dominance for a number of ultimately right hemisphere skills (e.g., map walking, face recognition, tone perception) may evolve throughout childhood, first dominated by the left hemisphere and ultimately by the right, with the transition occurring around puberty (Carey and Levine, 1980; Denckla, Rudel and Broman, 1980) (Fig. 6).

The maturation gradient pattern remains in dispute, proponents for both arguments presenting both theoretical and clinical support for their position. The possibility of mixed gradients for different functions and cerebral locations may act as a confound. In either case, rate of hemispheric maturation affects the extent of plasticity.

*Plasticity: age at injury*

Overall, focal cortical injury during childhood is less detrimental than injury in adulthood. The principle of Kennard (1940), the earlier the better, has long been a generally accepted corollary. Recently, however, the nature of the gradient underlying the effects of focal injury throughout the course of childhood has been further explored and debated. Specially, ques-

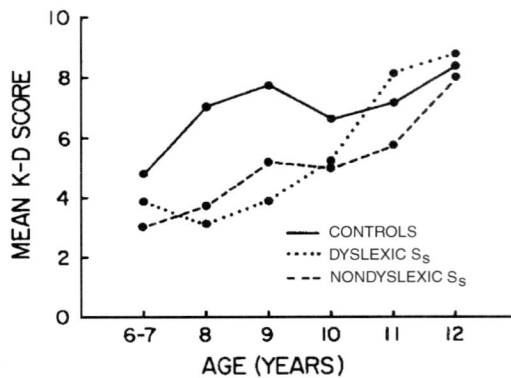

Fig. 6. Developmental dominance and map walking. Relationship of age to Kohn–Dennis route walking scores for dyslexic, non-dyslexic learning disabled and controls. During early development map walking (an ultimately right hemisphere dominated skill) is mediated by the left hemisphere. Around puberty, when the bulk of myelination of the corpus callosum is completed, the skill switches rightward. Non-dyslexic learning disabled and controls evidence a decline in performance during puberty when mediation of the task is probably shifting from left to right. By contrast dyslexic show no decline in performance since their relatively good right hemisphere has been mediating the task throughout. From Denckla et al., 1980, with permission

tions have been raised about whether a pre-perinatal injury is really less severe than an injury occurring at the age of 1 year or 5 years or at puberty. Questions have also been raised about the severity of the consequences of congenital pathology, even when focal.

In terms of general cognitive abilities, some early focal lesion studies suggest that the best outcome occurs with pre-perinatal injury, while other support better outcome from injuries occurring around age one year compared with those occurring pre-perinatally. Yet other studies appear to demonstrate that insults occurring between 1 and 4 years have the most severe effects, relatively speaking (Fig. 7). Ultimately a large sample of seizure-free children with comparable lesions incurred at different ages will be required to provide a clear answer to this question

With respect specifically to language, likelihood of recovery and speed of recovery from acquired aphasia in childhood due to stroke does not change between the ages of 1 and 15 years (see Nass, 1999, for review). When children with pre- and post-language acquisition left hemisphere injury are assessed with the same language battery (measuring phonics, semantics, syntax, reading, and spelling)

there is little long-term deficit in either group (Woods and Carey, 1979). By contrast, Vargha-Khadem, Isaacs, Papaleloudi et al. (1991) found that left hemispherectomy patients had severe impairments in language processing whether the insults occurred during early, middle and late childhood. In the paired right hemispherectomy group only the child with the early childhood injury had a language deficit. In another case study follow-up of a child with a left hemispherectomy at the age of 10 years revealed a language deficit pattern similar to that of children with developmental language disorders, while follow-up of a child with a right hemispherectomy at the age of 10 years did not (Stark and McGregor, 1997). Studies of patients with partial epilepsy (as opposed to those with clear structural pathology) suggest that the more immature brain is capable of greater reorganization of language. Naming is less affected after left temporal lobectomy the younger the patient at onset of epilepsy (Davis, Kiss, Luo et al., 1998; Saykin, Gur, Sussman et al., 1989). These discrepancies highlight the need to look at lesion type and seizure status when examining age effects.

Different degrees of reorganization of language have been demonstrated at different ages at injury. Rasmussen and Milner (1977) found (based on carotid amytal testing) a high likelihood of reorganization of language with transfer to the right hemisphere only when the left hemisphere injury occurred before versus after the age of 6 years. (Of note, most patients in the age group of less than 6 years were under 2 years of age at the time of injury.) Muller, Behen, Rothermel et al. (1999a) documented a greater rightward shift of language (PET imaging) among children with injuries prior to 6 years compared with those who sustained their injury after the age of 10 years (Fig. 8), as well as among children with injuries prior to the age of 5 years versus after the age of 20 years (Muller, Behen, Rothermel et al., 1999b). In patients with partial epilepsy without apparent lesions, the earlier the onset of epilepsy the more right hemisphere language is seen with left hemisphere epilepsy and the more left hemisphere language is seen with right hemisphere epilepsy (Helmstaedter et al., 1997b). Presumably, the greater capacity of the less mature nervous system for reorganization of language localization underlies the greater recovery.

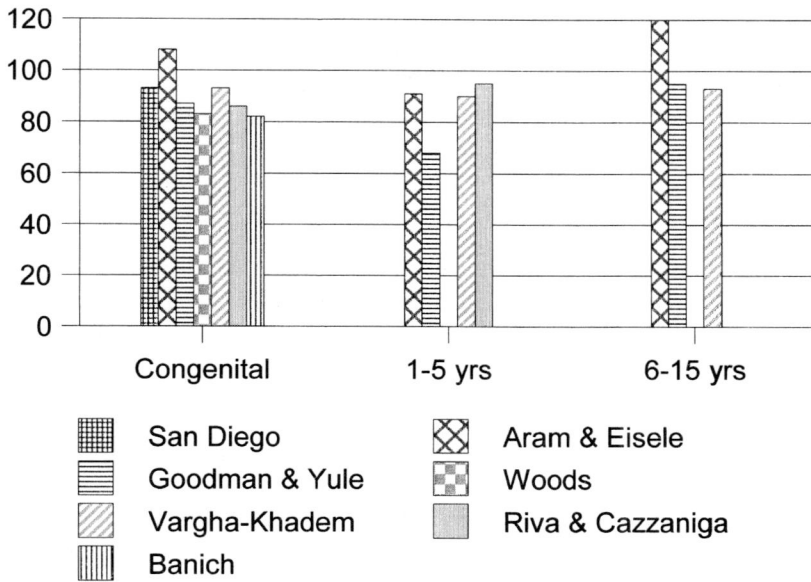

Fig. 7. Effects of age at lesion on IQ. Data modified from Aram and Eisele, 1994a; Banich et al., 1990; Bates, 1999; Bates and Roe, 2001; Goodman and Yude, 1996; Riva and Cazzaniga, 1986; Vargha-Khadem et al., 2000; Woods, 1980.

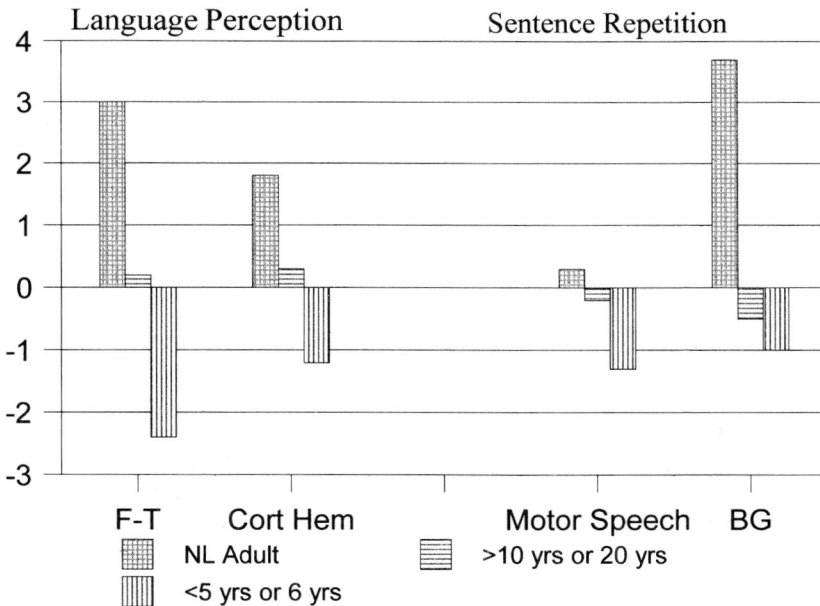

Fig. 8. Effects of age at lesion on language reorganization. Negative changes reflect shift in function to the right hemisphere. Modified from Muller et al., 1998b, 1999a.

The effect of age at injury on outcome after a diffuse insult highlights the evident competition between early vulnerability (Taylor and Ounsted, 1971) and plasticity. The traumatic brain injury literature offers consistent support for greater deficits after insults in infancy and early childhood than in adolescence and adulthood, and for greater deficits in adulthood than in adolescence (Levin, Ewing-Cobbs and Eisenberg, 1995). Early disruption of the developmental process may have a more deleterious impact because of the greater number of skills yet to be acquired that are vulnerable to the insult (Dennis, 1989). By contrast, both the adolescent and the adult have consolidated knowledge, but the adolescent brain is more plastic than the adult one and thus recovery is better.

Based on data from a 48-patient hemispherectomy cohort Curtiss and colleagues (Curtiss and De Bode, 1999; De Bode and Curtiss, 2000) portray the relationship between age at insult and resultant outcome in terms of critical impact points. Using this paradigm, early insults could have as equally deleterious effects as later insults, depending on the point in both neurological and functional maturation at which the insult is sustained. If an insult occurs at some critical impact point in maturation, during which both the subsequent neurological and cognitive development requisite to support normal or relatively intact function are affected, a poor outcome may be predicted, despite the early occurrence of the insult. In Curtiss and De Bode's (1999) cohort those with congenital disorders did less well than those with acquired disorders. This difference reflects the fact that those with congenital disorders had developmental brain anomalies which affected the development of the entire hemisphere.

The critical impact points hypothesis is in keeping with Kolb's (Kolb and Gibb, 2001) findings (Fig. 9) of different effects of an insult relating more to physiologic/cellular events than age per se. Despite very early brain damage, at a time just after neural proliferation is complete, but when neural migration and differentiation are still ongoing, there is marked generalized atrophy of dendritic arborization and a decrease in spine density in neurons throughout the cortical mantle (Kolb and Gibb, 2001), reminiscent of some abnormalities seen in the mentally retarded (Purpura, 1974). These diffuse changes underlie the poor functional outcome. In contrast, when the cortical mantle is damaged later, during the period of rapid dendritic growth and synaptic formation, there is a generalized enhancement of dendritic arborization and/or spine density throughout the remaining cortex. Enhanced dendritic response correlates with

better functional recovery. Earlier is not necessarily better. The specific maturational events occurring at the time of injury determine outcome by differentially effecting cellular events that influence plasticity.

*Plasticity: time since injury/duration of recovery period*

The effect of time since injury is inevitably confounded with the age at injury. The earlier the insult, the longer the likely recovery period. Thus, reviewing hemispherectomy data, St. James-Roberts (1981) concluded that differences in recovery after injury to the immature versus mature nervous system are not due solely to age at lesion, but also reflect length of recovery period (as well as etiology of lesion and types of tests used). Follow-up in adults is shorter because of their more limited life expectancy. Any cohort that includes patients with brain tumors automatically alters the potential duration of the recovery period.

On the other hand, cognitive deficits can at times be more prominent among children with very early injury, as opposed to children with later injury, despite longer time since injury/duration of potential recovery period. Deficits among children with congenital abnormalities can become more prominent over time despite what should serve as a longer recovery period. For example, younger children with congenital hydrocephalus perform better than older children with congenital hydrocephalus on tasks measuring efficiency of word finding, grammatical comprehension and metalinguistic awareness (Dennis and Barnes, 1993). IQ scores of children with perinatal focal injuries often decline over time (Aram, 1999). Educational progress slows down as children with early generalized injury grow older. Suppression of the normal cognitive growth rate could reflect deterioration of skills, failure to develop the skills at an age-appropriate rate, or effects of age-related changes in task complexity (Taylor and Alden, 1997) and/or limitations of plasticity.

Nevertheless, declining plasticity over time does not mean that reorganization cannot be a prolonged process. For example, in the Sturge–Weber syndrome progressive calcification is nevertheless associated with continuing reorganization of language

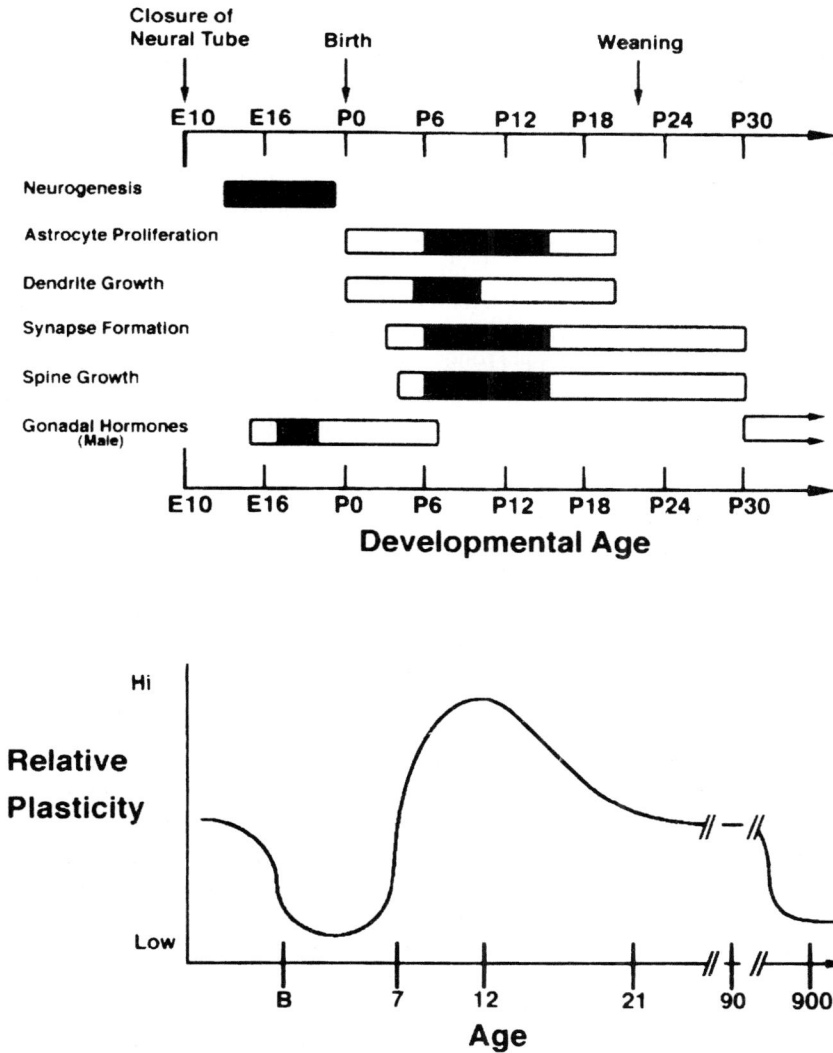

Fig. 9. Top: main cellular events related to cortical plasticity. Bars mark the beginning and end of the different processes. The shaded area illustrates the time of maximum activity. Bottom: summary of the time-dependent differences in cortical plasticity. E = embryologic day; P = postnatal day. From Kolb and Gibb, 2001, with permission.

which extends into late childhood (Muller, Chugani, Muzik et al., 1997a). The recovery period after left hemisphere injury during which the right hemisphere continues to take over the more subtle aspects of language and verbal memory, can be quite prolonged (Ogden, 1989). Acquisition of language by patients who are not exposed to language or who do not speak by the end of the first decade also attests to the prolonged period during which reorganization can occur (Curtiss, 1977; Grimshaw, Adelstein, Bryden et al.,

1998; Vargha-Khadem, Carr, Isaacs et al., 1997). Transfer of language from right to left can occur in a time frame generally considered to exceed the usual duration of cerebral plasticity (Helmstaedter et al., 1997a).

*Plasticity: effect of age at testing*

Both age at injury and time since injury interact with effect of age at testing. The age at testing ef-

45

fect reflects on several issues (1) whether there is a developmental complexity threshold beyond which compensation is not possible, (2) whether the effects of decreased neural capacity increase over time, and (3) whether deficits could actually appear due to changes in the area of brain mediating a particular cognitive function at different ages. Exemplifying the first principle, children with early focal lesions and right hemispherectomy, while able to perform simple spatial tasks, are ultimately unable to perform spatial tasks normally acquired after the age of 10 years (Kohn and Dennis, 1974). Decline in cognitive performance over time and in the older patients with early focal lesions (Aram, 1999; Banich et al., 1990; Levine et al., 1987) corroborates the second principle. The concept of progressive encephalization speaks to the third principle (Goldman and Isseroff, 1983). In animal studies caudate lesions impair the performance of both infant and adult monkeys on a delayed alternation task. Prefrontal cortex lesions produce greater impairment in the adult than the infant. The caudate participates in the mediation of delayed alternation during infancy and adulthood. Its status changes overtime: it loses its autonomy. The prefrontal cortex does not participate in the mediation of delayed alternation until adulthood. At that time it augments rather than replaces the caudate contribution. Hence deficits can 'appear to appear', although they have always been present, i.e., in the monkey with a prefrontal lesion. Longitudinal follow-up studies of preterm infants with caudate injury demonstrate changing deficit patterns (on delayed alternation tasks) depending on the age at testing, suggesting that the role of the caudate nucleus changes over time here too (Ross, Boatwright, Auld et al., 1996; Ross, Tessler, Auld et al., 1992).

*Plasticity: etiology of lesion*

Etiology of lesions affects plasticity, because it determines both the focal versus diffuse nature of injury and the time course of the damage (acute versus chronic versus progressive). Whether all types of generalized insults (e.g., meningitis/encephalitis, hydrocephalus, early central nervous system irradiation, traumatic brain injury, malnutrition, congenital 'treatable' metabolic disorders like hypothyroidism or phenylketonuria) affect plasticity similarly re-

mains to be determined. Etiology of injury interacts with length of recovery period, e.g., neoplastic lesions curtailing survival. Etiology even of very early focal lesions affects plasticity. Prenatal developmental lesions (with early-onset seizures) often do not displace language from the left hemisphere (Duchowny, Jayakar, Harvey et al., 1996), whereas lesions acquired during the perinatal period generally result in transfer of language. Contrasting two congenital and focal disorders — hemimegalencephaly and Sturge–Weber — Curtiss and De Bode (1999) suggest that the abnormalities during intrahemispheric cortical organization and during the early period of interhemispheric connectivity that occur in hemimegalencephaly, but not in Sturge–Weber, explain the difference in severity of the two disorders. Despite the congenital occurrence of both, the outcome of hemimegalencephaly is worse. The critical impact point affected by the later is more important than that affected by the former.

*Plasticity: extent of lesion*

Bilateral lesions limit plasticity more than focal lesions. This is particularly true for the infant whose recovery after diffuse brain injury is limited. By contrast, the older child is less vulnerable to diffuse injury especially when the etiology of the damage is trauma (Levin et al., 1995), possibly because cognitive skills had crystallized before the injury.

Not surprisingly, multilobar congenital disorders of one hemisphere have a better prognosis that congenital disorders involving the whole hemisphere (Curtiss and De Bode, 1999). Although the size of an early focal lesion appears to affect overall functioning (Banich et al., 1990; Levine et al., 1987; Vargha-Khadem, O'Gorman and Watters, 1985), no clear left- versus right-sided differences or differential effects on language based on lesion size have been found (Rasmussen and Milner, 1977). Degree of plasticity for language appears unaffected by large lesion size, even to the point of hemispherectomy. Bates (1997) has termed this a fresh start effect. A U-shaped outcome curve reflects the fact that (1) residual brain can be inhibitory, and (2) intra- versus inter-hemispheric reorganization may be variously advantageous. More damage would result in a better outcome than a little damage. On the other hand small differences in lesion size could theoretically produce large differences as the developing brain may act as an amplifier for the development of other brain regions (Kornhuber et al., 1985). If true, this is another possible explanation for greater deficits after small than large lesions.

*Location of lesion*

An adult-like anterior–posterior dichotomy of a language deficit pattern is not found after pre-language acquisition focal lesions (see below for discussion), whereas this dichotomy characterizes the acquired aphasias of childhood (Van Hout, 1997). Transfer of language to the right hemisphere does not occur unless the early lesion is in primary language cortex (regardless of size of lesion), and transfer rarely occurs if handedness does not shift, i.e., the lesion involved/extended into the motor cortex (Rasmussen and Milner, 1977). Subcortical lesions may have a more detrimental effect on language acquisition than cortical lesion (Janowsky and Nass, 1987; Nass, 1999; Staudt, Grodd, Niemann et al., 2001). More primitive structures are probably less plastic than neocortical regions. Frontal lesions regardless of side may be particularly detrimental to language development as well (Bates, 1999; Dennis and Barnes, 2001). Thus, the location of a lesion has some effect on the extent of recovery, i.e., is a factor in the extent plasticity.

Further, the apparent location of a lesion may not reflect the entirety of the injury. Metabolic imaging studies demonstrate effects remote from the lesion itself, as well as different remote effects of the same structural lesion in different patients (Kerrigan, Chugani and Phelps, 1991). Remote effects may diminish over time, changing the 'location' of the lesion.

*Other factors: epilepsy*

Epilepsy has a detrimental effect on all aspects of cognitive development (Vargha-Khadem, Isaacs, Van der Werf et al., 1992; Vargha-Khadem, Isaacs, Watkins et al., 2000). Curtiss and De Bode (1999) found that in their 48-patient hemispherectomy cohort those with later-onset seizures tended to have better language outcome regardless of the side

of hemispherectomy than those with earlier-onset seizures. This likely represents differing underlying etiology in the two groups. Vargha-Khadem et al. (2000) found that with congenital, early (1–5 years) or late lesions (5–15 years) those with seizures had a poorer outcome. This was particularly true for those with congenital left lesions and all age groups with right hemisphere lesions. Approximately 25% of the congenital focal lesion population have neonatal seizures and/or develop seizures. Thus, a sizeable proportion may have deficits that extend beyond the bounds of the lesion itself. In a sense epilepsy turns a focal lesion into a more diffuse lesion. Epilepsy alters the extent of remote effects seen on metabolic imaging in patients with focal lesion. What effect epileptiform discharge has on plasticity is yet to be determined. Although controversial, the data from patients with the Landau–Kleffner syndrome suggest that epileptiform discharge alone interferes with language acquisition and thus, by extrapolation, with plasticity (Tuchman, 1997).

The specific effects of epilepsy in children with focal pathology has been best studied for language. Children with left frontal seizures followed from ages of 3 to 8 years evidenced catch-up in receptive, but not in expressive language skills (see below for a contrast with those with left hemisphere structural pathology) (Cohen and Le Normand, 1998). Rosenblatt, Vernet, Montes et al. (1998) describe a child with continuous epileptiform activity whose language improved rapidly and dramatically after left hemispherectomy at the age of 2 years. Vargha-Khadem et al. (1997) described a young child with Sturge–Weber and significant language delays who made dramatic gains in the years following a left hemispherectomy for seizure control at the age of 8 years. Indeed, his ultimate language capacity did not differ from other children with early left hemispherectomies who had not had major early delays in language acquisition suggesting that the brain remains plastic despite interference by seizures.

## Learning: plasticity in action

Everyday learning dramatizes the rapidity with which central nervous system changes can occur. Examples of learning and the underlying mechanisms in several cognitive domains are presented below.

*Visual–perceptual learning*

During visual–perceptual learning neuronal number and interconnections, as well as neuronal sensitivity and selectivity can change. Some visual neurons respond dynamically to both context and experience suggesting that certain visual areas are not hard-wired for particular perceptual tasks (Chelazzi, Miller, Duncan et al., 1993; Moran and Desimone, 1985); thus learning occurs fluidly. Competition contributes to cortical plasticity; representational translocations and substitutions occur constantly. Different brain regions mediate a visual–perceptual task during versus after learning. For example, the right parietal cortex is involved in novel (assessed by PET scanning) (Corbetta, Shulman, Miezin et al., 1995), but not learned, visual search (assessed by transcranial magnetic stimulation inhibition) (Walsh, Ashbridge and Cowey, 1998).

*Somatosensory learning*

Experience-dependent neuronal plasticity has been studied by assessing (magnetic source imaging) performance before and after training on a unilateral tactile discrimination task of sequentially applied multi-finger stimuli. Subjects show rapid improvement in performance and complete transfer of the learned task to the untrained hand. Physiologic changes are documented in associative rather than in primary sensory cortex. Higher level structures are not surprisingly engaged during the learning process (Wang, Merzenich, Sameshima et al., 1995).

*Motor learning*

Experience-dependent plasticity has been studied by examining the modification of neural structures which results from the acquisition of new motor skills. For example, training on a simple thumb movement task (Classen, Liepert, Wise et al., 1998) rapidly, but transiently, changes the cortical network representing the thumb kinematics. Examining the acquisition of complex fine motor skills, Pascual-Leone, Nguyet, Cohen et al. (1995a) mapped (transcranial magnetic stimulation) the cortical motor areas targeting the hand muscles in subjects learning a one-handed, five-finger piano exercise. Over the course of 5 days, as subjects learned the exercise through daily 2-h manual practice sessions, the cortical motor areas targeting the contralateral hand muscles enlarged. In control subjects who played the piano for 2 h each day but did not practice a specific exercise, the cortical changes were similar, but less pronounced. Thus, cortical changes can occur rapidly and are more dramatic when a specific learned skill is involved. In another study of complex finger movements cortical motor output maps (generated using transcranial magnetic stimulation) of the reading hand in blind proficient braille readers obtained on a day in which they worked as braille proofreaders were compared with the maps obtained on a day when they did not work. The maps of the reading hand were significantly larger after a work shift than after two days off. These results illustrate the rapidity of modulation in motor cortical outputs relative to the preceding activity and highlight the importance of timing for elucidating the correlates of skill acquisition (Pascual-Leone, Wassermann, Sadato et al., 1995b).

## Plasticity: specific skill systems

*Language*

The extent of plasticity varies for different neurologic/cognitive functions. Plasticity manifested as reorganization of function, generally with transfer of function to the intact hemisphere, is more pronounced for language than for other cognitive and neurologic functions (Muller et al., 1998a,b; Muller, Rothermel, Behen et al., 1998c). This is true despite the fact that language is strongly lateralized to the left hemisphere from the outset.

*Patterns of reorganization of language after early injury*

A seminal study of Rasmussen and Milner (1977) (based on carotid amytal testing) of language organization in patients with early focal brain injury and epilepsy documented that (1) transfer of language to the intact right hemisphere was the most common recovery pattern, (2) transfer did not occur unless the lesion involved primary language

TABLE 1

Relationship between handedness and language dominance in patients with epilepsy as documented by carotid amytal testing

| Handedness | Language dominance | | | |
|---|---|---|---|---|
| | right dominant | left dominant | incompletely left dominant | strongly bilateral |
| Right | 5 | 110 | 19 | 8 |
| Left | 10 | 4 | 8 | 3 |
| Ambidexter | 0 | 3 | 1 | 2 |
| Total | 15 | 117 | 28 | 13 |

Modified from Kurthen (1994).

cortex, regardless of size, and (3) transfer rarely occurred if handedness did not switch, i.e., the lesion involved/extended into motor cortex. Recently, Staudt et al. (2001) have shown that transfer of language to the right hemisphere after early left periventricular injury did not occur unless the left facial motor tract was involved, suggesting that the impairment of speech motor output from the left hemisphere is a prerequisite to alteration of language representation. Subsequent studies of children with congenital, early pre-language acquisition and post-language acquisition (acquired aphasia in childhood) left hemisphere injury and/or hemispherectomy corroborate reorganization of language by transfer to the intact right hemisphere as the most common 'recovery' pattern and document that language development/recovery is generally good (Bates, 1999; Nass, 1997; Van Hout, 1997). In epileptic patients without definable lesions, transfer of language to the right hemisphere is more often incomplete (Kurthen, 1994) (Table 1). In some patients language is reorganized within the left hemisphere, generally at the periphery of the lesion. In such patients less language recovery and lower Verbal IQ has been documented by some investigators (Lansdell, 1969; Ojemann and Creutzfeldt, 1987). Although recovery by reorganization of language into the right hemisphere has been considered the most common mechanism in adults as well, some recent studies (utilizing dynamic imaging techniques) of adults with acquired aphasia demonstrate that recruitment of the right hemisphere for recovering language may actually be less effective than restitution of function in the left perisylvian region (superior temporal cortex) of the left hemisphere (Karbe, Thiel and Weber-Luxenburger et al., 1998).

Recent dynamic imaging studies provide further details about patterns of intra- and inter-hemispheric language reorganization after early injury. Muller et al. (1998c) examined the organization of language (positron emission tomography imaging, PET) in a 6-year-old boy who had a right functional hemispherectomy [1] at the age of 3 years. Tasks measuring receptive language and prosody activated left perisylvian cortices. Activation was also seen in residual cortical and subcortical areas on the right, surprisingly suggesting some right hemisphere involvement in language mediation. Studying children with early focal lesions during language tasks (PET imaging), Muller and colleagues (Muller, Rothermel and Behen, 1997b; Muller, Rothermel, Muzik et al., 1997c; Muller et al., 1997a, 1998a,b, 1998c, 1999a) demonstrated both additive (activation in regions not normally involved in language processing) and subtractive (lack of activation in left hemisphere regions normally activated by language tasks) activity. A rightward shift of language activation occurred in the patients with early left perisylvian temporal–parietal lesions. Right hemisphere involvement in language perception included homologous regions (similar to those ordinarily activated in the left

---

[1] Total hemispherectomy is associated with serious morbidity and mortality in the short and long term. Alternatives include: hemidecortication, removal of most of one cerebral hemisphere including the insular cortex and portions of the basal ganglia; subtotal hemispherectomy, removal of two thirds to four fifths of the cortex of the affected hemisphere; functional hemispherectomy, removal of the central cortical region, including the parasaggital region and the cingulate gyrus, a temporal lobectomy including amygdala and hippocampus, transection of the white matter connections to frontal, parietal and occipital lobes, disconnecting the involved hemisphere from the brain stem and opposite hemisphere.

49

hemisphere): inferior frontal; superior temporal and non-homologous regions: anterior, inferior, middle temporal; cingulate; basal ganglia. Right hemisphere involvement in sentence repetition included predominantly the non-homologous premotor cortex. These results not only confirm recruitment of the right hemisphere for language after left hemisphere lesions, but delineate its intrahemispheric localization. There was little intrahemispheric reorganization in the left lesion group. In essence outcome reflects the relative import of the loss of left hemisphere language cortex versus the gain of right hemisphere cortex. Surprisingly the number of brain regions activated by language processing tasks was greater in the right than the left lesion group. Language perception activated regions in both perisylvian and extraperisylvian cortex. There is also greater subcortical and cerebellar language involvement after right hemisphere lesions. These results are consistent with the clinical findings (see below) that the right hemisphere plays a role in language acquisition. Thus, after an early right hemisphere lesion, atypical areas within the left hemisphere need to be recruited for language processing. Involvement in language acquisition after an early focal lesion could cause an increase in compensatory spread of language. The subtractive effects documented in the early focal lesion population reflected structural problems in the area of damage, diaschisis in anatomically connected sites remote from damaged areas during resting state (resulting from a loss of afferent input to the remote site), and functional diaschisis occurring in areas remote from damage during activation tasks.

Another study (Muller et al., 1999b) compared the responses to language stimuli of 13 patients with early (prior to age five years) and 10 with late-onset (after 20 years of age) left hemisphere lesions. While listening to sentences the normal asymmetry (increased left frontal–temporal blood flow) was reduced in those with late left lesions and reversed in those with early left lesions. During sentence repetition the findings were similar, but reached significance only in the basal ganglia, but not for the (pre)motor and insular regions. Thus, reorganization after early left hemisphere injury tended to enlist the right hemisphere to a far greater degree than later injury. Extrasylvian areas were enlisted for language processing in both age groups.

*Patterns of language acquisition after early focal injury*

In their seminal studies of school-age hemispherectomy patients (early focal lesion with intractable seizures requiring hemispherectomy), Dennis and Whitaker (1976) demonstrated differential linguistic abilities in the left and right hemispheres — the solo right hemisphere lacking the "analytic, organizational, syntactic, and hierarchical competence" necessary to deal with taxing linguistic problems. Follow-up studies during the teen-age years documented that those with left hemisperectomy were inferior at complex syntactic tasks, contextual semantic analysis, and written language (Dennis, 1980; Dennis, Lovett and Wiegel-Crump, 1981; Lovett et al., 1986; Vargha-Khadem and Polkey, 1992). In addition, individual left hemisperectomy patients showed different strengths and weaknesses, suggesting that 'right hemispheres' do not mediate language in uniform fashion. These studies provided both initial and continuing support for the theory of innate specialization of the left hemisphere for language and secondarily for limited plasticity — lack of complete right hemisphere take over of language.

Other studies of hemisperectomy patients produce somewhat different results or have been differently interpreted. Smith and Sugar (1975) demonstrated supra-normal catchup language development between 8 and 11 years of age in a single patient with a congenital left hemisphere lesion (and subsequent hemisperectomy). Kohn (1980) reported, examining a small group of adolescents with congenital left hemisphere lesions (and later hemisperectomy) and well documented right hemisphere language dominance, that only those with seizure onset prior to the age of 7 years performed poorly on complex syntactic tasks. Rosenblatt et al. (1998) described a child with continuous epileptiform activity whose language after left hemisperectomy at the age of 2 years improved rapidly and dramatically. In another case study Vargha-Khadem et al. (1997) described a patient with Sturge–Weber syndrome affecting the left hemisphere who failed to develop speech throughout early childhood and whose comprehension of single words and simple commands remained at an age equivalent to 3–4 years. Following left hemisperectomy at the age of 8 years and discontinuation of anticonvulsants when he was 9 years old, he acquired expressive language rapidly. At the age of 15 years receptive and expressive language were at an 8–10 year age equivalent. (Notably, this patient acquired language at a relatively late age, when plasticity/recovery is generally thought to be more limited/adult-like.) Thus, Kohn's position that language can develop normally in the right hemisphere if 'interference' (seizures) from the left does not occur is corroborated at least in part by a number of other investigators.

The language outcome of children with congenital focal lesions (generally pre-perinatal middle cerebral artery territory infarctions) who often do not have seizures (or at least intractable seizures) and therefore do not undergo hemispherectomy, has been a focus of study for the past decade. In general, longitudinal follow-up beginning as early as 6 months of age reveals that initial language acquisition is mildly to moderately delayed after both congenital left and right hemisphere lesions, albeit in different ways. Catch-up in language skills in both groups occurs around school age. Thus, by the age 5–7 years language problems are barely, if at all, detectable, in either lesion group (Bates, 1999; Bates et al., 1997; Bates and Roe, 2001). Other studies do, however, continue to document subtle language and language-based academic skill deficits particularly after early left hemisphere injury (Aram, 1999).

Different aspects of language are affected by early left versus right hemisphere lesions, and lesions in different locations produce different effects. Infants with congenital focal injury (3 right, 2 left) assessed from the onset of babbling through the age of 2 years were initially delayed in the production of gestures and words. Towards the end of the second year, word production normalized, as reported by parents, for those with anterior lesions, but not for the two patients with left posterior lesions. Spontaneous speech during free play was normal in quantity, but vocalizations were phonologically deviant (Marchman, Miller and Bates, 1991). Early delays in single word use and in multi-word sentences occurred, but catch-up in syntax occurred at 2 years of age in most of a group of 15 toddlers studied (Feldman, 1994; Feldman, Holland, Kemp et al., 1992a). Left hemisphere injury was not invariably associated with language delay; indeed, the most competent speaker in this cohort had a left hemisphere lesion. In a case study a child with a left hemisphere lesion evidenced normal development of Hebrew morphology (Levy and Amir, 1994). Another child with a left lesion, however, had a documented period of jargon aphasia during language acquisition (Feldman, Holland and Brown, 1992b). Right hemisphere lesions were sometimes associated with significant delays in acquisition (Feldman, 1994; Feldman et al., 1992a). Longitudinal assessment of 27 children between the ages of 1 and 3 years revealed expressive language delays regardless of lesion side or site throughout the age range tested (Thal, Marchman, Stiles et al., 1991). Comprehension delays occurred only in the youngest children. The most significant comprehension delays occurred in the right lesion group. Phonological delays and expressive vocabulary delays were most persistent in the subgroup with left posterior lesions. Detailing parent reports and spontaneous speech data on 55 children with focal lesions between the ages of 10 and 44 months, Bates et al. (1997) confirmed their prior finding that children with right hemisphere lesions were at greater risk for delays in word comprehension and communicative gesture between 10 and 17 months. Children with left temporal lobe involvement showed greater delays in expressive vocabulary and grammar acquisition throughout the study period of 10 to 44 months. Frontal lesions of either hemisphere affected language acquisition between 16 and 31 months. Reilly et al. (1998) found on a story telling task that between the ages of 3 and 5 years children with right lesions scored better in terms of grammatical diversity. Those with left temporal damage had particular difficulty with both morphologic (e.g., word endings like ed, ing) and syntactic measures. Side of lesion effects were not present in those over 5 years. Assessing preschool children longitudinally over a 2-year period, Muter, Taylor and Vargha-Khadem (1997) found no effects of side of lesion. Thus, during infancy and the toddler years intrahemispheric location of lesion (specifically frontal lesions) and side of lesion both affect language acquisition. Catch-up acquisition in those with both left and right lesion groups may occur by school age, i.e., language deficits can diminish over time, suggesting a positive interaction between plasticity and language development.

At school age some studies find no language deficits, some find subtle deficits in both lesion groups, some find subtle deficits only in those with left lesions, and some find deficits only in those with seizures. Evaluating the early left focal lesion population at school age, Woods and Carey (1979), assessing semantics, syntax and language-based academics, found no difference as compared with IQ-matched controls, except in spelling. (This contrasts with still subtle, but more marked deficits in a group tested on the same measures, whose left hemisphere insults occurred after language acquisition and caused an apparent initial aphasia.) Reilly et al. (1998) found that both lesion groups were equally delayed on a story telling task in terms of narrative length and complexity compared with controls. Notably, both lesion groups did better than children with developmental language disorders. Bates, Reilly, Wulfect et al. (2001) found that from the age of 5–8 years there was no difference between the right and left lesion groups in spontaneous speech collected during biographical interviews. Vargha-Khadem et al. (1985) found only minimal language deficits in those with left lesions, regardless of the extent of the lesion. In a later study with a larger cohort, Vargha-Khadem et al. (1992) found no language deficits related to the side of lesion. Indeed, no deficits were apparent except in those with seizures, and these deficits were non lateralizing.

Other investigators have found subtle but greater language deficits at school age in those with left lesions (Aram, 1999; Aram and Ekelman, 1987; Aram, Ekelman and Whitaker, 1986, 1987; Aram, Meyers and Ekelman, 1990b; Eisele and Aram, 1993, 1994; Eisele, Lust and Aram, 1998). Spontaneous speech samples revealed that left lesion children had more difficulty producing both simple and complex sentences. On grammatical imitation and comprehension tasks of complex coordinate, passive, and relative clause structures, children with left lesions evidenced relatively impaired imitation coupled with relatively preserved (but nonetheless impaired) comprehension. Right lesion children also had difficulty, but to a lesser degree. The results were interpreted as consistent with an early and continuous left hemisphere specialization for expressive syntax (Eisele and Aram, 1994). Left lesion, but not right lesion, children had difficulties on the Token Test. (Memory

difficulty was, however, a bigger factor in impairing performance than linguistic complexity.) Left lesion children were marginally impaired, compared with right lesion children, on measures of lexical retrieval, comprehension and production. Both left and right lesion children had difficulties inferring the truth or falseness of implicative sentences, but only those with left lesion had difficulty with presupposition. Whereas left lesion children had difficulty with both lexical and syntactic forms of negation, those with right lesions were only impaired on the lexical part of the task (Eisele et al., 1998). Evaluating children at the age of 5 years with congenital unilateral lesions but without hemiparesis, Glass (1998) found adult-like deficit patterns for receptive language. (Notably, most of these studies differ from the longitudinal focal lesion studies because the comparison group is matched controls, as opposed to contrasting the two lesion groups.)

These data bring up several issues with regard to the extent and mechanisms of plasticity, as well as its interaction with timing of and the reason(s) for hemispheric specialization. The presence of early deficits after pre-language acquisition insults to either hemisphere can be interpreted as reflecting insufficient plasticity of the immature central nervous system to fully spare language during its early development. The fact that most deficits diminish over time suggests that multiple/alternative routes to language acquisition exist and/or can evolve if needed and trade on/require both hemispheres.

That there are alternative routes to language acquisition is consistent with normative data documenting different styles of early language learning (analytic versus holistic speakers). Normative data also demonstrate that different areas of brain (both inter- and intra- hemispheric) are involved in different aspects of language acquisition at different points in early development (Mills, Coffey and Neville, 1993a,b). They are also consistent with the speculation of Bates et al. (1997) that hemisphere-specific computational biases — detail left, integration right — predominate at various stages in the language learning process and are thereby responsible for deficit patterns (see above). Based on such a model, critical period effects derive not only from endogenously determined maturational changes, but also reflect the learning history in relation to the characteristics of the language to be learned (March-man, 1993). Based on early language development in Hebrew, Levy and Amir (1994) suggest that simpler, more autonomous systems (Hebrew as opposed to English, morphology as opposed to syntax) are more robust and thus less susceptible to the effects of early lesions on innately programmed linguistic skills. Such systems would arguably be more plastic. With regard to intra-hemispheric specialization, it is notable that posterior lesions and frontal lesions of either hemisphere have non-adult-like effects on early language acquisition. Neville and colleagues found that 13 to 20 month olds with left lesions displayed a reversed lateral distribution of evoked potentials, consistent with the hypothesis that neural systems linked to good language probably initially develop bilaterally and can become stabilized in either an intact left or right hemisphere and support good language comprehension. This also is a form of plasticity.

Thus, there is evidence from the studies of children with congenital unilateral lesions of both innate specialization, emergent specialization and plasticity. Whether plasticity actually increases over time (evidenced as catch-up by school age) or whether this is an artifact of the different stages in language development, perhaps interacting with specialization (*intra*hemispheric as well as *inter*hemispheric), remains to be determined. Early brain damage may counteract the genetic disposition by affecting and modifying the neural activity/plasticity interaction (Bates, 1999; Vargha-Khadem et al., 2000). Hemispheric computational biases (aspects of language acquisition that reflect hemispheric processing style rather than linguistics per se) may also be relevant here.

*Patterns of language-based academic skills after early focal lesions*
Language-based academic skills are also affected by early focal lesions. As children with 'recovered aphasia' have persistent academic difficulties (Van Hout, 1997; Woods and Carey, 1979), academic problems would also be predicted for the congenital focal lesion population if innate specialization and computational biases prevail and plasticity is limited. Overall, studies in this area document greater reading and spelling difficulties in children with congenital

left hemisphere lesions (Aram, Gillespie and Yamashita, 1990a; Kershner and King, 1974; Kiessling, Denckla and Carlton, 1983; Ogden, 1996; Vargha-Khadem et al., 1997; Woods and Carey, 1979). The right hemisphere is at a significant disadvantage compared with the left in the comprehension of abstract, low frequency words, in phonetic feature analysis, and in the subtleties of grammar, such as the comprehension of passive negative constructions and the correct use of morphological markers in unfamiliar contexts (e.g., application of comparative and superlative forms of an adjective to nonwords) (Vargha-Khadem and Polkey, 1992). Such studies can be interpreted as supporting the view that plasticity is limited by the complexity of the task, as well as innate specialization, age at lesion and age at testing.

*Lessons about plasticity: developmental language disorders versus language disorders after focal lesions*
Unilateral left hemisphere damage does not work as an explanatory model of developmental language disorders. Although children with congenital and acquired unilateral brain lesions may have language difficulties, few (subcortical damage being a possible exception) have deficits as severe as those seen in children with developmental language disorders. Children with developmental language disorders and children with early unilateral lesions do share a similar developmental course. In both groups language onset and development is slow during the preschool years but tends to improve by school age. Those with early focal lesions, however, have minimal long-term language-based learning deficits (Aram and Eisele, 1994b), while those with developmental language disorders are at significant risk for long-term language-based learning deficits. One recent case study finds to the contrary. Follow-up of a child with a left hemispherectomy at the age of 10 years revealed a language deficit pattern similar to that of children with developmental language disorders (Stark and McGregor, 1997).

The lesions are by definition apparent in those with early hemispheric damage, but only minor anatomical (Selmud-Clikeman, 1997) (reversed planum temporale asymmetries) and metabolic abnormalities are found in most children with developmental language problems, and clear-cut left hemisphere pathology is rare. Bates' (1997) fresh start hypothesis (see above) may be relevant here. Large focal lesions permit reorganization, while language mediated by a more minor atypical anatomic substrate is more aberrant.

Plasticity may actually work to the disadvantage of the DLD child. By the time such a child enters school he/she has undergone several million practice trials, which result in brain remodeling that creates a representation of this atypical less adaptive language pattern. Some of these children have consistent, but abnormal temporal integration/segmentation abilities. They take in sound chunks without making rapid intrasyllabic distinctions. This atypical learned representation of language has ramifications for reading. It is an example of a maladaptive effect of plasticity. These children are working with functional but inefficient tools. Having the tools mitigates against normalization and change. Tallal and colleagues have used a "functional self creation plasticity process" (i.e., Fast Forward) to try to correct the abnormal learning pattern (Merzenich, Jenkins, Johnston et al., 1996a). With only 20 days of training some children with developmental language disorders switch from a non-phonologic mode of language processing to a phonologic one.

*Auditory perceptual system*

The auditory perceptual system provides the framework for the development of speech and language. Auditory cortex plasticity can be demonstrated during normal language acquisition, as well as in the context of sensory deprivation (deafness).

*Effects of sensory stimulation: normal development*
The ability to discriminate speech sounds is already present in the neonatal period (Cheour, Alho, Ceponiene et al., 1998; Pallier, Bosch and Sebastian-Galles, 1997), but the transformation of speech sounds into language is a dynamic process that depends on auditory cortex plasticity. Early language exposure affects the ability to discriminate between phonemes; infants can differentiate a wide range of sounds, but they gradually lose the ability to discriminate between sounds that are not relevant to or reinforced by their native language. This phe-

nomenon has been termed the 'perceptual magnet effect'; sounds sufficiently similar to a prototypic vowel or consonant are 'captured' and are perceived as examples of that sound, so that differences between them (which might be meaningful in another language) become undetectable. For example, when a series of repeated sounds is interrupted by an unexpected 'oddball', an evoked potential mismatch negativity signal results, which originates in primary auditory cortex and indicates a difference between the neural representations of the two sounds. At 6 months, Finnish children show mismatch negativity signaling a perceived difference between vowels. At 1 year they show a stronger response to the 'oddball' sound that is a vowel in their native language than to a vowel that is unique to another language, Estonian. By contrast, 1-year-old Estonian children, who have been exposed to both vowels, show 'oddball' responses to both vowels. Thus, the early phonetic environment has a strong influence on auditory perception and speech development, which is a reflection of changes in the auditory cortex.

Clinical examples of plasticity in the auditory perceptual system extend beyond infancy. A few studies document that perception of non-native speech sounds can be learned through training (Lively, Pisoni, Yamada et al., 1994) (as opposed to 'unlearned' during development). Auditory spatial perception is important to early language learning. The physical properties of the outer ear plays a role in calibrating the developing auditory cortex in this regard (Rauschecker, 1999). Investigators altering the adult human ear with plastic implants (Hofman, Van Riswick and Van Opstal, 1998; Wightman and Kistler, 1998) find that although the implants initially disrupt sound perception, subjects learn to localize sounds with their 'new ears' within a few weeks. Notably, subjects perform normally as soon as the implants are removed. Thus, unlike other forms of sensory adaptation (e.g., visual adaptation to prism glasses), the original auditory map appears to be preserved along side the new one. Musical training leads to an expansion in the representation of complex harmonic sounds in the auditory cortex. The development of perfect pitch also results in a concomitant expansion of auditory cortex. The critical period for the development of perfect pitch coincides with the critical period for acquiring a second language with a native accent (at about 8 years of age).

### Effects of sensory deprivation

Studies of the deaf (as well as the blind, see below) provide an opportunity to evaluate reorganization after auditory deprivation, with resulting compensatory visual and somatosensory changes (cross-modal plasticity) and to reassess the concept of critical periods, as new technology (cochlear implants) allows some deaf to gain some hearing.

### Cross-modal plasticity

Studies of the deaf demonstrate that the cortical regions involved in language processing depend more on the nature of the cognitive task than on the sensory modality used for communication. In the pre-lingual deaf, sign language activates the language areas (supratemporal gyri), but not primary auditory cortex (Nishimura, Hashikawa, Doi et al., 1999). Watching a video of sign-language words signed by a native signer activates (PET) the supratemporal gyri bilaterally, whereas watching a video showing someone moving both hands up and down in a meaningless manner activates the occipital lobe visual cortex (Nishimura et al., 1999). In bilinguals (those with sign and spoken language) sign language activates visual areas (Soderfeldt, Ingvar, Ronnberg et al., 1997), as well as Broca's and Wernicke's areas of the left hemisphere (Neville, Bavelier, Corina et al., 1998). Early exposure to American Sign Language in both hearing and deaf native signers increases the role of the right hemisphere in language processing (Bavelier, Corina, Jezzard et al., 1998; Neville and Bavelier, 1998). The reorganization pattern in signers is cross-modal; language cortex is activated by visual stimuli. Lack of cross-modal plasticity of the primary auditory cortex (Hickok, Bellugi and Klima, 1997) may be due to the relatively rigid organization of primary auditory cortex. In addition, non-visual areas not ordinarily involved in language processing are recruited when signing is a medium for language.

### Age effects

Studies of deaf subjects undergoing cochlear implantations provide a unique opportunity to examine critical periods in the development of linguistic auditory processing. The neural network that projects from the inner ear to the primary auditory cortex forms without any auditory input, but post-processing neurons require proper neural input to mature (cortical evoked potentials). The auditory system retains its plasticity for some time, however, as evidenced by the fact that the late introduction of auditory stimulation by a cochlear implant results in the resumption of the normal maturational sequence (Ponton, Don, Eggermont et al., 1996), but with a clear age effect. Deaf children implanted before the age of 5 years are likely to perform better on speech perception and speech production tasks than children implanted at an older age. Degree of prior exposure to language affects outcome as well. The pre-lingual deaf can hear sounds through a cochlear implant, but they do not understand the words without extensive training. In the pre-lingual deaf language stimulation through the cochlear implant only activates primary auditory cortex, whereas in the post-lingual deaf it activates both primary and secondary auditory cortices (Naito, Hirano, Honjo et al., 1997). Some degree of early language priming is required to recruit the full auditory cortex. Despite some plasticity for sounds, plasticity for language is limited by age and prior exposure (Robinson, 1998).

### Visual system

### Effects of sensory deprivation

Plasticity has been extensively investigated in the visual system by studying and comparing the patterns of reorganization that occur with congenital and acquired sensory deprivation (blindness).

### Cross-modal plasticity

As described above for the auditory system, impaired sensory functioning in one domain can result in enhanced function in another sensory domain. Blind subjects, for example, have better auditory localization (attending to sounds in peripheral auditory space (Roder, Teder-Salejarvi, Sterr et al., 1999b) and auditory discrimination (detecting a rare target tone among frequent standard tones (Roder, Rosler and Neville, 1999a)) abilities than sighted controls. The tactile perceptual abilities of blind subjects are also often superior to those of sighted controls (Cohen, Weeks, Sadato et al., 1999).

The neurophysiologic counterparts of these trade offs (enhanced abilities in the setting of visual deprivation) are being actively investigated. Although gross brain structure (MRI) does not differ (Buchel, Price, Frackowiak et al., 1998; Kujala, Alho, Huoti-lainen et al., 1997), occipital cerebral blood flow and metabolism in both primary and secondary visual cortices at rest and during tactile and auditory discrimination tasks is increased in blind subjects compared to sighted controls (Pons, 1996; Sadato, Pascual-Leone, Grafman et al., 1996). Stimulation of the right hand by touch in the blind causes bilateral activation of the visual cortex (Sadato et al., 1996). Braille reading by the blind activates the inferior parietal lobule, primary visual cortex, superior occipital gyri, fusiform gyri, ventral premotor area, superior parietal lobule, cerebellum and primary sensorimotor area bilaterally, as well as the right dorsal premotor cortex, right middle occipital gyrus and right prefrontal area. During non-braille discrimination tasks, in blind subjects, the ventral occipital regions, including the primary visual cortex and fusiform gyri bilaterally were activated while the secondary somatosensory area was deactivated. The reverse pattern was found in sighted subjects where the secondary somatosensory area was activated while the ventral occipital regions were suppressed. Thus, tactile processing pathways usually linked in the secondary somatosensory area appear to be rerouted in blind subjects to the ventral occipital cortical regions originally reserved for visual shape discrimination (Sadato, Pascual-Leone, Grafman et al., 1998). Areas ordinarily reserved for visual processing input can be reallocated for processing in other sensory modalities (auditory and tactile), i.e., cross-modal transfer.

Cross-modal plasticity is affected by features of the task. Braille reading results in greater activation in the primary visual cortex than other simple tactile discrimination tasks. This effect could be due to the increased complexity of the braille task, and/or the additional lexical component involved in braille reading (Sadato et al., 1996). The prolonged somatosensory tactile learning associated with braille reading may also enhance this effect (Sadato et al., 1996). Tactile imagery tasks (which have both cognitive and sensory components) recruit both visual cortex and parietal association cortex (evoked potential studies) (Uhl, Kretschmer, Lindinger et al., 1994).

On a selective auditory attention task (dichotic listening paradigm), reaction times for an ear attended to differed for the congenitally blind compared with controls (Liotti, Ryder and Woldorff, 1998). Progressive recruitment of parietal and then occipital cortex for auditory attention provides further evidence for cross-modal sensory reorganization in the blind (Liotti et al., 1998). The occipital cortex is activated during auditory discrimination tasks in blind subjects (evoked response potentials, magneto-encephalography, SPECT, fMRI) (Kujala et al., 1997; Sadato et al., 1996; Uhl, Franzen, Podreka et al., 1993). Abnormally high metabolism already observed in the occipital cortex of the early blind at rest (Veraart, De Volder and Wanet-Defalque et al., 1990) shows a trend to further increase during the use of a sensory/auditory substitution device (ultrasonic echolocation). The metabolic recruitment of the occipital cortex in early blind subjects using a substitution prosthesis could reflect concurrent stimulation of functional cross-modal sensory connections. Given the unfamiliarity of the task, it suggests that the period of plasticity is rather prolonged (De Volder, Catalan-Ahumada, Robert et al., 1999).

*Single versus dual sensory system processing*
In sighted subjects processing in one sensory modality may inhibit functioning in another. In normal controls (with no braille reading training), tactile discrimination is associated with a decrease in regional cerebral blood flow to primary visual cortex (Sadato et al., 1996). During visual tasks regional cerebral blood flow in the auditory and somatosensory cortices decreases. Even selective attention to one sensory modality can cause decreased metabolic activity in areas responsible for processing in another sensory modality (Haxby, Horwitz, Ungerleider et al., 1994). By contrast, in the blind tactile discrimination is not associated with decreased metabolic activity in visual cortex (the opposite occurs, see above). Processing in the tactile modality does not require selective attention in blind subjects since they do not have an alternative. Visual imagery is not an alternative sensory modality (which, in the sighted, could invoke the need for selective attention) in the congenitally blind. They have been shown to have little or no 'visual' memory, as documented by studies of features potentially facilitating braille reading. Thus,

the blind perform the same tasks in a different way and metabolic ramifications are demonstrable.

*Effects of age at blindness*
The effects of visual experience on the organization of visual cortex have been extensively studied. Experience-dependent cortical reorganization has been investigated through a comparison between subjects with congenital versus acquired blindness. Resting metabolic activity (PET) in occipital cortex differs in early versus late (after puberty) blind. Activation studies also reveal differences between these two groups which are task-specific. Congenitally blind subjects show task-specific activation of extrastriate (but not striate) visual areas and parietal association areas during braille reading, compared with auditory word processing. Blind subjects who lost their sight after puberty show additional activation in the primary visual cortex with the same tasks. Access to visual imagery in subjects with late blindness who have had early visual experience may explain the greater cross-modal activation (Buchel et al., 1998). Occipital cortex is strongly activated (PET) in the congenitally blind and early-onset blind groups, but not in the late-onset (after the age of 14 years) blind group during braille reading. Repetitive transcranial magnetic stimulation of occipital cortex disrupts the braille reading task in congenitally blind and early-onset blind subjects, but not in late-onset blind subjects. Based on these findings Cohen et al. (1999) suggest that there is a critical period for cross-modal plasticity that ends some time before the age of 14 years. (The lack of a more specific cut-off may well reflect the arbitrariness of the age range of the groups assessed.) The putative cut-off age for cross-modal transfer in the visual system may overlap that seen in the acquisition of native-like second languages and for rehabilitation of individuals with amblyopia. There is some evidence, however, of cross-modal reorganization in the mature as well as the immature brain. Both parietal and occipital cortex are activated during a pitch-change discrimination in individuals blinded after childhood (Kujala et al., 1997).

In summary, visual cortex appears to be quite plastic, allowing for significant cross-modal transfer of somatosensory/tactile and auditory information. Cross-modal plasticity is age-dependent, limited for the most part to those with pre-pubertal-onset blindness. Putative neuronal mechanisms of cross-modal plasticity, such as unmasking of ordinarily silent sensory inputs, stabilization of normally transient connections, or axonal sprouting, trade on the plasticity of both the visual cortex and neighboring cortical regions (Rauschecker, 1995).

*Somatosensory system*

The somatosensory system provides a forum for examining a number of principles of plasticity, including adaptive and maladaptive aspects, effects of central versus peripheral lesions on somatosensory function, and the rate at which change can occur.

*Effects of central hemispheric lesions/insults*
The motor, somatosensory, and language systems are not equally plastic, the somatosensory systems being the least plastic of the three. Sensory functions transferred from one hemisphere to the other in hemispherectomy patients (fMRI) are mediated by associative sensory areas in the intact hemisphere, as opposed to primary somatosensory cortex (Graveline, Mikulis, Crawley et al., 1998), which is not sufficiently plastic to permit interhemispheric relocation of hand somatosensory cortex after unilateral brain damage. Consistent with less somatosensory plasticity, all the adults in one series showed interhemispheric reorganization of motor function, but only half showed interhemispheric reorganization of sensory functions as well (Cao, Vikingstad, Huttenlocher et al., 1994). Children with early focal injury generally have bilateral deficits in cortical somatosensory functions (stereoagnosis and graphesthesia) (Cooper, Majnemer, Rosenblatt et al., 1995). Sensory stimulation (measured by fMRI) in congenital hemiplegics produces activation in the ipsilateral hemisphere in one third, in the contralateral hemisphere in one third, and results in no activation in the hand area in one third. The more severe the sensory deficit, the more likely there is to be interhemispheric reorganization. This association, however, rather than signifying greater plasticity after greater insult, may reflect a 'barrier' to ipsilateral somatosensory connections.

One explanation for differential reorganization in different cortical modalities could be the degree of crossed versus uncrossed representation. Somatosensory pathways are almost completely crossed, while motor and auditory pathways are predominantly crossed but have a significant uncrossed component. Degree of uncrossed representation cannot be the sole explanation, however, as language which is completely lateralized shows the greatest interhemispheric reorganization potential among the cortical modalities. Plasticity appears to be modular; association cortex is more plastic than primary sensory cortex (Graveline et al., 1998). The relative lack of plasticity of the somatosensory system likely reflects a number of factors possibly driven by the comparative lack of need for sophisticated somatosensory skills.

*Effects of peripheral injury — early and late*
In contrast to the lack of somatosensory reorganization after cortical lesions, peripheral insults stimulate central somatosensory reorganization. After amputation in both children and adults, somatosensory cortex previously devoted to the amputated area frequently mediates inputs from areas near the stump, often enlarging and/or shifting their cortical representation (Elbert, Flor, Birbaumer et al., 1994; Sica, Sanz, Cohen et al., 1984). In a sense, plasticity allows the brain to re-constructs a 'body image' (Ramachandran and Hirstein, 1998).

Amputees often have the feeling that the missing limb is still present. Because of the reorganization of somatosensory cortex, phantom sensations can be evoked by touching 'trigger zones' on other parts of the body. Touching the face or remaining upper arm on the side of an amputated arm may, for example, produce sensations both of those body parts and of the missing hand (Ramachandran and Hirstein, 1998). Trigger zones presumably activate neurons in the arm or the face territories in the brain, as well as the territories previously devoted to the amputated area. Phantom sensations may result from stimulation of preserved/reorganized representation of the missing limb in the somatosensory cortex or by an inappropriate interpretation of the afferent signal possibly by experience-based recalibration (Cohen, Brasil-Neto, Pascual-Leone et al., 1993b). Reorganization is not necessarily beneficial, however, since it causes a misperception, i.e., that the phantom limb is being touched (Kaas, 1998).

Phantom limb phenomena and cortical reorganization are highly correlated. Cortical reorganization (measured by magnetic source imaging) is more extensive in individuals with phantom limb pain than in those with non-painful phantom phenomena (Flor, Elbert, Muhlnickel et al., 1998). The amount of cortical invasion of the deafferented cortex and the amount of pain-evoked sensation mislocalized to the phantom limb also correlate strongly (Grusser, Winter, Muhlnickel et al., 2001).

Contrasting with many settings in which there is more reorganization when insults occur early rather than late, painful and non-painful phantom limb phenomena are generally absent in congenital amputees. Scalp transcranial magnetic stimulation does not induce a sensation of movement in patients with a congenitally missing hand (Cohen, Brasil-Neto, Pascual-Leone et al., 1993a,b). Sensory discrimination is normal and mislocalization (referral of stimulation-induced sensation to a phantom limb) is generally absent (Flor et al., 1998). Upper extremity limb amputation during childhood can shift limb representation in somatosensory cortex, but unlike adults there is no association between reorganization and presence of phantom pain. Patients with congenital absence of the hand (congenital aplasia) may never have developed an area of sensory representation for the absent hand (Cohen, Bandinelli, Topka et al., 1991b; Cohen, Roth, Wassermann et al., 1991c). Gallagher, Butterworth and Cole (1998) speculate that aplasic phantoms are absent because they depend on the existence of specific neural circuits resulting from innate motor schemas, like the hand–mouth coordination demonstrable in utero. By contrast, the presence of any phantom experiences in patients with congenital aplasia (Melzack, Israel, Lacroix et al., 1997) provides evidence of a distributed neural representation of the body that is in part genetically determined.

The topography of referred sensation can change over a few weeks. While the overall extent of reorganization is stable, the concomitant changes in the pattern of sensory processing are not. Alterations of cortical sensory processing may not be hard-wired, but mediated instead by a fluctuating, extensive and interconnected neural network (Knecht, Henningsen, Hohling et al., 1998). Relevance for neurological rehabilitation programs is obvious. In sum, peripheral injury produces significant central somatosensory re-organization that is age-dependent and reflects in clinical phenomena.

*Effects of special skills*

Like peripheral injury special skills can cause significant reorganization. The somatosensory cortical representation of the fingers expands when the amount of sensory input increases. For example, the somatosensory cortical representation of the left hand of string players, the hand responsible for complex and demanding fingering of the strings, is expanded (Elbert, Pantev, Wienbruch et al., 1995). Significant enlargement of sensorimotor cortex representation (transcranial magnetic stimulation mapping) has also been demonstrated for braille readers' reading finger (Pascual-Leone, Cammarota, Wassermann et al., 1993) and serves to enhance this specialized hand skill. Braille readers also lack the expected homuncular pattern in one or both hemispheres (Sterr, Muller, Elbert et al., 1998). The resulting 'smearing' of the digital cortical representation is adaptive for three-finger braille readers (three fingers are more efficient than one) because it fuses inputs transmitted over different fingers so that the incoming information can be processed as a whole (Sterr et al., 1998).

Enlarged representation is not always advantageous, however. Enlargement of sensorimotor cortex sometimes occurs at the expense of the representation of other fingers in braille readers. Cortical reorganization can result in misperceptions which can be maladaptive. Three-finger braille readers (in contrast to one-finger readers) misidentify which finger is being touched during tactile sensory threshold determination, although they have no difficulty in determining that one of the fingers has been touched. The topographic reorganization of finger representation (measured by magnetic source imaging) correlates with the mislocalization of tactile stimulation of the fingers (Sterr et al., 1998).

*Motor system*

Study of the motor system also provides a forum for examining a number of principles of plasticity including: efficacy of various mechanisms of plasticity (Muller et al., 1997c); relative effects of central and peripheral lesions/insults on motor cortex functioning; the rate at which plasticity changes can occur; the levels of the central nervous system at which they occur; when rehabilitation affects motor recovery; and the potential for maladaptive reorganization (mirror movements).

*Effects of peripheral lesions*

Amputation is a strong stimulus for motor, as well as somatosensory, reorganization (Chen, Corwell, Yaseen et al., 1998), and there is a difference between congenital and acquired lesions. Muscles in amputees can be activated with transcranial magnetic stimulation of cortical regions several centimeters wider than in controls. Muscles proximal to the stump are activated from more scalp positions than those contralateral to the stump. Congenital amputations also result in reorganization of motor outputs targeting muscles immediately proximal to the stump in both congenital and acquired amputees. However, magnetic scalp stimulation induced a sensation of movement in the missing hand or fingers of patients with acquired amputation, but did not do so in patients with congenital absence of a limb (Cohen, Bandinelli, Findley et al., 1991a; Cohen et al., 1991b,c).

*Effects of central lesions*

Similar to the somatosensory cortex, interhemispheric homotopic reorganization involving the primary motor cortex in the nonlesioned hemisphere is limited. In contrast to the somatosensory cortex, metabolic imaging documents lesion-induced activation in both secondary motor areas (both in the lesioned and contralateral hemisphere) and in remote areas not normally directly involved in motor control, such as prefrontal, anterior cingulate, inferior parietal cortices and other associative motor areas (fMRI) (Chugani, Muller and Chugani, 1996; Graveline et al., 1998; Muller et al., 1998a,b). Because the motor system has relatively greater uncrossed representation, lesions of one cerebral hemisphere can have extralesional and bilateral consequences for motor control (Benechke, Meyer and Freund, 1991; Brown, Schumacher and Rohlmann, 1989; Colebatch and Gandevia, 1989; Jones, Donaldson and Parkin, 1989). Progressive derangement of cortex around injured areas, i.e., damage extending into healthy cortex, can occur (Freund, 1996). Recovery/reorganization that involves both hemispheres is not always completely adaptive.

Mirror movements (Chen, Gerloff, Hallett et al., 1997; Farmer, Harrison, Ingram et al., 1991; Nirkko, Rosler, Ozdoba et al., 1997) epitomize a potentially maladaptive effect of reorganization occurring during recovery, particularly after injury to the immature nervous system (Muller, 1997; Nass, 1985). Mirror movements probably reflect a compensatory elaboration of ipsilateral motor tracts from the intact hemisphere to the impaired/contralesional hand (Eyre, Taylor, Villagra et al., 2001). Mirror movements are common and persistent in the early focal lesion population. Two thirds of subjects (21 of 33) with hemiplegic cerebral palsy in the cohort of Carr, Harrison, Evans et al. (1993) showed evidence of reorganization of central motor pathways. In both forms novel ipsilateral motor pathways projected from the undamaged motor cortex to the hemiplegic hand. There were no ipsilateral projections from the damaged motor cortex. Eleven subjects had intense mirror movements. Cross-correlation analysis and reflex testing suggested that corticospinal axons had branched abnormally and projected bilaterally to homologous motor neuron pools on both sides of the spinal cord in these subjects. The remaining ten subjects did not have intense mirror movements; in these subjects reflex testing revealed no evidence for last order branching of corticospinal axons. Good function of the hemiplegic hand was associated with the presence of muscle responses in that hand following magnetic stimulation of the contralateral motor cortex. When muscle responses were absent, hand function was poor unless the subject had intense mirror movements. Cohen et al. (1991a,c); Cohen, Ziemann, Chen et al. (1998) demonstrated that patients with mirror movements had a marked derangement of the map of outputs of distal hand muscles with enlarged and ipsilateral representations. Thus, the pathophysiology underlying mirror movements reflects both positive and negative reorganizational effects.

Patterns of motor reorganization are affected by relatively minor differences in age at injury. Muller et al. (1997c) explored the effects of maturation on motor activation (PET) of the affected hand in patients with unilateral lesion involving the Rolandic cortex. Patients with early lesions (onset <4 years), patients with late lesions (onset 10 years or more), and normal adults were studied. Activations in the contralesional Rolandic region were enhanced in both patient groups when compared to normal adults. Secondary motor and frontal–parietal non-motor cortices showed greater activation in the early than in the late lesion group, suggesting a greater potential for reorganization during very early development. Cerebellar activation was similar in late lesion patients and normal adults, but significantly weaker in early lesion patients. Despite differences in reorganization patterns once the insult has occurred, age at hemispherectomy and type of hemispherectomy (anatomical, functional, modified) do not affect motor outcome (Peacock, Wehby-Grant, Shields et al., 1996)

Several anatomical factors affect degree of motor recovery. Better motor function is associated with topographically differentiated ipsi- and contralateral representations in the remaining hemisphere (Pascual-Leone, Tarazona, Keenan et al., 1999). In animal models sparing of contralesional motor function is greater if the caudate and putamen are intact. Clinically improved metabolic function in deafferented caudate can occur as late as 1–2 years after hemispherectomy (Chugani, 1994). Preservation both of parts of the pyramidal tract and of the thalamic circuitry determines the quality of hand motor recovery following acute stroke in the adult (Binkofski, Seitz, Arnold et al., 1996). Return of caudate function may be responsible for late motor improvement in childhood hemiplegia.

A few studies speak to the issue of remediation and plasticity. Subsequent loss of hand representation after stroke has been forestalled in some cases by intensive remediation, particularly when it is of a stereotyped repetitive nature (Butefisch, Hummelsheim, Denzler et al., 1995; Nudo, 1997). Retraining of skilled hand use after stroke can prevent the loss of adjacent hand territory. In some instances, hand representation expanded into regions formerly occupied by representations of the elbow and shoulder. Functional reorganization in the undamaged motor cortex is accompanied by recovery of skilled hand function. These results suggest that after local damage to the motor cortex, rehabilitative training can shape subsequent reorganization in the adjacent intact cortex, and that the undamaged motor cortex may play an important role in motor recovery (Merzenich, Wright, Jenkins et al., 1996b; Nudo, 1997). However, there is also theoretical support for the view that starting remediation too soon or making remediation too intensive may actually have a negative effect on outcome (Kozlowski, James and Schallert, 1996).

## Conclusion

Overall, the accumulating data about plasticity suggest that it is more extensive in the mature nervous system than Kennard's (1940) seminal studies suggested. And changes can occur with great speed. However, plasticity is also more limited in the immature nervous system than Kennard's data suggested. Furthermore, plasticity can be maladaptive. Generalized pathology may be more detrimental when the nervous system is immature than when it is mature. Innate specialization, hemispheric maturational gradient effects and hemispheric computational biases may play roles in limiting plasticity. Different cognitive systems seem to be variably plastic. Visuospatial skills appear to be less plastic than language abilities. Language is used to express meaning and experiences derived from widely distributed neural systems. Hence, a number of different solutions may be possible (Bates et al., 1997). On the other hand visuospatial problems may be amenable to only a single clearly best solution. In the face of sensory deprivation, like deafness, the immature nervous system is able to coopt other brain regions to subserve the lost function. Clearly, the dynamic events involved in maturation represent complex phenomena ripe for further investigation.

## References

Akshoomoff NA, Feroleto CC, Doyle RE et al.: The impact of early unilateral brain injury on perceptual organization and visual memory. Neuropsychologia: 40(5); 539–561, 2002.

Amaducci LS, Sorbi S, Albanese A: CAT activity differs in right and left temporal lobe. Neurology: 31; 799–805, 1981.

Aram D: Neuroplasticity: Evidence from unilateral brain lesions in children. In Broman SH, Fletcher JM (Eds.), The Changing Nervous System: Neurobehavioral Consequences of Early Brain Disorders. New York: Oxford Press, Ch. 11, pp. 254–273, 1999.

Aram D, Eisele J: Intellectual stability in children with unilateral brain lesions. Neuropsychologia: 32; 85–95, 1994a.

Aram D, Eisele J: Limits to a left hemisphere explanation for specific language impairment. Journal of Speech Hearing Research: 37(4); 824–830, 1994b.

Aram D, Ekelman BL: Unilateral brain lesions in childhood: Performance on the revised Token Test. Brain and Language: 32; 137–158, 1987.

Aram D, Ekelman BL, Whitaker H: Spoken syntax in children with acquired unilateral hemisphere lesions. Brain and Language: 27; 75–100, 1986.

Aram D, Ekelman B, Whitaker H: Lexical retrieval in left and right brain lesioned children. Brain and Language: 28; 61–87, 1987.

Aram D, Gillespie L, Yamashita T: Reading among children with left and right brain lesions. Developmental Neuropsychology: 6; 301–317, 1990a.

Aram D, Meyers S, Ekelman B: Fluency of conversational speech in children with unilateral brain lesions. Brain and Language: 38; 105–122, 1990b.

Bach-y-Rita P: Brain plasticity as a basis for recovery of function in humans. Neuropsychologia: 28; 547–554, 1990.

Banich M, Levine S, Kim H et al.: The effects of developmental factors on IQ in hemiplegic children. Neuropsychologia: 28; 35–45, 1990.

Bates E: Origins of language disorders: A comparative approach. Developmental Neuropsychology: 13(3); 447–476, 1997.

Bates E: Plasticity, localization and language development. In Broman SH, Fletcher JM (Eds), The Changing Nervous System: Neurobehavioral Consequences of Early Brain Disorders. New York, NY: Oxford Press, pp. 214–253, 1999.

Bates E, Reilly J, Wulfect B et al.: Differential effects of unilateral lesions on language production in children and adults. Brain and Language: 79; 223–265, 2001.

Bates E, Roe K: Language development in children with unilateral brain injury. In Nelson CA, Luciana M (Eds), Handbook of Developmental Cognitive Neuroscience. Cambridge, MA: MIT Press, Ch. 20, pp. 281–308, 2001.

Bates E, Thal D, Aram D et al.: Language acquisition — from first words to grammar — after congenital focal lesion. Developmental Psychology: 13; 530–546, 1997.

Bavelier D, Corina D, Jezzard P et al.: Hemispheric specialization for English and ASL: Left invariance–right variability. Neuroreport: 9(7); 1537–1542, 1998.

Benechke R, Meyer BU, Freund HJ: Reorganization of descending motor pathways in patients after hemispherectomy and severe hemispheric lesions demonstrated by magnetic brain stimulation. Experimental Brain Research: 83; 419–426, 1991.

Best, C.T. (Ed), 1985: Hemispheric Function and Collaboration in the Child. Orlando, FL: Academic Press, 1985.

Best CT: The emergence of cerebral asymmetries in early human development: A literature review and neuroembryological model. In Molfese DL, Segalowitz SJ (Eds), Brain Lateralization in Children. New York, NY: Guilford Press, pp. 5–34, 1988.

Binkofski F, Seitz RJ, Arnold S et al.: Thalamic metabolism

and corticospinal tract integrity determine motor recovery in stroke. Annals of Neurology: 39(4); 460–470, 1996.

Birbaumer K, Lutzenberger N, Cohen W et al.: Reorganization of motor and somatosensory cortex in upper extremity amputees with phantom limb pain. Journal of Neuroscience: 21(10); 3609–3618, 2001.

Brown J, Schumacher U, Rohlmann A: Aimed movements to visual targets in hemiplegic and normal children: Is the good hand normal? Neuropsychologia: 27; 283–302, 1989.

Buchel CC, Price R, Frackowiak S et al.: Different activation patterns in the visual cortex of late and congenitally blind subjects. Brain: 121(3); 409–419, 1998.

Burkland C, Smith A: Language and the cerebral hemispheres. Neurology: 27; 627–633, 1977.

Butefisch C, Hummelsheim H, Denzler P et al.: Repetitive training of isolated movements improves the outcome of motor rehabilitation of the centrally paretic hand. Journal of the Neurological Sciences: 130(1); 59–68, 1995.

Cao Y, Vikingstad E, Huttenlocher P et al.: fMRI studies of reorganization of the human hand somatosensory area after unilateral brain injury in the perinatal period. Proceedings of the National Academy of Sciences of the United States of America: 91; 9612–9616, 1994.

Carey S, Levine, S: Development of right hemisphere skills: U-Curves. In Caplan D (Ed), Biological Studies of Human Processes. Cambridge, MA: MIT Press, 1980, pp. 55–67.

Carr LJ, Harrison L, Evans A et al.: Patterns of central motor reorganization in hemiplegic CP. Brain: 116; 1223–1247, 1993.

Chelazzi L, Miller EK, Duncan J et al.: A neural basis for visual search in inferior temporal cortex. Nature: 363(6427); 345–347, 1993.

Chen R, Corwell B, Yaseen Z et al.: Mechanisms of cortical reorganization in lower-limb amputees. Journal of Neuroscience: 18(9); 3443–3450, 1998.

Chen R, Gerloff C, Hallett M et al.: Involvement of the ipsilateral motor cortex in finger movements of different complexities. Annals of Neurology: 41(2); 247–254, 1997.

Cheour M, Alho K, Ceponiene R et al.: Maturation of mismatch negativity in infants. International Journal of Psychophysiology: 29(2); 217–226, 1998.

Chi JD, Dooling EC, Gilles FH: Gyral development of the human brain. Annals of Neurology: 1; 86–93, 1977.

Chiron C, Jambaque I, Nabbout R et al.: The right hemisphere is dominant in human infants. Brain: 120; 1057–1065, 1997.

Chiron C, Raynaud C, Maziere B et al.: Changes in regional cerebral blood flow during brain maturation in children and adolescents. Journal of Nuclear Medicine: 33; 696–703, 1992.

Chugani HT: Development of regional glucose metabolism in relation to behavior and plasticity. In Dawson G, Fischer K (Eds), Human Development and the Developing Brain. New York, NY: Guilford Press, pp. 153–175, 1994.

Chugani HT, Muller RA, Chugani DC: Functional brain reorganization in children. Brain and Development: 18; 347–356, 1996.

Chugani HT, Phelps ME: Maturational changes in cerebral func-

tion in infants determined by FDG positron emission tomography. Science: 231; 840–843, 1986.

Classen J, Liepert J, Wise SP et al.: Rapid plasticity of human cortical movement representation induced by practice. Journal of Neurophysiology: 79(2); 1117–1123, 1998.

Cohen H, Le Normand MT: Language development in children with simple-partial left-hemisphere epilepsy. Brain and Language: 64(3); 409–422, 1998.

Cohen LG, Bandinelli S, Findley TW et al.: Motor reorganization after upper limb amputation in man. A study with focal magnetic stimulation. Brain: 114; 615–627, 1991a.

Cohen LG, Bandinelli S, Topka HR et al.: Topographic maps of human motor cortex in normal and pathological conditions: Mirror movements, amputations and spinal cord injuries. Electroencephalography and Clinical Neurophysiology B, Supplement: 43; 36–50, 1991b.

Cohen LG, Brasil-Neto JP, Pascual-Leone A et al.: Plasticity of cortical motor output organization following deafferentation, cerebral lesions, and skill acquisition. Advances in Neurology: 63; 187–200, 1993a.

Cohen LG, Brasil-Neto JP, Pascual-Leone A et al.: Plasticity of cortical motor output organization following deafferentation, cerebral lesions, and skill acquisition. In Devinsky O, Beric A, Dogali M (Eds), Electrical and Magnetic Stimulation of the Brain and Spinal Cord. New York, NY: Raven Press, pp. 187–200, 1993b.

Cohen LG, Roth BJ, Wassermann EM et al.: Magnetic stimulation of the human cerebral cortex: An indicator of reorganization in motor pathways in certain pathological conditions. Journal of Clinical Neurophysiology: 8(1); 56–65, 1991c.

Cohen LG, Weeks RA, Sadato N et al.: Period of susceptibility for cross-modal plasticity in the blind. Annals of Neurology: 45(4); 451–460, 1999.

Cohen LG, Ziemann U, Chen R et al.: Studies of neuroplasticity with transcranial magnetic stimulation. Journal of Clinical Neurophysiology: 15(4); 305–324, 1998.

Cohen M, Holmes G, Campbell R et al.: Memory performance following unilateral electrical stimulation of the hippocampus in a child with right temporal lobe epilepsy. Epilepsy: 3; 115–122, 1994.

Cohen S, Huttenlocher P, Banich M et al.: Factors affecting cognitive functioning in hemiplegic children. Developmental Medical Child Neurology: 29; 27–35, 1987.

Colebatch JG, Gandevia SC: The distribution of muscular weakness in upper motor neuron lesions affecting the arm. Brain: 112; 749–63, 1989.

Cooper J, Majnemer A, Rosenblatt B et al.: The determination of sensory deficit in children with hemiplegic cerebral palsy. Journal of Child Neurology: 10; 300–309, 1995.

Corballis M, Morgan M: On the biological basis of human laterality, evidence for a maturational left right gradient. Behavioral Brain Science: 2; 261–336, 1978.

Corbetta M, Shulman GL, Miezin FM et al.: Superior parietal cortex activation during spatial attention shifts and visual feature conjunction. Science: 270(5237); 802–805, 1995.

Curtiss SR: Genie: A Psycholinguistic Study of a Modern Day 'Wild Child'. New York, NY: Academic Press, 1977.

Curtiss S, De Bode S: Age and etiology as predictors of language outcome after hemispherectomy. Developmental Neuroscience: 21; 174–181, 1999.

Davis KD, Kiss ZH, Luo L et al.: Phantom sensations generated by thalamic microstimulation. Nature: 391(6665); 385–387, 1998.

De Bode S, Curtiss SR: Language after hemispherectomy. Brain and Cognition: 43; 135–139, 2000.

Denckla M, Rudel R, Broman M: The development of a spatial orientation skill in normal, learning disabled, and neurologically impaired children. In Caplan D (Ed), Biological Studies of Human Processes. Cambridge, MA: MIT Press, 1980, pp. 22–29.

Dennis M: Capacity and strategy for syntactic comprehension after left or right hemidecortication. Brain and Language: 10(2); 287–317, 1980.

Dennis M: Language and the young damaged brain. In Boll TJ, Bryant BK (Eds), Clinical Neuropsychology and Brain Function: Research, Measurement, and Practice. Washington, DC: American Psychiatric Association, pp. 89–112, 1989.

Dennis M, Barnes MA: Oral discourse after early-onset hydrocephalus: Linguistic ambiguity, figurative language, speech acts, and script-based inferences. Journal of Pediatric Psychology: 18(5); 639–652, 1993.

Dennis M, Barnes M: Speech acts after mild or severe childhood head injury. Aphasiology: 14; 391–405, 2001.

Dennis M, Lovett M, Wiegel-Crump CA: Written language acquisition after left or right hemidecortication in infancy. Brain and Language: 12(1); 54–91, 1981.

Dennis M, Whitaker H: Language acquisition following hemidecortication. Brain and Language: 3; 404–433, 1976.

Di Piero V, Chollet F, Dolan RJ et al.: The functional nature of cerebellar diaschisis. Stroke: 21(9); 1365–1369, 1990.

Duchowny M, Jayakar P, Harvey S et al.: Language cortex representation: Effects of developmental versus acquired pathology. Annals of Neurology: 40; 31–38, 1996.

De Volder AG, Catalan-Ahumada M, Robert A et al.: Changes in occipital cortex activity in early blind humans using a sensory substitution device. Brain Research: 826(1); 128–134, 1999.

Eisele J, Aram DM: Differential effects of early hemisphere damage on lexical comprehension and production. Aphasiology: 7(5); 513–523, 1993.

Eisele J, Aram D: The comprehension and imitation of syntactic structures in left and right hemisphere injured children. Brain and Language: 46; 212–231, 1994.

Eisele J, Lust B, Aram D: Presupposition and implication of truth: Linguistic deficits following early brain lesions. Brain and Language: 61; 376–394, 1998.

Elbert T, Flor H, Birbaumer N et al.: Extensive reorganization of the somatosensory cortex in adult humans after nervous system injury. Neuroreport: 5(18); 2593–2597, 1994.

Elbert T, Pantev C, Wienbruch C et al.: Increased cortical representation of the fingers of the left hand in string players. Science: 270(5234); 305–307, 1995.

Elbert T, Sterr A, Flor H et al.: Input-increase and input-decrease types of cortical reorganization after upper extremity amputation in humans. Experimental Brain Research: 117(1); 161–164, 1997.

Eriksson P, Perfilieva E, Björk-Eriksson T et al.: Neurogenesis in the adult human hippocampus. Nature Neuroscience: 4; 1313–1317, 1998.

Eyre J, Taylor J, Villagra F et al.: Evidence of activity dependent withdrawal of corticospinal projections during human development. Neurology: 57; 1543–1554, 2001.

Farmer SF, Harrison LM, Ingram DA et al.: Plasticity of central motor pathways in children with hemiplegic cerebral palsy. Neurology: 41(9); 1505–1510, 1991.

Feldman H: Language development after early unilateral brain injury: A replication study. In Tager-Flusberg H (Ed), Constraints on Language Acquisition: Studies of Atypical Children. Hillsdale, NJ: Lawrence Erlbaum Associates, pp. 75–90, 1994.

Feldman H, Holland A, Brown R: A fluent language disorder following antepartum left-hemisphere brain injury. Journal of Communication Disorders: 25(2–3); 125–142, 1992b.

Feldman HM, Holland AL, Kemp SS et al.: Language development after unilateral brain injury. Brain and Language: 42(1); 89–102, 1992a.

Flor H, Elbert T, Muhlnickel W et al.: Cortical reorganization and phantom phenomena in congenital and traumatic upper-extremity amputees. Experimental Brain Research: 119(2); 205–212, 1998.

Freund HJ: Remapping the brain. Science: 272; 1754, 1996.

Fujiki N, Naito Y, Nagamine T et al.: Influence of unilateral deafness on auditory evoked magnetic field. Neuroreport: 9(14); 3129–3133, 1998.

Gallagher S, Butterworth G, Cole L: Hand mouth coordination, congenital absence of limb, and evidence for innate body schema. Brain and Cognition: 38; 53–65, 1998.

Geschwind N, Galaburda A: Cerebral Lateralization. Cambridge, MA: MIT Press, 1987.

Glass P: Patterns of neuropsychological deficit at age five years following neonatal unilateral brain injury. Brain and Language: 63; 346–356, 1998.

Goldman P, Isseroff A: The neurobiology of cognitive development. In Mussen P (Ed), Handbook of Child Psychology. New York, NY: Wiley, pp. 281–344, 1983.

Goodman R, Yude C: IQ and its predictors in childhood hemiplegia. Developmental Medicine and Child Neurology: 38; 881–890, 1996.

Graveline CJ, Mikulis DJ, Crawley AP et al.: Regionalized sensorimotor plasticity after hemispherectomy fMRI evaluation. Pediatric Neurology: 19(5); 337–342, 1998.

Grimshaw GS, Adelstein A, Bryden MP et al.: First-language acquisition in adolescence: Evidence for a critical period for verbal language development. Brain and Language: 63; 237–255, 1998.

Grusser SM, Winter C, Muhlnickel W et al.: The relationship of perceptual phenomena and cortical reorganization in upper extremity amputees. Neuroscience: 102(2); 263–72, 2001.

Guerreiro M, Castro-Caldas A, Martins I: Aphasia following right hemisphere lesion in a woman with a left hemisphere injury in childhood. Brain and Language: 49; 288–298, 1995.

Hardie H: The consequences of deafness and chronic intra-cochlear electrical stimulation on the central auditory pathways. Clinical and Experimental Pharmacology and Physiology: 25(5); 303–309, 1998.

Haxby JV, Horwitz B, Ungerleider LG et al.: The functional organization of human extrastriate cortex: A PET-rCBF study of selective attention to faces and locations. Journal of Neuroscience: 14; 6336–6353, 1994.

Hellige JB: Hemispheric asymmetry: What's right and what's left. Cambridge, MA: Harvard University Press, 2001.

Helmstaedter C, Kurthen M, Gleibner U et al.: Natural atypical language dominance and language shifts from the right to the left hemisphere in right hemisphere pathology. Die Naturwissenschaften: 84; 250–253, 1997a.

Helmstaedter C, Kurthen M, Linke DB et al.: Right hemisphere restitution of language and memory functions in right hemisphere language-dominant patients with left temporal lobe epilepsy. Brain: 117; 729–737, 1994.

Helmstaedter C, Kurthen M, Linke DB et al.: Patterns of language dominance in focal left and right hemisphere epilepsies: Relation to MRI findings, EEG, sex, and age at onset of epilepsy. Brain and Cognition: 33(2); 135–150, 1997b.

Helmstaedter C, Pohl C, Elger CE: Relations between verbal and nonverbal memory performance: Evidence of confounding effects particularly in patients with right temporal lobe epilepsy. Cortex: 31(2); 345–355, 1995.

Hickok G, Bellugi U, Klima ES: The basis of the neural organization for language: Evidence from sign language aphasia. Reviews in the Neurosciences: 8; 205–222, 1997.

Hofman PM, Van Riswick JG, Van Opstal AJ: Relearning sound localization with new ears. Nature Neuroscience: 1(5); 417–421, 1998.

Huttenlocher P: Synaptogenesis, synapse elimination and neural plasticity in human cerebral cortex. In Nelson C (Ed), Threats to Optimal Development. Hillsdale, NJ: Lawrence Erlbaum Associates, pp. 36–54, 1994.

Isaacs E, Chrisie D, Vargha-Khadem F et al.: Effects of hemispheric side of injury, age at injury, and presence of seizure disorder on functional ear and hand asymmetries in hemiplegic children. Neuropsychologia: 34(2); 127–137, 1996.

Jacobs B, Schall M, Scheibel A: A quantitative dendritic analysis of Wernicke's area: Gender hemispheric, and environmental factors. Journal of Comparative Neurology: 237; 97–111, 1993.

Janowsky J, Nass R: Early language development in children with cortical and subcortical perinatal injury. Journal of Behavior and Developmental Pediatrics: 8; 3–7, 1987.

Jeeves MA: Compensatory mechanisms — neural and behavioral: Evidence from prenatal damage to the forebrain commissures. In Rose FD, Johnson DA (Eds), Recovery from Brain Damage: Reflections and Directions. New York, NY: Plenum Press, pp. 153–168, 1992.

Jones RD, Donaldson IM, Parkin PJ: Impairment and recovery of ipsilateral sensory–motor function following unilateral cerebral infarction. Brain: 112; 113–132, 1989.

Kaas JH: Neurobiology: Phantoms of the brain. Nature: 391; 331–333, 1998.

Kagan J: Continuity and discontinuity in development. In Brauth SE, Hall WS, Dooling RJ (Eds), Plasticity of Development. Cambridge, MA: MIT Press, pp. 11–40, 1991.

Karbe H, Thiel A, Weber-Luxenburger G et al.: Brain plasticity in poststroke aphasia: What is the contribution of the right hemisphere? Brain and Language: 64(2); 215–30, 1998.

Kennard M: Relation of age to motor impairments in humans and subhuman primates. Archives of Neurology and Psychiatry: 44; 377–397, 1940.

Kerrigan J, Chugani H, Phelps M: Regional cerebral glucose metabolism in clinical subtypes of cerebral palsy. Pediatric Neurology: 7; 415–425, 1991.

Kershner J, King A: Laterality in achieving hemiplegic children. Perceptual Motor Skills: 39; 1283–1289, 1974.

Kiessling LS, Denckla M, Carlton M: Evidence for differential hemispheric function in children with hemiplegic cerebral palsy. Developmental Medicine and Child Neurology: 25; 727–734, 1983.

Kilgard M, Merzenich M: Plasticity of temporal information processing in the primary auditory cortex. Nature Neuroscience: 8; 727–731, 1998.

Knecht S, Henningsen H, Hohling C et al.: Plasticity of plasticity? Changes in the pattern of perceptual correlates of reorganization after amputation. Brain: 121; 717–724, 1998.

Kohn B: Right hemisphere speech representation and comprehension of syntax after left cerebral injury. Brain and Language: 9; 350–361, 1980.

Kohn B, Dennis M: Selective impairments of visuo-spatial abilities in infantile hemiplegics after right cerebral hemidecortication. Neuropsychologia: 12; 505–512, 1974.

Kolb B, Gibb R: Early brain injury, behavior and plasticity. In Nelson C, Luciana M (Eds), Handbook of Developmental Cognitive Neuroscience. Cambridge, MA: MIT Press, pp. 175–190, 2001.

Kornhuber HH, Bechinger D, Jung H et al.: A quantitative relationship between the extent of localized cerebral lesions and the intellectual and behavioral deficiency in children. European Archives of Psychiatry and Neurological Science: 235; 129–133, 1985.

Kozlowski DA, James DC, Schallert T: Use-dependent exaggeration of neuronal injury after unilateral sensorimotor cortex lesions. Journal of Neuroscience: 16(15); 4776–4786, 1996.

Kujala T, Alho K, Huotilainen M et al.: Electrophysiological evidence for cross-modal plasticity in humans with early- and late-onset blindness. Psychophysiology: 34(2); 213–216, 1997.

Kurthen M: Quantitative and qualitative evaluation of patterns of cerebral language dominance. Brain and Language: 46; 536–564, 1994.

Lansdell H: Verbal and non verbal factors in right hemisphere speech, relation to early neurologic history. Journal of Comparative Physiological and Psychology: 69; 734–738, 1969.

Leiner HC, Leiner AL, Dow RS: The human cerebro-cerebellar system: Its computing, cognitive and language skills. Behavioral and Brain Research: 44; 113–128, 1991.

Lenneberg EH: Foundations of Language. New York, NY: Wiley, 1965.

Levin H, Ewing-Cobbs L, Eisenberg H: Neurobehavioral outcome of pediatric closed head injury in children. In Broman SH, Michel ME (Eds), Traumatic Head Injury in Children. New York, NY: Oxford University Press, pp. 70–94, 1995.

Levine S, Huttenlocher P, Banich M et al.: Factors effecting cognitive functioning of hemiplegic children. Developmental Medicine and Child Neurology: 29; 27–35, 1987.

Levy Y, Amir N: Morphology in a child with a congenital left hemisphere brain lesion: implications for normal acquisition. In Tager-Flusberg H (Ed), Constraints on Language Acquisition: Studies of Atypical Children. Hillsdale, NJ: Lawrence Erlbaum Associates, pp. 49–74, 1994.

Liotti M, Ryder K, Woldorff M: Auditory attention in the congenitally blind: Where, when and what gets reorganized? Neuroreport: 9(6); 1007–1012, 1998.

Lively SE, Pisoni DB, Yamada RA et al.: Training Japanese listeners to identify English /r/ and /l/. Long-term retention of new phonetic categories. Journal of the Acoustical Society of America: 96(4); 2076–2087, 1994.

Lovett MW, Dennis M, Newman JE: Making reference: The cohesive use of pronouns in the narrative discourse of hemidecorticate adolescents. Brain and Language: 29(2); 224–251, 1986.

Mancini J, De Schonen S, Deruelle C, Massoulier A: Face recognition in children with early right or left brain damage. Developmental Medicine and Child Neurology: 36; 156–167, 1994.

Marchman V: Constraints on plasticity in a connectionist model of the English past tense. Journal of Cognitive Neuroscience: 5; 215–234, 1993.

Marchman V, Miller R, Bates E: Babble and first words in children with focal brain injury. Applied Psycholinguistics: 12; 1–22, 1991.

Melzack R, Israel R, Lacroix R et al.: Phantom limbs in people with congenital limb deficiency or amputation in early childhood. Brain: 120; 1603–1620, 1997.

Merzenich M, Jenkins W: Cortical plasticity, learning and learning dysfunction. In Julesz B, Kovacs I (Eds), Maturational Windows and Adult Cortical Plasticity. New York, NY: Addison-Wesley, pp. 247–269, 1995.

Merzenich M, Jenkins WM, Johnston P et al.: Temporal processing deficits of language-learning impaired children ameliorated by training. Science: 271(5245); 77–81, 1996a.

Merzenich M, Wright B, Jenkins W et al.: Cortical plasticity underlying perceptual, motor, and cognitive skill development: Implications for neurorehabilitation. Cold Spring Harbor Symposia on Quantitative Biology: 61; 1–8, 1996b.

Mills D, Coffey S, Neville H: Variability in cerebral organization during primary language acquisition. In Dawson G, Fischer K (Eds), Human Behavior and the Developing Brain. New York, NY: Guilford Publications, pp. 427–455, 1993a.

Mills D, Coffey S, Neville H: Language acquisition and cerebral specialization in 20 month old infants. Journal of Cognitive Neuroscience: 10; 111–115, 1993b.

Molfese D, Segalowitz S: Brain Lateralization in Children. New York, NY: Guilford Press, 1988.

Moran J, Desimone R: Selective attention gates visual processing in the extrastriate cortex. Science: 229; 782–784, 1985.

Morgan MJ: Molyneux's Question: Vision, Touch, and the Philosophy of Perception. New York, NY: Cambridge University Press, 1977.

Muller RA: Ontogeny of ipsilateral corticospinal projections: A developmental study with TMS. Annals of Neurology: 42; 703–711, 1997.

Muller RA, Behen ME, Rothermel RD et al.: Brain organization for language in children, adolescents, and adults with left hemisphere lesion: A PET study. Progress in Neuro- Psychopharmacology and Biological Psychiatry: 23(4); 657–68, 1999a.

Muller RA, Behen ME, Rothermel RD et al.: Language organization in patients with early and late left-hemisphere lesion: A PET study. Neuropsychologia: 37(5); 545–557, 1999b.

Muller RA, Chugani HT, Muzik O et al.: Brain organization of motor and language functions following hemispherectomy: A [(15)O]–water positron emission tomography study. Journal of Child Neurology: 13(1); 16–22, 1998a.

Muller RA, Chugani HT, Muzik O et al.: Language and motor functions activate calcified hemisphere in patients with Sturge–Weber syndrome: A positron emission tomography study. Journal of Child Neurology: 12(7); 431–437, 1997a.

Muller RA, Rothermel RD, Behen ME: Receptive and expressive language activations for sentences: A PET study. Neuroreport: 8(17); 3767–3770, 1997b.

Muller RA, Rothermel R, Behen M et al.: Brain organization of language after early unilateral lesion: A PET study. Brain and Language: 62; 422–451, 1998b.

Muller R, Rothermel R, Behen M et al.: Differential patterns of language and motor reorganization following early left hemisphere lesion: A PET study. Archives of Neurology: 55(8); 1113–1119, 1998c.

Muller RA, Rothermel RD, Muzik O et al.: Plasticity of motor organization in children and adults. Neuroreport: 8(14); 3103–3108, 1997c.

Muter V, Taylor S, Vargha-Khadem F: A longitudinal study of early intellectual development in hemiplegic children. Neuropsychologia: 35(3); 289–298, 1997.

Naito Y, Hirano S, Honjo I et al.: Sound-induced activation of auditory cortices in cochlear implant users with post- and pre-lingual deafness demonstrated by positron emission tomography. Acta Oto-Laryngologica: 117(4); 490–496, 1997.

Nass R: Mirror movement asymmetries after congenital unilateral brain injury. Neurology: 35; 1059–1062, 1985.

Nass R: Language development after early focal lesions. In Nass R, Rapin I (Eds), Seminars in Pediatric Neurology: Developmental Language Disorders. Philadelphia: Saunders, pp. 36–42, 1997.

Nass, R: Developmental speech and language disorders. In Berg B (Ed), Principles of Child Neurology (2nd ed.). New York, NY: McGraw-Hill, pp. 220–226, 1999.

Nass R, Peterson H, Koch D: Differential effects of congenital left versus right brain damage on intelligence. Brain and Cognition: 9; 258–266, 1989.

Nass R, Sadler A, Sidtis J: Dichotic listening performance after congenital unilateral brain injury: Evidence for crowding. Neurology: 42; 1960–1965, 1992.

Nass R, Stiles J: Complication of the perinatum: Congenital focal lesions. In Frank Y (Ed), Pediatric Behavioral Neurology. Boca Raton, FL: CRC Press, pp. 55–64, 1996.

Nelson C, Luciana M (Eds): Handbook of Developmental Cognitive Neuroscience. Cambridge, MA: MIT Press, 2001.

Neville HJ, Bavelier D: Neural organization and plasticity of language. Current Opinion in Neurobiology: 8(2); 254–258, 1998.

Neville HJ, Bavelier D, Corina D et al.: Cerebral organization for language in deaf and hearing subjects: Biological constraints and effects of experience. Proceedings of the National Academy of Sciences of the United States of America: 95(3); 922–929, 1998.

Neville HJ, Coffey SA, Lawson DS et al.: Neural systems mediating American sign language: Effects of sensory experience and age of acquisition. Brain and Language: 57(3); 285–308, 1997.

Niimura K, Chugani DC, Muzik O et al.: Cerebellar reorganization following cortical injury in humans: Effects of lesion size and age. Neurology: 52(4); 792–797, 1999.

Nirkko AC, Rosler KM, Ozdoba C et al.: Human cortical plasticity: Functional recovery with mirror movements. Neurology: 48; 1090–1093, 1997.

Nishimura H, Hashikawa K, Doi K et al.: Sign language 'heard' in the auditory cortex [letter]. Nature: 397(6715); 116, 1999.

Nitkin R: Dendritic mechanisms in brain function and developmental disabilities. Cerebral Cortex: 10; 925–926, 2000.

Nudo RJ: Remodeling of cortical motor representations after stroke: Implications for recovery from brain damage. Molecular Psychiatry: 2(3); 188–191, 1997.

Ogden JA: Language and memory functions after long recovery periods in left hemispherectomized subjects. Neuropsychologia: 26(5); 645–659, 1988.

Ogden JA: Visuospatial and other 'right-hemispheric' functions after long recovery periods in left- hemispherectomized subjects. Neuropsychologia: 27(6); 765–776, 1989.

Ogden JA: Phonological dyslexia and phonological dysgraphia following left and right hemispherectomy. Neuropsychologia: 34(9); 905–918, 1996.

Ojemann G, Creutzfeldt O: Language in humans and animals: Contribution of brain stimulation and recording. In Plum F (Ed), Handbook of Physiology. Bethesda, MD: American Physiological Society, pp. 675–700, 1987.

Pallier C, Bosch L, Sebastian-Galles N: A limit on behavioral plasticity in speech perception. Cognition: 64(3); B9–B17, 1997.

Pascual-Leone A, Cammarota A, Wassermann EM et al.: Modulation of motor cortical outputs to the reading hand of braille readers. Annals of Neurology: 34(1); 33–37, 1993.

Pascual-Leone A, Nguyet D, Cohen LG et al.: Modulation of muscle responses evoked by transcranial magnetic stimulation during the acquisition of new fine motor skills. Journal of Neurophysiology: 74(3); 1037–1045, 1995a.

Pascual-Leone A, Peris M, Tormos JM et al.: Reorganization of human cortical motor output maps following traumatic forearm amputation. Neuroreport: 7(13); 2068–2070, 1996.

Pascual-Leone A, Tarazona F, Keenan J et al.: Transcranial magnetic stimulation and neuroplasticity. Neuropsychologia: 37(2); 207–217, 1999.

Pascual-Leone A, Wassermann EM, Sadato N et al.: The role of reading activity on the modulation of motor cortical outputs to the reading hand in Braille readers. Annals of Neurology: 38(6); 910–915, 1995b.

Peacock WJ, Wehby-Grant MC, Shields WD et al.: Hemispherectomy for intractable seizures in children: A report of 58 cases. Childs Nervous System: 12(7); 376–384, 1996.

Pons T: Novel sensations in the congenitally blind. Nature: 380(6574); 479–480, 1996.

Ponton CW, Don M, Eggermont JJ et al.: Auditory system plasticity in children after long periods of complete deafness. Neuroreport: 8(1); 61–65, 1996.

Purpura D: Dendritic spine 'dysgenesis' and mental retardation. Science: 186; 1126–1128, 1974.

Raichle ME, Fiez JA, Videen TO et al.: Practice-related changes in human brain functional anatomy during nonmotor learning. Cerebral Cortex: 4(1); 8–26, 1994.

Rakic P: Young neurons for old brains? Nature Neuroscience: 8; 645–647, 1998.

Ramachandran V: Perceptual correlates of massive cortical reorganization. Neuroreport: 3; 583–586, 1992.

Ramachandran VS, Hirstein W: The perception of phantom limbs. The D.O. Hebb Lecture. Brain: 121(9); 1603–1630, 1998.

Rasmussen T, Milner B: The role of early left brain injury in determining lateralization of cerebral speech functions. In Dimond SJ, Blizard D (Eds), Evolution and Lateralization of the Brain (Vol. 299). New York, NY: New York Academy of Sciences, pp. 255–269, 1977.

Rausch R, Boone K, Ary CM: Right-hemisphere language dominance in temporal lobe epilepsy: Clinical and neuropsychological correlates. Journal of Clinical and Experimental Neuropsychology: 13(2); 217–231, 1991.

Rauschecker JP: Compensatory plasticity and sensory substitution in the cerebral cortex. Trends in Neurosciences: 18(1); 36–43, 1995.

Rauschecker JP: Auditory cortical plasticity: A comparison with other sensory systems. Trends in Neurosciences: 22(2); 74–80, 1999.

Reilly J, Bates E, Marchman V: Narrative in children with focal lesions. Brain and Language: 61; 335–375, 1998.

Riva D, Cazzaniga L: Late effects of unilateral brain lesions before and after the first year of life. Neuropsychologia: 24; 423–428, 1986.

Robinson K: Implications of developmental plasticity for the language acquisition of deaf children with cochlear implants. International Journal of Pediatric Otorhinolaryngology: 46; 71–80, 1998.

Roder B, Rosler F, Neville HJ: Effects of interstimulus interval on auditory event-related potentials in congenitally blind and normally sighted humans. Neuroscience Letters: 264; 53–56, 1999a.

Roder B, Teder-Salejarvi W, Sterr A et al.: Improved auditory spatial tuning in blind humans. Nature: 400(6740); 162–166, 1999b.

Rosenblatt B, Vernet O, Montes J et al.: Continuous unilateral epileptiform activity and language delay: Effect of functional hemispherectomy on language acquisition. Epilepsia: 39; 787–792, 1998.

Ross G, Boatwright S, Auld P et al.: Effects of prematurity and germinal matrix hemorrhage on frontal function at age 2 years. Brain and Cognition: 32; 1–13, 1996.

Ross G, Tessler J, Auld P et al.: Effects of prematurity and germinal matrix hemorrhage on frontal function. Developmental Psychology: 28; 1067–1074, 1992.

Rossi P, Parmeggiani A, Santucci M: Neuropsychological and psychiatric findings in cerebral cortex dysplasias. In Guerrini, R. et al. (Eds), Dysplasias of Cerebral Cortex and Epilepsy. Philadelphia: Lippincott Raven, pp. 345–351, 1996.

Ryals BM, Rubel EW, Lippe W: Issues in neural plasticity as related to cochlear implants in children. American Journal of Otology: 12(22); 43–47, 1991.

Sadato N, Pascual-Leone A, Grafman J et al.: Activation of the primary visual cortex by Braille reading in blind subjects. Nature: 380(6574); 526–528, 1996.

Sadato N, Pascual-Leone A, Grafman J et al.: Neural networks for Braille reading. Brain: 121; 213–29, 1998.

Sadato N, Zeffiro TA, Campbell G et al.: Regional cerebral blood flow changes in motor cortical areas after transient anesthesia of the forearm. Annals of Neurology: 37(1); 74–81, 1995.

Sandson T, Manoach D, Price B et al.: Right hemisphere learning disability associated with left hemisphere dysfunction: Anomalous dominance and development. Journal of Neurology, Neurosurgery and Psychiatry: 57; 1129–1133, 1994.

Sass K, Silberfein C, Platis J et al.: Right hemisphere mediation of verbal learning and memory in acquired right hemisphere speech dominant patients. Journal of the International Neuropsychology Society: 1; 554–560, 1995.

Saykin AJ, Gur RC, Sussman NM et al.: Memory deficits before and after temporal lobectomy: Effect of laterality and age of onset. Brain and Cognition: 9(2); 191–200, 1989.

Scheibel AB: Quantitative studies of dendritic complexity: Effects of experience. Brain and Cognition: 12; 85–101, 1990.

Scheibel AB, Conrad T, Perdue S et al.: A quantitative study of dendrite complexity in selected areas of the human cerebral cortex. Brain and Cognition: 12(1); 85–101, 1990.

Schneider G: Is it really better to have your brain lesion early? A revision of the 'Kennard Principle'. Neuropsychologia: 17; 557–584, 1979.

Selmud-Clikeman M: Developmental language disorders. In Nass R, Rapin I (Eds), Seminars in Pediatric Neurology, Language Disorders in Children. Philadelphia: Saunders, pp. 85–92, 1997.

Shamoto H, Chugani HT: Glucose metabolism in the human cerebellum: An analysis of crossed cerebellar diaschisis in children with unilateral cerebral injury. Journal of Child Neurology: 12; 407–414, 1997.

Shewmon DA, Holmes GL, Byrne PA: Consciousness in congenitally decorticate children: Developmental vegetative state as self-fulfilling prophecy. Developmental Medicine and Child Neurology: 41(6); 364–374, 1999.

Sica RE, Sanz OP, Cohen LG et al.: Changes in the N1-P1 component of the somatosensory cortical evoked response in patients with partial limb amputation. Electromyography and Clinical Neurophysiology: 24(5); 415–427, 1984.

Simonds RJ, Scheibel AB: The postnatal development of the motor speech area: A preliminary study. Brain and Language: 37(1); 42–58, 1989.

Skoyles JR: Evolution's 'missing link': A hypothesis upon neural plasticity, prefrontal working memory and the origins of modern cognition. Medical Hypotheses: 48(6); 499–501, 1997.

Smith A: On the organization, disorganization and reorganization of language and other brain functions. In LeBrun Y, Zangwell O (Eds), Lateralization of Language in the Child. Lisse: Swets and Zeitlinger, pp. 241–266, 1981.

Smith A, Sugar O: Development of above normal language and intelligence 21 years after hemispherectomy. Neurology: 25; 813–818, 1975.

Soderfeldt B, Ingvar M, Ronnberg J et al.: Signed and spoken language perception studied by positron emission tomography. Neurology: 49(1); 82–87, 1997.

Stark R: Follow-up study of a right and a left hemispherectomized child: Implications for localization and impairment of language in children. Brain and Language: 60(2); 222–243, 1997.

Stark RE, Bleile K, Brandt J et al.: Speech-language outcomes of hemispherectomy in children and young adults. Brain and Language: 51; 406–421, 1995.

Stark R, McGregor K: Followup study of a right and a left hemispherectomized child: Implications for localization and impairment of language in children. Brain and Language: 60; 222–242, 1997.

Staudt M, Grodd W, Niemann G et al.: Early left periventricular brain lesions induce right hemispheric organization of speech. Neurology: 57(1); 122–5, 2001.

Sterr A, Muller MM, Elbert T et al.: Changed perceptions in Braille readers. Nature: 391(6663); 134–135, 1998.

Stiles J: Spatial cognitive development. In Nelson C, Luciana M (Eds), Handbook of Developmental Cognitive Neuroscience. Cambridge, MA: MIT Press, pp. 399–414, 2001.

Stiles J, Nass R: Spatial grouping activity in young children with congenital right or left brain damage. Brain and Cognition: 15; 201–223, 1991.

Stiles J, Stern C, Trauner D et al.: Developmental changes in spatial grouping activity in children with early focal injury: Evidence from a modeling task. Brain and Cognition: 31; 46–62, 1996.

Stiles J, Trauner D, Engel M et al.: The development of drawing in children with congenital focal brain injury: Evidence for limited functional recovery. Neuropsychologia: 35; 299–312, 1997.

Stiles-Davis J, Janowski J, Engel M et al.: Drawing skills after congenital left versus right brain injury. Neuropsychologia: 26; 359–371, 1988.

Stiles-Davis J, Sugarman S, Nass R: Spatial constructions in children with early right hemisphere damage. Brain and Cognition: 4; 388–412, 1985.

St. James-Roberts I: A reinterpretation of hemispherectomy data without functional plasticity of brain. Brain and Language: 13; 31–53, 1981.

Strauss E, Satz P, Wada J: An examination of the crowding hypothesis in epileptic patients who have undergone the carotid amytal test. Neuropsychologia: 28(11); 1221–1227, 1990.

Studer L: Neural potential of human embryonic stem cells. Nature Biotechnology: 19; 1117–1118, 2001.

Tapp TD: Blindsight in hindsight. Consciousness and Cognition: 6(1); 67–74, 1997.

Taylor DC, Ounsted C: Biological mechanisms influencing the outcome of seizures in response to fevers. Epilepsia: 12; 33–45, 1971.

Taylor HG, Alden J: Age-related differences in outcomes following childhood brain insults: An introduction and overview. Journal of the International Neuropsychological Society: 3(6); 555–567, 1997.

Teuber HL: Why two brains? In Schmitt F, Worden F (Eds), The Neurosciences: Third Study Program. Cambridge, MA: MIT Press, pp. 71–74, 1974.

Thal D, Marchman V, Stiles J et al.: Early lexical development in children with focal brain injury. Brain and Language: 40; 491–527, 1991.

Thatcher R: Cyclic cortical reorganization: Origins of human cognitive development. In Dawson G, Fischer F (Eds), Development and Cognition. New York, NY: Academic Press, pp. 232–266, 1994.

Thatcher R, Walker R, Giudice S: Human cerebral hemispheres develop at different rates and ages. Science: 236; 1110–1113, 1987.

Truy E: Neuro-functional imaging and profound deafness. International Journal of Pediatric Otorhinolaryngology: 47(2); 131–136, 1999.

Tuchman R: Epileptic aphasia. In Rapin I, Nass R (Eds), Seminars in Neurology. New York, NY: Saunders, pp. 76–84, 1997.

Turkewitz G: A prenatal source for the development of hemispheric specialization. In Molfese D, Segalowitz S (Eds), Brain Lateralization in Children. New York, NY: Guilford Press, pp. 73–81, 1988.

Uhl F, Franzen P, Podreka I et al.: Increased regional cerebral blood flow in inferior occipital cortex and cerebellum of early blind humans. Neuroscience Letters: 150(2); 162–164, 1993.

Uhl F, Kretschmer T, Lindinger G et al.: Tactile mental imagery in sighted persons and in patients suffering from peripheral blindness early in life. Electroencephalography and Clinical Neurophysiology: 91(4); 249–255, 1994.

Van Hout A: Acquired aphasia in childhood. In Rapin I, Nass R(Eds), Seminars in Neurology. New York, NY: Saunders, pp. 69–75, 1997.

Vargha-Khadem F, Carr LJ, Isaacs E et al.: Onset of speech after left hemispherectomy in a nine-year-old boy. Brain: 120(1); 159–182, 1997.

Vargha-Khadem F, Isaacs EB, Papaleloudi H et al.: Development of language in six hemispherectomized patients. Brain: 114; 473–495, 1991.

Vargha-Khadem F, Isaacs EB, Van der Werf S et al.: Development of intelligence and memory in children with hemiplegic cerebral palsy: The deleterious consequences of early seizures. Brain: 115(1); 315–329, 1992.

Vargha-Khadem F, Isaacs EB, Watkins R et al.: Ontogenetic specialization of hemispheric function. In Oxbury J, Polkey C, Duchowny M, Intractable Focal Epilepsy. London: Saunders, pp. 406–417, 2000.

Vargha-Khadem F, O'Gorman AM, Watters GV: Aphasia and handedness in relation to hemispheric side, age at injury and severity of cerebral lesion during childhood. Brain: 108; 677–696, 1985.

Vargha-Khadem F, Polkey CE: A review of cognitive outcome after hemidecortication in humans. Advances in Experimental Medicine Biology: 325; 137–151, 1992.

Veraart C, De Volder A, Wanet-Defalque M et al.: Glucose utilization in human visual cortex is, respectively, elevated and decreased in early versus late blindness. Brain Research: 510; 115–121, 1990.

Walsh V, Ashbridge E, Cowey A: Cortical plasticity in perceptual learning demonstrated by transcranial magnetic stimulation. Neuropsychologia: 36(4); 363–367, 1998.

Wanet-Defalque MC, Veraart C, De Volder A et al.: High metabolic activity in the visual cortex of early blind human subjects. Brain Research: 446(2); 369–373, 1988.

Wang X, Merzenich MM, Sameshima K et al.: Remodelling of hand representation in adult cortex determined by timing of tactile stimulation. Nature: 378(6552); 13–14, 1995.

Weinberger NM: Learning-induced changes of auditory receptive fields. Current Opinion in Neurobiology: 3; 570–577, 1993.

Wightman F, Kistler D: Of vulcan ears, human ears and 'earprints'. Nature Neuroscience: 1; 337–339, 1998.

Woods BT: The restricted effects of right-hemisphere lesions after age one: Wechsler test data. Neuropsychologia: 18(1); 65–70, 1980.

Woods BT, Carey S: Language deficits after apparent clinical recovery from childhood aphasia. Annals of Neurology: 6; 405–409, 1979.

Woods BT, Teuber HL: Early onset of complementary specialization of cerebral hemispheres in man. Transactions of the American Neurological Association: 98; 113–117, 1973.

Woods BT, Teuber HL: Changing patterns of childhood aphasia. Annals of Neurology: 3; 273–280, 1978.

Yamada H, Sadato N, Konishi Y et al.: A milestone for normal development of the infantile brain detected by functional MRI. Neurology: 55(2); 218–23, 2000.

Ziemann U, Corwell B, Cohen LG: Modulation of plasticity in human motor cortex after forearm ischemic nerve block. Journal of Neuroscience: 18(3); 1115–1123, 1998.

*Handbook of Neuropsychology*, 2nd Edition, Vol. 8, Part I
S.J. Segalowitz and I. Rapin (Eds)

CHAPTER 4

# Epidemiologic perspectives on neuropsychological disorders in children

David C. Bellinger [a,*], Leonard A. Rappaport [b,c], Michael D. Weiler [d] and
Nathaniel B. Beers [c]

[a] *Departments of Neurology, Children's Hospital and Harvard Medical School, Boston, MA, USA*
[b] *Department of Medicine, Children's Hospital, Boston, MA, USA*
[c] *Department of Pediatrics, Harvard Medical School, Boston, MA, USA*
[d] *Departments of Psychiatry, Children's Hospital and Harvard Medical School, Boston, MA, USA*

## Introduction

Epidemiology is "the study of the distribution and determinants of health-related states or events in specified populations, and the application of this study to control of health problems" (Last, 1988, p. 42). It consists of a relatively small set of concepts that bear on the design, analysis, and interpretation of studies of disease occurrence. The ease with which the concepts can be stated belies the seriousness of the consequences that may result from their misapplication. Indeed, what might seem like a trivial limitation of a study may have profound implications for the inferences that can be drawn from it (Feinleib, 1987; Sackett, 1979).

The primary contributions that epidemiology can make to the study of higher cortical disorders in children are to provide the tools needed (1) to specify the prevalence (or incidence) of different disorders (as well as variations among population subgroups defined, for example, by age, race, sex, and socioeconomic status), and (2) to identify antecedents and correlates of disease occurrence or of its natural history. Epidemiologic methods are primarily designed to identify and, to the extent possible, reduce the many potential threats to the internal and external validity of studies designed to address these issues. In this chapter, we describe some of the methodologic principles that are pertinent to the conduct and interpretation of studies of child neuropsychology. We explore, in particular, issues relating to study design (e.g., case definition, sampling, bias, selection of a control group), data analysis (e.g., statistical power, confounding bias), and study inferences. More detailed and comprehensive discussion of epidemiologic concepts and methods is provided in textbooks such as Elwood (1998), Gordis (1996), Kelsey, Whittemore, Evans and Thompson (1996), MacMahon and Trichopoulos (1996) and Rothman and Greenland (1998).

## Study design issues

### Classification of designs

Although epidemiologists argue, seemingly endlessly, about nosologies and classifications of research design (Kramer and Boivin, 1987), several types of studies can be readily discerned, and their application to a research question tends to follow a fairly stereotypical sequence. First, a hypothesis is generated on the basis of clinical observation, fol-

* Corresponding author. Tel.: +1 (617) 355-6565;
E-mail: david.bellinger@al.tch.harvard.edu

lowed by case series (e.g., a report on a group of patients seen in a particular hospital clinic). Use of such convenience samples as bases for drawing inferences can be problematic. The referral mechanisms that generate such samples are usually poorly characterized, so generalizations about disease etiology and natural history will be biased to the extent that the patients in the case series are not representative of all individuals with the disease.

Following case series reports, case-control (or case-referent), cross-sectional, and retrospective or prospective cohort studies are conducted, depending on the specific hypothesis being tested and the resources available. The case-control design is especially useful to child neuropsychologists because it involves comparing children with a particular diagnosis of interest (the 'cases') to children who do not meet diagnostic criteria ('the controls') for differences in the frequency of exposures, conditions, or events thought to be etiologically related to the diagnosis. For instance, a variety of potential causes of attention deficit hyperactivity disorder have been investigated by means of case-control studies, including maternal cigarette smoking during pregnancy (Milberger, Biederman, Faraone et al., 1996) and prenatal/perinatal events (Milberger, Biederman, Faraone et al., 1997). ADHD cases and their controls have also been compared in terms of their performance on a battery of tests of executive functions (Pennington and Ozonoff, 1996) or automatic information processing (Hazell, Carr, Lewin et al., 1999). In another application of a case-control design, children with chronic health conditions have been compared to children without chronic health conditions in terms of their personal adjustment and mental health risk (Stein, Westbrook and Silver, 1998).

After case series or case-control studies have suggested that individuals with a disease or condition experienced some exposure or event more frequently than did individuals without the disease or condition, investigators typically mount cross-sectional or cohort studies to explore this association in greater detail. In studies of this type, children are selected for inclusion in the study sample based on whether or not they experienced the exposure or event of interest rather than based on whether they have a particular disease or condition. The study question then becomes: Do the 'exposed' and 'unexposed'

children develop some outcome of interest at significantly different rates? For example, to study the impact of in utero cocaine exposure on child development, an investigator might assemble a cohort of women who, at the time of delivery, admitted using cocaine during pregnancy and compare the neurobehavioral test scores of their children to the scores of children whose mothers denied using cocaine during pregnancy (e.g., Espy, Kaufmann and Glisky, 1999).

Whether a case-control or a cohort study is the most appropriate choice of design for a particular study question depends on several considerations. A case-control study tends to be less expensive and quicker to conduct and is the most efficient way to study the epidemiology of a rare disease. On the other hand, use of a cross-sectional or cohort design provides an opportunity to study more than one outcome in relation to a particular exposure. In addition, such a design may be the only way to study the sequelae of a rare exposure.

*Incidence versus prevalence samples*

The prevalence of a disease refers to the number of cases that exist at a given time in a specified population. It is essentially a cross-sectional measure in that it is usually calculated with respect to a hypothetical 'instant in time', generating a point prevalence estimate. Other time frames are sometimes used, however, especially for diseases in which symptom severity may wax and wane (Kessler, McGonagle, Zhao et al., 1994). Thus, the lifetime prevalence of depression refers to the number of individuals who meet diagnostic criteria for depression at any point in their lifetime. In contrast, the incidence of the disease refers to the number of new cases that occur within a specified population within a specified period of time. Because incidence is referenced to a particular period of time, it can be used to calculate rates of occurrence (e.g., the number of new cases of a particular cancer that are diagnosed within a given year may be 1/500,000 individuals). The distinction between prevalence and incidence, although subtle and sometimes blurred, is a critical one.

The validity of both case-control and cross-sectional/cohort studies requires that cases selected for study be representative of the population of all cases. One important strategy for achieving this (and other goals) is to consider as eligible for inclusion in a study only incident cases. Assembling a sample of incident cases usually requires population screening and/or the cooperation of all individuals and/or institutions expected to provide services to those with the outcome. Although it is easier to assemble a cohort of prevalent cases (e.g., all children in a specified population who meet diagnostic criteria for a learning disability), important disadvantages to this approach limit it as a basis for drawing generalizations. In the interval between the time a child's disorder is identified and information on exposure is collected, processes associated with the child's handicap or deficit may alter the distribution of exposures among the cases (e.g., did marital discord and emotional disturbance of the child contribute to a learning disability or are such difficulties a consequence of the handicap?).

In general, researchers tend to study incident cases and clinicians prevalent cases, a difference that may lead to discrepant conclusions about the antecedents, correlates, and prognosis of a disorder. This is because prevalence samples generally include patients with more serious cases of disease, more treatment resistant cases, or cases of longer duration. In a prevalence sample, factors that are found to correlate with disease may actually be correlates not of the occurrence of the disease, per se, but correlates of the duration of the disease, or correlates of referral for the disease. Not surprisingly, studying such samples typically leads to less sanguine judgments about the long-term prognosis associated with a disease. The label 'clinician's illusion' has been suggested (by researchers) for this form of referral or reporting bias (Cohen and Cohen, 1984). For instance, cases ascertained from clinics or hospitals tend to have different characteristics from cases ascertained from the general population. The estimate of the frequency with which febrile seizures in children are associated with neurological sequelae is substantially higher in clinic-based samples of children than it is in samples consisting of all children within a completely enumerated population who have a history of febrile seizures (Ellenberg and Nelson, 1980). Similarly, children with ADHD who are cared for by specialists in child and adolescent psychiatry tend to be more severely impaired and are more likely to have significant comorbid conditions

than are children with ADHD who are in the care of general psychiatrists (Zarins, Suarez, Pincus et al., 1998).

An implication of the above is that, for many diseases, studies limited to cases referred to specialized treatment centers will produce biased estimates of even such basic statistics as disease prevalence, let alone etiology, natural history, or comorbidities. For example, Mason, Banerjee, Eapen et al. (1998) used a two-stage procedure (informant, followed by interview) for investigating the prevalence of Tourette's syndrome (TS) among all 13–14 year old children attending a randomly selected mainstream secondary school in West Essex, England. The prevalence estimate they calculated, 3%, was four times greater than the next largest estimate reported in the literature, and several hundred times higher than the estimates deriving by asking health care providers to identify cases known to them, or by soliciting self- and parent-reports of TS cases. This reflects the difference between what might be called the 'ascertained' prevalence rate, which has its uses (e.g., for planning of service needs), and the 'true' prevalence rate (Roeleveld, Zielhuis and Gabreels, 1997). As another example, system-identified samples of learning-disabled children may differ substantially from children identified as learning-disabled by the application of well-defined research criteria. The contrast appears to be especially striking for females (Bussing, Zima, Perwein et al., 1998; Shaywitz, Shaywitz, Fletcher and Escobar, 1990).

The importance of the distinction between incidence and prevalence samples will be reduced when the disease under study is one for which most individuals with the disease would be expected to come to medical attention for diagnosis or treatment. A prime example is autism (Angold, Costello and Erkanli, 1999). In addition, assembling a prevalence or clinic-based sample would be appropriate if that is the population to which one wishes to generalize, or when the disease is so rare that it would take a very long time to accrue an adequate number of incident cases for study. Although complete ascertainment and recruitment of cases should be the goal, it is important to recognize that failure to achieve perfection in this effort will not invariably lead to bias in study inferences (e.g., Goodman and Yude, 1996).

*Selection bias*

One of the greatest threats to study validity, selection bias exists if a study sample is not representative of the source population from which it was drawn and to which the investigator wishes to generalize the results (Ellenberg, 1994). It can affect the validity of studies of any design type, often exerting its influence even prior to the enrollment of subjects in a study. In a case-control study, selection bias may occur if the likelihood of an individual's identification as a case depends on his or her status with respect to the antecedent or correlate being evaluated. When such a bias exists, the distribution of that factor will differ among those who participate in a study and those who are eligible but who do not participate or are not selected, potentially biasing any estimate of the association between the factor and 'caseness'. One form of this is the familiar self-selection, participation, or volunteer bias, in which the subset of individuals who agree to participate differs in key respects from the entire target or source population (Betan, Roberts and McCluskey-Fawcett, 1995; Noll, Zeller, Vannatta et al., 1997; Stein, Bauman and Ireys, 1991). In a study involving several phases of participation, Larroque, Kaminski, Bouvier-Colle and Hollebecque (1999) found that respondents differed from non-respondents at each stage of the study, with individuals who were late or sporadic respondents having characteristics that were intermediate between those of full or early respondents and complete non-respondents.

A more subtle form of selection bias is diagnostic bias. Early case-control studies of the association between oral contraceptive (OC) use and venous thromboembolism recruited women who were hospitalized with this condition. It was later demonstrated that the reason why some women with this disease were hospitalized was due to their physicians' knowledge that they were taking OCs and the physicians' suspicions, based on early anecdotal reports, that this behavior increased the risk of thromboembolism (Rothman, 1986). Obstetric malpractice cases are preferentially seen in developmental evaluation clinics, often at the request of attorneys who want an independent documentation of damages. Investigators who draw their cases of delayed development, mental retardation, or other dysfunction from a highly selected referral

source such as this are at risk of making errors in inference about the role of perinatal events in causing later developmental problems.

A major source of bias in case-control studies results from the fact that information about exposure history must be collected retrospectively. Its value may be limited by recall bias (differential quality of recall depending on outcome status) or by the unavailability of adequate records (Joffe and Grisso, 1985; Thomas, Chess and Birch, 1966; Tilley, Barnes, Bergstralh et al., 1985). The extent of recall bias depends on a variety of factors, including the time interval involved, the perceived significance of the past events at issue, the wording of questions, and the social desirability of the events or activities (e.g., alcohol and drug use during pregnancy) (Coughlin, 1990).

The difficulty of maintaining a cohort over a period of years, and the bias that may be introduced by selective lost-to-follow-up, is a major drawback of the prospective cohort design (Aylward, Hatcher, Stripp et al., 1985). Follow-up studies of prenatal exposure to lead and cocaine provide examples of this challenge. In a study of low-level prenatal lead exposure, children in the low-lead group who dropped out of the cohort over the course of the follow-up period had achieved higher developmental scores during the time that they participated than had the children in the low-lead group who participated throughout the study. The opposite pattern held among the children in the high-lead group. Children who dropped out during the follow-up period had achieved lower scores than had the children who participated throughout (Bellinger and Stiles, 1993). The impact of this biased attrition was to produce an attenuation, over the course of the study, in the association between children's lead burdens and their developmental scores.

Mayes and Cicchetti (1995) suggested that bias resulting from cohort attrition may be responsible, in part, for inconsistencies reported in studies of the long-term developmental outcomes of infants prenatally exposed to cocaine. As evidence that attrition was unbiased, investigators frequently report the absence of statistically significant differences in the baseline characteristics of participants who were retained in a cohort and those who were lost (Vestbo and Rasmussen, 1992). Apart from the fact that the results of a test of significance are not germane in this context, such an analysis does not address the essential question: 'had it been possible to follow the entire cohort, would the estimate of the association between the independent and dependent variables differ meaningfully from the estimate that was obtained based only those in the original cohort who were retained through the follow-up period? When viewed in these terms, the relevant comparison for assessing the bias introduced by attrition is the following. Among the original participants who were eventually lost-to-follow-up, were the associations between the independent and dependent variables that were estimated prior to lost-to-follow-up similar to those associations estimated among the original participants who were retained in the cohort? In more concrete terms, was the slope of the regression line relating lead level to cognitive development based on children who later dropped out of the study cohort different from the slope of the regression line calculated based on children who remained members of the study cohort?

### Competing risks

An issue that can limit the value of a case-control study involves the concept of competing risks. This is a particular problem for studies of disorders and outcomes that may reflect the influences of many different factors, i.e., that represent final common pathways. For some diseases, the known causes are so few in number that a case-control design is useful for estimating the risk of the disease associated with a particular exposure or event. For example, to the best of our knowledge, angiosarcoma of the liver is caused almost exclusively by exposure to the industrial chemical vinyl chloride, so a case-control study can provide a valid estimate of the population attributable risk associated with vinyl chloride. When the outcome of interest can be caused by many different exposures or events, however, a case-control approach to studying its antecedents and correlates may be relatively uninformative because the increase in risk associated with any one risk factor may be small relative to the aggregate risk associated with other causal influences. In a recent study investigating the cognitive effects of low-level lead exposure, investigators specifically chose as their

sampling frame 9 to 12 year old children with learning problems who were attending special education schools (Minder, Das-Smaal and Orlebeke, 1998). The authors argued that this choice increased their likelihood of detecting an association between low-level lead burden and neuropsychological outcomes, should one exist. When no such association was found, the authors concluded that lead exposures of the magnitude represented in the sample are unlikely to cause poor learning outcomes. Why was this sampling strategy probably a poor choice for testing the study hypothesis? All the children in the study sample had learning problems attributable to some factor, whether this was elevated lead exposure, an intraventricular hemorrhage due to prematurity, a congenital heart lesion that resulted in chronic hypoxemia, or any number of other insults. Thus, a variety of factors combined to generate the study sample. It should not be too surprising, therefore, that the 'signal' due to one particular risk factor, an elevated lead level, was weak (not statistically significant) in the face of a very high background rate of poor outcomes due to many other competing risk factors. In effect, the hypothesis actually tested in this study was that elevated lead exposure is such a strong determinant of learning problems that its signal can be perceived even amid the substantial 'noise' in the outcome that is attributable to the many other determinants of these outcomes, and that the severity (rather than merely the presence) of a learning problem varies with lead level. A cohort study is likely to provide a better approach to this issue, as it would test the more reasonable hypothesis that children with higher lead burdens are at higher risk of having a learning problem than are children with lower lead burdens.

An investigator interested in assessing the contribution of a particular risk factor to an outcome that has multiple determinants will often define the sampling frame in such a way as to exclude individuals who possess other strong risk factors for the outcome of interest (Rothman and Poole, 1988). Thus, the association between air pollution and lung function might best be studied by limiting the study sample to nonsmokers, eliminating by sample restriction a substantial portion of the variability in the outcome of interest that is unrelated to the exposure of interest. Similarly, the inverse association between prenatal lead exposure and birth weight is stronger among women who do not smoke cigarettes during pregnancy than it is among women who do smoke, most likely because this activity is itself inversely related to infants' birth weights, making it difficult, statistically, to appreciate the smaller effect on birth weight that may be due to lead (Bornschein, Grote, Mitchell et al., 1989). Although multivariate statistical methods can often be helpful in taking account of outcome variability that is related to factors other than the one of primary interest, their utility is reduced when the contributions of these other factors are much greater than that of the primary factor (Bellinger, Leviton and Waternaux, 1989).

*Selection of a control group*

Selection of an adequate control group can pose some of the most difficult problems involved in conducting an epidemiological study. The purpose of a control group is to provide an accurate estimate of the background prevalence of the exposure of interest, that is to provide an estimate of the expected frequency of a given exposure among cases if, in fact, that exposure is not associated with the likelihood that an individual will become a case. An appropriate control is thus an individual who would have been included in the case group, that is would have been identified by the case sampling mechanism, had he or she manifested the disease of interest. Some investigators select as controls individuals who not only do not have the disorder of interest (i.e., the disorder warranting classification as a case), but individuals who are without other types of pathology as well. For instance, an investigator interested in the association between ADHD and some perinatal event might restrict the control group to children who do not meet criteria for depression, conduct disorder, or oppositional defiant disorder. A problem arises, however, if the same restrictions are not imposed on the ADHD cases, many of whom may also have one (or more) of these comorbid conditions. Such a strategy is generally motivated by a concern that because different disorders may share etiologies, 'purifying' the control group by screening out individuals with other disorders potentially related to the risk factor of interest will produce a more valid estimate of the association between the risk factor and the disorder of primary interest. Because

this asymmetry in the method for selecting cases and controls selectively eliminates individuals with exposure to the risk factor from the control group, the result will be a bias towards finding such an association. This bias has been called the 'well control' artefact (Schwartz and Link, 1989). It represents a selection bias insofar as an individual's likelihood of being included as a control is related to exposure status. Thus, it is important that a difference in case status is the only reason that one individual ends up in the case group and another in the control group. Any restrictions applied to membership in one group must be applied equally to the other.

Matching of cases and controls (in a case-control study setting) or of exposed and unexposed individuals (in a cohort study setting) on variables thought to be associated with the outcome of interest will reduce potential confounding by these variables, although matching can be difficult to implement and is inefficient if the number of matching factors is large (McKinlay, 1977). It is especially useful, however, when the effect of the factor of interest is relatively weak compared to other causal factors. For instance, the use of sibling controls in evaluating pre- and perinatal antecedents of a developmental handicap would insure similarity between cases and controls in terms of social class, the home environment, and other strong predictors of child development. On the other hand, choosing as a control a subsequently born sibling can create problems as well, attributable to the fact that having a handicapped child may affect family culture in subtle ways. Women who have had intra-partum problems are likely to be monitored more closely throughout pregnancy than are women without previous difficulties, potentially resulting in a 'diagnostic suspicion bias' and thus the identification of conditions in subsequent offspring that would not have been identified had the preceding child not been a case (Sackett, 1979). In addition, the sibling born after a handicapped child may be invested with greater parental expectations and thus treated in ways that differ substantially from the way in which the handicapped child was treated.

*Misclassification*

The major source of bias or imprecision in assessing exposure and outcome in an epidemiologic study is misclassification, specifically an error in determining whether a child experienced some event or exposure and in determining whether the child has a certain disease or condition. Misclassification of exposure is random (or non-differential) if the likelihood of such error is not systematically related to a child's outcome status (and vice versa). Because random misclassification simply introduces additional variability into the data, it usually, although not invariably (Sorohan and Gilthorpe, 1994), leads to an underestimate of the association between an exposure and an outcome, that is bias towards the null hypothesis. When misclassification is systematically different among study groups, however (usually called differential misclassification), it can be a major threat to study validity. Such differential misclassification can introduce bias either toward or away from the null hypothesis depending on the specific circumstances. In this section, we focus on issues pertaining to the classification of study subjects with respect to outcome.

Epidemiology began as a discipline with the study of infectious disease epidemics. Identifying 'cases' was relatively straightforward, as a person did or did not have a disease such as cholera or tuberculosis. Case definition is more problematic for diseases in which the clinical presentation varies widely (e.g., Alexander's Disease; Herndon, 1999). With new developments in diagnostic imaging or genetic analysis it sometimes becomes apparent that conditions previously regarded as separate entities are variations in the expression of a single entity. For example, in the last decade, velo-cardio-facial syndrome, DiGeorge syndrome, and conotruncal anomaly face syndrome were all recognized as being the result of the same genetic anomaly, what is now called the chromosome 22q11 deletion syndrome (Thomas and Graham, 1997). As with the blind men and the elephant, these three syndromes had previously been described independently by investigators who emphasized different aspects of the complex, variable presentation of these patients (e.g., immunological and endocrine abnormalities, patalal and facial dysmorphologies, congenital heart defects, learning disabilities).

Diagnosis is even less straightforward in the domain of developmental neuropsychology, psychiatry, and neurology, in which criteria often refer solely to behavioral presentation and history rather than to laboratory test results. Thus, the statement that ". . . disease classification is not only a prerequisite of epidemiologic study, but also one of its goals" (MacMahon and Pugh, 1970) is more applicable to this class of disorders than it is to diseases to which Koch's classic postulate (one disease-one pathogen) apply. Much of the epidemiological work in this field thus involves efforts, such as the successive revisions of the Diagnostic and Statistical Manual of the American Psychiatric Association, to refine the criteria for defining the occurrence of a disorder. Thus, McBurnett, Pfiffner, Willcutt et al. (1999) reported that DSM-IV criteria for ADHD are superior to those of DSM-III-R in terms of 'subcategorical homogeneity', e.g., in identifying distinct subtypes of children with ADHD. One implication of this evolutionary process of refinement, however, is that the diagnostic criteria for some diseases represent a moving target, with shifts in practice potentially vitiating the validity of prior efforts to establish incidence and prevalence and to identify disease antecedents and correlates. Cerebral palsy, a group of non-progressive motor disorders generally diagnosed on the basis of clinical signs, illustrates this problem. Advances in brain imaging, methods for identifying metabolic disorders, and karotyping have led to the identification of many distinct syndromes among the group of children who were formerly identified as having cerebral palsy (Mutch, Alberman, Hagberg et al., 1992), e.g., X-linked hydrocephalus syndrome, lysosomal storage disorder, Rett syndrome, and trisomy 4p syndrome, to name only a few (Badawi, Watson, Petterson et al., 1998). Whether such cases are included or excluded will clearly have substantial impact on estimates of prevalence (Williams and Alberman, 1998). Considerable effort, therefore, has been invested in standardizing inclusion criteria for this diagnosis to facilitate inter-study comparisons (e.g., insuring the comparability of cases included in registers, the validity of assessments of time trends in prevalence estimates, efforts to replicate investigations of hypotheses about etiology) (see Badawi et al., 1998).

Reading disability illustrates the principle that a prevalence estimate can vary depending on the specific case definition employed. It is a disorder that was previously widely believed to represent an 'all or none' phenomenon, evident as a distinct bump in the distribution of children's reading scores (Rutter and Yule, 1975). Later studies failed to support this conceptualization, suggesting instead that reading scores are essentially normally distributed so that the prevalence of reading disorder is heavily dependent on the cut-off (e.g., 1 SD, 2 SDs) used to define it (Shaywitz, Escobar, Shaywitz et al., 1992). The choice of cut-off may also affect the likelihood that a child classified as reading-disabled at one age will be similarly classified at a later age. Waters (1973) cautioned that, ". . . it is important not to readily accept as a definite clinical entity, something that we cannot readily define."

To illustrate some of the issues in applying epidemiologic concepts such as case definition, prevalence, and screening to conditions with neuropsychological involvement, we discuss in the following section two disorders: ADHD and autism.

*Attention deficit hyperactivity disorder*
ADHD can be used to illustrate many of the issues involved in epidemiologic studies of neuropsychological disorders. Because the prevalence of ADHD in the general population is relatively low (approximately 5%) (American Psychiatric Association, 1994), many children must be screened in order to identify a sufficient number to study. Assessment of ADHD is thought to be best accomplished by a time- and resource-intensive multimodal approach (Barkley, Fischer, Newby and Breen, 1988). In real-world studies, however, compromises are often made in the number of children assessed and the methods used to collect these data. In order to assemble subjects who are representative of the entire population of children with ADHD, care must be taken in choosing the source from which the study sample is drawn. Restricting the sampling frame to children in public schools will miss those in institutions (Szatmari, 1992) or those in special schools specifically for children with severe forms of ADHD. Examining children in medical outpatient clinics might over-identify children who are accident prone, while studying children referred to psychiatric outpatient clinics might over-identify children with comorbid symptoms (Biederman, Faraone, Doyle et al., 1993). Because ADHD is associated with poorer socioeconomic status (Velez, Johnson and Cohen, 1989), selecting subjects from a center serving only one so-

cioeconomic class could result in a distorted estimate of symptom prevalence in the general population.

Once an appropriate population from which to draw a study sample is identified, a mechanism for identifying the cases of children with ADHD must be specified. One of the greatest challenges in integrating the vast database on ADHD is the fact that in recent decades the criteria for diagnosing ADHD have been modified on repeated occasions as a result of shifts in nosological approach. Moreover, clinicians still cannot refer to any laboratory, neuroimaging, or electroencephalographic finding as a 'gold standard' to validate a diagnosis of ADHD (Tannock, 1998).

The presumed presentation of ADHD has changed markedly. In DSM-II (American Psychiatric Association, 1968), the diagnosis of the 'hyperkinetic reaction' required abnormal levels of inattention, impulsivity, and motor activity. In DSM-III (American Psychiatric Association, 1980), attention and impulse control problems were emphasized, eliminating hyperactivity as a necessary finding. In DSM-III-R, the three sets of symptoms of inattention, over-activity, and impulsivity were combined, with the presence of symptoms of hyperactivity required for a diagnosis of ADHD (Lahey, Applegate, McBurnett et al., 1994). The current system of DSM-IV permits the diagnosis to be assigned to a child who presents with attention symptoms alone or with hyperactivity–impulsivity symptoms alone. A diagnosis of ADHD-combined type can be assigned to a child who shows both inattention and hyperactivity–impulsivity. The implications of these changes in diagnostic criteria for prevalence estimates are substantial, as demonstrated by comparisons of the results of applying DSM-III-R and DSM-IV criteria to teachers' ratings of students' behavior. Because of the addition of the predominately inattentive type category to the ADHD typology in DSM-IV, the prevalence of all types of ADHD diagnoses using DMS-IV criteria were 57% and 64% higher than the prevalences based on DSM-III-R criteria, based on data collected in Tennessee and Germany, respectively (Baumgaertel, Wolraich and Dietrich, 1995; Wolraich, Hannah, Pinnock and Baumgaertel, 1996).

ADHD is similar to reading disability and other diagnoses that are made solely on the basis of clinical presentation in that it is not clear the extent to which it represents the severe end of a continuous range of functioning and the extent to which children with ADHD are qualitatively different from children without ADHD (Biederman et al., 1993). As noted, DSM-IV relies on categorical criteria in that a child must display six or more symptoms in order to be assigned the diagnosis. Without a means of verifying the diagnosis (i.e., independent of parent and teacher information), the mechanism for determining the number of diagnostic symptoms needed must be considered somewhat arbitrary. In the DSM-IV field trials for ADHD, it was found that requiring five symptoms resulted in the best agreement with independent clinical diagnoses and estimates of impairment on a functional assessment scale. Nonetheless, to guard against over-diagnosis (i.e., false positives), a more conservative, but nevertheless arbitrary, cut-off of six symptoms was selected for inclusion in the final version of DSM-IV (Lahey et al., 1994).

Although many studies have relied on structured interviews of parents and children to verify the diagnosis of ADHD (e.g., Biederman et al., 1993; Chen, Faraone, Biederman and Tsuang, 1994; Rey, Morris-Yates and Stainslaw, 1992; Shekim, Cantwell, Kashani et al., 1986; Steingard, Biederman, Doyle and Sprich-Buckminster, 1992), use of structured interviews alone may result in overdiagnosis (Carlson, Kashani, Thomas et al., 1987; Welner, Reich, Herjanic et al., 1987) Moreover, information derived from child interviews may not be reliable, or at least may be unstable across the critical age range (Edelbrock, Costello, Dulcan et al., 1985). DSM-IV criteria stipulate that ADHD symptoms must be evident in multiple settings (i.e., home, work, school). This requirement has not always been applied in recent epidemiologic studies, possibly because of the lower prevalence of cross-situational problems and the difficulties of combining data across observers and setting. For example, should the total number of ADHD symptoms be pooled, should some threshold number of symptoms be required for behaviors in different settings, or should only those symptoms endorsed in both settings be considered (Szatmari, 1992)? Anderson, Williams, McGee and Silva (1987) found that the prevalence of ADD symptoms dropped by 34% when symptoms had to be endorsed by at least two respondents (i.e., teacher, child, parent). Using DSM-IV-based questionnaire data, Weiler, Waber, Bellinger et al. (1999) found that 12% of children met diagnostic criteria for ADHD (i.e., six or more symptoms) by parent report alone, 15% met criteria by teacher report alone, but only 6% met criteria if 6 or more DSM-IV symptoms were necessary both by parent and teacher report.

The high prevalence of comorbidity among children with ADHD (50% to 80%) (Tannock, 1998) calls into question the extent to which ADHD and the cormorbid conditions are independent, specifically raising the issue of whether these other conditions have the same etiology as the ADHD symptoms. Different nosologies reflect different ways of resolving this issue. Whereas DSM-IV permits multiple, concurrent diagnoses, the ICD system favored in Europe tends towards a single diagnosis, thus differentiating among the varieties of comorbid combinations (Tannock, 1998). This may account, at least part, for the differences in prevalence estimates between North America and Europe. Certainly some findings support the validity of the ICD approach. Comorbid types of ADHD differ not only in the severity of their symptoms (Biederman et al., 1993; Steingard et al., 1992) but also in their response to medication (Tannock, Fine, Heintz and Schachar, 1995; Tannock, Ickowicz and Schachar, 1995).

Estimating the prevalence of low base-rate disorders can be problematic. As an example, let us make three assumptions: (1) there is an independent, completely reliable (but costly) method of making an ADHD diagnosis that would allow independent verification of the accuracy of a second diagnostic regime (e.g., questionnaire); (2) the true base rate of ADHD in the population is 5%; (3) the sensitivity and specificity of the questionnaire are both 95% (see Table 1). Despite the high levels of sensitivity and specificity of the questionnaire, a prevalence estimate that is based on it may be misleading. If we administered our hypothetical questionnaire with very high (i.e., 95%) sensitivity and specificity to the parents of 1000 children in a population with a 5% base rate of ADHD, 47 or 48 of the 50 children with ADHD would be diagnosed, on the basis of the questionnaire, as having ADHD (i.e., 95% sensitivity). Nine hundred and two of the 950 children without ADHD would be diagnosed, on the basis of the questionnaire, as not having ADHD (i.e., 95% specificity) and 48 of the children with-

TABLE 1

Screning test characteristics

| Screening result | Disease status | |
|---|---|---|
| | Yes | No |
| Positive | A | B |
| Negative | C | D |

The *sensitivity* of a screening test is defined as the percentage of individuals who truly have an outcome of interest who are also positive on the screening test (i.e., true positives). The *specificity* of a screening test is defined as the percentage of individuals who truly do not have the outcome of interest who are also negative on the screening test (i.e., true negatives). Sensitivity = A/(A + C). Specificity = D/(B + D). Other useful characteristics of a screening test include: *positive predictive value*, the percentage of individuals who screen positive who actually have the disease, i.e., A/(A + B), and the *negative predictive value*, the percentage of individuals who screen negative who are actually without the disease, i.e., D/(C + D).

out ADHD would be positive on the questionnaire (i.e., 1–specificity × 950). Combining the true positives (48) with the false positives (also 48 in this example) would lead to an estimated base rate of 9.6, nearly double the actual rate. In other words, to get an accurate estimate of the prevalence of low base-rate conditions, the specificity of a test must be extraordinarily high. This can be achieved by raising the cutoff level, although this will invariably result in fewer children with true ADHD being identified (i.e., lower sensitivity). For example, Chen et al. (1994) compared the Attention Problems scale of the parent-completed Child Behavior Checklist (CBCL; Achenbach, 1991) and structured interviews with mothers and children (over 11 years of age). Using a *T* score cutoff of 1 standard deviation (60), the sensitivity of the CBCL was 70%. When a *T* score of 70 was used, the sensitivity of the CBCL in the cross-validation sample fell to 23%. If we use these figures of sensitivity and specificity in our hypothetical example, the resulting prevalence estimate of 3% is closer to the 'true' 5% base rate. A problem remains, however. Only 39% of the children identified on the questionnaire as having ADHD were true positives, so the majority of the children constituting the 3% prevalence represent false positives. In other words, in the context of a low base rate, a screening instrument that has what appears to be satisfactory sensitivity and specificity will nevertheless have a low positive predictive value, and thus yield an inaccurate estimate of prevalence (Clark and Harrington, 1999).

*Autism*

The controversy over whether the prevalence of autism has changed in recent years illustrates the principle that, for conditions diagnosed exclusively on the basis of behavior, case counting can be affected by a variety of factors, including whether or not effective interventions are available.

The name and core diagnostic signs and symptoms of ADHD have changed repeatedly since this disorder was first described. In contrast, autism has retained the same name and core symptoms since Kanner first described it in 1943: (1) onset during infancy, (2) delayed language acquisition, (3) language that is often echolalic, unusual and non-communicative, (4) difficulty in establishing reciprocal relationships with others, (5) a tendency to engage in stereotyped, repetitive, non-imaginative play, and (6) a need for sameness. DSM-IV does distinguish 5 subtypes, however, depending on clinical presentation and natural history (American Psychiatric Association, 1994). Significant changes have occurred in the nature of the hypotheses advanced regarding its etiology. An estimated 20% of cases are now thought to have a biological cause, such as a viral infection (e.g., rubella, herpes encephalitis), a drug exposure (e.g., thalidomide, valproate), or a gene defect (Rapin, 1999).

Historically the prevalence of autism has been estimated to be 4–5 per 10,000. Despite the consistency over time in core characteristics, it is not clear whether the prevalence of autism has increased. Several studies suggest that it has not (Fombonne and Du Mazaubrun, 1992; Fombonne, Du Mazaubrun, Cans and Grandjean, 1997; Sponheim and Skjeldal, 1998), while others suggest that it has increased markedly (Gillberg, Steffenburg and Schaumann, 1991; Honda, Shimizu, Misumi et al., 1996; Tanoue, Oda, Asano and Kawashima, 1988; Webb, Lobo, Hervas et al., 1997; ). A variety of hypotheses have been proposed to explain this secular trend. For example, Gillberg et al. (1991) studied the incidence of autism in Göteborg, Sweden, and explained an apparent increase in prevalence in terms of an over-representation of immigrant populations in the study sample. Honda et al. (1996) suggested that an apparent increase in Japan was the result of classifying as autistic higher functioning individuals who had not been included in previous study samples. Fombonne et al. (1997) suggested that the prevalence of autism has remained approximately 5/10,000, but that including children with other pervasive developmental disorders and Asperger syndrome among the cases increases the prevalence estimate to approximately 16/10,000. Indeed, studies of the prevalence of Asperger syndrome alone yielded a prevalence higher than the 4–5/10,000 attributed to autism (Ehlers and Gillberg, 1993).

Many clinicians in the United States would probably offer the opinion that the prevalence of autism is increasing because they are diagnosing it more frequently. For example, in our infant diagnostic programs at Children's Hospital (Boston), it was formerly not unusual to go three months, seeing four infants and toddlers per week, without seeing a new patient who we considered to be autistic. Currently, however, we make a new diagnosis of autism at least twice per week. Rather than speaking to the prevalence of autism, the experience presumably largely reflects changes in the referral patterns to our programs. Although the reasons for these changes are not entirely clear, several hypotheses to explain increased early referral come to mind. First, as suggested above, it is possible, although difficult to prove, that diagnostic criteria for autism have been expanded, so that children with other disorders are counted as cases when the prevalence of autism is estimated. Children who were formerly classified as 'atypical', showing variations on Kanner's core characteristics, may now be diagnosed as autistic. Second, tertiary programs may be seeing more infants and toddlers with autism because pediatricians are more skilled in identifying children with developmental problems and make earlier referrals to specialty clinics. Pediatric resident training in the United States must now include Developmental and Behavioral Pediatrics, presumably increasing pediatricians' knowledge in this area. Third, the recently enacted Individuals with Disabilities Education Act (USA) mandates services for infants and toddlers with developmental problems, resulting in an increased availability of early intervention programs. In addition, recent research suggests that some in-terventions, such as Applied Behavior Analysis, can make a difference in children's outcomes (Lovaas, 1987; Lovaas, Smith and McEachin, 1989), with positive effects maintained through the elementary school years (McEachin, Smith-Tristram and Lovaas, 1993). The availability of services for very young children and the recognition that these services are efficacious might encourage pediatricians to recognize potential developmental problems earlier and to tolerate a higher rate of false positive referrals. In contrast, in the recent past, when intervention alternatives for young children were limited and more generic, with little differentiation between interventions for mental retardation and autism, it was not as essential for the clinician to come to a specific diagnosis.

## Analytic strategies

### Statistical power

The power of a statistical test refers to the probability that the null hypothesis (i.e., that an exposure and an outcome are not associated with one another) will be rejected, given that in fact it is false (see Table 2). Being a probability, power varies between 0 and 1, with higher values being more desirable. Thus, one minus power equals the probability of committing an error of inference, specifically a Type II or false negative error. A Type I error represents a false positive error, that of concluding that the null hypothesis is false when in fact it is true. Ideally, the calculation of power should be considered an essential step in the design of a study. Power is especially pertinent with regard to studies in which a purported risk factor is found not to be associated with an outcome, i.e., when the null hypothesis is not rejected. If the power of the statistical test of this hypothesis is low, the study's scientific contribution and its implications for clinical practice must be viewed as minimal.

Power is a function of several aspects of study design. For both case-control and cohort studies, power depends on (1) sample size, (2) the Type I error rate considered acceptable ($\alpha$, chosen by the investigator and conventionally set at 0.05), and (3) the target effect size that the investigator wishes to be able to detect (if the exposure and outcome are, in fact,

TABLE 2

Type I and Type II errors, statistical power

| Results in the study sample | Truth in the population | |
|---|---|---|
| | Exposure and disease are truly associated | Exposure and disease are truly not associated |
| Null hypothesis is rejected | Correct | Type I error |
| Null hypothesis is not rejected | Type II error | Correct |

Type I and II errors are errors in drawing inferences about 'truth' in the population based on the results observed in a study sample. The probability of committing a Type I error (rejecting the null hypothesis when, in fact, it is true) is referred to as $\alpha$. By convention, $\alpha$ is usually set by the investigator at 5% (the familiar 0.05 level of statistical significance). The probability of committing a Type II error is referred to as $\beta$. $1 - \beta$ thus corresponds to the statistical power of the hypothesis test. It represents the likelihood, for a given $\alpha$, of observing an association between the exposure and the outcome in the study sample if one actually exists in the population from which the study sample was drawn.

TABLE 3

Sample size requirements for case-control studies of exposure–outcome associations [a]

| Relative risk [b] | Prevalence of exposure | | | |
|---|---|---|---|---|
| | 0.01 | 0.05 | 0.10 | 0.15 |
| 1.5 | 7954 [c] | 1687 | 910 | 465 |
| 2.0 | 2394 | 515 | 282 | 152 |
| 2.5 | 1245 | 271 | 151 | 84 |
| 3.0 | 803 | 176 | 99 | 58 |
| 4.0 | 448 | 100 | 58 | 36 |
| 5.0 | 304 | 69 | 41 | 26 |
| 10.0 | 112 | 27 | 17 | 13 |
| 20.0 | 50 | 14 | 10 | 9 |

[a] Assumptions: $\alpha = 0.05$ (two-sided) ($\varepsilon$ is the risk of making a Type I error, i.e., rejecting the null hypothesis when it is true); $\beta = 0.20$ ($\beta$ is the risk of making a Type II error, i.e., failing to reject the null hypothesis when it is false).
[b] Relative risk of disease associated with exposure.
[c] Sample size needed in each group (cases and controls).

TABLE 4

Sample size requirements for cohort studies of exposure–outcome associations [a]

| Relative risk [b] | Incidence of outcome among non-exposed group | | | |
|---|---|---|---|---|
| | 0.01 | 0.025 | 0.05 | 0.10 |
| 1.5 | 7741 [c] | 3037 | 1469 | 685 |
| 2.0 | 2316 | 904 | 434 | 199 |
| 2.5 | 1197 | 465 | 221 | 99 |
| 3.0 | 767 | 297 | 140 | 62 |
| 4.0 | 423 | 162 | 75 | 31 |
| 5.0 | 284 | 108 | 49 | 19 |
| 10.0 | 99 | 36 | 14 | – [d] |
| 20.0 | 40 | 12 | – | – |

[a] Assumptions $\alpha = 0.05$ (two-sided) ($\alpha$ is the risk of making a Type I error, i.e., rejecting the null hypothesis when it is true), $\beta = 0.20$ ($\beta$ is the risk of making a Type II error, i.e., failing to reject the null hypothesis when it is false).
[b] Relative risk of disease associated with exposure.
[c] Sample size needed in each group (exposed and non-exposed).
[d] Fewer than 5 individuals per group are needed.

associated). In addition, the power of a case-control study depends on the prevalence of the exposure of interest in the target population, while the power of a cohort study depends on the incidence of the outcome of interest among unexposed. The target effect size may be phrased in terms of the difference between groups in terms of a binary, categorical, or continuously distributed variable. If an exposure or disease is infrequent or the relative risk of disease associated with the exposure is modest, the number of subjects required to insure that a statistical test of the association will be informative (i.e., has adequate power) can be surprisingly large (Tables 3 and 4). A study comparing 20 autistic children and 20 non-

autistic controls, conducted to evaluate a prenatal or perinatal event that occurs with a frequency of less than 10%, has insufficient power to detect risks of the magnitude that would be reasonable to expect. For example, only if autistic children were 10 times more likely to have experienced the exposure would the power of the study be adequate (i.e., >0.8).

It is not uncommon for power estimates for a study to be calculated based on the primary hypothesis, but for investigators to test other, more complex hypotheses in the course of data analysis. These may involve comparisons of alternative models of a dose–response relationship or different models for characterizing the joint impact of two factors on the outcome (e.g., synergism, antagonism, additivity). It is important to recognize that the statistical power of such ancillary analyses of more complex patterns in the data may be considerably lower than the power of the tests of the main study hypotheses insofar as they often involve analyses of subsets of the study sample (Lubin and Gail, 1990).

It is impossible to state firm rules about the effect size that a study should have adequate power to detect. Any non-zero effect size will be statistically significant if the sample size is large enough. Thus this is not solely, or even primarily, a statistical question and requires the weighing of clinical, economic, and ethical considerations. An investigator might be interested in detecting only large treatment effects if the risks of the treatment are substantial or if the treatment is very expensive (e.g., extracorporeal membrane oxygenation therapy) (Raju, Langenberg, Sen and Aldana, 1992). On the other hand, it might be important, both clinically and economically, to detect a small effect of a therapy that is cheap, relatively harmless, and successful in reducing the morbidity associated with a prevalent disease (e.g., common cold).

Calculating power in neuropsychological research can be difficult because of the frequency with which experimental measures are used. Accurate estimates of the variances of scores on such measures are often not available. Furthermore, the variance estimate that is available may not be appropriate if the subjects under study were not drawn from the same population as the one on which the estimate was derived. The influence of test reliability (i.e., measurement error) on statistical power is particularly relevant to neuropsychological research (Charter, 1997), particularly in light of the substantial heterogeneity in the sensitivity of tests purporting to assess the same domain (Chouinard and Braun, 1993). The greater the variability in the outcome that is attributable to random measurement error, the larger the critical treatment or group difference needs to be in order to maintain a given level of statistical power (Boyle and Pickles, 1998). The reduction in power is a particular problem when the exposure of primary interest accounts for a relatively small amount of outcome variance (Soper, Cicchetti, Satz et al., 1988). It can also be a problem when an investigator's goal is to draw

inferences about the pattern of strengths and weaknesses associated with a particular exposure (e.g., methyl mercury) or diagnosis (e.g., Williams syndrome). In order to draw such inferences, the tests used to assess different domains should be equivalent in their discriminating power, specifically their true-score variance (Chapman and Chapman, 1978). If they are not, differential performance across domains may not be due to differential ability across domains. Deficits may appear to lie in a particular domain simply because the instrument used to assess that domain is technically superior to the instruments used to assess other domains.

The entertaining personal and historical perspectives on power analysis and null hypothesis testing of Cohen (1990) are highly recommended.

### Confounding bias

Unrecognized confounding bias is a major threat to study validity, potentially resulting in erroneous inferences. A confounding variable is associated with both the exposure and the outcome, although not in the putative causal pathway linking them. For example, in unadjusted (often referred to as 'crude') analyses, coffee consumption tends to be associated with an increased risk of lung cancer. This is (presumably) not because of any biological process linking the two, but because cigarette smoking, a major cause of lung cancer, tends to be more common among coffee drinkers than it is among individuals who do not drink coffee. Thus failure to take account of cigarette smoking in the analysis would result in an error of inference. If one were to stratify the study sample into smokers and nonsmokers and examine the association between lung cancer incidence and coffee consumption separately within each of these strata, it is likely that no association would be found in either. The disappearance of an association when analyses are stratified in this way is a reliable clue that the stratification variable is a bone fide confounder.

In general, confounding is study-specific, a product of a particular study design (i.e., sampling strategy) and is reflected in the pattern of covariance among exposures in the particular cohort assembled. The extent to which is it a problem will differ even among studies that share a focus on the same exposure and outcome. Confounding can lead to either a Type I error (by creating spurious association between an exposure and an outcome) or a Type II error (obscuring a true association). With regard to the latter, in one study of lead exposure and child development, children's blood lead levels and their social class standing were confounded in an unusual way (Wasserman, Liu, Lolacono et al., 1997). Because executives of a smelting operation were provided with exclusive housing in proximity to the smelter, the blood lead levels of their children were much higher than the levels of the children of smelter laborers, who lived father away and thus were less exposed to airborne lead from stack emissions. Because high social class was associated both with higher lead exposure and with higher IQ scores, the failure to adjust for social class resulted in an underestimate of the association between blood lead level and child IQ.

In a non-experimental study, confounding can be reduced, although rarely completely eliminated, at the time of study design, data analysis, or both. The choice depends partly on an investigator's prior knowledge about the patterns of association among the pertinent variables. Restricting the sample to individuals with the same value on a known confounder (e.g., gestational age, gender, social class, race) will reduce confounding by that variable, although it will restrict the opportunity to evaluate the extent to which the exposure–outcome association varies among strata of that variable (i.e., effect modification). Sample restriction can also limit the generalizability of study findings.

If confounding is addressed at the stage of data analysis, an investigator's choice is largely between stratification and multivariate modeling. Stratified analysis is straightforward but becomes less feasible when it is necessary to stratify simultaneously on several confounders. Multivariate modeling (e.g., multiple linear or logistic regression) permits estimation of an exposure–outcome association that is adjusted simultaneously for multiple confounders. In both approaches to regression, the coefficient assigned to the exposure of interest represents a conditional estimate of the association, that is conditional on adjustment for the other predictor variables included in the model. Linear regression methods are used when the dependent variable is continuously

distributed (e.g., $T$ score for Total Problems score on the Child Behavior Checklist). Logistic regression methods are used when the dependent variable is categorical and, most commonly, binary (e.g., when Total Problems score on the CBCL is classified as 'normal' or 'abnormal'). In linear regression, the coefficient assigned to a predictor represents the estimated change in the dependent variable for each unit change in the predictor. In logistic regression, the coefficient assigned to a predictor represents the natural logarithm of the odds of the outcome associated with each unit change in the predictor (i.e., ln odds ratio $= \beta$). Thus, the coefficient $\beta$ can be transformed to the more familiar form of an odds ratio or a relative risk, by raising e, the base of the natural logarithm (2.718), to the power $\beta$.

It is important to recognize the limitations of multivariate analysis. As Leon (1993) noted, "Results of epidemiologic studies often refer to 'adjusted effects' as if to imply that, the statistical wand having been waved, the adjusted estimates are free from confounding" (p. 479). Present-day computing resources make multivariate techniques easy to implement, but there are many pitfalls in their use. For example, most methods require rather strict and sometimes unrealistic assumptions about the univariate and joint distributions of the variables included in a model, their independence of one another, and their relationships with the outcome (i.e., additive in linear regression, multiplicative in logistic regression). The use of algorithms that add or delete variables from a regression model in stepwise fashion can be misleading because precision of estimation rather than validity is the criterion for variable selection (Kleinbaum, Kupper and Morgenstern, 1982). That is, such algorithms focus on the $p$-value of the association between a candidate variable and the outcome rather than on the impact that adjustment for that variable has on the association of primary interest. (This distinction is only relevant when the goal of model building is to adjust for confounding. When the goal is to identify the model that best predicts the outcome, variable selection methods based solely on $p$-values are appropriate.) Because a true confounder may not meet the $p$-value-based criterion for retention or inclusion in the model, a biased estimate of the association between the outcome and the exposure of interest may result. Head-to-head comparison of alternative approaches to confounder selection, using the criteria of power, bias, mean-squared error, and coverage of the confidence interval, suggests that under most circumstances, a 'change-in-estimate' criterion is superior to methods based solely on *p*-values. In such an approach, a variable is included in a multivariate model if its omission results in more than some specified change in the estimated coefficient of the exposure of interest (Mickey and Greenland, 1989). A 10% change rule is frequently applied. For instance, one might be interested in the association between parenting stress and children's adaptation. Assume that the crude coefficient for parenting stress, generated in a bivariate regression analysis, is 2.0, meaning that a unit change in parent stress is associated with a change of 2 units in the measure of childhood adaptation. In constructing a multivariate model using a 'change in estimate approach', the variables included in the model would be those that, when added to parenting stress in a multiple linear regression model, result in the parenting stress coefficient increasing to more than 2.20 or decreasing to 1.80 or less (i.e., changes of 10% or more). A potential drawback of this 'change in estimate' approach is that potential confounders are usually considered one at a time, whereas it is sometimes the joint presence of two or more additional variables that induces a substantial change in the effect estimate of primary interest. The amount of change that should be used as the criterion for variable selection is a matter of judgment, with the criterion selected representing an analyst's balancing of the relative costs associated with imprecision and bias in estimation.

Subject matter considerations are paramount in constructing multivariate models (Robins and Greenland, 1986). As noted, relying on inferential statistical tests (i.e., *p*-values) to select variables to be considered as potential confounders may result in invalid estimates (if bona fide confounders are overlooked) or less precise estimates if variables that are not true confounders are included in the model (Dales and Ury, 1978). If *p*-values are used, $\alpha$ should be considerably larger than the conventional 0.05 level, perhaps as large as 0.25, in order to avoid missing true confounders (Bellinger, Leviton, Waternaux and Allred, 1985; Mickey and Greenland, 1989). Requiring that the theoretical bases for including a variable in a model be made explicit may reduce the likelihood that an invalid model is proposed. An 'iatrogenic bias' (Bulterys and Morgenstern, 1993), will be introduced (and the probability of a Type II error increased) if a variable that is intermediate in a hypothetical causal pathway between an exposure and an outcome is treated as though it were simply a confounder and the association 'adjusted for' this variable. For instance, it is conventional in studies of low-level lead exposure and children's cognitive function to adjust for children's social class. Although lead exposure does tend to co-occur with other social class-related developmental risk factors, social class standing may be, to some extent, a proxy measure for lead exposure opportunities (e.g., housing with old lead-based paint in poor condition, proximity to industrial point sources). What is needed, therefore, is a way to distinguish these two components of the variance that social class shares with children's development, because adjustment should properly be made only for that portion that reflects risk factors other than lead (Bellinger et al., 1989). In practical terms, of course, this may be extremely difficult to accomplish.

The omission of a variable that does not meet the definition of a confounder will not bias estimation, but its inclusion in a model may be important if it is strongly associated with the outcome. By reducing substantially the amount of unexplained variance in the outcome, its inclusion will increase the power of the test of the main study hypothesis. Greene and Ernhart (1991) offered the example of a randomized trial evaluating the effect of a nutritional supplement on children's vigilance scores. Randomization produced equivalent distributions of child age in the two treatment groups, but vigilance scores increased significantly with child age. In crude analyses, the variability in vigilance scores attributable to child age obscured a beneficial effect of nutritional supplementation on scores. This was evident only when age was included in the regression model, allowing the supplement effect to be estimated with much greater precision.

### Missing data

It is almost inevitable that data will not be obtained from some subjects on key study variables, especially in the setting of a longitudinal design. Much has been written about how to approach this problem in the data analysis phase (Little and Rubin, 1989). Restricting analyses to subjects for whom complete data are available is inefficient and, because of the reduced sample size, is likely to result in less precise effect estimates. Of greater concern, however, is the fact that data are usually not missing 'at random', resulting in effect estimates that are biased, differing from those that would have been calculated based on 100% complete data. One commonly used method for addressing this problem is to include in regression models indicator variables that code 'missingness' on a given variable. Another method is to impute missing data using regression methods. The drawback of this approach, which essentially entails filling in average values calculated on the basis of the available data, is that the resulting standard errors of the estimated coefficients are smaller than they should be, increasing the likelihood of Type I errors. A variety of more sophisticated, computationally intensive, approaches have recently been developed, including multiple imputation methods, maximum likelihood methods, and weighted estimating equation methods (Greenland and Finkle, 1995).

## Causal inferences

The goal of much of epidemiological research is to identify antecedent conditions or events whose elimination or abatement would reduce the occurrence of disease or dysfunction. This requires that causal inferences be drawn from epidemiologic studies, most of which are observational in design rather than randomized clinical trials. Because of the large number of potential biases to which epidemiologic studies are subject, no study, by itself, can provide an adequate basis for concluding that Exposure A 'causes' Outcome X. Considerable thought, therefore, has been devoted to establishing guidelines for drawing causal inferences about an association from a collection of imperfect epidemiologic studies (Greenland, 1987). One approach focuses on the designs of the studies on which the evidence of an association is based, establishing a hierarchy of rigor (Sackett, Richardson, Rosenberg and Haynes, 1997). Sackett and colleagues, for instance, recognize five levels: (1) large randomized trials with results that

have a high degree of statistical certainty, (2) small randomized trials with results of low statistical certainty, (3) non-randomized prospective studies of concurrent treatment and control groups, (4) non-randomized historical cohort comparisons, and (5) case series that lack controls. This system clearly reflects its origins in clinical medicine and the need to evaluate alternative therapies for diseases such as hypertension and depression. It is less applicable to the behavioral sciences, where randomized trials are less often a reasonable option. The relative merit of alternative study designs is not absolute but situation-specific, so that a case-control design might be the best choice for pursuing one research question, a randomized trial the best choice for another, and a qualitative design the best choice for another (Sackett and Wennberg, 1997).

Hill (1965) offered an alternative approach to evaluating the likelihood that an observed association reflects a causal process. He recommended that nine aspects of the association be considered. At best, these should be viewed as heuristic rather than as hard-and-fast rules.

### Strength

The greater the increase in the risk of disease that is associated with an exposure, the less likely it is that a third variable, a confounder, is responsible for the association. Of course, a true causal exposure may produce only a modest increase in risk if there are many other factors that also cause the outcome. Thus, the strength criterion pertains more to the statistical aspects of the association than to its biological underpinnings.

### Consistency

Have different investigators observed a similar association in different populations at different times using different methodologies? If so, "we can justifiably infer that the association is not due to some constant error or fallacy that permeates every inquiry" (Hill, 1965, p. 296). On the other hand, a lack of consistency in findings across study settings cannot necessarily be interpreted as strong evidence that the association, when observed, is not causal insofar as disease occurrence generally reflects the joint influence of more than one component cause (Pearce, 1989; Rothman, 1986). The distribution of the other component causes may differ across settings, resulting in different degrees of association between the health endpoint and the exposure of primary interest.

## Specificity

Some rare outcomes occur almost exclusively in association with a particular exposure, such as the link, mentioned earlier, between occupational exposure to vinyl chloride and angiosarcoma of the liver. This tends to be the exception, however. Many common exposures, such as cigarette smoking and obesity, tend to be associated with multiple organ dysfunctions. There is no compelling logical reason why the breadth of an exposure's adverse effects on physiologic processes should affect the decision as to whether the link to any particular dysfunction reflects a causal process. For this reason, specificity tends to be accorded little weight in assessing whether an association is likely to reflect a causal association.

## Temporality

In order to conclude that an exposure caused an outcome, one must be confident that the exposure occurred before the outcome occurred. This is perhaps the most fundamental of Hill's criteria.

## Biological gradient

The hypothesis of a causal relationship is strengthened if the risk or severity of the outcome increases as exposure increases (i.e., a dose–response or dose–effect relationship). By itself, this does not implicate causality insofar as confounding could also account for an apparent dose–response. Moreover, the absence of dose–response cannot be interpreted as strong evidence against a causal relationship if the underlying biological mechanisms, including the threshold dose required to produce the response, are not well understood.

## Plausibility and coherence

The hypothesis of causality is supported if the association is consistent with existing biological knowl-

edge. This guideline also should not be given inordinate weight because what is biologically implausible today may become plausible as additional knowledge is accumulated. In 19th century London, John Snow identified water taken from the Broad Street pump as the likely source of a cholera epidemic long before the vibrio bacillus was identified as the water-borne pathogen that causes this disease.

## Analogy

Evidence that exposures similar to Exposure A cause outcomes similar to Outcome X may increase an investigator's willingness to accept the hypothesis that Exposure A causes Outcome X.

## Experiment

On rare occasions, it may be possible to study a 'natural' experiment, involving a reduction in the prevalence or intensity of the exposure in a given population. Correlated changes in the pattern of the outcome in this population may be interpreted as supporting a causal interpretation. Such data, referred to as 'ecologic', are considered to be weak insofar as, in contrast to the typical cohort study, information on exposure and outcome is known only at the population level rather than at the level of individual members of the population (Comstock, 1988). Moreover, other factors causally related to the outcome may also have changed over the same period. For instance it is difficult to answer the question of whether children's SAT scores increased as population exposures to the neurotoxicant lead declined over the last two decades as the use of lead as a gasoline additive was phased out. This is because many other societal changes that could plausibly affect SAT scores also occurred over this period and are thus confounded with the changes in lead exposure.

Even rarer in child neuropsychology are true experiments or randomized clinical trials. Such studies generally involve the use of child development as endpoints in the evaluation of new treatment or intervention modalities (e.g., Bellinger et al., 1999; McCarton, Brooks-Gunn, Wallace et al., 1997; TLC Trial Group, 1998).

## Conclusion

With respect to the small clinical investigations that are typical of research studies in child neuropsychology, greater attention to issues such as the representativeness and comparability of patient and control groups and the adequacy of sample size will return dividends in the form of increased study validity and generalizability. Epidemiologists are trained to draw attention to potential biases and weaknesses in study design and execution. Among the many jokes about this field is one that goes, 'Show me a child who is a nit-picker and I'll show you a child at risk of becoming an epidemiologist'. In evaluating a study, it is important to go beyond identifying potential weaknesses to consider whether they are sufficiently important to invalidate the study results. Usually this is accomplished by means of qualitative analysis or expert judgment, the results of which are likely to be affected by the expert's own biases regarding the phenomenon under study. Greenland (1996) recently described some simple methods for approaching this process on a more quantitative basis. These methods essentially correspond to sensitivity analyses in which the key analyses are repeated incorporating a range of assumptions about the extent of confounding by unmeasured variables, or about the extent of error in the classification or measurement of exposure and disease. Using such an approach, one can determine how large the association between a disease and some potential but unmeasured confounder would have to be in order to account completely for an observed association between the disease and the exposure of interest. With respect to misclassification, one can recalculate the associations of interest assuming different values for the sensitivity and specificity of the exposure and disease measurements. The results should effectively bracket the 'truth' by providing the range of plausible outcomes. These methods are conceptually similar to those used in meta-analysis to evaluate publication bias, the 'file drawer problem', whereby one calculates the number of unpublished studies with null findings that would have to exist in order to render the association of interest nonsignificant (Rosenthal, 1979).

In the end, of course, the methods Greenland describes only improve the quality of the data summaries that provide the basis for drawing inferences. There is no substitute for sound scientific judgment.

## Acknowledgements

Preparation of this chapter was supported, in part, by grants P50 HD33803, P30 HD33803, and MCJ009163010.

## References

Achenbach T: Manual for the Child Behavior Checklist/4-18 and 1991 Profile. Burlington: University of Vermont, Department of Psychiatry, 1991.

American Psychiatric Association: Diagnostic and Statistical Manual of Mental Disorders, 2nd ed. (DSM-II). Washington, DC: American Psychiatric Association, 1968.

American Psychiatric Association: Diagnostic and Statistical Manual of Mental Disorders, 3rd ed. (DSM-III). Washington, DC: American Psychiatric Association, 1980.

American Psychiatric Association: Diagnostic and Statistical Manual of Mental Disorders (3rd ed. revised). Washington, DC, 1987: American Psychiatric Association, 1987.

American Psychiatric Association: Diagnostic and Statistical Manual of Mental Disorders, 4th ed. (DSM-IV). Washington, DC: American Psychiatric Association, 1994.

Anderson J, Williams S, McGee R, Silva P: DSM-III disorders in preadolescent children. Archives of General Psychiatry: 44; 69–76, 1987.

Angold A, Costello E, Erkanli A: Comorbidity. Journal of Child Psychology and Psychiatry: 40; 57–87, 1999.

Aylward G, Hatcher R, Stripp B, Gustafson N, Leavitt L: Who goes and who stays: subject loss in a multicenter, longitudinal follow-up study. Journal of Developmental and Behavioral Pediatrics: 6; 3–8, 1985.

Badawi N, Watson L, Petterson B, Blair E, Slee J, Haan E, Stanley F: What constitutes cerebral palsy? Developmental Medicine and Child Neurology: 40; 520–527, 1998.

Barkley R, Fischer M, Newby R, Breen M: Development of a multimethod clinical protocol for assessing stimulant drug response in children with attention deficit disorder. Journal of Clinical Child Psychology: 17; 14–24, 1988.

Baumgaertel A, Wolraich M, Dietrich M: Comparison of diagnostic criteria for attention deficit disorders in a German elementary school sample. Journal of the American Academy of Child and Adolescent Psychiatry: 34; 629–638, 1995.

Bellinger D: Effect modification in epidemiologic studies of low-level neurotoxicant exposures and health outcomes. Neurotoxicology and Teratolgy: 22; 133–140, 2000.

Bellinger D, Leviton A, Waternaux C: Lead, IQ, and social class. International Journal of Epidemiology: 18; 180–185, 1989.

Bellinger D, Leviton A, Waternaux C, Allred E: Methodological issues in modeling the relationship between low-level lead exposure and infant development: Examples from the Boston Lead Study. Environmental Research: 38; 119–129, 1985.

Bellinger D, Leviton A, Sloman J: Antecedents and correlates of improved cognitive performance in children exposed in utero to low levels of lead. Environmental Health Perspectives: 89; 5–11, 1990.

Bellinger D, Stiles K: Epidemiologic approaches to assessing the developmental toxicity of lead. Neurotoxicology: 14; 151–160, 1993.

Bellinger D, Wypij D, Kuban K, Rapaport L, Hickey P, Wernovsky G, Jonas R, Newburger J: Developmental and neurologic status of children at four years of age after heart surgery with hypothermic circulatory arrest or low-flow cardiopulmonary bypass. Circulation: 100; 526–532, 1999.

Betan E, Roberts M, McCluskey-Fawcett K: Rates of participation for clinical child and pediatric psychology research: Issues in methodology. Journal of Clinical Child Psychology: 24; 227–235, 1995.

Biederman J, Faraone S, Doyle A, Lehman K, Kraus I, Perrin J, Tsuang M: Convergence of the child behavior checklist with structured interview-based psychiatric diagnoses of ADHD children with and without comorbidity. Journal of Child Psychology and Psychiatry: 34; 1241–1251, 1993.

Bornschein R, Grote J, Mitchell T, Succop P, Dietrich K, Krafft K, Hammond P: Effects of prenatal lead exposure on infant size at birth. In Smith M, Grant L, Sors A (Eds), Lead Exposure and Child Development: An International Assessment. Boston, MA: Kluwer, pp. 307–319, 1989.

Boyle M, Pickles A: Strategies to manipulate reliability: Impact on statistical associations. Journal of the American Academy of Child and Adolescent Psychiatry: 37; 1077–1084, 1998.

Bryson S, Clark B, Smith I: First report of a Canadian epidemiological study of autistic syndromes. Journal of Child Psychology and Psychiatry: 29; 433–435, 1988.

Bulterys M, Morgenstern H: Confounding or intermediate effect? An appraisal of iatrogenic bias in perinatal AIDS research. Paediatric and Perinatal Epidemiology: 7; 387–394, 1993.

Bussing R, Zima B, Perwein A, Belin T, Widawski M: Children in special education programs: Attention deficit hyperactivity disorder, use of services, and unmet needs. American Journal of Public Health: 88; 800–886, 1998.

Carlson G, Kashani J, Thomas M, Valdya A, Daniel A: Comparison of two structured interviews on a psychiatrically hospitalized population of children. Journal of the American Academy of Child and Adolescent Psychiatry: 26; 645–648, 1987.

Chapman L, Chapman J: The measurement of differential deficit. Journal of Psychiatric Research: 14; 303–311, 1978.

Charter R: Effect of measurement error on tests of statistical significance. Journal of Clinical and Experimental Neuropsychology: 19; 458–462, 1997.

Chen W, Faraone S, Biederman J, Tsuang M: Diagnostic accuracy of the child behavior checklist scales for Attention-Deficit Hyperactivity Disorder: A receiver-operating characteristic analysis. Journal of Consulting and Clinical Psychology: 62; 1017–1025, 1994.

Chouinard M-J, Braun C: A meta-analysis of the relative sensitivity of neuropsychological screening tests. Journal of Clinical and Experimental Neuropsychology: 591–607, 1993.

Clark A, Harrington R: On diagnosing rare disorders rarely: Appropriate use of screening instruments. Journal of Child Psychology and Psychiatry: 40; 287–290, 1999.

Cohen J: Things I have learned (so far). American Psychologist: 45; 1304–1312, 1990.

Cohen P, Cohen J: The clinician's illusion. Archives of General Psychiatry: 41; 1178–1182, 1984.

Comstock G: Soft water/hard arteries: An interpretation of ecologic findings. In Gordis L (Ed.) Epidemiology and Health Risk Assessment. New York: Oxford University Press, pp. 248–255, 1988.

Coughlin S: Recall bias in epidemiologic studies. Journal of Clinical Epidemiology: 43; 87–91, 1990.

Dales L, Ury H: An improper use of statistical significance testing in studying covariables. International Journal of Epidemiology: 4; 373–375, 1978.

Edelbrock C, Costello A, Dulcan M, Kalas R, Conover N: Age differences in the reliability of the psychiatric interview of the child. Child Development: 56; 256–275, 1985.

Ehlers S, Gillberg C: The epidemiology of Asperger syndrome. Journal of Child and Adolescent Psychology and Psychiatry and Allied Disciplines: 34; 1327–1350, 1993.

Ellenberg J: Selection bias in observational and experimental studies. Statistics in Medicine: 13; 557–567, 1994.

Ellenberg J, Nelson K: Sample selection and the natural history of disease: Studies of febrile seizures. Journal of the American Medical Association: 243; 1337–1340, 1980.

Elwood M: Critical Appraisal of Epidemiological Studies and Clinical Trials, 2nd ed. New York: Oxford University Press, 1998.

Espy K, Kaufmann P, Glisky M: Neuropsychological function in toddlers exposed to cocaine in utero: A preliminary study. Developmental Neuropsychology: 15; 447–460, 1999.

Feinleib M: Biases and weak associations. Preventive Medicine: 16; 150–164, 1987.

Fombonne E: Is the prevalence of autism increasing? Journal of Autism and Developmental Disorders: 26; 673–676, 1996.

Fombonne E, Du Mazaubrun C: Prevalence of infantile autism in four French regions. Social Psychiatry and Psychiatric Epidemiology: 27; 203–210, 1992.

Fombonne E, Du Mazaubrun C, Cans C, Grandjean H: Autism and associated medical disorders in a French epidemiological survey. Journal of the American Academy of Child and Adolescent Psychiatry: 36; 1561–1569, 1997.

Gillberg C, Steffenburg S, Schaumann H: Is autism more common now than ten years ago? British Journal of Psychiatry: 158: 403–409, 1991.

Goodman R, Yude C: Do incomplete ascertainment and recruitment matter? A study of childhood hemiplegia. Developmental Medicine and Child Neurology: 38; 156–165, 1996.

Gordis L: Epidemiology. Philadelphia, PA: W.B. Saunders Company, 1996.

Greene T, Ernhart C: Adjustment for cofactors in pediatric research. Journal of Developmental and Behavioral Pediatrics: 12; 378–386, 1991.

Greenland S: Evolution of Epidemiologic Ideas: Annotated Readings on Concepts and Methods. Chestnut Hill, MA: Epidemiology Resources Inc., 1987.

Greenland S: Basic methods for sensitivity analysis of biases. International Journal of Epidemiology: 25; 1107–1116, 1996.

Greenland S, Finkle W: A critical look at methods for handling missing covariates in epidemiologic regression analyses. American Journal of Epidemiology: 142; 1255–1264, 1995.

Hazell P, Carr V, Lewin T, Dewis S, Heathcote D, Brucki B: Effortful and automatic information processing in boys with ADHD and specific learning disorders. Journal of Child Psychology and Psychiatry: 40: 275–286, 1999.

Herndon R: Is Alexander's Disease a nosologic entity or a common pathologic pattern of diverse etiology? Journal of Child Neurology: 14; 275–276, 1999.

Hill A: The environment and disease: association or causation? Proceedings of the Royal Society of Medicine: 58; 295–300, 1965.

Honda H, Shimizu H, Misumi K, Niimi M, Ohashi Y: Cumulative incidence and prevalence of childhood autism in children in Japan. British Journal of Psychiatry: 169; 228–235, 1996.

Joffe M, Grisso J: Comparison of antenatal hospital records with retrospective interviewing. Journal of Biosocial Science: 17; 113–119, 1985.

Kanner L: Autistic disturbances of affective contact. Nervous Child: 2; 217–250, 1943.

Kelsey J, Whittemore A, Evans A, Thompson D: Methods in Observational Epidemiology, 2nd ed. New York: Oxford University Press, 1996.

Kessler R, McGonagle K, Zhao S, Nelson C, Hughes M, Eshleman S, Wittchen H, Kendler K: Lifetime and 12-month prevalence of DSM-III-R psychiatric disorders in the United States. Archives of General Psychiatry: 51; 8–19, 1994.

Kleinbaum D, Kupper L, Morgenstern H: Epidemiologic Research: Principles and Quantitative Methods. Toronto, ON: Lifetime Learning Publications, 1982.

Kraemer H: Evaluating Medical Tests. London: Sage Publications, 1992.

Kramer M, Boivin J-F: Toward an 'unconfounded' classification of epidemiologic research design. Journal of Chronic Disease: 40; 683–688, 1987.

Lahey B, Applegate B, McBurnett K, Biederman J, Greenhill L, Hynd G, Barkley R, Newcorn J, Jensen P, Richters J, Garfinkle B, Kerdyk L, Frick P, Ollendick T, Perez D, Hart E, Waldman I, Shaffer D: DSM-IV field trials for attention deficit hyperactivity disorder in children and adolescents. American Journal of Psychiatry: 151; 1673–1685, 1994.

Larroque B, Kaminski M, Bouvier-Colle M-H, Hollebecque V: Participation in a mail survey: Role of repeated mailings and characteristics of nonrespondents among recent mothers. Paediatric and Perinatal Epidemiology: 13; 218–233, 1999.

Last J: A Dictionary of Epidemiology, 2nd ed. New York: Oxford University Press, 1988.

Leon D: Failed or misleading adjustment for confounding. Lancet: 342; 479–481, 1993.

Lindsay R, Tomazic T, Whitman B, Accardo P: Early ear problems and developmental problems at school age. Clinical Pediatrics: 38; 123–132, 1999.

Little R, Rubin D: Statistical Analysis with Missing Data. New York: Wiley, 1989.

Lovaas O: Behavioral treatment and normal education and intellectual functioning in young autistic children. Journal of Consulting Clinical Psychology: 55; 3–9, 1987.

Lovaas O, Smith T, McEachin J: Clarifying comments on the young autism study: Reply to Schopler. Journal of Consulting and Clinical Psychology: 57; 165–167, 1989.

Lubin J, Gail M: On power and sample size for studying features of the relative odds of disease. American Journal of Epidemiology: 131; 552–556, 1990.

MacMahon B, Trichopoulos D: Epidemiology: Principles and Methods, 2nd ed. Boston, MA: Little, Brown and Company, 1996.

Mason A, Banerjee S, Eapen V, Zeitlin H, Robertson M: The prevalence of Tourette syndrome in a mainstream school population. Developmental Medicine and Child Neurology: 40; 292–296, 1998.

MacMahon B, Pugh TF: Epidemiology: Principles and Methods. Boston: Little, Brown and Company, 1970.

Mayes L, Cicchetti D: Prenatal cocaine exposure and neurobehavioral development: How subjects lost to follow-up bias study results. Child Neuropsychology: 1; 128–139, 1995.

Mayes L, Kirk V, Haywood N, Buchanan D, Hedvall G, Stahlman M: Changing cognitive outcome in preterm infants with hyaline membrane disease. American Journal of Diseases of Children: 139; 20–24, 1985.

McBurnett K, Pfiffner L, Willcutt E, Tamm L, Lerner M, Ottolini Y, Furman M: Experimental cross-validation of DSM-IV types of attention-deficit/hyperactivity disorder. Journal of the American Academy of Child and Adolescent Psychiatry: 38; 17–24, 1999.

McCarton C, Brooks-Gunn J, Wallace I, Bauer C, Bennett F, Bernbaum J, Broyles R, Casey P, McCormick M, Scott D, Tyson J, Tonascia J, Meinert C: Results at age 8 years of early intervention for low-birth-weight premature infants. Journal of the American Medical Association: 277; 126–132, 1997.

McEachin J, Smith-Tristram T, Lovaas I: Long-term outcome for children with autism who received early intensive behavioral treatment. American Journal of Mental Retardation: 97; 359–372, 1993.

McKinlay S: Pair matching — a reappraisal of a popular technique. Biometrics: 33; 725–735, 1977.

Mickey R, Greenland S: The impact of confounder selection criteria on effect estimation. American Journal of Epidemiology: 129; 125–137, 1989.

Milberger S, Biederman J, Faraone S, Chen L, Jones J: Is maternal smoking during pregnancy a risk factor for attention deficit hyperactivity disorder in children? American Journal of Psychiatry: 153; 1138–1142, 1996.

Milberger S, Biederman J, Faraone S, Guite J, Tsuang M: Pregnancy, delivery and infancy complications and attention deficit hyperactivity disorder: Issues of gene-environment interactions. Biological Psychiatry: 41; 65–75, 1997.

Minder B, Das-Smaal E, Orlebeke J: Cognition in children does not suffer from very low lead exposure. Journal of Learning Disabilities: 31; 494–502, 1998.

Mutch L, Alberman E, Hagberg B, Kodama K, Perat M: Cerebral palsy epidemiology: Where are we and where are we going?

Developmental Medicine and Child Neurology: 34; 547–555, 1992.

Noll R, Zeller M, Vannatta K, Bukowski W, Davies W: Potential bias in classroom research: Comparison of children with permission and those who do not receive permission to participate. Journal of Clinical Child Psychology: 26; 36–42, 1997.

Pearce N: Analytical implications of epidemiologic concepts of interaction. International Journal of Epidemiology: 17; 976–980, 1989.

Pennington BF, Ozonoff S: Executive functions and developmental psychopathology. Journal of Child Psychology and Psychiatry: 37; 51–87, 1996.

Raju T, Langenberg P, Sen A, Aldana O: How much 'better' is good enough? American Journal of Diseases in Children: 146; 407–411, 1992.

Rapin I: Autism in search of a home in the brain. Neurology: 52; 902–904, 1999.

Rey J, Morris-Yates A, Stainslaw H: Measuring the accuracy of diagnostic tests using receiver operating characteristics (ROC) analysis. International Journal of Methods in Psychiatric Research: 2; 39–50, 1992.

Robins J: The control of confounding by intermediate variables. Statistics in Medicine: 8; 679–701, 1989.

Robins J, Greenland S: The role of model selection in causal inference from nonexperimental data. American Journal of Epidemiology: 123; 392–402, 1986.

Roeleveld N, Zielhuis G, Gabreels F: The prevalence of mental retardation: A critical review of the literature. Developmental Medicine and Child Neurology: 39; 125–132, 1997.

Rosenthal R: The 'file drawer problem' and tolerance for null results. Psychological Bulletin: 86; 638–641, 1979.

Rothman K: Modern Epidemiology. Boston, MA: Little, Brown and Company, 1986.

Rothman K, Poole C: A programme for strengthening weak associations. International Journal of Epidemiology: 319; 955–959, 1988.

Rothman K, Greenland S: Modern Epidemiology, 2nd ed. Philadelphia, PA: Lippincott-Raven, 1998.

Rutter M, Gould M: Classification. In Rutter M, Hersov L (Eds), Child and Adolescent Psychiatry, 2nd ed. Boston, MA: Blackwell, pp. 304–321, 1985.

Rutter M, Yule W: The concept of specific-reading retardation. Journal of Child Psychology and Psychiatry: 16; 181–197, 1975.

Sackett D: Bias in analytic research. Journal of Chronic Disease: 32; 51–63, 1979.

Sackett D, Richardson W, Rosenberg W, Haynes R: Evidence-Based Medicine: How to Practice and Teach EBM. New York: Churchill and Livingstone, 1997.

Sackett D, Wennberg J: Choosing the best research design for each question. British Medical Journal: 315; 1636, 1997.

Schwartz S, Link B: The 'well control' artefact in case/control studies of specific psychiatric disorders. Psychological Medicine: 19; 737–742, 1989.

Shaywitz S, Shaywitz B, Fletcher J, Escobar M: Prevalence of reading disability in boys and girls: Results of the Connecticut Longitudinal Study. Journal of the American Medical Association: 264; 998–1002, 1990.

Shaywitz S, Escobar M, Shaywitz B, Fletcher J, Makuch R: Evidence that dyslexia may represent the lower tail of a normal distribution of reading ability. New England Journal of Medicine: 326; 145–150, 1992.

Shekim W, Cantwell D, Kashani J, Beck N, Martin J, Rosenberg J: Dimensional and categorical approaches to the diagnosis of attention deficit disorder in children. Journal of the American Academy of Child Psychiatry: 25; 653–658, 1986.

Soper H, Cicchetti D, Satz P, Light R, Orsini D: Null hypothesis disrespect in neuropsychology: Dangers of alpha and beta errors. Journal of Clinical and Experimental Neuropsychology: 10; 255–270, 1988.

Sorohan T, Gilthorpe M: Non-differential misclassification of exposure always leads to an underestimate of risk: An incorrect conclusion. Occupational and Environmental Medicine: 51; 839–840, 1994.

Sponheim E, Skjeldal O: Autism and related disorders: epidemiological findings in a Norwegian study using ICD-10 diagnostic criterion. Journal of Autism and Related Disorders: 28; 217–227, 1998.

Stein R, Bauman L, Ireys H: Who enrolls in prevention trials? Discordance in perception of risk by professionals and participants. American Journal of Community Psychology: 19; 603–617, 1991.

Stein REK, Westbrook LE, Silver EJ: Comparison of adjustment of school-age children with and without chronic conditions: Results from community-based samples. Journal of Developmental and Behavioral Pediatrics: 19; 267–272, 1998.

Steingard R, Biederman J, Doyle A, Sprich-Buckminster S: Psychiatric comorbidity in attention deficit disorder: Impact on the interpretation of Child Behavior Checklist results. Journal of the American Academy of Child and Adolescent Psychiatry: 31; 449–454, 1992.

Strauss M, Allred L: Methodological issues in detecting specific long-term consequences of perinatal drug exposure. Neurobehavioral Toxicology and Teratology: 8; 369–375, 1986.

Szatmari P: The epidemiology of Attention-Deficit Hyperactivity disorders. Child and Adolescent Psychiatric Clinics of North America: 1; 361–371, 1992.

Tannock R: Attention Deficit Hyperactivity Disorder: Advances in cognitive, neurobiological, and genetic research. Journal of Child Psychology and Psychiatry: 39; 65–99, 1998.

Tannock R, Fine J, Heintz T, Schachar R: A linguistic approach detects stimulant effects in two children with attention deficit hyperactivity disorder. Journal of Child and Adolescent Psychopharmacology: 5; 177–189, 1995.

Tannock R, Ickowicz A, Schachar R: Differential effects of methylphenidate on working memory in ADHD children with and without comorbid anxiety. Journal of the American Academy of Child and Adolescent Psychiatry: 34; 886–888, 1995.

Tanoue Y, Oda S, Asano F, Kawashima K: Epidemiology of infantile autism in southern Ibaraki, Japan: Differences in prevalence birth cohorts. Journal of Autism and Developmental Disorders: 18; 155–166, 1988.

Thomas S, Chess S, Birch H: Distortions in developmental reporting made by parents of behaviorally disturbed children. Journal of the American Academy of Child Psychiatry: 5; 226–234, 1966.

Thomas J, Graham J: Chromosome 22q11 Deletion syndrome: An update and review for the primary pediatrician. Clinical Pediatrics: 36; 253–266, 1997.

Tilley B, Barnes A, Bergstralh E, Labarthe D, Noller K, Colton T, Adam E: A comparison of pregnancy history recall and medical records. American Journal of Epidemiology: 121; 269–281, 1985.

Treatment of Lead-exposed Children Trial Group: The Treatment of Lead-exposed Children (TLC) trial: Design and recruitment for a study of the effect of oral chelation on growth and development in toddlers. Paediatric and Perinatal Epidemiology: 12; 313–333, 1998.

Velez C, Johnson J, Cohen P: A longitudinal analysis of selected risk factors for childhood psychopathology. Journal of the American Academy of Child and Adolescent Psychiatry: 28; 861–864, 1989.

Vestbo J, Rasmussen F: Baseline characteristics are not sufficient indicators of non-response bias in follow-up studies. Journal of Epidemiology and Community Health: 46; 617–619, 1992.

Wasserman G, Liu X, Lolacono N, Factor-Litvak P, Kline J, Popovac D, Morina N, Musabegovic A, Vrenezi N, Capuni-Paracka S, Lekic V, Preteni-Redjepi E, Hadzialjevic S, Slavkovich V, Graziano J: Lead exposure and intelligence in 7-year-old children: The Yugoslavia Prospective Study. En-vironmental Health Perspectives: 105; 956–962, 1997.

Waters W: The epidemiological enigma of migraine. Journal of Epidemiology: 2; 189–194, 1973.

Webb E, Lobo S, Hervas A, Scourfield J, Fraser W: The changing prevalence of autistic disorder in a Welsh health district. Developmental Medicine and Child Neurology: 39; 150–152, 1997.

Weiler M, Waber D, Bellinger D, Marmor J, Wypij D, Rancier S: Mother and teacher reports of ADHD symptoms: DSM-IV questionnaire data. Journal of the American Academy of Child and Adolescent Psychiatry: 38; 1139–1147, 1999.

Welner Z, Reich W, Herjanic B, Jung K, Amado H: Reliability, validity, and parent–child agreement studies of the Diagnostic Interview for Children and Adolescents (DICA). Journal of the American Academy of Child and Adolescent Psychiatry: 26; 649–653, 1987.

Williams K, Alberman E: The impact of diagnostic labeling in population-based research into cerebral palsy. Developmental Medicine and Child Neurology: 40; 182–185, 1998.

Wolraich M, Hannah J, Pinnock T, Baumgaertel A: Comparison of diagnostic criteria for attention-deficit hyperactivity disorder in a county-wide sample. Journal of the American Academy of Child and Adolescent Psychiatry: 35; 319–324, 1996.

Zarins D, Suarez A, Pincus H, Kupersanin E, Zito J: Clinical and treatment characteristics of children with attention-deficit/hyperactivity disorder in psychiatric practice. Journal of the American Academy of Child and Adolescent Psychiatry: 37; 1262–1270, 1998.

*Handbook of Neuropsychology*, 2nd Edition, Vol. 8, Part I
S.J. Segalowitz and I. Rapin (Eds)

CHAPTER 5

# Electrophysiology in developmental neuropsychology

Mitchell Steinschneider [a,b,*] and Michelle Dunn [a]

[a] *Department of Neurology, Rose F. Kennedy Center, Albert Einstein College of Medicine, Bronx, NY 10461, USA*
[b] *Department of Neuroscience, Rose F. Kennedy Center, Albert Einstein College of Medicine, Bronx, NY 10461, USA*

## Introduction: concepts and methods in developmental neuropsychology

It is a testament to the explosive growth in developmental neuropsychology that recent advances pertaining to the use of event-related potentials (ERP), event-related magnetic fields (ERMF) and the electroencephalogram (EEG) cannot be thoroughly summarized in a single chapter. Instead, key issues related to their use will be stressed, and some of the major findings utilizing these techniques highlighted. Two main themes will dominate this chapter. The first emphasizes that the design and implementation of ERP/ERMF studies must incorporate evolving concepts of brain organization and development in order to maximize its relevance to the field of cognitive neuroscience. The second, intimately interwoven with the first, promotes the benefits of interpreting ERP studies in light of integrated results acquired from other physiological and psychological disciplines. Too often, ERP studies can be criticized for 'preaching to the choir', interpreting results and formulating hypotheses solely in the light of similar work. Limiting the audience of these studies, and failing to discuss ERP results in a broader neuroscience context, dampens the enthusiasm for these techniques by researchers in allied fields. This is unfortunate, because many of the evolving concepts in cognitive neuroscience emphasize the importance of coordinated activity by widely distributed neuronal ensembles, a subject that is highly suited for non-invasive, electrophysiological analysis. Equally important, cognitive neuropsychology needs to embrace the ramifications of the revolutionary advances in molecular neurobiological knowledge related to normal and aberrant brain and cognitive development.

*Importance of distributed neural networks for relating brain activity to perception, cognition and memory*

A key concept of brain organization that must be appreciated for electrophysiological studies of development is that sensory perception and cognitive functions are derived from the activity of distributed networks of neurons located both within and across functional and cytoarchitectonic fields (e.g., Bartels and Zeki, 1998). In the visual system, which is the most extensively studied sensory system, this organization is broadly divided into two processing streams: a dorsal, or parietal stream, that is intimately involved in the processing of spatial information, motion and eye movements, and a ventral, or temporal stream, that is specialized for perception of the form and color of objects (e.g., Tootell, Dale, Sereno and Malach, 1996). This organization predicts that perception of visual objects, and even the basic attributes making up these objects (e.g., color, form, location, motion and depth), requires the long-range interaction of neuronal ensembles spanning multiple brain regions (e.g., Spillmann and

* Corresponding author. Tel.: +1 (718) 430-4115; Fax: +1 (718) 430-8588; E-mail: steinsch@aecom.yu.edu

Werner, 1996). These phenomena are likely based on several mechanisms that include converging feed-forward projections onto higher brain centers, with the development of new and more complex stimulus dimension maps, and feedback connections that may help associate the higher-order responses with cellular activity pertaining to more specific stimulus features represented in lower centers (e.g., Spillmann and Werner, 1996).

These considerations have profound implications for developmental ERP studies. The extensive cortical activation that occurs during even basic sensory processing requires that these studies identify ERP components emanating from the different brain regions. Synchronization of higher-order activity with that of lower-level sensory centers, which subserves the process of binding multiple stimulus attributes into a single perceptual object (Spillmann and Werner, 1996), complicates the problem, as a strictly hierarchically arranged sequence of ERP components generated by primary, secondary and finally tertiary areas becomes untenable. Thus, developmental ERP studies must incorporate technical advances that assist in the spatial and temporal dissection of the brain potentials contributed by each activated brain region. Unfortunately, most studies to date have focused primarily on peak latency and amplitude measurements obtained from only a limited number of electrode sites. This precludes a detailed analysis of the neural activity patterns predicted by complementary studies using functional neuroimaging techniques and those obtained in experimental animals. Clarification of relevant neural mechanisms associated with cognitive development, and studied by ERPs, will be severely encumbered until these concerns are adequately addressed.

*The importance of dynamic brain development for ERP studies*

The difficulties enunciated above are compounded in developmental neuropsychology by the obvious fact that brain development is a dynamic state, and thus it is not necessarily appropriate to extrapolate ERP findings obtained in adults to those acquired at younger ages. First, marked changes occur at the anatomical level of development, indicating that the interpretation of brain potentials observed at one age

may not be applicable to those obtained at another. For instance, while the volume of primary visual cortex (V1, area 17) reaches adult values by 4 months of age, synaptic density continues to rapidly rise until 8 months of age and subsequently decreases (Huttenlocher, De Courten, Garey and Van Der Loos, 1982). Because ERP amplitude is influenced by both generator size and the number of synaptic potentials activated within that generator, visual-evoked potentials (VEPs) will reflect a complex summation of both these developmentally changing factors. Visual cortical values cannot be extrapolated to other regions, as synaptic density within primary auditory cortex (Heschl's gyrus) reaches peak values at 3 months postnatal age, and that occurring in portions of prefrontal cortex do not reach peak synaptic density levels until after 15 months (Huttenlocher and Dabholkar, 1997). Net synapse elimination also varies across regions, and is completed by 12 years of age in auditory cortex but continues until mid-adolescence in prefrontal areas. Concurrent with these changes are additional features of axonal and dendritic growth and subcortical myelination that will alter the timing and patterns of brain potentials. Moreover, since learning modulates not only the strength of specific synaptic connections but even transforms the spatio-temporal patterns of receptive field maps (e.g., Cruikshank and Weinberger, 1996; Kilgard and Merzenich, 1998; Recanzone, Schreiner and Merzenich, 1993; Weinberger, 1997), it becomes evident that ERP studies must incorporate longitudinal testing in order to better assess the maturational changes that occur with development.

Newer conceptual frameworks, which are partly driven by the progress made in molecular biology, amplify the importance of longitudinal studies in developmental neuropsychology. Cognitive neuropsychology typically involves inferring normal cognitive functions from analysis of patterns observed in subjects with dysfunctional brain processes (Bishop, 1997; Temple, 1997). Cognitive functions are envisioned as being based on innately pre-programmed modules, with a module defined as a brain system responsible for the rapid and rather automatic processing associated with a specific cognitive operation. Detailed analysis of cognitive capacities and deficiencies in individuals with acquired brain damage help define the nature of the processing modules. Much of the groundwork for developmental neuropsychology is based on this view of intrinsic modularity in brain function (Temple, 1997).

However, newer frameworks stress that these acquired disorders are inadequate models of normal and abnormal developmental neuropsychological constructs (see Bishop, 1997; Karmiloff-Smith, 1998). In contrast to focusing on ideas that modules are pre-programmed innate systems, and that primary causes of deficits can be identified through the patterns of subject deficits, these modern models argue that elementary features of biology interact with development itself to mold the phenotypical outcomes. Many of the developmental disorders most avidly studied, such as developmental language disorders and attention deficit–hyperactivity disorder (ADHD), have, at least in part, a genetic component. The genetic defect, in turn, will cause production of a gene product abnormal in quality or quantity. It is unrealistic to assume that these primary causes, which result in defects of essential building blocks for cell structure and function, could be discerned from the ultimate cognitive deficit patterns (Flint, 1999). Further, the development of normal pathways and circuits would be likewise specified by the complex interactions of genetically determined biological constraints with the environment through experience.

This controversy is most apparent in the theories surrounding developmental language disorders (DLD). At one extreme are theories based on phonological processing deficits inherent in language-specific modules (for review see Rosen, 1999). At another extreme are theories that basic sensory–motor deficits pertaining to the rapid temporal processing of sensory information, and the production of rapid sequential movements, underlie the deficits seen in DLD (e.g., Tallal, 1999; Tallal, Miller and Fitch, 1993; Tallal, Merzenich, Miller and Jenkins, 1998; Wright, Lombardino, King et al., 1997). While a thorough critique of this controversy is beyond the scope of this chapter (e.g., see Bishop, Carlyon, Deeks and Bishop, 1999b; Cacace and McFarland, 1998; Studdert-Kennedy and Mody, 1995), it is likely that the complexity of language development allows for multiple different combinations of biological or environmental deficits to be responsible for DLD, and that one subset of this broadly based ab-

normality is associated with deficiencies in rapid temporal processing of sensory stimuli (Bishop, Bishop, Bright et al., 1999a; Dougherety, Cynader, Bjornson et al., 1998; Hari and Kiesilä, 1996; Heath, Hogben and Clark, 1999; Helenius, Utuela and Hari, 1999a). A key unresolved question is whether temporal processing deficiencies are causal for DLD, or whether they represent a parallel deficit in additional sensory/motor tasks (Rosen, 1999). Furthermore, the specific temporal processing deficits might abate as compensatory brain mechanisms are constructed, leaving behind language-processing abnormalities that are more resistant to change (Bishop, 1997; Karmiloff-Smith, 1998). These considerations highlight the importance of longitudinal ERP studies, as examination in only older age children might fail to observe abnormalities in basic sensory processing that would be evident in the youngest age groups.

## Event-related potentials: definition and classification

ERPs result from the net electrical activity of neuronal ensembles time-locked to an externally observable event, such as a stimulus or a motor response. While certain potentials can occasionally be observed superimposed upon the on-going EEG recorded from scalp electrodes, ERPs generally require averaging a number of EEG samples time-locked to the observed event in order to be visualized. When the background EEG is randomly related to the event and the ERPs are stable in waveform, then the signal-to-noise ratio is improved in proportion to the square root of the number of averaged epochs. Sufficient averaging allows even very small signals, on the order of a fraction of a microvolt, to be recorded reliably. This resolution enables the synchronized activity of far-field brainstem structures to be accurately obtained from scalp electrodes, and forms the basis for the clinically important brainstem auditory and somatosensory potentials. In contrast, most cortical potentials of interest are an order of magnitude larger than their brainstem counterparts and require the averaging of substantially fewer samples to obtain a consistent waveform.

ERPs are conveniently divided into three major categories: sensory-evoked, movement-related, and processing-contingent potentials. Sensory-evoked potentials are obligatory responses evoked by the physical attributes of the stimulus. With proper recording parameters and placement of electrodes, neural activation evoked by visual, auditory and somatosensory stimuli can be traced from periphery, through subcortical pathways, to cortex. Thus, sensory-evoked potentials can provide an objective measure of the integrity of sensory pathways and structures, and because these responses are sensitive to the physical characteristics of the stimuli, can offer some measure of sensory threshold independent of the cooperation of the subject. This feature has been extensively exploited in the evaluation of sensory functioning (e.g., hearing threshold) in infants, young children, and subjects who are otherwise unable to cooperate with behavioral test paradigms. At this date, most of the studies relevant for developmental neuropsychology have been performed in the visual and auditory modalities, and we will focus later discussion only on these two sensory-evoked responses. In contrast to sensory-evoked potentials, which are evoked following the delivery of a stimulus, movement-related potentials have components that both precede the movement and follow it. Unfortunately, movement-related potential studies in children remain severely limited in number, and we will not deal with them at any length (for reviews, see Deecke, 1996; McCallum, 1988; Starr, Sandroni and Michalewski, 1995; Vaughan and Arezzo, 1988).

Processing-contingent potentials (PCPs) are a wide-ranging group of potentials that reflect further perceptual or cognitive processing of stimuli beyond that associated with obligatory sensory-evoked activity. PCPs are often termed 'endogenous potentials' to differentiate them from obligatory 'exogenous' ERP components that are principally elicited by physical properties of the stimulus. These potentials include automatic discriminative responses such as the mismatch negativity (MMN), discussed later in the context of auditory ERPs, and potentials generally regarded as reflecting active, attention-dependent processing. However, this distinction is often blurred, as certain potentials indexing higher perceptual operations (e.g., MMN) may occur automatically in the absence of attention, and exogenous potentials can be strongly modulated by attentional factors (e.g., Woldorff, Hillyard, Gallen et al., 1998).

This modulation of ERPs that index more automatic processing by attention has occasionally been overlooked in studies that compare these automatic potentials across subject populations (e.g., ADHD versus control children) where attention may be an important variable.

## Event-related potentials as tools in neuropsychology

ERPs can be utilized in developmental neuropsychology at various levels of analysis. Sensory-evoked potentials serve as a probe of the anatomical integrity of the sensory pathways, yield objective measures of system sensitivity to changes in stimulus parameters and thresholds of activity, and identify normal and aberrant maturational changes in the responses. PCPs index features of selective attention, and processes associated with discriminative functions and other cognitive operations. Behavioral performance is the end result of a complex sequence of serial and parallel brain events that cannot be directly inferred from the behavioral data alone. A strength of ERP studies is that the intermediate neural steps in this complex sequence can be dissected out, yielding data that can extend beyond quantitative measures and which can identity qualitative changes in neural functions associated with changes in behavioral tasks, and that occurring with developmental maturation and in different subject populations.

Thus, an ultimate goal of ERP investigations is to identify those intermediate stages of neural processing that directly relate to the distributed neural networks underlying complex perceptual and cognitive functions. This goal entails two phases of analysis. The first stage requires that the ERP generators be defined in terms of their location and timing. Frequently, ERPs are recorded from only a very limited number of scalp electrodes, and the focus of the investigations are directed at quantification of a limited number of ERP amplitude and latency measurements. This procedure does not adequately consider the mechanisms generating the evoked potentials that must be accounted for in order to maximize the interpretation of the results. For instance, it is often assumed that increased amplitude of an ERP component directly reflects a greater amount of neural activation. However, since ERP waves are derived from the summation of volume-conducted field potentials generated by multiple neural sources, this finding could be the result of the decrease in amplitude of a concurrent potential with an opposite polarity. Likewise, apparent changes in the peak latency of an ERP component, often interpreted as representing faster processing, might result from its truncation by the modulation of a subsequent wave. The problem is especially acute with PCPs, since ERPs associated with higher perceptual and cognitive processes are typically derived from spatially and temporally overlapping evoked fields generated by multiple brain regions whose individual contributions to the surface-recorded data are unknown. The second stage of analysis entails establishing the relationship between specific physiological mechanisms and their reflection in the surface-recorded data. This problem is especially challenging, as non-invasive techniques are severely limited in their capacity to directly identify neural processes, and requires for its resolution integration with more physiologically specific, invasive studies in humans and experimental animals.

## Neural basis of event-related potentials

*Non-invasive methods of event-related potential generator localization*

Scalp-recorded ERPs have specific limitations that need to be recognized when they are applied to studies of developmental neuropsychology. First, not all active brain regions yield field potentials that can easily be detected at the scalp. This is especially true for brain structures such as the basal ganglia that do not possess a directionally coherent architecture capable of generating dipolar electrical fields that would volume conduct to the brain surface. Small cortical fields anatomically located deep within sulci or at the ventral surface of the brain may also generate difficult-to-record electrical fields. Second, the details of neural activity within a given structure are lost with summation of activity from subregions of that tissue. Third, voltages recorded from scalp locations represent the difference in potential between each site and a reference electrode. Thus, the timing, waveshape and amplitude of the resultant wave may be significantly altered by the choice of refer-

ence electrode site. Despite limitations such as these, surface-recorded ERPs can provide relevant, temporally dynamic profiles of cortical activity patterns when data are adequately handled.

Surface potential topography provides the only non-invasive data set from which the anatomical localization of ERP generators can be obtained. Initial steps in analysis usually include creating isopotential maps of the ERP voltage distribution from amplitude measurements at each electrode site. This procedure emphasizes the requirement that sufficient recording locations be utilized. The electrode site yielding the maximum amplitude of the ERP wave is not necessarily at the location of the component generator. Components of the cortical auditory-evoked potential generated within primary cortex or the planum temporale lying on the temporal lobe produce amplitude maxima overlying the frontal convexity (Arezzo, Pickoff and Vaughan, 1975; Wood and Wolpaw, 1982), visual-evoked potentials evoked by hemifield stimulation are sometimes maximal overlying the occipital hemisphere opposite to the activated visual cortex (Celesia, 1988), and somatosensory-evoked potentials evoked by leg stimulation are maximal overlying the hemisphere ipsilateral to the stimulus (Emerson, 1988). These 'paradoxical' distributions are based on the specific dipolar orientations of the activated cellular elements or their mesial location, and highlight the need to consider the spatial geometry of the activated tissue when relating voltage distributions to generator sources. Furthermore, choice of reference electrode may significantly bias voltage distributions.

One method to eliminate the contribution of the reference electrode to the ERP waveforms, as well as to sharpen voltage maps distorted by the high-resistance skull which leads to low-pass filtering and subsequent blurring of the potential distribution, is to compute a second spatial derivative (Laplacian) of the raw data (Gevins, Smith, McEvoy et al., 1999; Perrin, Bertrand and Pernier, 1987). The second spatial derivative is proportional to the magnitude of current flow perpendicular to the surface of the scalp, and therefore provides an estimate of the transcranial current flow entering and leaving the skull directly beneath the recording electrode. These computational maps are independent of the reference electrode used, and are also insensitive to lateral current flow within the skull and scalp. This procedure emphasizes the high spatial frequencies characteristic of local field potentials, enhancing the ability to make inferences regarding the generator sources of the potentials. Despite these improvements, the Laplacian derivation is still constrained by the possible overlapping of currents generated by concurrent generators.

Event-related magnetic fields (ERMFs) are a complementary method for examining surface-recorded neural activity and determining the localization of intracranial generators (see Hari, 1999 and Reite, Teale and Rojas, 1999 for recent reviews). Though the same synaptically driven transmembrane current flows generate both the voltage and magnetic fields, ERPs are derived from extracellular volume currents, while ERMF result from net intraneuronal current flows. The dipolar fields recorded by the two techniques are rotated 90° from each other, resulting in a pronounced sensitivity in the ERMF for currents tangential to the cortical surface. In contrast, ERPs are especially sensitive to current flows that are radially oriented with respect to the brain surface. This difference makes ERMF relatively insensitive to generators located over the surface of cortical gyri (radial orientation), and most sensitive to neuronal activity buried within sulci (tangential orientation). ERMFs do not involve referential recordings, a distinct advantage over ERP requirements. Furthermore, electrical conductivity differences between brain, skull, and scalp do not distort the induced magnetic fields. This leads to greater spatial resolution of the isomagnetic flux lines than the isopotential contours obtained in ERPs. Better spatial resolution in turn provides greater accuracy in modeling the localization of generators (Crouzeix, Yvert, Bertrand and Pernier, 1999; Leahy, Mosher, Spencer et al., 1998).

Processing methods used to localize ERP/ERMF generators utilize mathematical approaches to attempt the solution of the 'inverse' problem, which is a description of the location, orientation and temporal activation patterns of intracranial generators from the measured surface ERP or ERMF distribution. The main impediment to this procedure is that there are theoretically an infinite number of possible solutions to explain a given voltage or magnetic surface distribution pattern. In contrast, the 'forward' problem is a resolvable calculation that determines the surface potential or magnetic field distribution generated by known generators with specific locations, orientations and strengths (e.g., Crouzeix et al., 1999; Koles, 1998; Leahy et al., 1998).

The equivalent current dipole (ECD) is a key construct for most 'inverse problem' methods (e.g., Miltner, Braun, Johnson et al., 1994; Reite et al., 1999. Generators are viewed as time varying dipoles with various locations, orientations and strengths that model the summed activity within a circumscribed region of brain. One popular and commercially available method that permits the localization of dipole generators is called Brain Electrical Source Analysis (BESA, e.g., Miltner et al., 1994; Scherg, Vajsar and Picton, 1989). BESA calculates the best fitting locations, orientations and strengths for multiple ECDs based on a reiterative process that attempts to decrease the variance, using a least-squares fitting algorithm, between the predicted surface distributions computed from a 'forward' model and the actual distributions recorded from the scalp. The procedure systematically varies the position, orientation, and strength of a selected number of ECD generators in order to produce a best-fit solution. Thus, BESA decomposes the ERP into a sequence of source waveforms that offer the best statistical fit to the empirical data for an assumed number of dipoles. Similar methods are available for analysis of ERMF data (e.g., see Ahlfors, Simpson, Dale et al., 1999; Liu, Belliveau and Dale, 1998). Results of these methods are dependent on user-determined parameters, including the number of dipoles to be allowed, and as such are subject to significant error introduced by the investigator (Miltner et al., 1994). Under optimal conditions, typical error for ECD-based modeling is at least several mm for ERMFs and up to several cm for ERPs (e.g., Crouzeix et al., 1999; Krings, Chiappa, Cuffin et al., 1999; Leahy et al., 1998; Yvert, Bertrand, Thévenet et al., 1997). As a rule, error is greater for generators deep in the brain or in ventral locations, and is reduced with an increased number of recording electrodes. Thus, a more suitable interpretation of a calculated ECD is that it represents a 'center of gravity' for activity within a given brain region (Gevins et al., 1999). Details of neuronal responses within that area are inaccessible by ECD-based analysis.

A major problem inherent in all source localization models is that the data cannot specify the actual location and extent of neuronal activation. Thus, anatomical constraints need to be introduced in order to limit the possible loci of activation and determine their contribution to the surface data (see Liu et al., 1998; Luck, 1999). One straightforward method utilizes known neuroanatomy and physiology of a neural system to facilitate generator localization. Thus, modeling of early auditory cortical responses could restrict a single ECD in each hemisphere to be located in the superior temporal plane in the region of primary auditory cortex. Increasingly, structural MRIs of the subjects are used in conjunction with the ERP/ERMFs to further refine this process, with the added benefit that individual variations in cortical anatomy can be visualized and incorporated into the source identification procedure. More sophisticated methods include the combination of functional neuroimaging techniques (e.g., functional MRI) and ERP/ERMF data to both quantify the number of ECD sources required in a given paradigm and to qualify their location in the brain. This combined approach is especially powerful when evaluating ERP/ERMF field data evoked during complex perceptual or cognitive tasks, when it is likely that widespread parallel and serial activations occurring within close temporal succession will contribute to the field responses. For instance, combined fMRI and ERP/ERMF procedures have been implemented to examine the spatio-temporal patterns of activation within dorsal and ventral streams of visual cortex that arise from processing complex spatial and visual form stimuli (e.g., Ahlfors et al., 1999; Wang, Zhou, Qui et al., 1999a). While the addition of fMRI studies offer anatomical constraints for localizing generators of ERP/ERMF data, there are several important caveats that need to be appreciated (e.g., Liu et al., 1998; Luck, 1999). First, these techniques measure different aspects of neural function, and it would be unrealistic to assume a direct one-to-one correspondence between metabolic or blood flow indices and ERP/ERMF responses. Thus, fMRI activation may not be associated with ERPs, and the latter may not always be associated with fMRI changes. Further, ERP/ERMF responses reflect phasic changes in neural activity, whereas functional neuroimaging methods examine more tonic changes and require longer integration times. These considerations emphasize the importance of more direct and invasive procedures that can support, or modify the proposed generators obtained using non-invasive techniques.

*Invasive methods of event-related potential generator localization*

Additional evidence is needed to confirm the generator locations estimated from surface-recorded ERPs/ERMFs. Intracranial recordings are the only unambiguous way for determining if a structure contributes to the generation of an ERP/ERMF component (Halgren, Marinkovic and Chauvel, 1998). These recordings are obtained from patients undergoing evaluation and treatment for medically intractable problems, such as focal onset epilepsy unresponsive to anticonvulsant drugs. While these recording opportunities offer a unique window into human brain functions, there are multiple constraints that limit comprehensive investigations. These include restricted occasions for recording, access confined to neural structures directly relevant for patient care, and limited time for recordings. Furthermore, the structures being examined are often dysfunctional, precipitating the clinical investigations in the first place. Optimally, demonstrating that a neural structure contributes to a surface-recorded ERP/ERMF component involves directly tracing that component from the presumed generator to the surface of the head. However, electrode orientation may not be properly aligned with the angle of the dipole generator, and the extent of recordings may be insufficient to trace the components. At these times, animal models may afford insights into the propagation of ERP components to the brain surface. Old-world monkeys serve as the most useful animal model for examining ERP generation and propagation, as their gross brain anatomy, geometry and cytoarchitectonic organization are closest in approximation to that of the human brain (e.g., Galaburda and Sanides, 1980). The similar geometry in turn leads to comparable relationships between intracranial generators and surface ERP topography. The monkey model has contributed to the definition of ERP generators in multiple sensory and motor systems (for reviews see Schroeder, Steinschneider, Javitt et al., 1995; Vaughan and Arezzo, 1988).

Benefits of monkey model recordings for tracing ERP components from presumed generators to

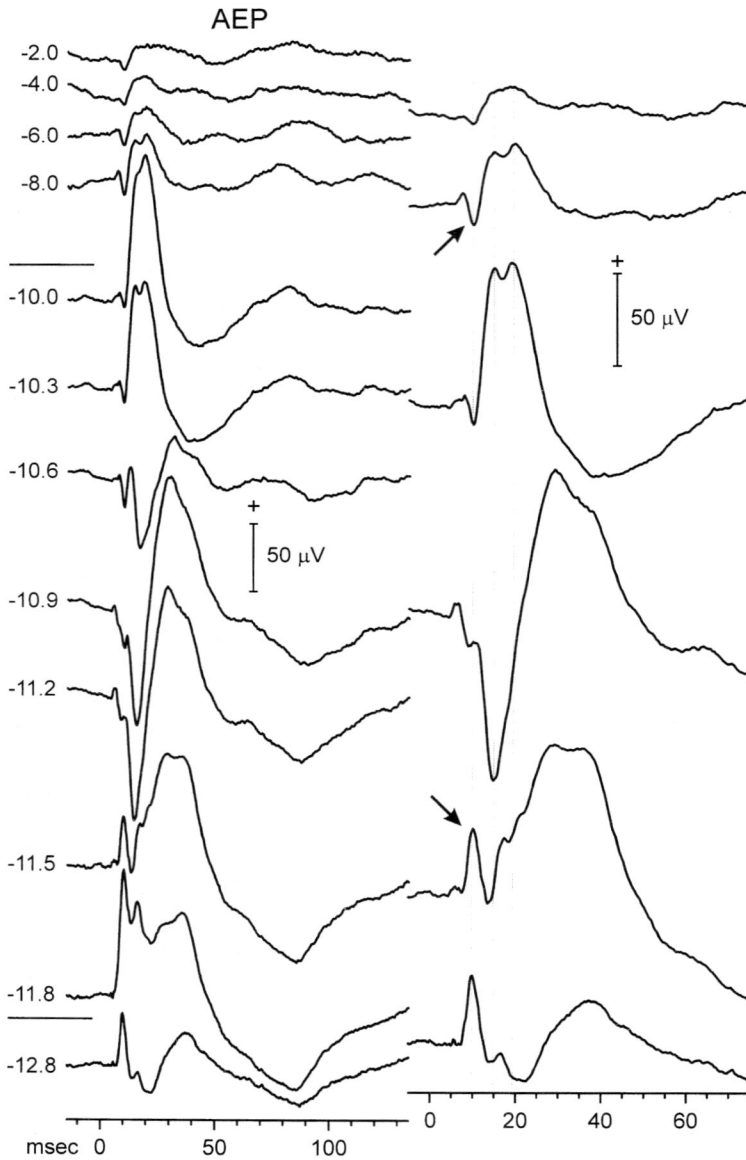

Fig. 1. Click-evoked auditory-evoked potentials (AEP) recorded from intracortical electrode sites in an old-world monkey. The left-hand column illustrates the AEPs recorded at various depths below the dural surface of the dorsolateral convexity of the brain. Depths in mm are shown at the far left, and the boundaries of primary auditory cortex (A1) are demarcated by horizontal bars. There is a marked increase in amplitude of the AEP as the electrode sites approach A1 from the dorsolateral surface, followed by a complex pattern of polarity inversion within the active tissue. The right-hand column illustrates an expanded view of the early cortical AEP, demonstrating inversion of the initial response within primate A1 (arrows). This surface negative wave is likely generated in part by the depolarization of distal segments of thalamocortical afferent fibers.

the brain surface are exemplified in Fig. 1, which illustrates click-evoked auditory-evoked potentials recorded both within primary auditory cortex (A1,

demarcated by horizontal bars shown at the far left) and at various depths below the dura overlying the dorsolateral convexity of the brain (listed at the far left). Orientation of the electrode was orthogonal to the surface of A1. As the recording depth increases, there is a marked increase in the amplitude of the potentials, culminating in a complex inversion in polarity of the various response components within A1 (left-hand column).

General waveshape of the response is preserved in the volume-conducted potentials, indicating that surface recordings over the dorsal scalp can index activity in auditory cortex located on the superior surface of the superior temporal gyrus.

Intracranial recordings in humans illustrate that caution is needed so as not to overinterpret dipole-modeling results obtained from non-invasive studies. For example, Howard MA, Volkov, Mirsky et al. (2000) identified functional connectivity from Heschl's gyrus to the posterior portion of the superior temporal gyrus (PSTG) with a latency of only several milliseconds using electrical stimulation procedures. This indicates that primary and at least one secondary auditory field will have tightly overlapping patterns of activity in the temporal domain, and that single dipole models of auditory cortical activity will be inadequate to define these response profiles. The problem is compounded by the demonstration that auditory cortical regions have different sensitivities to stimulus parameters, and that even closely spaced recording sites exhibit differential processing of sound stimuli (Howard et al., 2000; Steinschneider, Volkov, Noh et al., 1999). Thus, the basic tenet of dipole source localization techniques that extended regions of activated cortex can be modeled by a single dipole must be interpreted with great caution. Fig. 2 illustrates some of these complex aspects of auditory cortical processing. Two consonant–vowel syllables that differ in their voice onset time, /ba/ and /pa/, were presented to a patient with medically intractable epilepsy. Two electrode sites positioned within Heschl's gyrus and two subdural electrode sites in PSTG, each separated by about 1 cm, are illustrated. Responses from the different sites were recorded simultaneously. Marked temporal overlap between activity generated in Heschl's gyrus and that in PSTG is observed. Further, activity patterns from the closely spaced sites also differ significantly from each other. Responses to the unvoiced consonant–vowel syllable /pa/ from the deeper Heschl's gyrus electrode (site 1) and that from the PSTG electrode

directly lateral to Heschl's gyrus (PSTG 1) contain components time-locked to voicing onset (arrows) that are absent in the responses from the other two sites.

Similar findings are present when responses in the anterior and posterior Heschl's gyri are compared, with primary auditory cortex lying at the medial end of the anterior gyrus (Fig. 3). AEPs evoked by the stimulus /ta/ with an 80 ms VOT are illustrated from 8 simultaneously recorded electrode sites. Channel 1 of both electrodes were most medial and were low-impedance EEG electrodes, while the remainder were higher-impedance wire electrodes whose distances from channel 1 are denoted at the left of the figure. Channels 2 and 3 were adjacent to each other. Activity from all recorded channels overlap in time. Despite the larger amplitude AEPs recorded from the more posterior electrode, there is less stimulus detail represented by the responses. Thus, discrete components time-locked to voicing onset (solid arrows) and to the offset of the syllables (unfilled arrows) are only observed in the anterior electrode. These patterns, and those illustrated in Fig. 2, clearly highlight the hurdles facing the development of models of cortical processing based solely on non-invasive techniques (for additional comments see Schreiner, 1998). Furthermore, important suggestions for organization of human sensory cortices, exemplified by dipole modeling studies in auditory cortex, should be interpreted cautiously until confirmed by direct intracranial recordings (e.g., Langner, Sams, Heil and Schulze, 1997; Pantev, Bertrand, Eulitz et al., 1995; Pantev, Elbert, Ross et al., 1996; Poeppel, Phillips, Yellin et al., 1997; Simos, Breier, Zouridakis and Papanicolaou, 1998a; Simos, Diehl, Breier et al., 1998b).

*Neuronal mechanisms of event-related potential generation*

ERPs are generated by synchronized transmembrane current flows within neuronal ensembles, produced by synaptic activity or the coordinated action potential activity in axonal pathways. Synaptic activity is the predominant determinant of cortically generated ERPs, while synchronized action potentials are a major source of spinal cord and brainstem components in the brainstem auditory and somatosensory-evoked

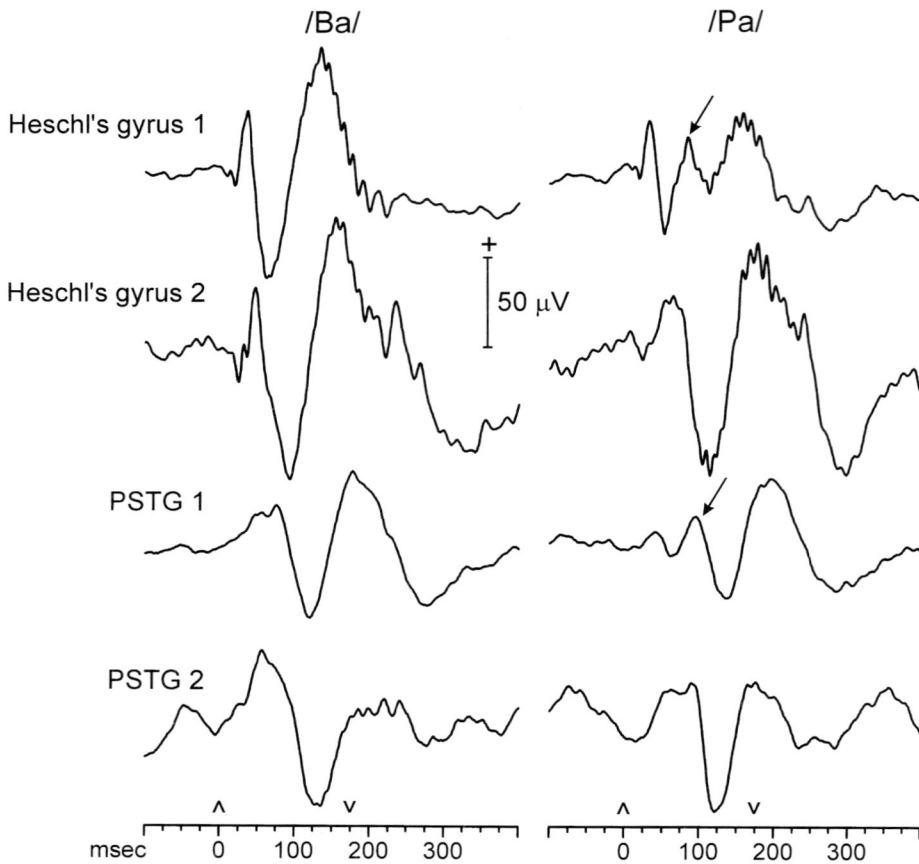

Fig. 2. AEPs evoked by the syllables /ba/ and /pa/, and simultaneously recorded directly from the human brain by two intracortical electrodes in Heschl's gyrus and two subdural electrodes located on the surface of the posterior superior temporal gyrus (PSTG). There is marked temporal overlap in the responses from Heschl's gyrus and the lateral convexity of the temporal lobe, as well as the differential representation of the syllables at the two sites in the same tissue. Only Heschl's gyrus site 1 and PSTG site 1 contain response components time-locked to the onset of voicing to /pa/. The arrowheads above the time lines denote syllable duration. See text for details.

potentials. When transmembrane current flows occurring in neuronal populations have a similar asymmetrical spatial orientation, as in the synaptic activity occurring on the apical dendrites of cortical pyramidal cells or similarly timed action potentials in a brainstem sensory pathway, they act as dipolar generators that produce volume currents within the brain and its coverings. For instance, net depolarization produced by excitatory postsynaptic potentials leads to current flow into the cells at the site of the synaptic activity, and passive circuit-completing capacitive currents flowing out of the neurons at adjacent sites. The location where current enters the cells, and

removed from the extracellular space, is termed a current sink. Likewise, a location where current is injected into the extracellular space from transmembrane capacitive flow is termed a current source. A positive voltage potential will be recorded in the extracellular space at the current source and negativity will be seen at the current sink. Net hyperpolarization of neurons will induce a pattern of sources and sinks reverse from that of excitatory synaptic activity. Thus, the overall pattern of extracellular currents, and resultant voltage and magnetic flow changes that are measured in ERP/ERMF studies, are determined by the type and locations of synaptic events and the

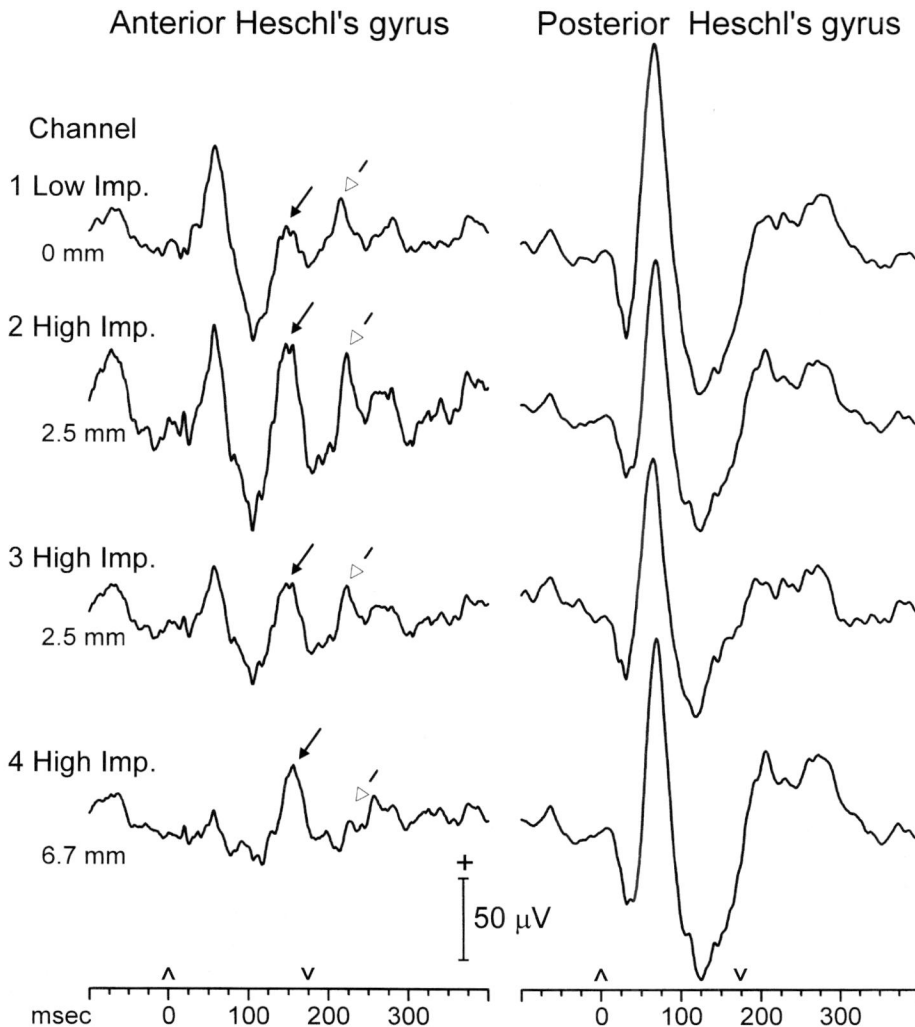

Fig. 3. AEPs evoked by the syllable /ta/ and simultaneously recorded directly from the human brain by four intracortical electrodes in the anterior Heschl's gyrus and four electrodes in the posterior Heschl's gyrus. Despite the larger responses recorded from the posterior electrodes, the AEPs do not represent detailed features of the stimulus that are observed in the smaller responses recorded from the anterior sites. These details include voicing onset (solid arrows) and stimulus offset (unfilled arrows). The marked temporal overlap of the AEPs recorded from the two gyri, and the non-uniformity of temporal response patterns when complex stimuli are presented, highlight the difficulties inherent in equivalent current dipole modeling obtained from non-invasively acquired data.

distribution of the passive current returns on adjacent portions of the neuronal populations.

The pattern of extracellular current sources and sinks can be defined by current source density (CSD) analysis (e.g., Freeman and Nicholson, 1975; Nicholson and Freeman, 1975; Vaughan and Arezzo, 1988), which reflects the second spatial derivative of the intracortical potential distribution. CSD analysis determines net transmembrane current flow by calculating whether a recording site acts as a current source or sink at each time point in the evoked response. A sink can index a site of net depolarization or it can represent passive current drawn to balance hyperpolarization at an adjacent site. A source can occur at a site of net hyperpolarization or represent circuit-completing current flow for an adjacent excitatory postsynaptic potential (EPSP). These possibilities can be distinguished by using multi-unit activity (MUA) as an independent measure of cellular excitation and inhibition. A sink coincident with increased unit activity indicates that the sink represents excitatory activity, while a source colocated with a reduction in unit activity suggests hyperpolarization.

This method of analysis is exemplified by the laminar profiles of AEPs, CSD and MUA concurrently recorded at 150-μm intervals to a 900-Hz best-frequency tone in A1 of an awake monkey (Fig. 4). Approximate boundaries for laminae III and IV, and

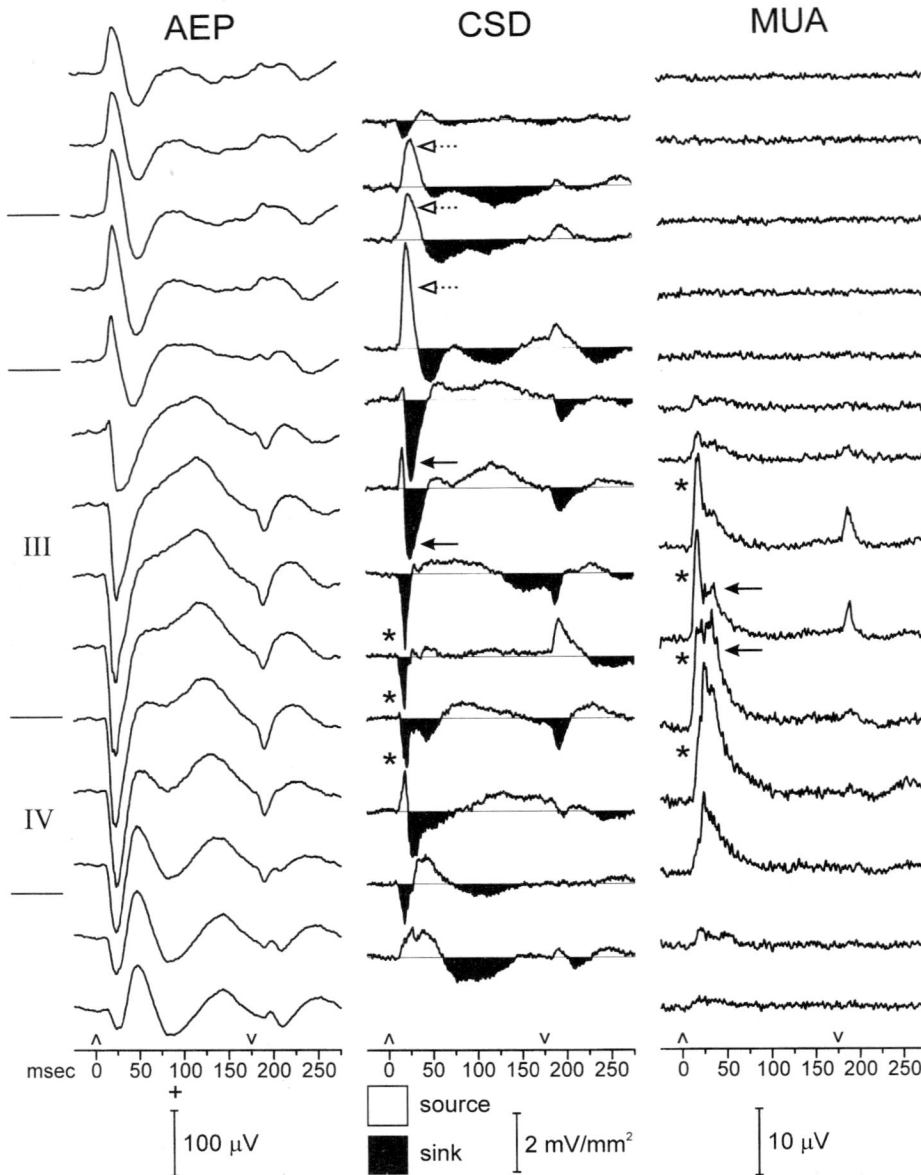

Fig. 4. Laminar profiles of AEPs, current source density (CSD), and multi-unit activity (MUA) simultaneously recorded from 14 sites in primate A1 at 150-μm intervals. The stimulus was a 900-Hz best frequency tone presented at 60 dB SPL. See text for details.

the top of lamina I, are shown at the far left. The AEP in A1 contains a prominent surface positivity that inverts in polarity within lamina III and is associated with superficial laminae sources (unfilled arrows) and deeper current sinks. The earlier of the associated sinks is located in lamina IV and lower lamina III (asterisks), while a somewhat later current sink is centered in more superficial regions of lamina III (solid arrows). An initial burst of MUA (asterisks) is coincident with the first of the sinks, and represents the initial activation of A1 (Steinschneider, Tenke, Schroeder et al., 1992). The later, more superficial, sink is coincident with the persistent increases in MUA after the initial burst (solid arrows) and likely reflects excitation induced by additional intracortical synaptic processing (e.g., Steinschneider, Schroeder, Arezzo and Vaughan, 1994). Thus, the initial cortical positivity is generated by multilaminar events that reflect both mono- and polysynaptic activation of A1 neuronal ensembles. Later AEP components are also generated by the contributions of activity in multiple laminae, though the surface response is dominated in morphology by the CSD patterns observed superficially. Recent uses of this procedure include the clarification of A1 organizational features (Fishman, Reser, Arezzo and Steinschneider, 2000; Reser, Fishman, Arezzo and Steinschneider, 2000), plasticity in somatosensory cortex (Schroeder, Seto and Garraghty, 1997), and streaming and effects of selective attention within the visual system (Mehta, Ulbert and Schroeder, 2000a,b).

## Auditory event-related potentials

### General use

Given that normal language development is dependent upon adequate hearing and central auditory processing, it is crucial that sensitive methods be available for the evaluation of auditory system integrity in infants and children. Electrophysiological assessment of the auditory system using ERPs offers a means by which the functional integrity of the auditory system can be assessed from periphery to cortex. Several of these procedures have become standard means by which auditory system functions are examined in infants at high risk for hearing deficits and later language abnormalities.

Auditory ERPs are divided into four categories based upon differences in their timing, brain structures assessed, and auditory processes engaged. These categories are: (1) the auditory brainstem response (ABR) that occurs within the first 15 ms after the onset of a sound stimulus and examines the integrity of the auditory periphery and brainstem pathways, (2) the middle latency response (MLR) that occurs between 15 and 50 ms after sound onset and represents the initial activation of auditory cortex, (3) the obligatory cortical auditory-evoked potential (CAEP) that consists of ERP components with latencies up to several hundred milliseconds after a sound and index later auditory cortical processes, and (4) auditory processing-contingent potentials (PCPs) which overlap and follow other CAEPs and are elicited when physical sound features are changed or when sound stimuli are actively discriminated.

### Auditory brainstem response

ABRs are the most clinically useful auditory ERP, and are routinely used in the assessment of hearing functions such as auditory sensitivity (threshold) in the very young and in those subjects who are incapable of participating in behavioral audiological tests (see Celesia and Brigell, 1999; Krumholz, 1999 for detailed reviews). ABRs are composed of seven component waves, labeled I to VII, and in normal adults occur within about 12 ms after stimulus onset. Waves I, III, and V are the most reliable, and can be recorded in infants as young as 30 weeks postconceptual age. The ABR subsequently undergoes marked maturational changes that are characterized by a decrease in absolute and interpeak latencies. Wave I reaches adult values by 1–2 months of age and wave V rapidly decreases in latency over the first 3 months after birth, and then more slowly until it reaches adult values by 3–5 years of age (Eggermont, 1989; Salamy, 1984). These early rapid changes mandate the use of age-specific norms for their accurate assessment.

The sequence of ABR components generally reflects the anatomical course of the auditory pathways through the brainstem (for review see Celesia and Brigell, 1999; Legatt, Arezzo and Vaughan, 1988). Thus, wave I is elicited by activity in the auditory nerve, wave III by activity in the lower pons in the region of the superior olivary complex, and wave V by activation of the upper pons and lower midbrain in the region of the inferior colliculus. While each wave of the ABR likely represents activity at multiple stages in the auditory pathway, these simplifications allow reasonable estimates for the maturation of relevant neuronal elements and localization of possible pathology. This localization is based on the specific pattern of ABR abnormalities observed. For instance, normal waves I and III with an absent wave V or prolonged wave III–V interpeak latency indicate dysfunction in the upper pons or lower midbrain, whereas abnormalities in earlier ABR components suggest dysfunction at more caudal locations.

ABR protocols in the newborn usually include stimulation with click stimuli presented at rates of about 10–30 per second and at high intensity (60–80 dB above behavioral adult threshold, HL). This protocol elicits ABRs with a morphology that enables identification of the major response components and determination of interpeak intervals. Less intense stimuli are also presented to estimate hearing thresholds. The presence of wave V, which is the most reliable ABR component, at stimulus intensities of 20 dB nHL is normal in the young child, while 30 dB nHL is the usual cutoff for neonates. Latency-intensity functions for waves I and V are also routinely used to define whether hearing deficits are due to conductive disturbances or abnormalities in the cochlea, auditory nerve, or brainstem pathways (Celesia and Brigell, 1999). Comparison of ABRs obtained from air- and bone-conducted stimuli can also assess these patterns of hearing deficits (Stapells and Ruben, 1989).

A principal use of ABRs is the identification of young children with hearing loss at an age early enough so that intervention may ameliorate resultant impairment of language development. This is especially important in infants prone to the development of hearing loss, which occurs in 1–5% of these 'high-risk newborns', which in turn represent about 5% of all live births (American Academy of Pediatrics Joint Committee on Infant Hearing, 1995). Risk factors include a family history of hearing impairment, congenital infection, head and neck deformities, low birth weight, severe hyperbilirubinemia, use of ototoxic medications, neonatal meningitis and asphyxia.

An important concern is the relationship between ABRs obtained in the infant and behaviorally determined hearing thresholds obtained in later infancy. Generally, there is excellent agreement between significant abnormalities in ABRs obtained in the neonate and subsequent identification of hearing loss (Hyde, Riko and Malizia, 1990; Sasama, 1990). For example, in one study, 667 high-risk newborns were evaluated with ABRs (Kramer, Vertes and Condon, 1989). Severe sensorineural hearing impairment was accurately predicted in infants who failed the ABR at click intensities of 45 dB HL, and milder dysfunction was predicted in infants who passed the ABR at 45 dB but failed at 30 dB. Recently, a large investigation has supported the utility of ABRs in newborns for identification of hearing loss in children (Mason and Hermann, 1998). This report documents the routine use of automated click-evoked ABRs obtained in 10,372 infants prior to discharge from a neonatal nursery. Average time of test was 15 min. The authors identified 415 babies who failed the screening test using a criterion for ABR failure of absence of response at >35 dB. Of these babies, 3.6% were later found to have permanent bilateral hearing loss. It was concluded that the screening test, whose average cost was $17 per patient and was less expensive than other routinely performed newborn tests, was a cost-effective means to identify hearing loss in the young. While it is clear that newborn screening leads to excessive false-positive results, indicating low specificity, errors can be reduced by follow-up examinations (Krumholz, 1999). Thus, ABR screening of high-risk neonates appears justified, especially when the additional costs in terms of human morbidity and monetary expenses incurred when hearing loss is not rapidly identified is considered.

Although click-evoked ABRs are clearly useful in screening for potential hearing deficits, they do have important limitations. Clicks are broadband stimuli that activate a wide frequency region of the cochlea, and thus may underestimate frequency-specific threshold elevations (Stapells, 1989). Detailed testing of specific frequency regions can be accomplished through use of tones in notched noise. Notch-filtered noise, which is reduced in intensity near the frequency of a tone stimulus, reduces the general activation of the cochlea. Close correlations exist between ABRs evoked by brief tone pips placed at the noise notch, and frequency-specific hearing thresholds in both normal infants and young children and those with hearing loss (Stapells, Gravel and Martin, 1995). Thus, this technique can improve ABR accuracy for defining frequency-specific hearing impairment.

Finally, it is important to remember that the ABR is not a direct test of hearing, but instead measures several useful features of the physiological response sensitivities of peripheral and brainstem auditory structures. There are many circumstances where ABRs are abnormal, and yet hearing thresholds as tested by behavioral criteria are normal (Stapells and Kurtzberg, 1991). The ABR reflects only the fastest and most synchronized volleys of activity in the auditory system. Less synchronized activity, which also is important for normal hearing, is not indexed by the ABR. Conversely, normal ABRs and persistently abnormal behavioral thresholds can be obtained in children, suggesting deficits in more central auditory or even non-auditory brain structures (Werner, Folsom and Mancl, 1994). This finding reinforces the need to supplement the ABR with other physiological measures that evaluate higher auditory centers, and indeed, other cortical brain regions involved in higher cognitive functions.

*Middle latency responses (MLR)*

MLRs consist of a sequence of low-amplitude ERP components with a latency of about 12 to 50 ms after acoustic stimulation in the adult (Celesia and Brigell, 1999). Five potentials, labeled $N_o$, $P_o$, $N_a$, $P_a$, and $N_b$ to reflect their polarity, occur following transient stimulation. Two components, $N_a$ (peak latency 15–25 ms), and $P_a$ (peak latency 25–30 ms), are most reliably recorded in the adult, and are the MLRs most commonly studied. These components are best observed when the high-pass filters of the recording amplifiers are set to eliminate the lowest-frequency components ($<10$ Hz) of the ERP.

Converging sources of evidence indicate that these components are, at least in part, generated within primary auditory cortex located on Heschl's gyrus. Clicks or tone pips consistently evoke ERP/ERMF $N_a$ and $P_a$ components that are best localized using dipole source modeling to auditory cortex located in or near Heschl's gyrus (Kuriki,

Nogai and Hirata, 1995; Pantev et al., 1995; Scherg and Von Cramon, 1986). Intracranial recordings in Heschl's gyrus confirm these conclusions (Celesia, 1976; Liégeois-Chauvel, Musolino, Badier et al., 1994; Steinschneider et al., 1999). Fig. 5 illustrates the generation of MLR components within Heschl's gyrus with latencies compatible to $N_a$ and $P_a$.

The clinical utility of the MLR in evaluating auditory cortical function in younger children has been hampered by its variability and recording inconsistency (Kraus, Smith, Reed et al., 1985; Stapells, Galambos, Costello and Makeig, 1988). Presenting the MLR protocol only when the child is awake, in lighter stages of sleep, or in REM sleep can improve reliability (McGee, Kraus, Killion et al., 1993). Because of the difficulties involved with either recording from awake small children or monitoring sleep state, MLRs are not routinely performed in the clinical assessment of auditory system integrity. Nevertheless, if MLR components are present, they provide evidence for functional integrity of the auditory pathways at the initial levels of auditory cortical processing. Their absence, however, cannot be used to indicate dysfunction.

While technical considerations restrict the clinical use of MLRs in the evaluation of individual patients, their use as a research tool for examining specific hypotheses in subject populations may in fact be underutilized. One example of this is the use of a variant of the MLR termed the steady-state response (SSR) (Jacobson, 1994). The SSR is a quasi-sinusoidal response usually elicited by repetitive, amplitude- or frequency-modulated sounds. Stimulation with these sounds results in a response phase-locked to the stimulus repetition rate. Non-invasive studies have suggested an optimal repetition rate of 40 Hz (e.g., Forss, Mäkelä, McEvoy and Hari, 1993), though direct intracranial recordings suggest more low-pass response characteristics in primary auditory cortex (Lee, Lueders, Dinner et al., 1984; Steinschneider et al., 1999). In a provocative study, the SSR to frequency-modulated tones were examined in 11–16-year-old children with predominantly expressive or receptive language disorders, and a group of age-matched controls (Stefanatos, Green and Ratcliff, 1989). Children with receptive language dysphasia produced SSRs that were decreased in amplitude relative to the expressive language disorder group

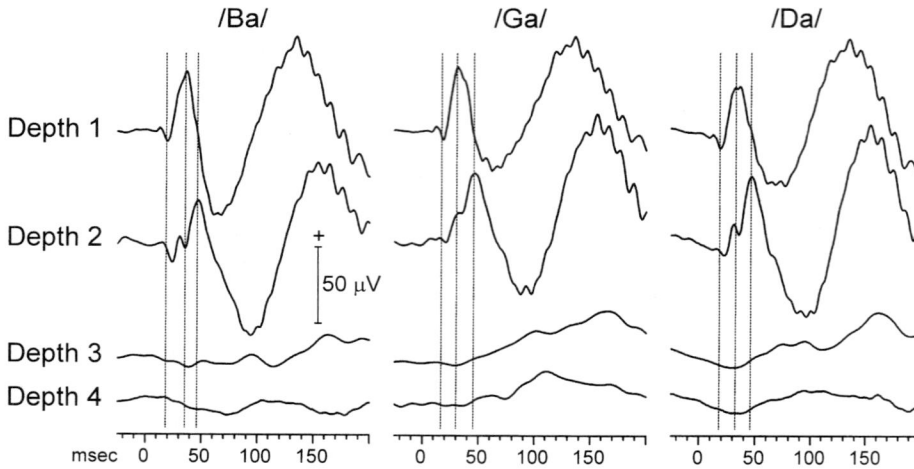

Fig. 5. AEPs evoked by three syllables and recorded by four electrode contacts (1 cm intervals) located in Heschl's gyrus. The early segments of the responses are shown, and drop lines help visualize the timing characteristics of the shortest latency components. Responses are restricted to the deepest and most posteromedial sites (Depths 1 and 2), with the deepest site exhibiting responses with slightly shorter latencies than those at Depth 2. These depths correspond to primary auditory cortex. See text for details.

and the controls. These response deficits were interpreted to suggest that there is a fundamental defect in the ability of auditory cortex to encode rapidly changing sounds in some children. A similar decrement has been reported for responses evoked by amplitude-modulated tones in a group of dyslexic adults compared to matched controls (McAnally and Stein, 1997). While the authors termed the response an amplitude modulation following response, they concluded from latency data that the evoked activity was likely generated in auditory cortex and not brainstem structures, suggesting that this response was an SSR. Thus, these findings suggest that a basic defect in processing rapidly changing sounds in auditory cortex could interfere with normal auditory processing of speech during development, leading to subsequent receptive dysphasia or later dyslexia. Although these findings need to be considered preliminary, they do indicate the relevance of SSRs in assessing early auditory cortical processing in various language-impaired populations, and argue for additional, related studies.

### Cortical auditory-evoked potentials (CAEP)

Larger and more reliably elicited cortical auditory-evoked responses (CAEP) follow the MLR. In adults, these potentials include a positivity that peaks at about 50 ms after stimulus onset, and has been termed the P1 or P50. It is followed by a large negativity (N1) and positivity (P2) that peak at about 100 and 200 ms, respectively. These components have been the subject of a considerable body of research investigating their relevance for auditory cortical processing of sound in both adults and children. This is especially true for the N1 component. In our opinion, the significance ascribed to changes in these components when they are modulated by experimental manipulations is often overinterpreted. Problems are particularly evident when detailed claims of auditory cortex organization are made that are based solely on amplitude and voltage distribution changes in the CAEP with variations in stimulus parameters. These problems arise primarily because it is underappreciated that the components that make up the CAEP are complex potentials generated within multiple cytoarchitectonic areas, and cannot be adequately modeled by single equivalent dipole source generators within each hemisphere (Liégeois-Chauvel et al., 1994; Steinschneider et al., 1999).

The P50 component is generated in part by activity in primary auditory cortex located on Heschl's gyrus. This conclusion rests partly on converging data acquired from topography of surface-recorded AEPs (Wood and Wolpaw, 1982) and dipole localization of magnetic responses (Huotilainen, Winkler,

Alho et al., 1998; Onitsuka, Ninomiya, Sato et al., 2000; Reite et al., 1988). The P50 has a voltage maximum fronto-centrally, and inverts in polarity to become negative ventral to the sylvian fissure, consistent with a generator located on the superior surface of the superior temporal gyrus. More definitive localization of the P50 to primary auditory cortex is based on intracranial measurements taken from Heschl's gyrus, where CAEP components of nearly identical latency are recorded (Liégeois-Chauvel et al., 1994; Liégeois-Chauvel, deGraaf, Laguitton and Chauvel, 1999; Steinschneider et al., 1999; see Fig. 5). CSD analysis of the probable analog of the P50 in a monkey model further suggests that this component is principally generated by synaptic activity on pyramidal cell elements in lamina III (Steinschneider et al., 1994). Additional contributions from non-primary auditory cortex to the P50 recorded at the scalp can be inferred by the human intracranial recordings, wherein overlapping activity occurs posterior to Heschl's gyrus on the planum temporale and lateral to the primary field on the posterior superior temporal gyrus (Howard et al., 2000; Liégeois-Chauvel et al., 1994; Liégeois-Chauvel et al., 1999; Steinschneider et al., 1999; see Figs. 2 and 3). Thus, even for this early CAEP, multiple areas of auditory cortex are activated in parallel.

Generators for the N1 component are even more diffuse. For instance, at least 3 generators of the N1 component have been proposed, one with vertically oriented dipoles located on the planum temporale, another in association auditory cortex located on the lateral surface of the posterior superior temporal gyrus, and a third likely located outside auditory cortex and possibly within motor or premotor cortex (Giard, Perrin, Echallier et al., 1994; Näätänen, 1990; Näätänen and Picton, 1987). Source analysis suggests that the N1 component generated on the superior temporal plane is in fact composed of at least 2 generators (Scherg et al., 1989). Intracortically acquired CAEPs suggest that the principal generator of the N1 is located in the planum temporale, posterior to Heschl's gyrus (Liégeois-Chauvel et al., 1994). This conclusion is supported by other intracortical studies that have also noted a large amplitude potential of similar latency within the planum temporale (Liégeois-Chauvel et al., 1999; Steinschneider et al., 1999; see Fig. 3). The latter studies also recorded components with latencies overlapping the N1 in Heschl's gyrus. Contributions to the N1 from lateral auditory association cortex is also indicated from source analysis of surface recorded data, and supported by intracranial recordings (Howard et al., 2000; Scherg et al., 1989; Steinschneider et al., 1999; see Fig. 2). The intracranial data also demonstrate that the P2 CAEP component is a composite waveform derived from activity in multiple auditory cortical fields.

*Cortical auditory-evoked potential maturation*
The CAEP undergoes marked changes in morphology, amplitude, component distribution and timing over the first decades of life. These features must be appreciated in order to appropriately interpret the CAEP in reference to normal cortical development and that occurring in developmental disorders. Developmental changes in the neonate and young infant can be tracked using a 5-stage classification scheme (Kurtzberg, Hilbert, Kreuzer and Vaughan, 1984). These stages, illustrated in Fig. 6, are based on the CAEP recorded over midline central and lateral temporal regions and include: (1) an immature phase characterized by negative waves recorded at both recording sites; (2) an intermediate phase with a poorly defined midline response and a persistent negative wave over the lateral cortex; (3) a positive midline response and a negative lateral response; (4) a second intermediate phase with a positive midline response and a poorly defined lateral response; and (5) positive midline and lateral components. Using speech sounds as stimuli, Novak, Kurtzberg, Kreuzer and Vaughan (1989) found that the CAEP was at stage 3 in most full-term infants, and progressed to stage 5 by 3 months of age. From 3 to 6 months, the positive waves over both the midline and lateral sites differentiated into 2 positive peaks with intervening troughs (Fig. 7). As is typical for ERPs, there was a decrease in latency of the CAEP with maturation, such that at term, peak latencies were between 150 and 325 ms for the positivity recorded at central sites, which decreased at 6 months of age to 120 ms. In contrast, latency of the positivity recorded at lateral temporal sites was delayed, peaking at 150 ms. While the specific maturational events driving these changes in the CAEP are unknown, the developmental sequence of these potentials suggests an earlier

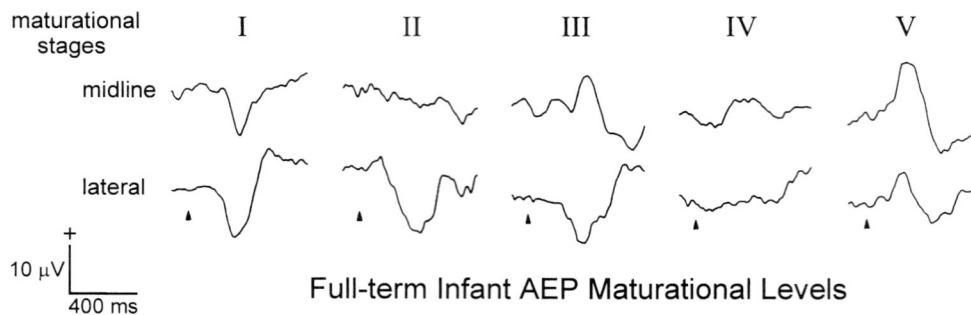

Fig. 6. Maturational levels of infant CAEPs, based upon polarity of responses recorded from midline and lateral electrode sites. Stage III, with a midline positivity and lateral negativity, is the most common pattern observed in term infants. Stage V is the most mature of these patterns, and is usually observed by 1 month of age. Stimulus eliciting these responses was the syllable /ta/, and its onset is denoted by the arrowheads.

maturation of primary auditory cortex, as indexed by the midline responses, from that in secondary auditory cortex located on the lateral temporal surface.

Changes in the CAEP continue through adolescence, indicating that caution is required when comparing potentials acquired at different ages. One developmental aspect of the CAEP is the dominance in early childhood of the P1 component at midline electrodes in comparison to the N1 wave, reversing the typical pattern observed in adults (Kraus, McGee, Carrell et al., 1993a; Sharma, Kraus, McGee and Nicol, 1997). This prominence persists through 10 years of age, when a rapid decrease in P1 amplitude occurs (Ponton, Eggermont, Kwong and Don, 2000). In parallel with the P1 decrement is a marked increase in N1 amplitude (Ponton et al., 2000). Peak latencies of both the P1 and N1 decrease with age. For P1, latencies in children about 5 years old range from 80 to 110 ms, slowly decreasing to reach adult values of 30–50 ms by 15 years of age (Ponton et al., 2000). These values represent a further decrease in latency from that observed in infancy, if the earlier positivity seen at 6 months of age can be equated with the P1 of early childhood (Novak et al., 1989). N1 peak latencies also decrease to adult values of 80–100 ms by middle teenage years, and range from 120 to 150 ms in younger children (Ponton et al., 2000). Estimates of a 2 ms/year decrease in N1 peak latency have been suggested for this age range (Tonnquist-Uhlén, Borg and Spens, 1995). Some variability in absolute values of P1 and N1 across different studies may reflect differences in stimulus type, intensity and interstimulus interval (e.g., Bruneau, Roux, Guérin et al.,

1997; Čeponienè, Cheour and Näätänen, 1998). In addition to the developmental changes observed for the N1 component recorded maximally over frontocentral regions, the N1 recorded from lateral temporal sites also exhibits maturational changes (Gomes, Dunn, Ritter et al., 2001). As expected, peak latency of the response decreases through childhood, though at all ages studied (6–12 years and adulthood), the response peaks after the centrally recorded activity. The amplitude of the temporal component also decreased with increasing age. Other studies have also reported the presence of a similarly timed negativity in younger children over temporal locations (Bruneau et al., 1997; Čeponienè et al., 1998), consistent with a lateral cortex generator. Maturation of the P2 CAEP component has been studied to a lesser degree, though it can be observed at least by the latter half of the first decade (Ponton et al., 2000).

It is tempting to speculate on the physiological significance of CAEP maturational features, as the responses may serve as markers for some of the underlying anatomical changes that occur with development. The first appearance of surface negative waves recorded in the premature infant coincides with the growth of thalamocortical fibers into auditory cortex and the development of a granular cell layer (Krmpotic-Nemanic, Kostovic, Kolovic et al., 1983; Krmpotic-Nemanic, Kostovic and Nemanic, 1984; Kurtzberg et al., 1984). Thus, negative waves at this developmental stage may reflect activity in the distal portions of thalamocortical fibers and in the granule layer 4 of the auditory cortex. This idea is consonant with analysis of the AEP recorded in mon-

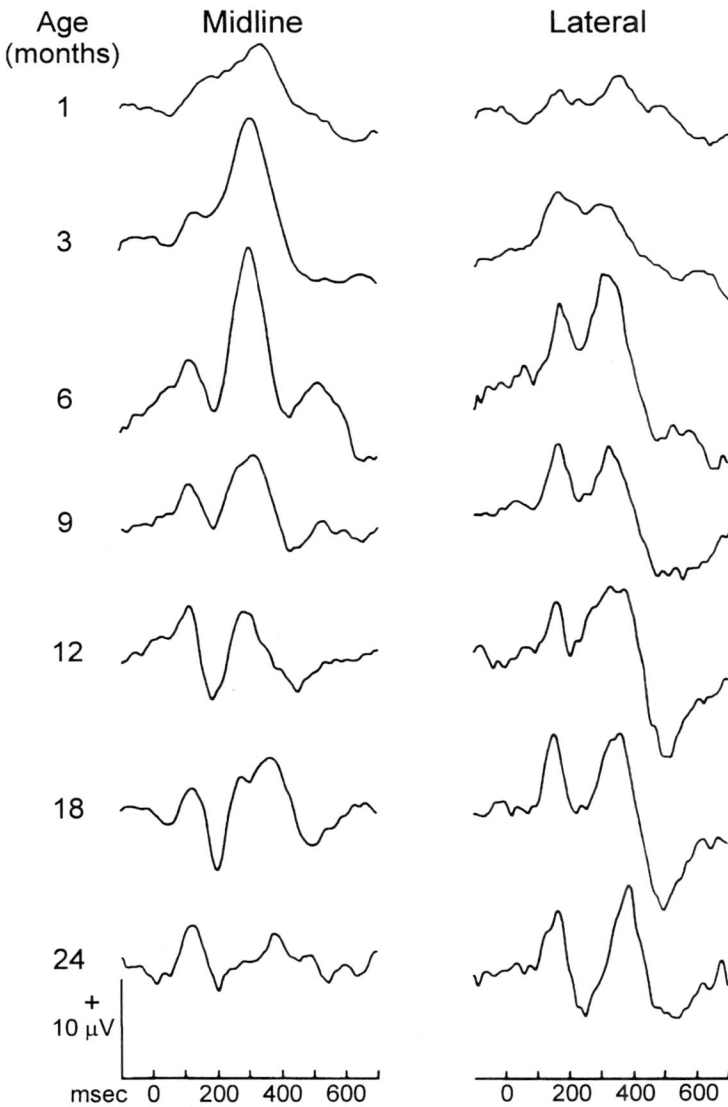

Fig. 7. Maturation of the CAEP through the first 2 years of life. Pronounced changes in timing and morphology of the responses recorded at midline and lateral electrodes emphasize that age-specific norms are required for analysis of the CAEP in normal development and in populations at risk for auditory cortical dysfunction.

key A1, as the profile for the initial surface negative wave is most consistent with a generator based on depolarization of thalamocortical fiber terminations and resultant EPSPs of postsynaptic stellate cells (Steinschneider et al., 1992). Surface positive waves in A1 are usually the result of EPSPs upon dendritic elements of pyramidal cells in supragranular layers (Steinschneider et al., 1994). Later dominance of sur-

face positive waves in the developing CAEP would thus represent the emergence of large-scale synaptic connections on pyramidal cells. This schema is consistent with data demonstrating that synaptic density in Heschl's gyrus reaches its peak at 3 postnatal months of age (Huttenlocher and Dabholkar, 1997), which would presumably include extensive synapses upon pyramidal cells. Later maturation of the CAEP is temporally associated with expansion of dendritic and axonal arbors, net synapse elimination that continues into the second decade, and with continued myelination that is probably a major contributor for the declining latencies of the responses (Huttenlocher and Dabholkar, 1997). The P1 component dominates N1 at central recording sites in early childhood. Given that P1 is primarily generated in Heschl's gyrus, while N1 has a major source more posterior on the planum temporale, the CAEP pattern in childhood may reflect a relative immaturity of these secondary cortical regions. This suggestion is consistent with earlier maturation of auditory cortex on Heschl's gyrus compared to other cortical regions (Huttenlocher and Dabholkar, 1997).

*Cortical auditory evoked potentials to speech sounds*
A key goal of developmental neuropsychology is to clarify the neural mechanisms associated with the emergence of language functions in infancy and childhood. To that end, a number of studies have examined the development of the CAEP using speech stimuli (e.g., Kraus et al., 1993a; Sharma et al., 1997). Generally, the obligatory components of the CAEP (i.e., P1 and N1) to speech sounds display maturational characteristics (e.g., decreasing latency with age and early P1 predominance) similar to those observed with non-speech stimuli (e.g., Bruneau et al., 1997; Ponton et al., 2000; Tonnquist-Uhlén et al., 1995). One limitation of these studies using speech stimuli is that they do not explicitly address obligatory aspects of auditory cortical processing more specific for language-related sounds or language development. Two lines of ERP research have examined more language-specific functions, and include studies evaluating hemispheric specificity in speech processing and the representation of phonetic features such as place of articulation and voice onset time (VOT). The latter line of investigation includes studies examining categorical perception of speech sounds, a cardinal feature of phonetic encoding.

Behavioral studies indicate that young infants already respond to phonetic stimuli in a categorical manner (Eimas, Siqueland, Jusczyk and Vigorito, 1971). These studies have focused on developmental features of the voicing contrast (e.g., /b/ versus /p/, /d/ versus /t/, /g/ versus /k/), based on the hypothesis that the VOT boundary is at least partially

determined by temporal processing mechanisms, and specifically, by the ability to identify the sequence of two acoustic events such as consonant release and voicing onset (e.g., Faulkner and Rosen, 1999; Formby, Barker, Abbey and Raney, 1993; Phillips, Taylor, Hall et al., 1997; Pisoni, 1977). This categorical boundary, which is around 20–30 ms, has been demonstrated in 2-month-old infants using a high-amplitude sucking procedure and various synthetic speech stimuli (Jusczyk, Rosner, Reed and Kennedy, 1989).

Behavioral findings have apparent physiological correlates in CAEP responses, suggesting that temporal processing constraints imposed on the neural representation of speech sounds are present in auditory cortex. In a series of experiments, Simos and colleagues examined the magnetic response counterparts of the CAEP in adults using consonant vowel (CV) syllables varying in their VOT, or two-tone analogs of the syllables varying in their tone onset time (TOT) (Simos et al., 1998a,b). The investigators found an abrupt decrease in the amplitude of the N1 ERMF component (N1m) as the VOT of the syllables or the TOT of the two-tone complexes increased from 20 to 40 ms. In parallel with these changes in the CAEP, the perception of the subjects abruptly changed from a voiced consonant (/g/) to an unvoiced consonant (/k/), and for the two-tone stimuli the subjects reported that they now heard two tone onsets instead of a single event. In a related study, Sharma and Dorman (1999) observed that as VOT increased and crossed the perceptual boundary from which adult subjects' perception changed from /d/ to /t/, there was the emergence of 2 discrete N1 components. The first N1 was evoked by consonant release, while the second was elicited by voicing onset. Interestingly, Simos and Molfese (1997) reported similar findings in the CAEP of newborn infants. They observed that the amplitudes of two negative waves peaking at 200 and 530 ms decreased as TOT increased from 20 to 40 ms.

Two intracortical studies recording the CAEP directly from auditory cortex extend the non-invasive findings that VOT is partially represented by responses time-locked to consonant release and voicing onset. The first study demonstrated the effect for natural speech in the left hemisphere and found VOT representation in Heschl's gyrus and planum temporale but not the posterior portion of the superior temporal gyrus (Liégeois-Chauvel et al., 1999). Steinschneider et al. (1999), observed CAEP components time-locked to VOT in the non-dominant Heschl's gyrus and posterior portion of the superior temporal gyrus but not the planum temporale. Furthermore, the effect showed categorical-like features, with a marked increase in the response evoked by voicing onset observed when the VOT was extended from 20 to 40 ms. Differences between the two studies may represent sampling biases from the limited recording sites necessitated by ethical restrictions. These studies clearly indicate, however, a representation of VOT that reflects temporal speech features in primary auditory cortex and at least several secondary auditory cortical fields. Of special note is the similarity of the physiological responses to those observed in animal models (e.g., Eggermont, 1999; McGee, Kraus, King and Nicol, 1996; Schreiner, 1998; Steinschneider et al., 1994; Steinschneider, Schroeder, Arezzo and Vaughan, 1995a). This similarity is illustrated in Fig. 8, which depicts the responses to four CV syllables varying in their VOT from 0 to 60 ms. CAEPs intracortically recorded from an electrode in Heschl's gyrus are shown in the left-hand column, and multi-unit activity recorded from a lower lamina III recording site in monkey A1 are shown in the right-hand column. The syllables with a VOT of 0 and 20 ms are generally perceived by listeners as /da/, while those with a VOT of 40 and 60 ms are perceived as /ta/. For the two unvoiced CV syllables with a VOT of 40 and 60 ms, there are responses to consonant release (onset) followed by time-locked bursts of activity evoked by voicing onset (solid arrows). In contrast, the responses to the voiced CV syllables only contain a prominent burst of activity evoked by consonant release. The expected locations of the responses to voicing onset for the 20 ms VOT stimulus are shown by the unfilled dotted arrows. The similarities in response patterns between human and animal emphasize that acoustic features of speech, and not some phonetic representation of the sounds, evoke the CAEP.

Developmental studies examining speech sound responses have been limited. Dehaene-Lambertz and Dehaene (1994) examined the CAEP from 16 three-month-old infants listening to syllables differing in their consonant place of articulation. The initial response, which peaked at 220 ms, was not sensitive to the varying characteristics of the consonants, whereas the second component peaking at 390 ms after stimulus onset did exhibit features modulated by phonetic change. Dipole analysis of this latter response, which was larger over the left hemisphere, suggested a generator in the posterior temporal lobe that likely reflected activity in a secondary auditory cortical field. The authors concluded that at this age, the infant brain detects a phonetic change in under 400 ms, though the nature of the change that is recognized remains unknown.

This study also suggests that differential processing of speech between the left and right temporal lobes could be identified using CAEP responses in early infancy (Dehaene-Lambertz and Dehaene, 1994). Furthermore, there appeared to be a left-sided predominance in the cortical activity, in keeping with left hemispheric dominance for language functions. Additional studies support the capacity of the CAEP to examine developmental aspects of hemispheric specialization. However, these studies do not uniformly indicate left hemispheric dominance for speech processing. In a series of investigations, Molfese and colleagues (Molfese, 1978, 1980; Molfese and Hess, 1978; Molfese and Molfese, 1988; Simos, Molfese and Brenden, 1997) have presented data that support an important role for the right hemisphere in the processing of the VOT phonetic parameter. Right-hemispheric ERP components that were categorically modified with changes in VOT, or tone-onset time of two-tone speech analogs, were observed in adults and children. These ERP components were generally recorded from sites overlying the lateral convexity of the right temporal lobe, suggesting that these categorical responses might be generated in 'non-dominant' secondary auditory cortical areas. A recent study examining developmental changes (age 3 to adult) in the amplitude and latency of the N1 components evoked by tones and syllables has demonstrated maturational differences in the responses recorded from the left and right hemispheres (Pang and Taylor, 2000). For components that are likely generated by auditory cortex located on the lateral convexity of the temporal lobe, there was earlier maturation to adult values in the responses from the left hemisphere, as well as earlier matura-

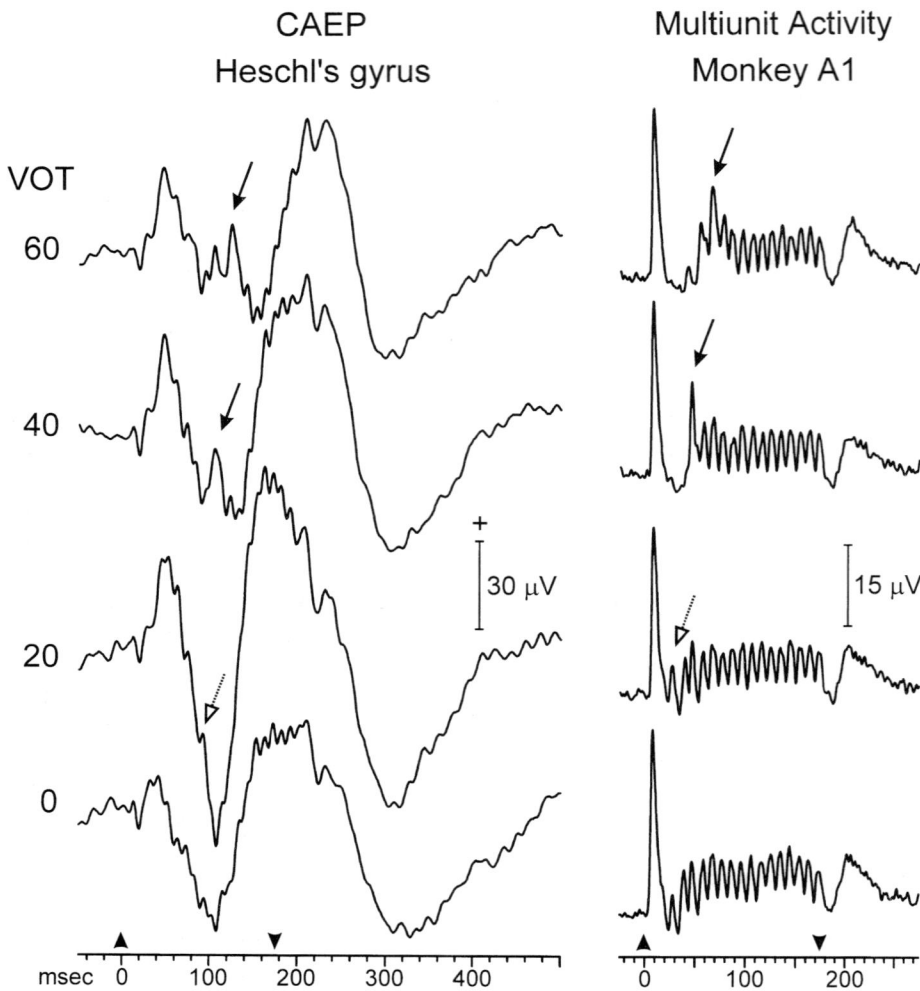

Fig. 8. Similarity in syllable-evoked response patterns between the CAEP recorded by an intracortical electrode in Heschl's gyrus and multi-unit activity in A1 of the monkey. The syllables, /da/ and /ta/, varied in their VOT from 0 to 60 ms. The syllables with a VOT of 40 and 60 ms contain prominent response bursts to both consonant onset and voicing onset (solid arrows), and are perceived by listeners as /ta/. The syllables with a VOT of 0 and 20 ms contain only a prominent response to consonant release. The location of the predicted response to voicing onset for the 20 ms VOT syllable is shown by the unfilled dotted arrows. The short-duration VOT syllables are generally perceived as /da/, suggesting that a temporal processing mechanism may facilitate categorical perception of this phonetic parameter. Suppression of multi-unit activity after the burst evoked by consonant release in the animal responses suggests that a refractory period diminishes the capacity to generate a second response burst for a time period approximating the VOT perceptual boundary. Arrowheads above the time lines mark stimulus onset and offset.

tion of the ERP to the syllable /da/ than to tones. While the significance of these findings remains to be elucidated, it is likely that they index some differences in the developmental trajectories of the two hemispheres in terms of acoustic and speech sound processing.

*Automatic discriminative responses*

The CAEP represents obligatory brain responses to acoustic stimuli. When two stimuli differing in some feature are presented in an 'oddball' paradigm, wherein a repetitively delivered stimulus (the standard) is occasionally replaced by a different stimulus (the deviant), new ERP components emerge that were not present when the stimuli were delivered in isolation. This new response, generally obtained by subtracting the ERP or MEG evoked by the standard stimulus from that elicited by the deviant, contains a negative deflection in the difference waveform that is termed the mismatch negativity (MMN). In unprocessed ERP waveforms the MMN can be seen superimposed upon the later portion of the N1 component and the initial part of the P2. The importance of the MMN for developmental neuropsychology is several fold (Cheour, Leppänen and Kraus, 2000). The MMN can be elicited without the active participation or attention of the subject. This makes the MMN an excellent physiological index for automatic detection of stimulus change by the brain. As such, the MMN is presumed to reflect disruption by a deviant stimulus of a short-term sensory memory trace induced by the preceding standard sounds (Näätänen, 1990). Duration of this short-term memory is brief, given that inter-stimulus intervals greater than several seconds preclude MMN generation. A large number of studies have examined the MMN as a measure of automatic discrimination of multiple sound attributes. These attributes range from simple differences in frequency, intensity or duration to complex differences in the phonetic content of speech and higher-order binding of stimulus patterns needed for acoustic scene analysis (e.g., Alain, Cortese and Picton, 1998; Desjardins, Trainor, Hevenor and Polak, 1999; Mathiak, Hertrich, Lutzenberger and Ackermann, 1999; Szymanski, Yund and Woods, 1999; Vaz Pato and Jones, 1999). MMN has also been used to examine auditory cortical organization as it relates to the processing of simple and more complex sound stimuli (e.g., Alho, Tervaniemi, Huotilainen et al., 1996; Tiitinen, Alho, Huotilainen et al., 1993). The second major advantage of the MMN is that, because it does not require the active participation of the subject, this physiological measure can be used to examine sensory discrimination in very young children and in those who are unable to cooperate with behavioral tasks.

Analyses of surface-recorded ERPs/ERMFs, supplemented by examination of intracortical field potentials, indicate that primary and multiple secondary auditory cortical fields on the supratemporal plane and lateral posterior temporal gyrus are generators of the MMN (Halgren et al., 1998; Kropotov, Alho, Näätänen et al., 2000; Näätänen, 1990). The specific locations of the dipoles are determined by the specific attributes of the stimuli being contrasted in the discrimination paradigms. Importantly, dipole sources computed from MMN topography cannot be considered as discrete foci of activity, but instead are best represented as centers of gravity for more widespread activity in the auditory cortex (Diesch and Luce, 1997). Frontal cortex has been suggested as an additional generator of MMN, and this potential may be involved in the orienting response (Näätänen, 1990). MMN-like activity in the animal model adds insight into the neural mechanisms associated with this automatic discriminative response. In the macaque monkey, a MMN has been observed both in far-field ERPs at the dorsal convexity and from direct recordings in primary auditory cortex (Javitt, Schroeder, Steinschneider et al., 1992; Javitt, Steinschneider, Schroeder et al., 1994; Javitt, Steinschneider, Schroeder and Arezzo, 1996). These responses are generated in supragranular laminae, superficial and later than the initial activation of primary cortex in lamina IV and lower lamina III. Furthermore, activity in NMDA channels partly generates MMN, an especially interesting finding given the putative role of NMDA receptors in learning and memory. Studies in the guinea pig model highlight the additional importance of non-lemniscal auditory thalamus and pathways in MMN generation (King, McGee, Rubel et al., 1995; Kraus, McGee, Littman et al., 1994; Kraus, McGee, Carrell and Sharma, 1995). These latter findings dovetail nicely with the hypothesis that non-lemniscal auditory thalamus activates nucleus basalis, which in turn initiates receptive field plasticity in primary auditory cortex via cholinergic inputs (e.g., Weinberger, 1997). Thus, It is likely that MMN is an index of intrinsic processing within auditory cortex modulated by more non-specific pathways that are involved in detecting potential behavioral relevance for incoming sensory stimuli.

*Mismatch negativity maturation*
Conflicting results attend developmental features of MMN. Several studies have reported that MMN is similar in latency and duration in young school-

A

B

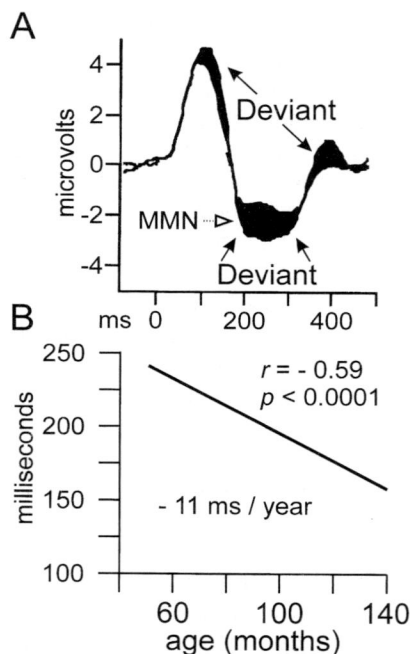

Fig. 9. (A) Schematic grand mean waveforms evoked by standard 1 kHz tones and 1.2 kHz deviant tones and recorded at Fz from 21 5- and 6-year-old children. Deviant tones, which occurred on 15% of the trials, elicited both larger positivities and an intervening negativity (MMN). Filled areas highlight waveform differences between the standard and deviant stimulus responses. (B) Regression line illustrating the decrease in peak MMN latency with increasing age in childhood. Adapted from Shafer et al. (2000).

age children and adults (Čeponienè et al., 1998; Kraus et al., 1993a; Kraus, McGee, Micco et al., 1993b), whereas a recent investigation documents a progressive decrease in latency through early school age (4–10 years) (Fig. 9; Shafer, Morr, Kreuzer and Kurtzberg, 2000). MMN has been reported in 30–35 week gestational age pre-term infants using vowel sounds as stimuli (Cheour, Alho, Čeponienè et al., 1998a), and its amplitude increases through the first year of postnatal life (Cheour et al., 2000). MMN is quite variable in this age group, and in one study that examined the response elicited by pure tone frequency change, only 57% of healthy newborn infants demonstrated the potential (Kurtzberg, Vaughan, Kreuzer and Fliegler, 1995). Furthermore, MMN, when present, may overlap with positive response components that appear to index more basic

refractory properties of the active tissue (Leppänen, Eklund and Lyytinen, 1997). In this study of 28 newborns, deviant tones elicited a positive wave peaking at 250–350 ms that was much smaller for the standard tones. A negative deflection consistent with a MMN was also recorded from fronto-central recording locations in half the subjects, a percentage similar to that reported by Kurtzberg et al. (1995). Studies in 3-month-old infants using an oddball paradigm and consonants differing in their place of articulation also report a positive wave in the response to the deviant stimulus, although acoustic change that crossed a phonemic boundary appeared to elicit a larger response than a similar acoustic change that did not straddle the boundary (Dehaene-Lambertz and Baillet, 1998; Dehaene-Lambertz and Dehaene, 1994). These findings indicate that while a true MMN that indexes a short-term sensory memory trace may be present in young infants, it is variably seen and often dominated by responses produced by stimulus change that denote release from habituation of neural activity. Thus, while MMN obtained from group data may yield valuable insight into neural processing in the very young, suggested by changing MMN scalp topography with age (Pang, Edmonds, Desjardins et al., 1998), its clinical role based on single subject responses is limited (Kurtzberg et al., 1995).

*Mismatch negativity stability and reliability*
Concerns about MMN stability and reliability, and its role in single case evaluations, persist through childhood. Kurtzberg et al. (1995) examined MMN in a frequency-dependent paradigm using young school-age children (mean age 8 years) and concluded that only group data yielded reliable data. In an extensive study of MMN stability in 7–11-year-old children, multiple oddball paradigms using tone frequency and duration, and consonant place of articulation as deviant stimuli were examined (Uwer and von Suchodoletz, 2000). In contrast to stable P1 and N1 CAEP components, MMN amplitude was stable only for duration and one of the phonetic contrasts. Replicability of MMN is less in children than in adults (Escera and Grau, 1996; Escera, Yago, Polo and Grau, 2000; Pekkonen, Rinne and Näätänen, 1995). There may be several reasons for the increased variability in the MMN in children. First, frequencies

are lower and amplitudes are higher in the EEG of children, thus worsening the signal-to-noise ratio for generation of the ERP. Second, attentional effects can modify the amplitude and stability of the MMN, even in adults (Kathmann, Frodl-Bauch and Hegerl, 1999; Szymanski et al., 1999; Woldorff et al., 1998), and this factor is likely more variable in children than in older subjects. Thus, test–retest protocols both within and across experimental sessions may need to be incorporated into developmental studies using MMN in order to assess the reliability of the findings and the applicability of the conclusions.

### *Mismatch negativity in the assessment of auditory system function*

One of the strongest uses of MMN to date has been its capacity to assess psychoacoustic hypotheses using physiological measures. With regard to speech processing, the MMN paradigm has been used to address the nature of the neural representation of speech sounds in auditory cortex. One extreme psychoacoustical hypothesis contends that speech is 'special', and that this type of acoustic stimulus is immediately encoded by specific mechanisms utilizing dedicated modules in the brain, which in turn preempt other forms of speech sound processing (e.g., Liberman and Mattingly, 1989). At the other extreme is the view that phonetic perception is based on more general properties of auditory system processing (e.g., Ohala, 1996). MMN can assess these hypotheses by examining whether acoustic or phonetic features of speech sounds are maintained in short-term memory of auditory cortex. In an excellent example of this type of investigation, Sharma, Kraus, McGee et al. (1993) presented synthetic stop consonant–vowel syllables varying in their formant transition frequencies in an oddball paradigm. They presented two pairs of stimuli, each equivalent in their acoustic differences. One pair was 'within' a phonemic category and both were perceived as /da/, while the other pair were identified as the different syllables /da/ and /ga/. These investigators found that the MMN in young adults was present for both contrasts, and did not significantly differ in latency, amplitude or area. From these data, the authors concluded that the speech sounds were pre-attentively represented in the auditory cortex as an acoustic signal and not according to phonemic categories. Later

work has expanded upon this protocol, and multiple studies have demonstrated that in young adults, the MMN is sensitive to both the acoustic and phonemic features of speech sounds (Sharma and Dorman, 1999; Szymanski et al., 1999; Winkler, Lehtokoski, Alku et al., 1999). Phonetic feature sensitivity is generally observed as an increased amplitude of the MMN when acoustic differences in the stimuli straddle perceptual boundaries. Thus, physiological investigations using MMN have suggested that auditory cortex represents acoustic and phonetic features of speech in parallel.

Similar studies have examined speech-evoked MMN in children, with special focus on the development of the enhanced amplitude in the response when stimuli straddle phonetic boundaries. Earlier work in school-age children has demonstrated that MMN can be elicited by small acoustic changes in a single phoneme (Kraus et al., 1993b). Recently, however, evidence obtained using MMN has suggested development of phonetically based discrimination in babies one year old (Cheour, Čeponiené, Lehtokoski et al., 1998b). In this study, the investigators took advantage of differences in the phonetic structure of vowels in Finnish and Estonian languages. The vowels /e/ and /ö/ occur in both languages, while only Estonian uses the vowel /õ/. At 6 months of age, the MMN was larger in amplitude for the vowel /õ/ than to /ö/ when compared against a standard stimulus /e/ in Finnish babies. The former vowel (/õ/) is acoustically more different from /e/ than /ö/, suggesting that at 6 months of age the MMN was elicited by acoustic features. However, at one year of age, the pattern of MMN amplitude was reversed for the vowels, so that now /õ/ evoked a smaller response than /ö/ in Finnish infants. Because this reversal was associated with a smaller acoustic difference, the authors concluded that the larger amplitude MMN to /ö/ was based on the fact that this vowel was phonemic in Finnish, while /õ/ was not. Furthermore, the pattern of MMN amplitude at one year of age in Finnish babies was reversed in Estonian infants. This profile was expected as both /õ/ and /ö/ are phonemic in Estonian, but the former vowel is acoustically more dissimilar to /e/ than /ö/. Thus, as in adults, MMN indexes both acoustic and phonetic discrimination by one year of age. At 6 months of age, the data suggest that discrimination is based on acoustical features of vowels, and that there is development of a phonetic module for perception in the latter half of the first year of life. Importantly, these electrophysiological findings parallel the development of language-specific phonetic discrimination capacities in young children (e.g., Pegg and Werker, 1997; Werker and Tees, 1999). The results of the study by Cheour et al. (1998b) in one-year old babies are similar to the results of an analogous study performed in adults (Näätänen, Lehtokoski, Lennes et al., 1997). Using the same stimuli, the adult study found native-language enhancement of the MMN to be localized to the left hemisphere, suggesting that language-specific memory traces are lateralized in auditory cortex.

*Cortical auditory-evoked potentials and mismatch negativity in developmental language disorders*
There has been a marked increase in the use of ERPs to examine the neural substrates of developmental language disorders (DLD) (for recent review see Leppänen and Lyytinen, 1997). DLD can be roughly divided into two main classes. The first class, termed specific language impairment (SLI), includes those children who have a deficit in language acquisition that cannot otherwise be attributable to an underlying problem such as mental retardation, hearing loss, or a specific neurological or psychiatric disorder. Developmental dyslexia is the second class of DLDs, and is defined as a deficit in reading skills despite adequate intelligence and socio-cultural/educational opportunities. The driving force behind many of these physiological investigations is the aforementioned hypothesis that abnormalities in rapid temporal processing of sensory information, and the production of rapid sequential movements, underlie the deficits seen in DLD (e.g., Tallal, 1999; Tallal et al., 1993; Tallal et al., 1998; Wright et al., 1997).

Several studies have examined the CAEP and MMN in the SLI population. No abnormalities have been identified in the P1 component of the CAEP (Korpilahti and Lang, 1994; Leppänen and Lyytinen, 1997). Given that a principal generator of the P1 is primary auditory cortex, this finding suggests that SLI is not determined by abnormalities at this early level in the auditory system. However, abnormalities in the middle latency, steady-state response evoked by frequency-modulated tones were reported to be markedly diminished in amplitude in a group of dysphasic children (Stefanatos et al., 1989), a finding supported by similar results in a group of dyslexic adults (McAnally and Stein, 1997). MLRs are likely generated at least in part by activity in primary auditory cortex, and thus it remains open as to the contribution of this cortical field in DLD. Either no changes in the N1 component of the CAEP have been reported in SLI children relative to controls, or a mild increase in peak latency or hemispheric asymmetry in the response has been observed (Korpilahti and Lang, 1994; Leppänen and Lyytinen, 1997; Tonnquist-Uhlén, Borg, Persson and Spens, 1996). Several investigations have consistently reported a decrease in amplitude of the MMN in SLI children in response to deviant tones differing in their frequency from the standards (Holopainen, Korpilahti, Juottonen et al., 1997; Holopainen, Korpilahti, Juottonen et al., 1998; Korpilahti and Lang, 1994). These abnormalities may reflect dysfunction in the SLI population at the level of auditory short-term memory. Unrecognized differences in attention to the stimuli in the passive oddball paradigm of these studies, however, could be the basis for the MMN findings, as increased attention leads to a more robust response.

One reason why many studies have failed to find consistent abnormalities in the N1 CAEP component may be based on their use of a limited number of fronto-central electrode sites. In an active auditory discrimination study of six young adults with varying degrees of auditory discrimination deficits who presented in childhood with verbal auditory agnosia, Klein, Kurtzberg, Brattson et al. (1995) observed a delayed latency in N1 recorded over lateral temporal sites, whereas the 'same' component recorded from fronto-central locations was not different from controls. This finding suggests dysfunction of secondary auditory cortical fields located on the lateral surface of the temporal lobes, and highlights the importance of using more complete electrode arrays in the assessment of auditory system function in normal subjects and those with DLD.

Several studies have compared auditory cortical ERMFs in dyslexic and normal individuals. In contrast to control subjects, a recent ERMF study of adult dyslexic individuals demonstrated that the N1m component evoked by the second of a pair of brief tone bursts that were either of the same or different frequency was significantly diminished in amplitude for interstimulus intervals (ISI) of 100 or 200 ms, but not for those presented 500 ms apart (Nagarajan, Mahncke, Salz et al., 1999). This physiological finding correlated with the capacity of subjects to temporally sequence the tones, and was interpreted as support for a temporal processing deficit in dyslexia. As in SLI subjects, four recent investigations have all reported abnormal MMN responses in dyslexic subjects compared to controls. In one study of adult dyslexic subjects, MMN was diminished in amplitude and increased in latency in a passive oddball paradigm using brief tone bursts of varying frequency (Baldeweg, Richardson, Watkins et al., 1999). MMN generated by tone duration differences were similar between the two groups. Furthermore, MMN latency evoked by frequency differences was correlated with reading errors for both regular words and non-words. The authors suggest that these findings indicate a deficit in frequency encoding at an early level in auditory cortex that might impact on acquisition of phonological skills. However, Schulte-Körne, Deimel, Bartling and Remschmidt (1998) failed to find a difference in MMN for frequency deviants between dyslexic children and age-matched controls, but did observe an attenuated MMN when stimuli were syllables differing in their consonant place of articulation. Additional MMN differences have been observed for more complex, tone pattern sequences, wherein the response was attenuated in amplitude in two different adult dyslexic groups relative to controls (Kujala, Myllyviita, Tervaniemi et al., 2000; Schulte-Körne, Deimel, Bartling and Remschmidt, 1999). Because the frequency content of the sequences was the same, these authors concluded that findings support a deficit in temporal processing.

Another way to assess whether auditory system abnormalities underlie DLD is to examine whether auditory-evoked ERPs recorded in pre-verbal infants can predict the development of language-related impairments. In one study, discriminative responses from 23 healthy newborns evoked by a short-duration syllable /ka/ deviant embedded in a series of long-duration syllable (/kaa/) standards were examined while the children were in quiet sleep (Leppänen, Pihko, Eklund and Lyytinen, 1999). About one half of these babies were from families with dyslexia (at-risk group). Of special note was that the response to the deviant was more negative in the control group than in the 'at-risk' subjects for dyslexia. The authors suggested that even in the neonatal period, acoustic stimulation is differentially processed in babies at special risk for developing dyslexia, and this difference may serve as a biological marker for the disorder. Molfese (2000) has recently reported complementary findings. He recorded the CAEP in 48 newborn infants, of which 17 were later characterized at 8 years of age as dyslexic, while an additional 7 were defined as poor readers. Stimuli used to elicit the CAEP in the newborns included two consonant–vowel syllables (/bi/ and /gi/) and pure tone analogs of the speech sounds. He used a discriminant function to differentiate response patterns between the three groups and found that about 81% of the sample was correctly classified using 6 neonatal CAEP response features. An easily interpretable profile of the CAEP response features that were predictive of later language dysfunction was not observed. For instance, several peak latency measures were found to be useful in the analysis: (1) the first large negative response evoked by the syllable /gi/ and recorded at the left frontal, left parietal, and right temporal electrode sites; (2) baseline-to-peak amplitude measures of the second large negative peak evoked by /gi/ at the right frontal site; (3) the first large negative peak recorded at the right temporal site in response to the non-speech analog of /bi/; and (4) the second large positive peak elicited by /bi/.

As evident by this brief summary of auditory-evoked ERPs in DLD, there is a bewildering complexity of the positive and negative findings that permeate this literature. Given the issues related to MMN reliability outlined in a previous section, recent ERP developmental investigations fall short of being able to reliably predict DLD with the goal of early intervention. What does appear from the data, however, is that physiological indices of auditory cortical dysfunction are associated with DLD. Especially interesting is the more consistent finding that MMN is abnormal in DLD, suggesting that neural mechanisms associated with short-term sensory memory, or those preceding memory storage, are dysfunctional. Less well studied is the possibility that initial states of auditory cortical processing are normal, but that later events occurring in secondary auditory cortex or even in traditional non-sensory areas such as frontal cortex are abnormal. A recent study by Bradlow, Kraus, Nicol et al. (1999) is instructive in this regard. They compared a group of normal school-age children with a group defined as learning impaired. The latter group encompassed a number of diagnoses, including learning impairment, attention deficit disorder, and dyslexia. The use of such a heterogeneous group was predicated on the previous finding of impaired behavioral discrimination of a rapid speech change (/da/ vs. /ga/) that was paralleled by diminished MMN amplitude in a similar cohort, suggesting that this population may have subtle auditory processing deficits relevant for the school difficulties (Kraus, McGee, Carrell et al., 1996). In the more recent study, lengthened formant transitions for the syllables /da/ and /ga/ (80 vs. 40 ms) did not improve discrimination thresholds for the learning impaired group (~50% worse). Despite this lack of behavioral improvement, MMN amplitude increased with the prolonged transition, approximating that of the normal controls. Thus, while preattentive indices of perceptual discrimination improved, supporting a role for a rapid temporal processing deficit in these children, it was not sufficient to facilitate behavioral measures. The latter likely requires improvements in a number of factors that extend beyond the functions of the classical auditory system.

## Visual-evoked potentials (VEP)

### Definition

The utility of VEPs for developmental neuropsychology parallel those described for auditory-evoked potentials, i.e., to assess the integrity and functional maturational of the visual system, as well as evaluate the system's sensitivity to multiple stimulus features. New interest in the maturation of complex visual processing that differentially engages ventral and dorsal streams of visual system networks makes this avenue of developmental neuropsychology both exciting and potentially quite provocative.

Transient and steady-state VEPs are the two main types of electrical responses recorded from the human scalp (for reviews see Celesia and Peachey, 1999; Krumholz, 1999). Transient VEPs

are generated by intermittent stimulation, such as visual checkerboard pattern reversals or diffuse light flashes, whereas steady-state VEPs are evoked by rapid repetitive stimulation (e.g., repetitive flash or rapid checkerboard reversals). The latter responses are sinusoidal deflections with a frequency equal to the rate of stimulation or a harmonic multiple of that rate. Transient VEPs consist of a characteristic sequence of ERP components recorded over the occipital scalp, including a P50, N70, P100 and N145 (letters and numbers designate wave polarity and average latency in adults, respectively). The P100 is the most reliable, and clinically most useful, response component. Response latencies and amplitudes are critically dependent on multiple stimulus parameters. For instance, checkerboard patterns of smaller check size elicit lower-amplitude and longer-latency VEP components. This characteristic enables pattern-reversal VEPs to serve as a physiological index of visual acuity. Fixation on the stimulus, however, is required. This constraint restricts the general utility of the pattern-reversal VEP to older, more cooperative children. Typically, flash-evoked VEPs are used in place of pattern-reversal stimuli in the very young. The principal benefits are that this stimulus does not require visual fixation and is less susceptible to state change. Conversely, sensitivity for assessing visual processing capacities is limited.

### Maturation

Flash VEPs can be recorded in premature infants as early as 24 weeks gestational age (Taylor, Menzies, MacMillan and Whyte, 1987). Early developmental features of the flash-evoked VEP have been documented in a large cohort of neurologically normal children without retinopathy (Pike, Marlow and Reber, 1999). Beginning at 27 weeks gestational age, a consistent negative–positive–negative response, termed N2, P2 and N3 by the authors, was observed. Latency of the components decreased through term, with the peak of the N2 component decreasing from about 300 ms to 250 ms. Beginning at approximately 32 weeks gestational age, a positivity termed P1 was evident. Latency of this wave did not significantly change over gestation, remaining at about 190 ms. A similar stability in P1 latency has been observed both for flash- and pattern-evoked VEPs during gestation in another large cohort of children (Kos-Pietro, Towle, Cakmur and Spire, 1997). However, there was a marked decrease in P1 latency over the first months after birth that was associated with a pronounced increase in P1 amplitude that peaked at about 1 year and then declined. Vaughan and Kurtzberg (1992) have reported a similar amplitude function of P1, except that the response peaked at 4 months and then declined to reach plateau levels in the latter half of the first year. Following infancy, P1 latency remains stable across school-age years, though pattern-reversal VEPs yield shorter latencies than flash-evoked responses (Tomoda, Tobimatsu and Mitsudome, 1999). Developmental features of the pattern-reversal VEP during infancy are illustrated in Fig. 10. Increased complexity and persistent shortening of response latency are characteristic of the VEP recorded at occipital sites. Maturation of the VEP overlying temporal and parietal sites lags behind occipital activity, first becoming evident several months after birth. This latter finding highlights the capacity to examine development of dorsal and ventral stream components.

Early changes in the VEP occurring during the first postnatal year parallel maturational changes in visual cortex anatomy (Burkhalter, 1993; Burkhalter, Bernardo and Charles, 1993; Huttenlocher and De Courten, 1987; Letinic and Kostovic, 1998), suggesting that VEPs may index important parameters of brain development. In concert with the amplitude increase in P1 is rapid synaptogenesis in striate cortex and formation of intracolumnar connections and feedforward connections from V1 to V2. These maturational features are associated with striate cortex reaching its normal adult volume by about 4 months of age. Since the homologue of P1 in monkey striate cortex is principally generated by depolarization of supragranular elements (Schroeder, Tenke, Givre et al., 1991), the increase in P1 amplitude likely reflects an increase in polysynaptic connections upon laminae 2/3 pyramidal cells. The subsequent decline in P1 amplitude is temporally coincident with synaptic pruning in striate cortex, and the establishment of intercolumnar horizontal connections within V1 and feedback connections from V2 to V1. This maturational scheme may reflect an initial development of processing mechanisms in-

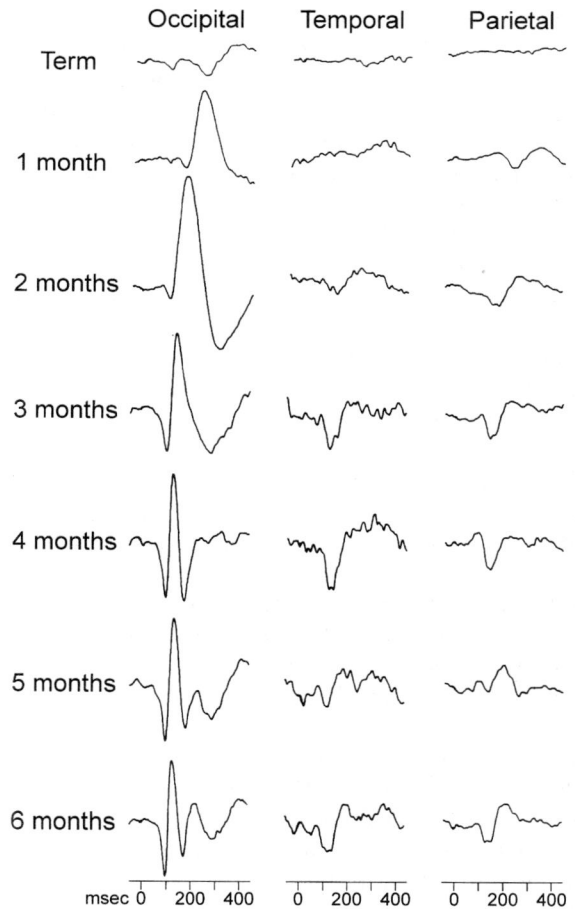

Fig. 10. Pattern-reversal VEPs obtained at sequential ages during infancy and recorded from occipital, temporal, and parietal sites. Maturation of the VEP at occipital sites includes emergence of new response components and reduction of latency for all evoked waves. Development of the VEP recorded from temporal and parietal sites lags behind activity recorded from occipital electrodes, with surface negativities becoming evident after several months of life.

volved in local features of visual scenes, followed by the longer-range connections necessary to integrate these features into a coherent whole (Burkhalter et al., 1993).

*Utility*

In addition to more typical uses of the VEP, such as for evaluation of demyelinating lesions in multiple sclerosis, several studies have examined the prognostic utility of this test in infants (e.g., Ekert, Keenan, Whyte et al., 1997; Shepherd, Saunders, McCulloch and Dutton, 1999; Whyte, 1993). Severe abnormalities in the VEP, such as absence or severely delayed components, are moderately predictive of abnormal neurological outcome. However, these studies have not adequately addressed whether the VEP can be used for predicting dysfunction specific for the visual system. Additionally, it is unclear whether the VEP offers any greater sensitivity for predictions of neurological outcome in neonates than longitudinal EEG studies. Overall, use of the VEP has less clinical utility than BAEPs in the assessment of sensory function in this population.

*Higher visual processing*

One of the most exciting frontiers for developmental neuropsychology is the potential to assess emergent brain functions involved in higher perceptual processing. Nowhere is this more evident than in the visual system, where anatomical and physiological studies are mapping out the roles of distributed neural networks, subsumed into dorsal and ventral streams of neural activity, involved in the representation of the visual world. The parallel nature of complex visual processing in dorsal and ventral visual streams has been studied in adults using ERP analysis (e.g., Martín-Loeches, Hinojosa and Rubia, 1999), and the expansion of this endeavor to studies of children offers the potential to assess the developmental maturation of these visual pathways. The best-studied higher visual process involves the specialized role of specific ventral brain regions for the recognition of faces. These studies exemplify the benefits of integrating multidisciplinary approaches toward the goal of understanding the neural bases and development of complex perceptual processes. Furthermore, they serve as a template upon which investigations of other complex visual phenomena can utilize.

*Face recognition*

Lesions in the inferior occipital and posterior temporal brain regions can produce a striking deficit in the ability to recognize faces (face agnosia or prosopagnosia; for review see Damasio, Tranel and Damasio, 1990). Functional MRI studies have refined localiza-

tion of face processing areas to the posterior fusiform gyrus and nearby structures, located at the junction of the inferior surfaces of the occipital and temporal lobes (e.g., Halgren, Dale, Sereno et al., 1999; Kanwisher, McDermott and Chun, 1997; Puce, Allison, Asgari et al., 1996). Intracortical ERP studies extend the fMRI findings by demonstrating the timing and characteristics of this activation (Allison, McCarthy, Nobre et al., 1994; Allison, Puce, Spencer and McCarthy, 1999; McCarthy, Puce, Belger and Allison, 1999; Puce, Allison and McCarthy, 1999). The first face-specific response is a negativity recorded over the ventral surface of extrastriate cortex with an onset of 140 ms and a peak at about 200 ms (N200). Similar to fMRI studies, there is a slight predominance of right hemispheric activation for faces that is particularly evident for upright (non-inverted) faces. N200 is relatively insensitive to multiple changes in the details of the faces and their familiarity, shows minimal habituation, is not affected by face–name learning, and does not demonstrate semantic priming. Later face-evoked ERP components are, however, variously affected by these factors (Puce et al., 1999).

Other sites located on more lateral aspects of the posterior temporal lobe and in the posterior superior temporal sulcus, as well as inferior temporal areas near face-specific sites, respond selectively to face parts (especially eyes and mouth), and other body parts (Allison, Puce and McCarthy, 2000; McCarthy et al., 1999; Puce, Allison, Bentin et al., 1998). This anatomical complexity may be responsible for a discrepancy in the latencies of the intracortically recorded responses and those recorded overlying the scalp. Face-specific responses with peak latencies of 160–170 ms can be recorded as negative potentials at lateral temporal sites and positive waves near the vertex (Eimer, 2000; George, Evans, Fiori et al., 1996; Halgren, Raij, Marinkovic et al., 2000; Rossion, Campanella, Gomez et al., 1999; Sams, Hietanen, Hari et al., 1997). While several equivalent current dipole models suggest that these responses are generated near the fusiform gyrus (Halgren et al., 2000; Sams et al., 1997), more recent work suggests that the ~30 ms discrepancy in peak latency can best be ascribed to somewhat earlier activation of a more lateral temporal region specific for the processing of eyes (Taylor, Edmonds, McCarthy and

Allison, 2001). Thus, ERP components evoked by whole faces and face parts likely overlap in scalp recordings, and appropriate control conditions are needed to dissect out the contributions of each stimulus feature to the total response evoked by faces.

It is with this fertile background that our understanding of face development is evolving. Perceptually, recognition of faces is superior to other objects even in the neonatal period (Carey, 1992). Improvement in face recognition occurs throughout childhood, and appears to involve enhanced holistic perception of facial attributes dominating over more piecemeal or featural information (Baenninger, 1994; Carey, 1992; Chung and Thomson, 1995). Aspects of face processing development are accessible to physiological investigation. This has been demonstrated in a group of 4–14-year-old children (Taylor, McCarthy, Saliba and Degiovanni, 1999). Stimuli were faces, cars, butterflies, and scrambled faces and cars. Butterflies were targets (12%), and all other stimuli were equally presented. An N170 was present maximally for faces and was best recorded from inferior temporal sites of the right hemisphere. While the N170 was present in all age groups, it was most prominent in adults. Furthermore, there was a gradual decrease in peak latency throughout childhood.

In a more extensive investigation, Taylor et al. (2001) have recently examined face and eye processing in a large group of 4–15-year-old children and adults. While latencies of the N170 decreased with increasing age, there was a dissociation in the rates of latency change between eye and whole face stimuli. Latencies of the N170 evoked by eyes were shorter in the younger age groups ad reached an asymptote at an earlier age than those evoked by whole faces. The N170 evoked by whole faces continued to shorten in latency into adulthood, at which time its latency was shorter than that to eyes. This dissociation in latency between stimuli supports the importance of eye (featural) processing in early childhood and a greater reliance on configural (holistic) processing in older individuals. It also demonstrates that these processes follow different maturational courses. N170 amplitude was always larger to eyes than to faces, and responses were always larger over the right hemisphere. In parallel with latency changes, eyes were the only stimuli presented to show an amplitude decrement with increasing age, again suggesting a greater reliance on configural processing in older subjects. Latency and amplitude changes with age were associated with pronounced differences in the voltage distribution of the potential, being maximal in more superior temporal electrodes in younger children and at inferior electrode sites in older children and adults. These distribution changes further support differential maturation of the various networks involved in the processing of faces and their components.

Later stages in the development of face recognition, possibly involving prefrontal cortex, may also be assessed. Six-month-old infants show an enhanced negative component (Nc) at fronto-temporal electrode sites when presented with familiar faces and toys (de Haan and Nelson, 1999). Topography of Nc was differentially affected by object type, and a right-hemisphere predominance for face processing was observed. The authors concluded that infants' experience with specific object categories, and recognized examples within those categories, influenced the electrocortical recording. Similar findings using geometric shapes as visual stimuli in an oddball paradigm have been obtained in 1–2-month-old infants (Karrer and Monti, 1995). Here, novel shapes evoked faster Nc amplitudes and higher-amplitude negative slow waves upon which the Nc was superimposed. This was associated with longer visual fixations upon the oddball stimuli, suggesting that Nc can serve as an index of attentional processes in infants.

These studies are at the leading edge of investigations into the development of higher visual processing mechanisms, and future studies examining the development of different visual attributes are on the horizon. Already, developmental studies for selective attention to color (Van der Stelt, Kok, Smulders et al., 1998) and visual motion detection (Hollants-Gilhuijs, De Munck, Kubova et al., 2000) have been initiated. For instance, the latter study has documented a negative surface component (N2) with a latency of about 180 ms in school-age children that is similar to adults, but with a hemispheric asymmetry differing from the older subjects, suggesting a continued immaturity in motion detection mechanisms. Combined fMRI and ERP/ERMF studies suggest that N2 is partly generated in area MT of the dorsal visual information stream (Ahlfors et al., 1999; Wang et al., 1999a). This indicates that development of both parietal and temporal pathways, differentially involved in the encoding of visual attributes, are accessible for analysis. Of special note is the similarity in polarity and latency of extrastriate activity for face, color and motion detection. In all cases, a negative component peaking at around 200 ms is observed with subtle differences in temporal–parietal–occipital topographies, suggesting that this activity is a marker for specific activation of different regions of extrastriate cortex (Hillyard and Anllo-Vento, 1998). A similar latency ERMF component evoked by letter strings and generated in the left inferior occipito-temporal cortex has been reported to be absent in dyslexic adults (Helenius, Tarkiainen, Cornelissen et al., 1999b), extending the role of ERP/ERMF studies to assess possible extrastriate system dysfunction in developmental disorders.

## Processing-contingent potentials (PCPS)

One of the most exciting applications of ERPs in developmental neuropsychology reflects the increased use of potentials associated with higher cognitive operations. Over the years, an increasingly complex array of PCPs has been identified in the setting of discriminative and selective attention tasks. These PCPs include multiple negative and positive components that overlap or follow earlier obligatory responses. The most prominent of these potentials include a host of processing negativities, P300, and long-latency positive PCPs (for reviews see Altenmüller and Gerloff, 1999; Hillyard, Mangun, Woldorff and Luck, 1997; Näätänen, 1990; Picton and Hillyard, 1988; Polich, 1999). Because PCPs frequently overlap with exogenous potentials, methods are required to separate activity associated with the different processes. Generally, a subtraction method is used, wherein ERPs evoked by a paradigm that requires some behavioral response or neural process has subtracted from it ERPs evoked when that response or process is not required. The difference waveform presumably reflects some measure of the brain activity specific for that behavioral response or neural process. Similar subtraction methods are used in functional neuroimaging studies to remove activation of brain regions engaged in simpler pro-

cesses from those associated with higher-level requirements. However, it would be premature from use of the subtraction method alone to conclude that the earlier processing areas were not directly involved in the higher-order processes, but only that additional regions became operational in the more demanding task. This methodological consideration highlights an important caveat for the subtraction technique, which is that it cannot always be assumed that the processes eliminated in the procedure remains stable across task conditions. The problem may be compounded in electrophysiological studies attempting to define generators for PCPs based upon surface ERP topography of difference waves. Now, flawed assumptions for the ERP subtractions will produce erroneous surface topographies, and result in faulty conclusions regarding potential generators.

### Processing negativities

#### Audition
Several processing negativities have been identified in discrimination and selective attention tasks. The latter is a more powerful paradigm, for it allows ERPs evoked by attended and unattended stimuli to be acquired in the same experimental run and compared (Fig. 11). Typically, two independent trains of stimuli are presented in a manner that facilitates selective attention to one stimulus set or another, as by dichotic stimulation. Rare target and frequent nontarget stimuli (e.g., tones of different frequencies) are embedded in both trains (i.e., double 'oddball' paradigm), and the task involves responding to the target stimulus in only the attended channel. Subtracting responses evoked by the unattended stimuli from those obtained to attended stimuli assesses attentional effects. A basic aspect of cognitive processes is the ability to focus on task-relevant stimuli and filter out stimuli irrelevant for the task (Berman and Friedman, 1995). Dysfunction of this process may be especially important in a number of developmental problems such as attention deficit hyperactivity disorder (ADHD), making this paradigm very relevant for developmental neuropsychology. Integrating ERPs into the selective attention paradigm facilitates examination of different hypotheses pertaining to attentional mechanisms (for review see Coull, 1998). This integration allows the assessment

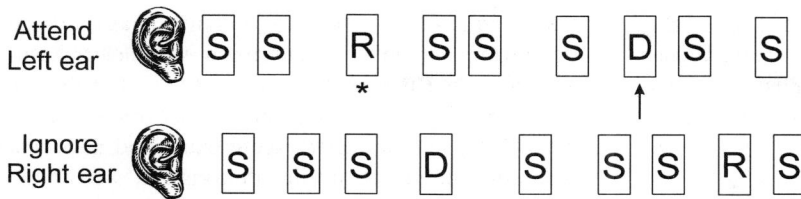

Fig. 11. Schematic for a typical selective attention paradigm performed in the auditory modality. Standard (S), deviant target (D), and occasionally rare (R) stimuli are presented in two different processing channels. Dichotic stimulation frequently serves as the medium for generating two channels. Location of stimulus presentation often serves as means by which several processing channels are initiated in the visual modality. Cross-modal stimulation (e.g., visual and auditory stimulation) can also be used as the two processing channels. The task of the subject is to respond to the deviant stimuli in the attended channel (arrow). Presentation of rare stimuli (asterisk) can evaluate the effects of novel stimuli on neural processing, and is frequently used to generate specific subcomponents of the P300 wave.

of whether selective attention is based on early gain control of incoming sensory input by comparing amplitudes of obligatory ERP components in the attended and unattended channels, or whether additional resources and neural events are engaged in the attentional process (Hillyard et al., 1997).

Using this powerful paradigm, it has been shown that attended stimuli evoke larger ERP/ERMF responses than unattended stimuli within the first 50 ms of stimulation (Woldorff, Gallen, Hampson et al., 1993; Woldorff et al., 1998). This enhancement extends to the N1 and MMN components (Coull, 1998; Hillyard et al., 1997; Trejo, Ryan-Jones and Kramer, 1995; Woldorff et al., 1998; Woods, Alho and Algazi, 1994), though additional processing negativities are also generated (see below). These findings indicate that one facet of selective attention is the enhancement of early sensory and short-term memory functions involved in the processing of attended stimuli. Since effects are noted in less than 50 ms after stimulus onset, within the range of the MLR of the AEP, this gain control appears to include primary auditory cortex.

Processing negativities that extend beyond enhancement of exogenous components of the CAEP are also generated by selective attention tasks, indicating that additional neural resources become active with attention. Both early and late processing negativities (also termed Nd) have been identified (Hillyard et al., 1997). The early Nd overlaps in time with the N1 and P2 CAEP components, and appears to be generated in multiple auditory cortical fields located both on the superior and lateral surfaces of the superior temporal gyrus (Alho, Teder, Lavikainen and Näätänen, 1994; Kasai, Nakagome, Itoh et al.,

1999; Woods et al., 1994). The specific fields that generate the early Nd may vary with the stimulus features that are being attended. Later Nd components peaking after 300 ms post-stimulus onset have a broader topographic distribution (Schröger, 1994). Generators include frontal cortex sites (Kasai et al., 1999), consistent with their roles in attention (e.g., Coull, 1998).

Additional processing negativities in the auditory modality include the N2, which is generated only to target stimuli in discrimination tasks (Alain, Achim and Richer, 1993; Ritter, Simson, Vaughan and Friedman, 1979). This component, which peaks between 200 and 300 ms, is maximal over lateral temporal and parietal sites, and shows clear hemispheric asymmetries when sound is processed in a phonetic context (Celsis, Doyon, Boulanouar et al., 1999; Kayser, Tenke and Bruder, 1998). Later left-hemisphere N2-like components associated with semantic classification and with a different topographic distribution than those associated with more general acoustic processing are also seen, suggesting that these negativities can examine sequential activations of auditory and language cortices (Lovrich, Novick and Vaughan, 1988; Novick, Lovrich and Vaughan, 1985).

Processing negativities related to selective attention undergo developmental changes typical of ERP components, with the early Nd amplitude becoming larger and the peak latency decreasing with increases in age (Berman and Friedman, 1995). These findings were interpreted as physiological support for the hypothesis that children have greater difficulty in attending to specific stimuli when confronted with competing inputs. More difficult to interpret changes in topography of processing negativities have also been observed with age (Oades, Dittmann-Balcar and Zerbin, 1997). Most likely, these changes partly represent differential maturation of the neural structures involved in selective attention.

*Vision*

Similar to the modulation of CAEPs by selective attention, the first effect on VEPs is an augmentation of the early P1 and N1 components when attention is directed to a specific location in visual space (reviewed in Hillyard et al., 1997; Hillyard and Anllo-Vento, 1998). While dipole modeling suggests that these effects occur in extrastriate visual cortex, fMRI findings support a similar location-dependent augmentation in striate cortex (Smith, Singh and Greenlee, 2000). Comparative effects are not observed when attention is focused on non-spatial location features, emphasizing the primacy of spatial attention in visual perception. Attention directed to non-spatial location features, such as color, shape or motion, lead to processing negativities and positivities, whose topographic distributions suggest differential activation of cortical regions involved in the encoding of specific visual attributes (Hillyard and Anllo-Vento, 1998; Martín-Loeches et al., 1999; Michie, Karayanides, Smith et al., 1999). Overall, these visual selective attention studies offer insight into the timing, and hierarchical organization, of visual perceptual processes.

As observed in the auditory modality, developmental studies also identify decreased latency and changes in topography of processing negativities that vary with age (DeFrance, Sands, Schweitzer et al., 1997; Taylor, 1993). Furthermore, these topographic changes are dependent on the specific visual processing task. For instance, processing negativities elicited by a task involving the detection of orthographic changes in the shapes of letters were different than those evoked by detection of visually presented letters that rhymed with the letter /v/ (Taylor, 1993). This difference indicates that ERPs can not only index the development of higher visual perceptual processes, but also access developmental changes that occur when visual stimuli initiate phonological processing mechanisms. In a similar vein, developmental features of number processing have been addressed using ERPs (Temple and Posner, 1998).

Here, the abstract concept of quantity was assessed by asking subjects to determine whether a visually presented number was larger or smaller than 5. Numbers closer to 5 evoke longer reaction times (distance effect). When ERPs were examined in 5-year olds and adults performing this task, it was found that both groups displayed longer reaction times, increased ERP negativities, and later positivities, when the comparison number was close to 5. ERP changes paralleled activation patterns obtained with functional neuroimaging studies (Dehaene, Tzourio, Frak et al., 1996), and were maximal in occipital regions and inferior parietal areas in both age groups. Findings thus support the suggestion that young children have an appreciation for basic number concepts that is more pronounced than previously thought.

*Semantic processing*

While not strictly limited as an index of semantic processing, a processing negativity that peaks at about 400 ms (N400) has been a powerful ERP measure of language functions, classically occurring when a sentence ends in a semantically incongruous manner (e.g., "I like milk and sugar in my *socks*": Kutas and Hillyard, 1980). N400 increases in amplitude as the incongruity in sentence meaning produced by the target word increases (Helenius, Salmelin, Service and Connolly, 1998). Similarly, a prominent N400 can be elicited when the second item in a pair of words is semantically unrelated to the first item. Conversely, the N400 diminishes as the degree of semantic relatedness increases between the two words. Therefore, this ERP component is an index of semantic priming, a process whereby identification of a word is easier when preceded by related words. This effect is thought to represent a means by which word meaning is represented in semantic memory, with automatic spread to other associated words occurring when a preceding word is semantically processed. N400-like components also appear to index phonological and orthographic processing mechanisms, as revealed by comparing ERPs elicited when word pairs either rhyme or do not rhyme, and when they share or do not share similar orthography (see McPherson, Ackerman, Holcomb and Dykma, 1998). Obviously, N400 might serve as a valuable vehicle by which to study features of normal and aberrant language development. As for all ERP components, its worth magnifies when the neural generators of the activation are identified.

N400 has a widespread topographic distribution over the scalp that is maximal over the vertex (Curran, Tucker, Kutas and Posner, 1993; Johnson and Hamm, 2000). Intracranial recordings performed during visual presentation of words suggest a generator in ventral extrastriate cortex, in the region of the collateral sulcus and anterior fusiform gyrus (McCarthy, Nobre, Bentin and Spencer, 1995; Nobre and McCarthy, 1995). ERMF recordings offer strong evidence that the superior temporal cortex, especially in the left hemisphere, is another prominent generator for this component (Helenius et al., 1998). Additional research suggests that N400 elicited by orthographic differences engages frontally predominant structures, while phonological components of the N400 are generated in more parietal regions (see McPherson et al., 1998). Thus, it is likely that N400 is a composite waveform generated by multiple structures involved in several facets of language decoding and perception.

Studies have begun to examine the utility of N400 in the assessment of language functions in children (Byrne, Connolly, MacLean et al., 1999). This study took advantage of the fact that N400 can also be generated when a word is semantically unrelated to a simultaneously presented picture. Using this paradigm, an N400 was obtained to semantically incongruous picture–word pairs in children from ages of 5 to 12. Importantly, this paradigm does not require the child to give a verbal or motor response, thus facilitating electrophysiological testing of language functions in subjects who have expressive or motor difficulties. Furthermore, this paradigm accurately estimated vocabulary capacities across age groups, enhancing the test's potential value as an adjunct for other forms of developmental language assessment.

N400 has also been used to compare language functions in normal reading adolescents and those with dyslexia (McPherson et al., 1998). The reading-impaired subjects were further subdivided into 2 groups based on their ability to decode visually presented non-words. Stimuli were word pairs that varied along the dimensions of rhyming and orthography, and the task was to determine whether the two words rhymed. Normal adolescent readers displayed a frontally predominant N400 for words that were orthographically dissimilar and a parietal N400 for non-rhyming words. A left-frontal motor preparedness potential, the contingent negative variation (CNV, see Starr et al., 1995), was also elicited in the time interval between the words in the pairs. Subjects with dyslexia and poor phonological skills differed from controls only in an aberrant N400 elicited in the rhyming task, while those subjects with dyslexia and better phonological skills had normal N400 components but a reduced amplitude CNV. The reduced CMV in this group was associated with slower reaction times when compared to the control group and the dyslexia group with poor phonological skills. The authors proposed that their results indicate that dyslexia can be subdivided into at least 2 subtypes, one deficient in the transformation of orthographic material into phonological units, and the other exhibiting abnormalities in processing speed. This hypothesis-driven study exemplifies the potential benefits in clarifying normal and dysfunctional higher-order processes when ERP analysis is thoughtfully integrated with detailed manipulation of stimulus parameters and well-characterized subject populations.

### Processing positivities

#### P300

P300 is the most intensely studied of all the endogenous potentials, and has generated the most interest, outside of the MMN, in terms of its potential clinical applications (for reviews see Hillyard and Picton, 1987; Polich, 1999). Significant confusion in the literature regarding the significance of this component is partly based on the P300 being a composite waveform generated by widespread brain regions. Intracranial recordings support the conclusion that at least three distinct neural systems are directly involved in the generation of P300 (Halgren et al., 1998). The first system is a specific activation of sensory cortex in response to the presentation of rare stimuli. Multiple components are evoked, regardless of the subject's attentional state, and include a MMN-like wave and later components that overlap in time with P300 recording at the scalp. While the intracortical data were obtained in auditory cortex, similar sensory-specific P300-like activity has been recorded in occipital cortex with visual stimuli (Rogers, Basile, Papanicolaou and Eisenberg, 1993). The second system is not modality specific and involves activation of prefrontal, anterior cingulate and inferior parietal cortices in response to rare stimuli. This activation occurs regardless of attention, and represents an automatic, physiological manifestation of an orienting response to external events. The dominant generator of this subcomponent of the P300, termed P3a, appears to be prefrontal cortex, given that this wave has a maximum amplitude overlying more frontal and central electrode sites at the scalp (Friedman, Kazmerski and Fabiani, 1997). P3a is associated with a preceding negativity (termed N2a) and a following negative slow wave, and its peak latency of about 300 ms is shorter than that of the other major subcomponent of P300, termed P3b. P3b, as recorded by intracranial electrodes (Halgren et al., 1998), is generated by a widespread ensemble of neural areas including the hippocampus and other limbic tissues, superior temporal sulcus, prefrontal cortex and intraparietal sulcus. It requires active discrimination of stimuli and is modality non-specific. Furthermore, P3b occurs at about the same time as the subject's response, suggesting that this component represents a physiological index for stimulus perception and completion of a cognitive task (Halgren et al., 1998). The latency of P3b is longer than P3a, and its scalp distribution shows a parietal maximum (Friedman et al., 1997).

## P300 maturation

The complex generator system of P300 predicts that its development likely represents modulation of multiple neural structures, each with its own time course of maturation. Thus, it is easy to envision that the timing, amplitude and spatial distribution of P300 will undergo complex changes with development. As expected, P300 latency decreases with age through childhood and adolescence (e.g., Taylor, 1993; Van der Stelt et al., 1998). While amplitude of P300 tends to be greater in children, the signal-to-noise ratio is worse than in adults (Miyazaki, Shibasaki, Suwazono et al., 1994), limiting its usefulness in the evaluation of individual subjects or in single trials. One of the more prominent aspects of P300 development is seen both in the young and in the

elderly. When presented with standard, novelty and oddball target stimuli, the P300 distribution in the elderly contains both parietal and frontal maxima. This distribution is similar for both the novel and target stimuli, and is associated with increased false-positive behavioral responses to the novel stimuli (Friedman et al., 1997). The authors interpreted this pattern as an indication that the elderly may not appropriately process stimuli that should have been previously well characterized, as manifested by an apparent P3a novelty response, and prefrontal cortex activation, to the targets. Similar findings appear to be a normal developmental finding in children. Target stimuli proceeded by a large number (>10) of standard sounds elicit a larger amplitude P300 with shorter latency and a more widespread voltage distribution into frontal areas in 9-year-old children when compared to targets occurring after a smaller number of standards (Kilpeläinen, Koistinen, Könönen et al., 1999a). This effect was greater than that occurring in adults, and was interpreted as the emergence of a P3a novelty response in children with long inter-target intervals. It was suggested that this represents a more rapid decay of the neural representation of target stimuli in children when compared to adults, and may represent an important index of memory and attention in the young.

Despite these developmental differences, other basic modulatory features of the P300 are similar across age groups. P3a amplitude decreases with repetition of identical rare stimuli across age groups (Cycowicz, Friedman and Rothstein, 1996; Cycowicz and Friedman, 1997), strengthening the hypothesis that this subcomponent in part represents an index for orientation to new environmental stimulation. Additionally, P300 voltage distributions change as a function of behavioral task (Taylor, 1993), indicating that it is not a unitary phenomenon in either children or adults. However, task-related voltage distributions are also modulated by subject age, suggesting maturation of processing strategies with development. In a similar vein, differences in processing strategies have been postulated between normal reading children and those who were born with very low birth weights, based on voltage distribution differences in P300-like ERP waves during lexical decision and semantic classification tasks (Khan, Frisk and Taylor, 1999).

## Event-related potentials in developmental disorders

### *Attention deficit/hyperactivity disorder (ADHD)*

ADHD is characterized by the core symptoms of childhood-onset inattention, impulsivity, and hyperactivity. It is a clinically heterogeneous disorder, with learning disabilities, conduct and other behavioral disorders, and tics often observed as associated features (Faraone and Biederman, 1998). Clinical heterogeneity is paralleled by genetic heterogeneity. Studies have also stressed the importance of environmental factors in the disorder (see Faraone and Biederman, 1998; Schulz, Himelstein, Halperin and Newcorn, 2000; Swanson, Castellanos, Murias et al., 1998). Genetic abnormalities have focused on dysfunction of several dopamine receptor genes and the dopamine transporter gene, the latter required for re-uptake of dopamine into presynaptic cells. Methylphenidate, a therapeutic mainstay for ADHD, blocks the dopamine transporter and increases the amount of dopamine present in the synapse, and also alters noradrenergic functions (Solanto, 1998). Effects on dopaminergic and noradrenergic functions are complex, and both increases and decreases in associated neural activity result from drug action. Complicating the ability to pinpoint discrete aspects of brain dysfunction in ADHD, both neurochemical systems are widely distributed in the brain, and both are hypothesized to be important in the pathogenesis of the disorder (see reviews in Faraone and Biederman, 1998; Schulz et al., 2000; Solanto, 1998; Swanson et al., 1998). However, most hypotheses envision abnormalities of attentional and other executive functions (planning and regulation of behavior) in prefrontal cortex. Prefrontal cortex is tightly connected to basal ganglia circuits and interconnected with parietal association cortex, which is involved with processing of behaviorally relevant stimuli. Thus, clinical, genetic, pharmacological and anatomical considerations highlight the complicated and multifaceted nature of ADHD.

It is therefore not surprising that related ERP studies often yield results that are contradictory and difficult to interpret. Amplitude of the P1 component of the CAEP has been reported as either smaller than controls (Kemner, Verbaten, Koelega et al.,

1996) or without change (Oades, Dittmann-Balcar, Schepker et al., 1996) in children with ADHD. The N1 component of the CAEP has been variously reported as without change (Kilpeläinen, Partanen and Karhu, 1999c), decreased in amplitude (Kemner et al., 1996; Kemner, Verbaten, Koelega et al., 1998; Satterfield, Schell and Nicholas, 1994), or decreased in latency from controls (Oades et al., 1996). The attentional state of the subjects is likely an important variable in the interpretation of these findings, as the decreased N1 amplitudes relative to controls may dissipate in passive listening conditions (Satterfield et al., 1994). Given that obligatory cortical responses are modified by attention, it is not clear whether the ERP effects are a true representation of specific deficits with regard to early sensory processing, or just a by-product of the attentional difficulties. A similar argument can be put forth in the evaluation of other sensory-evoked responses. Thus, low-amplitude MMN evoked by oddball auditory stimuli in children with ADHD (Kemner et al., 1996; Kilpeläinen et al., 1999c) may be a reflection of diminished attention to the stimuli. Other investigators have not observed an amplitude decrement in the MMN, but have reported an aberrant lateralization of the potential to the left hemisphere in this patient group (Oades et al., 1996). Also hard to interpret are reports that the P2 component of the CAEP is greater in amplitude and has a shorter peak latency in children with ADHD (Oades, 1998; Oades et al., 1996). While the authors propose that the enhanced P2 indexes increased inhibitory processes that decrease the ability of ADHD subjects to process new stimuli, this idea must be viewed with caution until confirmed by complementary data. Easier to incorporate into a scheme of attentional dysfunction in ADHD, the Nd difference wave, which is a measure of activity in attended auditory channels, is smaller in children with the disorder (Jonkman, Kemner, Verbaten et al., 1997a).

The best-characterized ERP component in the assessment of ADHD is P300. As discussed previously, an earlier subcomponent has a more frontally predominant voltage distribution that reflects an automatic orienting response to novel stimuli in prefrontal regions (P3a), while a later subcomponent has a posterior voltage maximum and indexes aspects of task-relevant cognitive processing. Despite the use of different visual, auditory or language-related tasks in multiple studies, a relatively consistent pattern has emerged, wherein the P3a component is larger in amplitude in children with ADHD, while simultaneously there is a reduction in size of P3b (e.g., Brandeis, Van Leeuwen, Rubia et al., 1998; Kilpeläinen, Partanen and Karhu, 1999b; Kilpeläinen, Partanen, Luoma et al., 1999d; Overtoom, Verbaten, Kemner et al., 1998; Robaey, Cansino, Dugas and Renault, 1995). Of special interest is the finding that in a standard auditory oddball paradigm, the P3a component fails to normally habituate in easily distractible children when examined at the beginning, middle and end of the behavioral task (Kilpeläinen et al., 1999d). In total, these findings suggest an abnormally enhanced orienting response to incoming stimuli, manifested by the increased P3a component, in children with ADHD. Stimuli that should have been categorized are processed in accentuated fashion as novel events in prefrontal brain regions. In parallel, the attenuated P3b ERP component implies deficiencies in the processing of behaviorally relevant stimuli in more posterior brain networks. These findings are congruent with most theories of ADHD, which promote the idea of abnormal sensory gating in prefrontal and parietal association cortices (Faraone and Biederman, 1998; Schulz et al., 2000; Swanson et al., 1998). Normalization of P3b has been reported with methylphenidate administration to children with ADHD (Jonkman, Kemner, Verbaten et al., 1997b; Taylor, Voros, Logan and Malone, 1993), supporting a role for electrophysiological measures in clarifying the effects of medication therapy on neural processing. However, improvements in electrophysiological indices are not uniformly present in studies examining the effects of medication therapy (Jonkman, Kemner, Verbaten et al., 1999), indicating that caution must be exercised when relating these measures to behavioral performance.

We predict that many of the inconsistencies present in the literature will be resolved with improved methodological experimental designs. The heterogeneous nature of ADHD may be responsible for some of the variability in the ERP data, and stricter exclusion criteria that limit investigations to specific subtypes of the disorder at specific ages, and using standardized behavioral tasks will likely improve the sensitivity and specificity of the re-

sults. Many studies have analyzed ERPs from only a few midline recording sites. Greater reliance on more extensive ERP mapping procedures incorporating sophisticated data sharpening techniques, dipole analysis paradigms, and co-registration with neuroimaging studies, should further refine and enrich the data sets.

*Autism*

Autism is a developmental syndrome characterized by severe impairments in social interaction, the presence of abnormal and restricted behavior patterns, and deficits in language acquisition and communication skills (e.g., Rapin, 1997; Volkmar, Cook, Pomeroy et al., 1999). It is a relatively common (~1 : 1000–2000) and genetically heterogeneous disorder (Lamb, Moore, Bailey and Monaco, 2000; Rutter, 2000; State, Lombroso, Pauls and Leckman, 2000). Pathological heterogeneity parallels the genetic variability, although megalencephaly, and varying degrees of cortical, brainstem and cerebellar dysgenesis have been fairly consistent findings (e.g., Bailey, Luthert, Dean et al., 1998; Courchesne, 1997; Hendren, De Backer and Pandina, 2000). Additionally, even when autistic individuals display adequate functional skills for a specific task, the brain regions activated, and by extension, the strategies utilized, may be different than controls (Ring, Baron-Cohen, Wheelwright et al., 1999). It is in this environment that ERP studies have been undertaken, with emphasis being placed on localizing the level of brain dysfunction that engenders the language abnormalities.

Children with autism are frequently characterized as having abnormalities in auditory processing, and often exhibit features characteristic of verbal auditory agnosia (e.g., Klein, Tuchman and Rapin, 2000). They may be under-reactive or hypersensitive to sound, and there is often poor auditory processing in the setting of significantly better visual–spatial processing (Ring et al., 1999). These observations have led most ERP studies examining language issues to focus on auditory system functions. Thus far, studies addressing auditory processing have provided fragmented evidence of normality or dysfunction at various levels of the neuroaxis. Studies examining ABRs have produced contradictory results, with some finding prolongation of central conduction time (McClelland, Eyre, Watson et al., 1992; Rosenhall, Johansson and Gillberg, 1988; Thivierge, Bedard, Cole and Maziade, 1990; Wong and Wong, 1991), and others observing no abnormality (Grillon, Courchesne and Akshoomoff, 1989; Rumsey, Grimes, Pikus et al., 1984). While abnormal ABRs suggest the intriguing prospect that they are a physiological marker for brainstem pathology in autism, critiques of these findings caution against their over interpretation (Klin, 1993). On the other hand, the variability in ABR findings across sample populations may reflect subtle group differences in the degree of brainstem pathology that was present in the subjects.

Inconsistency of results extends into investigations of auditory cortical functions. While the earliest auditory cortical activity, as indexed by the MLR, has been reported as normal in several studies (Buchwald, Erwin, Van Lancker et al., 1992; Grillon et al., 1989), the somewhat later P1 component has been described as either normal (Novick, Vaughan, Kurtzberg and Simson, 1980) or abnormally small in amplitude and without modulation by stimulus rate (Buchwald et al., 1992). Analysis of the N1 component in people with autism has also led to variable results. Normal amplitudes and latencies of N1b have been reported in two studies (Lincoln, Courchesne, Harms and Allen, 1995; Novick et al., 1980), although another has suggested smaller amplitudes (Bruneau, Roux, Adrien and Barthélémy, 1999) and a fourth has indicated that latencies may be shorter in children with autism (Oades, Walker, Geffen and Stern, 1988). This latter finding could conceivably reflect summation at the scalp with a smaller P1 (Buchwald et al., 1992), with no intrinsic abnormality of the processes underlying N1b generation. A suggestion that amplitude increments in the N1b component evoked by increases in stimulus frequency are absent in autistic subjects (Lincoln et al., 1995) has not been confirmed (Bruneau et al., 1999). In the only study to date examining MMN, a normal response was observed using speech sounds as the standard and deviant stimuli (Kemner, Verbaten, Cuperus et al., 1995).

In contrast to the highly variable response abnormalities observed in these early measures of auditory system integrity, more consistent dysfunction referable to higher auditory centers located on the lateral surface of the superior temporal gyrus has been demonstrated. This dysfunction has been indexed by evaluating the N1 component recorded from electrodes overlying the temporal lobes (N1c CAEP component). For instance, an older study with autistic subjects described a delay in the latency of N1c over the left hemisphere in response to speech stimuli (Narita and Koga, 1987). Furthermore, the longer-latency response was correlated with lower scores on the comprehension subtest of the Wechsler Intelligence Scale for Children. Klein et al. (1995) demonstrated that in some adults with autism and a history of severe receptive language impairment, there is a delayed N1c over temporal regions bilaterally in response to syllables and pure tones. Recently, both prolonged latencies and diminished amplitudes of bilaterally recorded N1c evoked by pure tones have been observed in the setting of a normal N1b latency and decreased amplitude (Bruneau et al., 1999). Finally, Dunn, Vaughan, Kreuzer and Kurtzberg (1999) reported that N1c was delayed in latency in a group of verbal, high-functioning children with autism (ages 7 to 11 years) in response to words presented during a semantic classification task. Mean delays in the peaks of the left temporal N1c and the following positivity were 43.5 and 70 ms, respectively. In this subject group, N1c in response to pure tones was not delayed (Table 1). Thus, while there appears to be variability across studies in latency comparisons of N1c when tonal stimuli are used, the overall pattern indicates dysfunction of auditory association cortex located on the lateral temporal cortex in people with autism.

Deficits pertaining to speech processing appear to extend beyond auditory regions into networks directly engaged in more complex language functions. Dunn et al. (1999) examined the modulation of the N400 processing negativity in higher functioning, verbal autistic children and age and non-verbal IQ matched controls (ages 7–11). This measure of semantic processing was examined by having the children behaviorally respond when an 'in-category' word was acoustically presented in a list of words. Subjects were required to identify any word belonging to the category 'animals'. While all subjects understood the task demand, the children with autism were slower in classifying targets and had a higher

TABLE 1

Event-related potential component N1c to word and tone stimuli in autistic versus control children

| Word stimuli | Left hemisphere | | Right hemisphere | |
|---|---|---|---|---|
| | C3 | T7 | C4 | T8 |
| *Targets* | | | | |
| Autistic | 114 (17) | 160 (26) | 114 (18) | 138 (33) |
| Control | 105 (13) | 120 (20) | 109 (13) | 118 (23) |
| *Non-targets* | | | | |
| Autistic | 119 (27) | 166 (23) | 117 (23) | 124 (27) |
| Control | 98 (9) | 119 (23) | 105 (10) | 119 (17) |
| Tone stimuli | | | | |
| *Targets* | | | | |
| Autistic | 88 (7) | 133 (6) | 88 (7) | 133 (7) |
| Control | 88 (5) | 134 (9) | 91 (4) | 131 (9) |
| *Non-targets* | | | | |
| Autistic | 87 (6) | 131 (4) | 87 (3) | 132 (5) |
| Control | 89 (6) | 131 (10) | 92 (5) | 127 (16) |

Group mean data in ms (s.d.). Adapted from Dunn et al., 1999.

error rate. As predicted, N400 was larger in amplitude for the non-target stimuli in the control group. This was anticipated as the instructional set given to the subjects and the word list composition (50% animal words) set up a semantic expectancy for animal words. Autistic children, however, showed no difference in N400 amplitude for the target and non-target words. This was interpreted as an indication that autistic children process semantic information differently than normal children, and to support the hypothesis that semantic processing deficits are a prominent component of the language abnormalities inherent to the autistic phenotype.

This physiological abnormality fits well with the language deficits delineated in autistic spectrum disorders. Verbal autistic children demonstrate two basic profiles of language impairment. The first pervasively affects all levels of language including phonology, syntax, semantics and pragmatics. The second involves circumscribed deficits in semantics and pragmatics (Tager-Flusberg, 1989). Deficits in semantics and pragmatics persist into adulthood even when other primary symptoms abate (Simmons and Baltaxe, 1975). Although verbal autistic children have categorical knowledge (Tager-Flusberg, 1985), they do not appropriately use that knowledge to support encoding or later recall of verbal

information (Fein, Dunn, Allen et al., 1996; Hermelin and O'Connor, 1970). There may also be an aberrant pattern of semantic distance between lexical concepts within a category (Dunn, Gomes and Sebastian, 1996; Wolff and Barlow, 1979). Thus, there appears to be a defect of selective lexical activation for word meaning that is consistent with semantic context over words that are inconsistent with that context. This abnormal selective lexical activation may be the basis for the absence of difference in the N400 wave observed in verbal autistic children when words are either part of, or distinct from, a predefined category (Dunn et al., 1999).

Dysfunction of executive functions, including attentional mechanisms, has also been explored by ERP studies in subjects with autism. While there is some inconsistency in the literature (see Kemner et al., 1995), most studies have observed abnormalities in the P300 potential. Using the oddball stimulus paradigm with additional novel stimuli, low-amplitude responses reflecting abnormalities of P3a and the subsequent, frontally predominant negativity termed Nc have been reported (Ciesielski, Courchesne and Elmasian, 1990; Courchesne, Lincoln, Kilman and Galambos, 1985; Kemner et al., 1995). These findings suggest dysfunction of prefrontal systems involved in detection and orientation to new stimuli of potential biological significance. The P3b subcomponent of P300, recorded optimally at midline parietal sites, is also reduced in amplitude in patients with autism (Ciesielski et al., 1990; Courchesne et al., 1985; Dunn et al., 1999; Novick et al., 1980). As P3b represents a physiological index for the successful completion of a cognitive task and is attention dependent, the diminished amplitude of the response could reflect malfunction of neural systems involved in the reallocation of attentional resources. Recently, differences in the P300 have been reported between patients with various subtypes of autistic-spectrum disorder (Kemner, Van der Gaag, Verbaten and Van Engeland, 1999). The authors report that in one subtype characterized by severe anxiety, termed multiple complex developmental disorder, the P3a response was significantly larger than in more typical autistic children, while the parietal P3b was reduced in amplitude. The enhanced P3a and apparent sensitivity to new stimuli may be a physiological marker for the anxious phenotype of this autistic subtype.

Furthermore, these findings emphasize the importance of examining ERPs in well-defined clinical groups, as variation in the phenotype of a disorder may be accompanied by marked differences in neural activation patterns and resultant ERP profiles. It is likely that progress in understanding the electrophysiology of autism will be greatly facilitated in the future when ERP results are correlated with abnormalities observed by neuroimaging and genetic studies. The prototype of the opportunities afforded by correlation of multiple disciplines is Williams syndrome.

*Williams syndrome*

Despite its rarity (1 : 20–30,000 live births), Williams syndrome stands at the forefront of delineating the relationship between genetics, cognitive development, and brain structure and function (Bellugi, Lichtenberger, Mills et al., 1999; Metcalfe, 1999). What makes this disorder so intriguing for developmental neuropsychology is its unique constellation of cognitive strengths and weaknesses, coupled to a restricted genetic abnormality and characteristic brain abnormalities. Genetically, Williams syndrome is a sporadic, autosomal dominant disorder with a submicroscopic deletion on the long arm of chromosome 7 affecting about 20 genes. Variability in the specifics of the deletion pattern determine phenotypic outcome. At the center of the deletion is the gene for elastin, and this abnormality is responsible for the classic cardiovascular anomalies typical of the disorder. Surrounding the elastin gene is a sequence of additional genes whose differential defects appear to be the genetic etiology for many of the other phenotypic features of Williams syndrome. Furthermore, the typical phenotype of Williams syndrome includes a distinctive pattern of brain anomalies. Some of the more germane findings include overall cerebral hypoplasia with an additional decrease in the size of the occipital and posterior parietal lobes, and a normally sized Heschl's gyrus.

The unique cognitive profile of Williams syndrome is highlighted by relatively well-preserved language/verbal and face recognition skills in the overall setting of a diminished full-scale IQ and severe deficits in visuo-spatial processing (Bellugi et al., 1999; Clahsen and Almazan, 1998; Jarrold,

Baddeley and Hewes, 1999). Expressive language skills are unusually strong in older children with Williams syndrome, especially those involved with use of grammar and morphosyntactical rules, which contrasts with the capabilities of children with specific language impairment or those with Down's syndrome (Bellugi et al., 1999; Clahsen and Almazan, 1998). Language abnormalities are present, however, and are especially evident in the lexical and semantic features of speech. Face processing, even on complicated tasks such as the Benton face recognition test which requires subjects to identify the same face under different lighting and orientation conditions, is normal or near normal when compared to age-matched controls. Again, this skill is superior to that displayed by children with other genetic conditions such as Down's syndrome (Bellugi et al., 1999). In contrast, visuo-spatial skills, such as those required to duplicate block-design patterns or judge line orientations, are markedly deficient in Williams syndrome (Bellugi et al., 1999). These deficits are further emphasized by the double dissociation in the strength of verbal working memory, as measured by digit span recall, and deficits in spatial memory between subjects with Williams and Down's syndrome (Jarrold et al., 1999). Additional features of the Williams syndrome cognitive profile include a friendly affect, affective speech patterns, and symptoms of ADHD.

While limited in number, ERP studies in subjects with Williams syndrome offer powerful insights into the neurophysiological underpinnings of cognitive development (Bellugi et al., 1999). Despite relatively well-preserved language functions, obligatory CAEP components and the N400 processing negativity show pronounced differences when compared with normal controls. In Williams syndrome, the P50 and P200 waves of the CAEP are accentuated in amplitude, while the N100 is diminished. The prominent P50 is consistent with its primary auditory cortical generator and the anatomical preservation of Heschl's gyrus in Williams syndrome despite hypoplasia of surrounding areas. Thus, one could hypothesize that there would be diminished overlap with concurrent negative waves generated by surrounding tissue, leading to the accentuated responses. The N400 potential, which indexes aspects of semantic processing, exhibits several anomalies in its voltage distribution. Open-class words (e.g., nouns and verbs) normally elicit a prominent N400 in the right posterior region of the brain, while closed-class words (e.g., articles and prepositions) evoke maximal excitation in the left frontal region. In subjects with Williams syndrome, the voltage distribution of N400 does not demonstrate the regional differences evoked by open- and closed-class words, and the N400 hemispheric asymmetry to closed-class words appears to be reversed. When ERPs were examined in a face identification paradigm, an N200 wave was markedly larger in amplitude in Williams syndrome subjects relative to controls. This amplitude discrepancy was not observed when subjects looked at pictures of objects. Also, a negativity at 320 ms elicited when there was a mismatch between face pairs did not exhibit the usual right frontal asymmetry seen in controls. These findings are important because they suggest that, even when cognitive skills approximate normal levels, it should not imply that the behavioral end results were obtained via similar neurophysiological processes. Furthermore, since the development of cognitive skills is dynamically changing in this population, it should not be assumed that associated neural processes are stable across time. Younger children with Williams syndrome perform better at tests of numerosity and poorer at tests examining vocabulary development, yet this cognitive pattern of skills reverses in later years (Paterson, Brown, Gsödl et al., 1999). These uneven developmental trajectories imply that the underlying neural mechanisms are also changing, and that one cannot infer substrates of neuropsychological development based solely on more mature levels of cognitive proficiency. This, in turn, highlights the importance of longitudinal ERP studies during development to assess the dynamic nature of neural mechanisms underlying perceptual and cognitive functions.

## Electroencephalography (EEG)

ERPs are time- and phase-locked indices of neural population activity superimposed upon on-going EEG rhythms. Averaging techniques improve the signal-to-noise ratio by diminishing EEG contamination of the ERP. However, the ever-present rhythms of the brain are important signals in their own right, and their analysis represents one of the most exciting topics in cognitive neuroscience. Measurement of the EEG is in the frequency domain, and changes in its complex spectral content are often time- but not phase-locked to both internal and external environmental events. This latter property of EEG dynamics means that directly averaging the time-varying signal, as for ERPs, will 'wash out' the non-phase-locked features of neural activity. Multiple spectral averaging techniques have been developed for examining EEG changes time-locked to definable events, and for removing the contribution of the ERP to these changes (for review see Pfurtscheller and Lopes da Silva, 1999).

EEG changes include increases and decreases of power in multiple frequency bands, which in turn reflect alterations in the synchronization of activity within neuronal populations of varying sizes (see Pfurtscheller and Lopes da Silva, 1999). These frequency bands extend from the lowest delta range (<4 Hz), through theta (4–8 Hz), alpha (8–13 Hz) and beta (13–30 Hz) frequencies, to the higher gamma range (>30 Hz). As a rule, synchronization within larger neuronal populations evokes frequency oscillations at lower frequencies and with greater amplitudes. A decrease of power within a specified frequency band elicited by an event is termed an event-related desynchronization (ERD), an increase of power is called an event-related synchronization (ERS). These oscillations are in turn generated, controlled and modulated by intrinsic membrane and synaptic properties of neurons, by the connections between excitatory and inhibitory neurons within neural networks, and by the effects of more diffuse subcortical neurotransmitter systems (e.g., Gray and McCormick, 1996; Hutcheon and Yarom, 2000; Metherate, Cox and Ashe, 1992; Munk, Roelfsema, König et al., 1996; Steriade, 1997; Traub, Spruston, Soltesz et al., 1998). Oscillations occur within neural structures located throughout the brain, and are thought to play central roles in sensory and motor functions, memory tasks and other cognitive processes. Dysfunction of these rhythms is also hypothesized to be an important contributor to multiple neurological diseases (Llinás, Ribary, Jeanmonod et al., 1999).

Complex changes of EEG rhythms occur in association with perceptual, motor, and cognitive tasks. These changes include periods of frequency restricted ERD and ERS that are often localized to discrete brain regions. ERD and ERS may occur simultaneously, forming complex spatio-temporal EEG patterns specific for the neurological function. Generally, ERD within frequency bands lower than the gamma range is associated with active neural processing within a brain region, while ERS reflects completion of a task, inhibition, or idling of that area (Pfurtscheller, 1992; Pfurtscheller and Lopes da Silva, 1999). EEG frequency content may also correlate with cognitive task performance. Fernández, Harmony, Silva-Pereyra et al. (2000) examined EEG patterns below the gamma frequency range in young adults performing verbal working memory, spatial working memory, and calculation tasks. Incorrect responses were associated with greater delta and beta activity, while accurate performance was associated with increased alpha frequencies. These changes were location specific. Other studies have shown that EEG changes associated with cognitive tasks are reproducible over time (McEvoy, Smith and Gevins, 2000), can be correlated with functional neuroimaging studies (Cook, O'Hara, Uijtdehaage et al., 1998), and are dysfunctional in neurological disorders such as stroke and Parkinson's disease (Pfurtscheller and Lopes da Silva, 1999).

Studies examining developmental features of quantitative EEG are limited, but the few studies performed suggest a fruitful ground for investigation. Maturational scales of the spectral content of the EEG and their correlation to chronological age have been proposed (Wackermann and Matoušek, 1998). Age-related changes in the latency of specific ERS rhythms occurring with cognitive tasks, and their relationship to cognitive ERPs have been observed (Yordanova and Kolev, 1997). In a study similar to that performed in adults (Fernández et al., 2000), EEG changes were related to task performance, with incorrect behavioral responses generally preceded by lower EEG frequencies (Fernández, Harmony, Silva et al., 1998). Brain areas demonstrating these changes were task specific, with incorrect responses occurring in a verbal word memory task associated with decreased alpha activity in frontal regions, while posterotemporal regions showed this pattern during errors in a color discrimination task, and activity in left-hemispheric sites were abnormal in a word categorization paradigm.

EEG abnormalities have been identified in developmental disorders. Comparing background EEG in 23 children with rolandic epileptic spikes versus the EEG in 39 controls, the group at risk for seizures had increased EEG power in most frequency ranges from ages 7 to 9, and increased delta and theta power from ages 10 to 12 (Braga, Manzano and Nóbrega, 2000). Findings suggest an immaturity of brain function in this population extending beyond the epileptiform activity. Decreased coherence of EEG rhythms in different cortical regions has been observed in children with learning disabilities, suggesting abnormalities in functional brain connections across areas (Marosi, Harmony, Sánchez et al., 1992). Two abnormal EEG patterns have been reported in children with ADHD (Chabot and Serfontein, 1996). In the first, there is focal slowing in frontal regions, while in the second, there is increased EEG power in the same cortical areas. These observations support frontal lobe dysfunction in ADHD. Hypercoherence or asymmetry of EEG patterns across hemispheres was also observed in children with ADHD. Finally, children with ADHD who responded behaviorally to methylphenidate had increased frontal lobe beta, and decreased central theta and alpha activity, during passive awake and vigilance conditions, when compared to children who did not benefit from medication therapy (Loo, Teale and Reite, 1999). Overall, these findings suggest that quantitative EEG can play an important role in defining features of neurophysiological disorders in children.

In contrast to ERD, which generally represents a marker for active cognitive processes, an increasing body of evidence indicates that ERS in the gamma frequency range reflects on-going information processing, and can be related to mechanisms of perceptual binding, motor coordination, and sensorimotor integration (for reviews see Pfurtscheller and Lopes da Silva, 1999; Sannita, 2000; Singer, 2000). Multiple studies have shown that using gamma oscillations, cortical neurons can synchronize responses both within cortical areas and over widely spaced brain regions with millisecond precision. Synchronization within an area facilitates transfer of information with minimal temporal dispersion to later processing stages. This population-based coding strategy compensates for the low firing rates and variability of single unit discharges, and raises the likelihood that neural processing at one level of the neuroaxis will impact on the activity at higher levels. Synchronization of neuronal activity across cortical regions facilitates perceptual binding by indicating that multiple attributes of a single object, which are represented in different cortical areas, are related. Non-synchronized neural discharges within these areas are interpreted as not reflecting characteristics of the same perceptual object. Indeed, given that many perceptual objects within any environment must be processed in parallel, the ability to synchronize activity suggests that temporal covariance of responses leads to perceptual grouping, with each represented object having its own time-locked signature. This process allows multiple objects to be simultaneously represented within the same neural tissue. Similar mechanisms are envisioned for encoding the coordinated activity of neuronal populations involved in discrete movements, and for integrating the relationships between sensory objects and motor responses. Representing a stimulus or motor act by synchronization of neuronal ensembles compensates for the fact that individual neurons are broadly tuned along multiple dimensions. Isolated neurons are incapable of encoding the limitless stimuli an individual may be confronted with, or the variations of movement that must be performed. Synchronization of neuronal populations permits flexible assembly formation capable of representing these almost limitless environmental stimuli or motor behaviors with limited neuronal numbers.

Developmental features of these exciting features of gamma-range EEG are just beginning to be explored. All that is required to study the development of oscillatory activity is to superimpose newer EEG data processing technologies upon pre-existing capabilities of performing EEG recordings and behavioral paradigms in children. Thus, it is almost certain that this field will become an active ground of investigation in the near future. Short-latency (within 120 ms post-stimulus onset) gamma band increases maximal in frontal electrode sites occur in children performing an auditory selective attention task (Yordanova, Banaschewski, Kolev et al., 2001). These increases are greater for target stimuli, but do not differentiate the attended from the unattended channel. This relationship with target stimuli suggests that gamma-band responses are involved in task-relevant stimulus evaluation. Abnormal gamma activity evoked by acoustic stimuli in an oddball task has been reported in patients with schizophrenia (Haig et al., 2000). Recently, gamma-range abnormalities have been identified in adults with Williams syndrome and autism (Grice, Spratling, Karmiloff-Smith et al., 2001). Normal adults showed a burst of frontally predominant gamma-band activity that was larger to upright versus inverted faces. This increase in gamma-band activity was not observed in the two patient populations. These findings suggest the exciting possibility that some of the cognitive dysfunctions present in developmental neuropsychological disorders may in part be based on abnormalities of gamma-range ERS both within and across brain regions.

**Concluding remarks**

The last decade has seen an explosive growth of physiological data that has markedly advanced our understanding of how the brain processes and stores sensory information, incorporates this with past experience, and initiates and carries out motor acts. The challenge for developmental neuropsychology is to integrate these evolving concepts of brain function with relevant experimental paradigms that can reliably assess maturational features of neural events and processes. As summarized in this chapter, use of electrophysiological techniques to examine neural development has all too frequently led to inconclusive and conflicting results. This is partly the logical outcome of using incomplete recording montages and relying on outdated and incorrect assumptions regarding the nature and significance of the ERP findings. Recordings obtained from limited electrode sites preclude topographical mapping of brain activity, and eliminate the possibility of relating data sets with current concepts of sensory streaming, and integration of perception with executive functions. We have illustrated that many of the exciting findings related to developmental ERP studies reflect activation or dysfunction within associative sensory fields or lateral frontal areas involved in executive functions. Sampling the activity from these regions requires a larger recording array than has often been often used in the past, coupled to more sophisticated analysis techniques. While these newer analysis methods are available for suggesting the location and timing of putative response generators, investigators' assumptions, such as modeling activity within extended brain regions by single equivalent current dipoles, are a gross simplification that frequently lead to inaccurate conclusions regarding neural organization. A greater reliance on complementary methodologies to assist in generator modeling is required in order to facilitate more precise determinations of the locations and functions of these neural generators. In this chapter, we have stressed the benefits that the complementary techniques of direct intracranial recordings in humans and experimental animals, supplemented by functional neuroimaging, can bring for refinement of the surface-recorded data and their analysis.

Finally, most physiological studies of development and its disorders have examined ERPs and ERMFs. A reemerging frontier of investigation is available through direct analysis of EEG. Regional variation in spectral content and coherence across brain areas appears to be a keen marker for the neural substrates underlying perception, learning, memory, motor planning, and action. Incorporation of these time-locked changes in neural rhythms with the phase-locked changes measured by ERPs/ERMFs offers a new opportunity to examine in greater breath the mechanisms and development of cognitive functions and related disorders.

## Acknowledgements

This work was supported by NIH grants DC-00657, DC-00120, DC-04290 and HD-36080. The authors gratefully acknowledge the collaboration with Dr. M.A. Howard, III and colleagues at the University of Iowa College of Medicine, for enabling the intracranial studies in human subjects to be carried out. Drs. J. Arezzo, Y. Fishman, and D. Reser were instrumental in the animal model studies. We thank Dr. V.L. Shafer for allowing us to display her data. Finally, we wish to thank Drs. D. Kurtzberg and H.G. Vaughan, Jr. for their co-authorship on the previous edition of this chapter, and for their continued support of this work.

## References

Ahlfors SP, Simpson GV, Dale AM, Belliveau JW, Liu AK, Korvenoja A, Virtanen J, Huotilainen M, Tootell RBH, Aronen HJ, Ilmoniemi RJ: Spatiotemporal activity of a cortical network for processing visual motion revealed by MEG and fMRI. Journal of Neurophysiology: 82; 2545–2555, 1999.

Alain C, Achim A, Richer F: Perceptual context and the selective attention effect on auditory event-related potentials. Psychophysiology: 30; 572–580, 1993.

Alain C, Cortese F, Picton TW: Event-related brain activity associated with auditory pattern processing. NeuroReport: 9; 3537–3541, 1998.

Alho K, Teder W, Lavikainen J, Näätänen R: Strongly focused attention and auditory event-related potentials. Biological Psychology: 38; 73–90, 1994.

Alho K, Tervaniemi M, Huotilainen M, Lavikainen J, Tiitinen H, Ilmoniemi RJ, Knuutila J, Näätänen R: Processing of complex sounds in the human auditory cortex as revealed by magnetic brain responses. Psychophysiology: 33; 369–375, 1996.

Allison T, McCarthy G, Nobre A, Puce A, Belger A: Human extrastriate visual cortex and the perception of faces, words, numbers, and colors. Cerebral Cortex: 5; 544–554, 1994.

Allison T, Puce A, McCarthy G: Social perception from visual cues: role of the STS region. Trends in Cognitive Science: 4; 267–278, 2000.

Allison T, Puce A, Spencer DP, McCarthy G: Electrophysiological studies of human face perception. I: Potentials generated in occipitotemporal cortex by face and non-face stimuli. Cerebral Cortex: 9; 415–430, 1999.

Altenmüller EO, Gerloff C: Psychophysiology and the EEG. In Niedermeyer E, Lopes Da Silva F (Eds), Electroencephalography: Basic Principles, Clinical Applications, and Related Fields. Philadelphia, PA: Lippincott Williams and Wilkins, pp. 637–655, 1999.

American Academy of Pediatrics Joint Committee on Infant Hearing: Joint committee on infant hearing 1994 position statement. Pediatrics: 95; 152–156, 1995.

Arezzo JC, Pickoff A, Vaughan HG Jr: The sources and intracerebral distribution of auditory evoked potentials in the alert rhesus monkey. Brain Research: 90; 57–73, 1975.

Baenninger M: The development of face recognition: featural or configurational processing? Journal of Experimental Child Psychology: 57; 377–396, 1994.

Bailey A, Luthert P, Dean A, Harding B, Janota I, Montgomery M, Rutter M, Lantos P: A clinicopathological study of autism. Brain: 121; 889–905, 1998.

Baldeweg T, Richardson A, Watkins S, Foale C, Gruzelier J: Impaired auditory frequency discrimination in dyslexia detected with mismatch evoked potentials. Annals of Neurology: 45; 495–503, 1999.

Bartels A, Zeki S: The theory of multistage integration in the visual brain. Proceedings of the Royal Society of London B: 265; 2327–2332, 1998.

Bellugi U, Lichtenberger L, Mills D, Galaburda A, Korenberg JR: Bridging cognition, the brain and molecular genetics:

evidence from Williams syndrome. Trends in Neurosciences: 22; 197–207, 1999.

Berman S, Friedman D: The development of selective attention as reflected by event-related brain potentials. Journal of Experimental Child Psychology: 59; 1–31, 1995.

Bishop DVM: Cognitive neuropsychology and developmental disorders: uncomfortable bedfellows. Quarterly Journal of Experimental Psychology: 50A; 899–923, 1997.

Bishop DVM, Bishop SJ, Bright P, James C, Delaney T, Tallal P: Different origin of auditory and phonological processing problems in children with language impairment: evidence from a twin study. Journal of Speech, Language, and Hearing Research: 42; 155–168, 1999a.

Bishop DVM, Carlyon RP, Deeks JM, Bishop SJ: Auditory temporal processing impairment: neither necessary nor sufficient for causing language impairment in children. Journal of Speech, Language, and Hearing Research: 42; 1295–1310, 1999b.

Bradlow AR, Kraus N, Nicol TG, McGee TJ, Cunningham J, Zecker SG; , Carrell TD: Effects of lengthened formant transition duration on discrimination and neural representation of synthetic CV syllables by normal and learning-disabled children. Journal of the Acoustical Society of America: 106; 2086–2096, 1999.

Braga NIO, Manzano GM, Nóbrega JAM: Quantitative analysis of EEG background activity in patients with rolandic spikes. Clinical Neurophysiology: 111; 1643–1645, 2000.

Brandeis D, Van Leeuwen TH, Rubia K, Vitacco D, Steger J, Pascual-Marqui RD, Steinhausen H-C: Neuroelectric mapping reveals precursor of stop failures in children with attention deficits. Behavioural Brain Research: 94; 111–125, 1998.

Bruneau N, Roux S, Adrien JL, Barthélémy C: Auditory associative cortex dysfunction in children with autism: evidence from late auditory evoked potentials (N1 wave – T complex). Clinical Neurophysiology: 110; 1927–1934, 1999.

Bruneau N, Roux S, Guérin P, Barthélémy C, LeLord G: Temporal prominence of auditory evoked potentials (N1 wave) in 4-8-year-old children. Psychophysiology: 34; 32–38, 1997.

Buchwald JS, Erwin R, Van Lancker D, Guthrie D, Schwafel J, Tanguay P: Midlatency auditory evoked responses: P1 abnormalities in adult autistic subjects. Electroencephalography and Clinical Neurophysiology: 84; 164–171, 1992.

Burkhalter A: Development of forward and feedback connections between areas V1 and V2 of human visual cortex. Cerebral Cortex: 3; 476–487, 1993.

Burkhalter A, Bernardo KL, Charles V: Development of local circuits in human visual cortex. Journal of Neuroscience: 13; 1916–1931, 1993.

Byrne JM, Connolly JF, MacLean SE, Dooley JM, Gordon KE, Beattie TL: Brain activity and language assessment using event-related potentials: development of a clinical protocol. Developmental Medicine and Child Neurology: 41; 740–747, 1999.

Cacace AT, McFarland DJ: Central auditory processing disorder in school-age children: a critical review. Journal of Speech, Language, and Hearing Research: 41; 355–373, 1998.

Carey S: Becoming a face expert. Philosophical Transactions of the Royal Society of London B: 335; 95–103, 1992.

Celesia GG: Organization of auditory cortical areas in man. Brain: 99; 403–414, 1976.

Celesia GG: Anatomy and physiology of visual evoked potentials and electroretinograms. In Gilmore R (Ed), Neurological Clinics, Evoked Potentials, Vol. 6. Philadelphia, PA: W.B. Sanders, pp. 657–680, 1988.

Celesia GG, Brigell MG: Auditory evoked potentials. In Niedermeyer E, Lopes Da Silva F (Eds), Electroencephalography: Basic Principles, Clinical Applications, and Related Fields. Philadelphia, PA: Lippincott Williams and Wilkins, pp. 994–1013, 1999.

Celesia GG, Peachey NS: Visual evoked potentials and electroretinograms. In Niedermeyer E, Lopes Da Silva F (Eds), Electroencephalography: Basic Principles, Clinical Applications, and Related Fields. Philadelphia, PA: Lippincott Williams and Wilkins, pp. 968–993, 1999.

Celsis P, Doyon B, Boulanouar K, Pastor J, Demonet J-F, Nespoulous J-L: ERP correlates of phoneme perception in speech and sound contexts. NeuroReport: 10; 1523–1527, 1999.

Čeponienè R, Cheour M, Näätänen R: Interstimulus interval and auditory event-related potentials in children: evidence for multiple generators. Electroencephalography and Clinical Neurophysiology: 108; 345–354, 1998.

Chabot RJ, Serfontein G: Quantitative electroencephalographic profiles of children with attention deficit disorder. Biological Psychiatry: 40; 951–963, 1996.

Cheour M, Alho K, Čeponienè R, Reinikainen K, Sainio K, Pohjavuori M, Aaltonen O, Näätänen R: Maturation of mismatch negativity in infants. International Journal of Psychophysiology: 29; 217–226, 1998a.

Cheour M, Čeponienè R, Lehtokoski A, Luuk A, Allik J, Alho K, Näätänen R: Development of language-specific phoneme representations in the infant brain. Nature Neuroscience: 1; 351–353, 1998b.

Cheour M, Leppänen PHT, Kraus N: Mismatch negativity (MMN) as a tool for investigating auditory discrimination and sensory memory in infants and children. Clinical Neurophysiology: 111; 4–16, 2000.

Chung M-S, Thomson DM: Development of face recognition. British Journal of Psychology: 86; 55–87, 1995.

Ciesielski KT, Courchesne E, Elmasian R: Effects of focused selective attention tasks on event-related potentials in autistic and normal individuals. Electroencephalography and Clinical Neurophysiology: 75; 207–220, 1990.

Clahsen H, Almazan M: Syntax and morphology in Williams syndrome. Cognition: 68; 167–198, 1998.

Cook IA, O'Hara R, Uijtdehaage SHJ, Mandelkern M, Leuchter AF: Assessing the accuracy of topographic EEG mapping for determining local brain function. Electroencephalography and Clinical Neurophysiology: 107; 408–414, 1998.

Coull JT: Neural correlates of attention and arousal: insights from electrophysiology, functional neuroimaging and psychopharmacology. Progress in Neurobiology: 55; 343–361, 1998.

Courchesne E: Brainstem, cerebellar and limbic neuroanatomical abnormalities in autism. Current Opinion in Neurobiology: 7; 269–278, 1997.

Courchesne E, Lincoln AJ, Kilman BA, Galambos R: Event-related brain potential correlates of the processing of novel visual and auditory information in autism. Journal of Autism and Developmental Disorders: 15; 55–76, 1985.

Crouzeix A, Yvert B, Bertrand O, Pernier J: An evaluation of dipole reconstruction accuracy with spherical and realistic head models in MEG. Clinical Neurophysiology: 110; 2176–2188, 1999.

Cruikshank SJ, Weinberger NM: Receptive-field plasticity in the adult auditory cortex induced by Hebbian covariance. Journal of Neuroscience: 16; 861–875, 1996.

Curran T, Tucker DM, Kutas M, Posner MI: Topography of the N400: brain electrical activity reflecting semantic expectancy. Electroencephalography and Clinical Neurophysiology: 88; 188–209, 1993.

Cycowicz YM, Friedman D: A developmental study of the effects of temporal order on the ERPs elicited by novel environmental sounds. Electroencephalography and Clinical Neurophysiology: 103; 304–318, 1997.

Cycowicz YM, Friedman D, Rothstein M: An ERP developmental study of repetition priming by auditory novel stimuli. Psychophysiology: 33; 680–690, 1996.

Damasio AR, Tranel D, Damasio H: Face agnosia and the neural substrates of memory. Annuual Review of Neuroscience: 13; 89–109, 1990.

Deecke L: Planning, preparation, execution, and imagery of volitional action. Cognitive Brain Research: 3; 59–64, 1996.

De Haan M, Nelson CA: Brain activity differentiates face and object processing in 6-month-old infants. Developmental Psychology: 35; 1113–1121, 1999.

DeFrance JF, Sands S, Schweitzer FC, Ginsberg L, Sharma JC: Age-related changes in cognitive ERPs of attention. Brain Topography: 9; 283–293, 1997.

Dehaene S, Tzourio N, Frak V, Raynaud L, Cohen L, Mehler J, Mazoyer B: Cerebral activations during number multiplication and comparison: a PET study. Neuropsychologia: 34; 1097–1106, 1996.

Dehaene-Lambertz G, Baillet S: A phonological representation in the infant brain. NeuroReport: 9; 1885–1888, 1998.

Dehaene-Lambertz G, Dehaene S: Speed and cerebral correlates of syllable discrimination in infants. Nature: 370; 292–295, 1994.

Desjardins R, Trainor LJ, Hevenor SJ, Polak CP: Using mismatch negativity to measure auditory temporal resolution thresholds. NeuroReport: 10; 2079–2082, 1999.

Diesch E, Luce T: Magnetic mismatch fields elicited by vowels and consonants. Experimental Brain Research: 116; 139–152, 1997.

Dougherety RF, Cynader MS, Bjornson BH, Edgell D, Giaschi DH: Dichotic pitch: a new stimulus distinguishes normal and dyslexic auditory function. NeuroReport: 9; 3001–3005, 1998.

Dunn M, Gomes H, Sebastian M: Prototypicality of responses of autistic, language disordered and normal children in a word fluency task. Journal of Child Neuropsychology: 2; 99–108, 1996.

Dunn M, Vaughan HG Jr, Kreuzer J, Kurtzberg D: Electro-physiologic correlates of semantic classification in autistic and normal children. Developmental Neuropsychology: 16; 79–99, 1999.

Eggermont JJ: The onset and development of auditory function: contribution of evoked potential studies. Journal of Speech-Language Pathology and Audiology: 13; 5–27, 1989.

Eggermont JJ: Neural correlates of gap detection in three auditory cortical fields in the cat. Journal of Neurophysiology: 81; 2570–2581, 1999.

Eilers RE, Morse PA, Gavin WJ, Oller DK: Discrimination of voice onset time in infancy. Journal of the Acoustical Society of America: 70; 955–965, 1981.

Eimas PD, Siqueland ER, Jusczyk P, Vigorito J: Speech perception in infants. Science: 171; 303–306, 1971.

Eimer M: Event-related brain potentials distinguish processing stages involved in face perception. Clinical Neurophysiology: 111; 694–705, 2000.

Ekert PG, Keenan NK, Whyte HE, Boulton J, Taylor MJ: Visual evoked potentials for prediction of neurodevelopmental outcome in preterm infants. Biology of the Neonate: 71; 148–155, 1997.

Emerson RG: Posterior tibial nerve somatosensory evoked potentials. In Gilmore R (Ed), Neurological Clinics, Evoked Potentials, Vol. 6. Philadelphia, PA: W.B. Sanders, pp. 735–750, 1988.

Escera C, Grau C: Short-term replicability of the mismatch negativity. Electroencephalography and Clinical Neurophysiology: 100; 549–554, 1996.

Escera C, Yago E, Polo MD, Grau C: The individual replicability of mismatch negativity at short and long inter-stimulus intervals. Clinical Neurophysiology: 111; 546–551, 2000.

Faraone SV, Biederman J: Neurobiology of attention-deficit hyperactivity disorder. Biological Psychiatry: 44; 951–958, 1998.

Faulkner A, Rosen S: Contributions of temporal encodings of voicing, voicelessness, fundamental frequency, and amplitude variation to audio-visual and auditory speech perception. Journal of the Acoustical Society of America: 106; 2063–2073, 1999.

Fein D, Dunn M, Allen D, Aram DM, Hall N, Morris R, Wilson BC: Neuropsychological and language data. In Rapin I (Ed), Preschool Children with Inadequate Communication: Developmental Language Disorder, Autism, Low IQ. Clinics in Developmental Medicine, London: MacKeith Press, pp. 123–154, 1996.

Fernández T, Harmony T, Silva-Pereyra J, Fernández-Bouzas A, Gersenowies J, Galán L, Carbonell F, Marosi E, Otero G, Valdés SI: Specific EEG frequencies at specific brain areas and performance. NeuroReport: 11; 2663–2668, 2000.

Fernández T, Harmony T, Silva J, Galán L, Díaz-Comas L, Bosch J, Rodrígues M, Fernández-Bouzas A, Yáñez G, Otero G, Marosi E: Relationship of specific EEG frequencies at specific brain areas with performance. NeuroReport: 9; 3681–3687, 1998.

Fishman YI, Reser DH, Arezzo JC, Steinschneider M: Complex tone processing in primary auditory cortex of the awake monkey. II. Pitch versus critical band representation. Journal of the Acoustical Society of America: 108; 247–262, 2000.

Flint J: The genetic basis of cognition. Brain: 122; 2015–2031, 1999.

Formby C, Barker C, Abbey H, Raney JJ: Detection of silent temporal gaps between narrow-band noise markers having second-formantlike properties of voiceless stop/vowel combinations. Journal of the Acoustical Society of America: 93; 1023–1027, 1993.

Forss N, Mäkelä JP, McEvoy L, Hari R: Temporal integration and oscillatory responses of the human auditory cortex revealed by evoked magnetic fields to click trains. Hearing Research: 68; 89–96, 1993.

Freeman JA, Nicholson C: Experimental optimization of current source-density technique for anuran cerebellum. Journal of Neurophysiology: 38; 369–382, 1975.

Friedman D, Kazmerski V, Fabiani M: An overview of age-related changes in the scalp distribution of P3b. Electroencephalography and Clinical Neurophysiology: 104; 498–513, 1997.

Galaburda AM, Sanides F: Cytoarchitectonic organization of the human auditory cortex. Journal of Comparative Neurology: 190; 596–610, 1980.

George N, Evans J, Fiori N, Davidoff J, Renault B: Brain events related to normal and moderately scrambled faces. Cognitive Brain Research: 4; 65–76, 1996.

Gevins A, Smith ME, McEvoy LK, Leong H, Le J: Electroencephalographic imaging of higher brain function. Philosophical Transactions of the Royal Society of London B: 354; 1125–1134, 1999.

Giard MH, Perrin F, Echallier JF, Thévenet M, Froment JC, Pernier J: Dissociation of temporal and frontal components in the human auditory N1 wave: a scalp current density and dipole model analysis. Electroencephalography and Clinical Neurophysiology: 92; 238–252, 1994.

Gomes H, Dunn M, Ritter W, Kurtzberg D, Brattson A, Kreuzer JA, Vaughan HG Jr: Spatiotemporal maturation of the central and lateral N1 components to tones. Developmental Brain Research: 129; 147–155, 2001.

Gray CM, McCormick DA: Chattering cells: superficial pyramidal neurons contributing to the generation of synchronous oscillations in the visual cortex. Science: 274; 109–113, 1996.

Grice SJ, Spratling MW, Karmiloff-Smith A, Halit H, Csibra G, de Haan M, Johnson MH: Disordered visual processing and oscillatory brain activity in autism and Williams syndrome. NeuroReport: 12; 2697–2700, 2001.

Grillon C, Courchesne E, Akshoomoff N: Brainstem and middle latency auditory evoked potentials in autism and developmental language disorder. Journal of Autism and Developmental Disorders: 19; 255–269, 1989.

Haig AR, Gordon E, De Pascalis V, Meares RA, Bahramali H, Harris A: Gamma activity in schizophrenia: evidence of impaired network binding? Clinical Neurophysiology: 111; 1461–1468, 2000.

Halgren E, Dale AM, Sereno MI, Tootell RBH, Marinkovic K, Rosen BR: Location of human face-selective cortex with respect to retinotopic areas. Human Brain Mapping: 7; 29–37, 1999.

Halgren E, Marinkovic K, Chauvel P: Generators of the late cognitive potentials in auditory and visual oddball tasks. Electroencephalography and Clinical Neurophysiology: 106; 156–164, 1998.

Halgren E, Raij T, Marinkovic K, Jousmäki V, Hari R: Cognitive response profile of the human fusiform face area as determined by MEG. Cerebral Cortex: 10; 69–81, 2000.

Hari R: Magnetoencephalography as a tool of clinical neurophysiology. In Niedermeyer E, Lopes Da Silva F (Eds), Electroencephalography: Basic Principles, Clinical Applications, and Related Fields. Philadelphia, PA: Lippincott Williams and Wilkins, pp. 1107–1134, 1999.

Hari R, Kiesilä P: Deficit of temporal auditory processing in dyslexic adults. Neuroscience Letters: 205; 138–140, 1996.

Heath SM, Hogben JH, Clark CD: Auditory temporal processing in disabled readers with and without oral language delay. Journal of Child Psychology and Psychiatry: 40; 637–647, 1999.

Helenius P, Salmelin R, Service E, Connolly JF: Distinct time courses of word and context comprehension in the left temporal cortex. Brain: 121; 1133–1142, 1998.

Helenius P, Tarkiainen A, Cornelissen P, Hansen PC, Salmelin R: Dissociation of normal feature analysis and deficient processing of letter-strings in dyslexic adults. Cerebral Cortex: 9; 476–483, 1999b.

Helenius P, Utuela K, Hari R: Auditory stream segregation in dyslexic adults. Brain: 122; 907–913, 1999a.

Hendren RL, De Backer I, Pandina GJ: Review of neuroimaging studies of child and adolescent psychiatric disorders from the past 10 years. Journal of the American Academy of Child and Adolescent Psychiatry: 39; 815–828, 2000.

Hermelin B, O'Connor N: Psychological Experiments with Autistic Children. Oxford: Pergamon Press, 1970.

Hillyard SA, Anllo-Vento L: Event-related brain potentials in the study of visual selective attention. Proceedings of the National Academy of Sciences of the USA: 95; 781–787, 1998.

Hillyard SA, Mangun GR, Woldorff MG, Luck SJ: Neural systems mediating selective attention. In Gazzanga MA (Ed-in-Chief), The Cognitive Neurosciences. Cambridge, MA: MIT Press, pp. 665–682, 1997.

Hillyard SA, Picton TW: Electrophysiology of cognition. In Mountcastle VB, Plum F, Geiger SR (Eds), Handbook of Physiology, Part 2, Higher Functions of the Brain. Baltimore: American Physiological Society, pp. 519–584, 1987.

Hollants-Gilhuijs MAM, De Munck J, Kubova Z, Van Royen E, Spekreijse H: The development of hemispheric asymmetry in human motion VEPs. Vision Research: 40; 1–11, 2000.

Holopainen IE, Korpilahti P, Juottonen K, Lang H, Sillanpää, M., 1997: Attenuated auditory event-related potential (mismatch negativity) in children with developmental dysphasia. Neuropediatrics: 28; 253–256, 1997.

Holopainen IE, Korpilahti P, Juottonen K, Lang H, Sillanpää, M., 1998: Abnormal frequency mismatch negativity in mentally retarded children and in children with developmental dysphasia. Journal of Child Neuropsychology: 13; 178–183, 1998.

Howard MA III, Volkov IO, Mirsky R, Garell PC, Noh MD, Granner M, Damasio H, Steinschneider M, Reale RA, Hind JE, Brugge JF: Auditory cortex on the human posterior superior temporal gyrus. Journal of Comparative Neurology: 416; 79–92, 2000.

Huotilainen M, Winkler I, Alho K, Escera C, Virtanen J, Ilmoniemi RJ, Jääskeläinen IP, Pekkonen E, Näätänen R: Combined mapping of human auditory EEG and MEG responses. Electroencephalography and Clinical Neurophysiology: 108; 370–379, 1998.

Hutcheon B, Yarom Y: Resonance, oscillation and the intrinsic frequency preferences of neurons. Trends in Neuroscience: 23; 216–222, 2000.

Huttenlocher PR, Dabholkar AS: Regional differences in synaptogenesis in human cerebral cortex. Journal of Comparative Neurology: 387; 167–178, 1997.

Huttenlocher PR, De Courten, C: The development of synapses in striate cortex of man. Human Neurobiology: 6; 1–9, 1987.

Huttenlocher PR, De Courten C, Garey LJ, Van Der Loos H: Synaptogenesis in human visual cortex — evidence for synapse elimination during normal development. Neuroscience Letters: 33; 247–252, 1982.

Hyde ML, Riko K, Malizia K: Audiometric accuracy of the click ABR in infants at risk for hearing loss. Journal of the American Academy of Audiology: 1; 59–66, 1990.

Jacobson GP: Magnetoencephalographic studies of auditory system functions. Journal Clinical Neurophysiology: 11; 343–364, 1994.

Jarrold C, Baddeley AD, Hewes AK: Genetically dissociated components of working memory: evidence from Down's and Williams syndrome. Neuropsychologia: 37; 637–651, 1999.

Javitt DC, Schroeder CE, Steinschneider M, Arezzo JC, Vaughan HG Jr: Demonstration of mismatch negativity in the monkey. Electroencephalography and Clinical Neurophysiology: 83; 87–90, 1992.

Javitt DC, Steinschneider M, Schroeder CE, Arezzo JC: Role of cortical N-methyl-D-aspartate receptors in auditory sensory memory and mismatch negativity generation: implications for schizophrenia. Proceedings of the National Academy of Sciences of the USA: 93; 11962–11967, 1996.

Javitt DC, Steinschneider M, Schroeder CE, Arezzo JC, Vaughan HG Jr: Detection of stimulus deviance within primary auditory cortex: intracortical mechanisms of mismatch negativity (MMN) generation. Brain Research: 667; 192–200, 1994.

Johnson BW, Hamm JP: High-density mapping in an N400 paradigm: evidence for bilateral temporal lobe generators. Clinical Neurophysiology: 111; 532–545, 2000.

Jonkman LM, Kemner C, Verbaten MN, Koelega, HS, Camfferman G, Van der Gaag R-J, Buitelaar JK, Van Engeland H: Event-related potentials and performance of attention-deficit hyperactivity disorder: Children and normal controls in auditory and visual selective attention tasks. Biological Psychiatry: 41; 595–611, 1997a.

Jonkman LM, Kemner C, Verbaten MN, Koelega, HS, Camfferman G, Van der Gaag R-J, Buitelaar JK, Van Engeland H: Effects of methylphenidate on event-related potentials and performance of attention-deficit hyperactivity disorder children in auditory and visual selective attention tasks. Biological Psychiatry: 41; 690–702, 1997b.

Jonkman LM, Kemner C, Verbaten MN, Van Engeland H, Kenemans JL, Camfferman G, Buitelaar JK, Koelega HS: Perceptual and response interference in children with attention-deficit hyperactivity disorder, and the effects of methylphenidate. Psychophysiology: 36; 419–429, 1999.

Jusczyk PW, Rosner BS, Reed MA, Kennedy LJ: Could temporal order differences underlie 2-month-olds' discrimination of English voicing contrasts? Journal of the Acoustical Society of America: 85; 1741–1749, 1989.

Kanwisher N, McDermott J, Chun MM: The fusiform face area: a module in human extrastriate cortex specialized for face perception. Journal of Neuroscience: 17; 4302–4311, 1997.

Karmiloff-Smith A: Development itself is the key to understanding developmental disorders. Trends in Cognitive Sciences: 2; 389–398, 1998.

Karrer R, Monti LA: Event-related potentials of 4–7-week-old infants in a visual recognition memory task. Electroencephalography and Clinical Neurophysiology: 94; 414–424, 1995.

Kasai K, Nakagome K, Itoh K, Koshida I, Fukuda M, Watanabe A, Kamio S, Murakami T, Hata A, Iwanami A, Hiramatsu K-I, Kato N: Electrophysiological evidence for sequential activation of multiple brain regions during the auditory selective attention process in humans. NeuroReport: 10; 3837–3842, 1999.

Kathmann N, Frodl-Bauch T, Hegerl U: Stability of the mismatch negativity under different stimulus and attention conditions. Clinical Neurophysiology: 110; 317–323, 1999.

Kayser J, Tenke CE, Bruder GE: Dissociation of brain ERP topographies for tonal and phonetic oddball tasks. Psychophysiology: 35; 576–590, 1998.

Kemner C, Verbaten MN, Cuperus JM, Camfferman G, Van Engeland H: Auditory event-related brain potentials in autistic children and three different control groups. Biological Psychiatry: 38; 150–165, 1995.

Kemner C, Verbaten MN, Koelega HS, Buitelaar JK, Van der Gaag RJ, Camfferman G, Van Engeland H: Event-related brain potentials in children with attention-deficit and hyperactivity disorder: effects of stimulus deviancy and task relevance in the visual and auditory modality. Biological Psychiatry: 40; 522–534, 1996.

Kemner C, Verbaten MN, Koelega HS, Camfferman G, Van Engeland H: Are abnormal event-related potentials specific to children with ADHD? A comparison with two clinical groups. Perceptual and Motor Skills: 87; 1083–1090, 1998.

Kemner C, Van der Gaag RJ, Verbaten MN, Van Engeland H: ERP differences among subtypes of pervasive developmental disorders. Biological Psychiatry: 46; 781–789, 1999.

Khan SC, Frisk V, Taylor MJ: Neurophysiological measures of reading difficulty in very-low-birthweight children. Psychophysiology: 36; 76–85, 1999.

Kilgard MP, Merzenich MM: Plasticity of temporal information processing in the primary auditory cortex. Nature Neurosciences: 1; 727–731, 1998.

Kilpeläinen R, Koistinen A, Könönen M, Herrgård E, Partanen J, Karhu J: P300 sequence effects differ between children and adults for auditory stimuli. Psychophysiology: 36; 343–350, 1999a.

Kilpeläinen R, Partanen J, Karhu J: What does the P300 brain response measure in children? New insight from stimulus sequence studies. NeuroReport: 10; 2625–2630, 1999b.

Kilpeläinen R, Partanen J, Karhu J: Reduced mismatch negativity (MMN) suggests deficits in preattentive auditory processing in distractible children. NeuroReport: 10; 3341–3345, 1999c.

Kilpeläinen R, Partanen J, Luoma L, Herrgård E, Yppärilä H, Karhu J: Persistent frontal P300 brain potential suggests abnormal processing of auditory information in distractible children. NeuroReport: 10; 3405–3410, 1999d.

King C, McGee T, Rubel EW, Nicol T, Kraus N: Acoustic features and acoustic change are represented by different central pathways. Hearing Research: 85; 45–52, 1995.

Klein SK, Kurtzberg D, Brattson A, Kreuzer JA, Stapells DR, Dunn MA, Rapin I, Vaughan HG Jr: Electrophysiologic manifestations of impaired temporal lobe auditory processing in verbal auditory agnosia. Brain and Language: 51; 383–405, 1995.

Klein SK, Tuchman RF, Rapin I: The influence of premorbid language skills and behavior on language recovery in children with verbal auditory agnosia. Journal of Child Neurology: 15; 36–43, 2000.

Klin A: Auditory brainstem responses in autism: brainstem dysfunction or peripheral hearing loss? Journal of Autism and Developmental Disorders: 23; 15–35, 1993.

Koles ZJ: Trends in EEG source localization. Electroencephalography and Clinical Neurophysiology: 106; 127–137, 1998.

Korpilahti P, Lang HA: Auditory ERP components and mismatch negativity in dysphasic children. Electroencephalography and Clinical Neurophysiology: 91; 256–264, 1994.

Kos-Pietro S, Towle VL, Cakmur R, Spire J-P: Maturation of human visual evoked potentials: 27 weeks conceptual age to 2 years. Neuropediatrics: 28; 318–323, 1997.

Kramer SJ, Vertes DR, Condon M: Auditory brainstem responses and clinical follow-up of high-risk infants. Pediatrics: 83; 385–392, 1989.

Kraus N, McGee T, Carrell T, Sharma A: Neurophysiologic bases of speech discrimination. Ear and Hearing: 16; 19–37, 1995.

Kraus N, McGee T, Carrell T, Sharma A, Micco A, Nicol T: Speech-evoked cortical potentials in children. Journal of the American Acaddemy of Audiology: 4; 238–248, 1993a.

Kraus N, McGee TJ, Carrell TD, Zecker SG, Nicol TG, Koch DB: Auditory neurophysiologic responses and discrimination deficits in children with learning problems. Science: 273; 971–973, 1996.

Kraus N, McGee T, Littman T, Nicol T, King C: Nonprimary auditory thalamic representation of acoustic change. Journal of Neurophysiology: 72; 1270–1277, 1994.

Kraus N, McGee T, Micco A, Sharma A, Carrell T, Nicol T: Mismatch negativity in school-age children to speech stimuli

that are just perceptibly different. Electroencephalography and Clinical Neurophysiology: 88; 123–130, 1993b.

Kraus N, Smith DI, Reed N, Stein L, Cartee C: Middle latency responses in children: effects of age and diagnostic category. Electroencephalography and Clinical Neurophysiology: 62; 343–351, 1985.

Krings T, Chiappa KH, Cuffin BN, Cochius JI, Connolly S, Cosgrove GR: Accuracy of EEG dipole source localization using implanted sources in the human brain. Clinical Neurophysiology: 110; 106–114, 1999.

Krmpotic-Nemanic J, Kostovic I, Kolovic Z, Nemanic D, Mrzljak L: Development of the human fetal auditory cortex: growth of afferent fibers. Acta Anatomy: 116; 69–73, 1983.

Krmpotic-Nemanic J, Kostovic I, Nemanic D: Prenatal and perinatal development of radial cell columns in the human auditory cortex. Acta Otolaryngology: 97; 489–495, 1984.

Kropotov JD, Alho K, Näätänen R, Ponomarev VA, Kropotova OV, Anichkov AD, Nechaev VB: Human auditory-cortex mechanisms of preattentive sound discrimination. Neuroscience Letters: 280; 87–90, 2000.

Krumholz A: Evoked potentials in infancy and childhood. In Niedermeyer E, Lopes Da Silva F (Eds), Electroencephalography: Basic Principles, Clinical Applications, and Related Fields. Philadelphia, PA: Lippincott Williams and Wilkins, pp. 1059–1072, 1999.

Kuhl PK, Williams KA, Lacerda F, Stevens KN, Lindblom B: Linguistic experience alters perception in infants by 6 months of age. Science: 255; 606–608, 1992.

Kujala T, Myllyviita K, Tervaniemi M, Alho K, Kallio J, Näätänen R: Basic auditory dysfunction in dyslexia as demonstrated by brain activity measurements. Psychophysiology: 37; 262–266, 2000.

Kuriki S, Nogai T, Hirata Y: Cortical sources of middle latency responses of auditory evoked magnetic field. Hearing Research: 92; 47–51, 1995.

Kurtzberg D, Hilbert PL, Kreuzer JA, Vaughan HG Jr: Differential maturation of cortical auditory evoked potentials to speech sounds in normal full term and very low-birthweight infants. Developmental Medicine of Child Neurology: 26; 466–475, 1984.

Kurtzberg D, Vaughan HG Jr, Kreuzer JA, Fliegel KZ: Developmental studies and clinical application of mismatch negativity: problems and prospects. Ear and Hearing: 16; 105–117, 1995.

Kutas M, Hillyard SA: Reading senseless sentences: brain potentials reflect semantic incongruity. Science: 207; 203–205, 1980.

Lamb JA, Moore J, Bailey A, Monaco AP: Autism: recent molecular genetic advances. Human Molecular Genetics: 9; 861–868, 2000.

Langner G, Sams M, Heil P, Schulze H: Frequency and periodicity are represented in orthogonal maps in the human auditory cortex: evidence from magnetoencephalography. Journal of Comparative Physiology A: 181; 665–676, 1997.

Leahy RM, Mosher JC, Spencer ME, Huang MX, Lewine JD: A study of dipole localization accuracy for MEG and EEG using a human skull phantom. Electroencephalography and Clinical Neurophysiology: 107; 159–173, 1998.

Lee YS, Lueders H, Dinner DS, Lesser RP, Hahn J, Klem G: Recording of auditory evoked potentials in man using chronic subdural electrodes. Brain: 107; 115–131, 1984.

Legatt AD, Arezzo JC, Vaughan HG Jr: Anatomic and physiologic bases of brain stem auditory evoked potentials. In Gilmore R (Ed), Neurologic Clinics, Vol. 6, Evoked Potentials. Philadelphia, PA: W.B. Sanders, pp. 681–704, 1988.

Leppänen PHT, Eklund KM, Lyytinen H: Event-related brain potentials to change in rapidly presented acoustic stimuli in newborns. Developmental Neuropsychology: 13; 175–204, 1997.

Leppänen PHT, Lyytinen H: Auditory event-related potentials in the study of developmental language-related disorders. Audiology and Neurootology: 2; 308–340, 1997.

Leppänen PHT, Pihko E, Eklund KM, Lyytinen H: Cortical responses of infants with and without a genetic risk for dyslexia: II. Group effects. NeuroReport: 10; 969–973, 1999.

Letinic K, Kostovic I: Postnatal development of calcium-binding proteins calbindin and parvalbumin in human visual cortex. Cerebral Cortex: 8; 660–669, 1998.

Liberman AM, Mattingly IG: A specialization for speech perception. Science: 243; 489–493, 1989.

Liégeois-Chauvel C, deGraaf JB, Laguitton V, Chauvel P: Specialization of left auditory cortex for speech perception in man depends on temporal coding. Cerebral Cortex; 9; 484–496, 1999.

Liégeois-Chauvel C, Musolino A, Badier JM, Marquis P, Chauvel P: Evoked potentials recorded from the auditory cortex in man: evaluation and topography of the middle latency components. Electroencephalography and Clinical Neurophysiology: 92; 204–214, 1994.

Lincoln AJ, Courchesne E, Harms L, Allen M: Sensory modulation of auditory stimuli in children with autism and receptive developmental language disorder: event-related brain potential evidence. Journal of Autism and Developmental Disorders: 25; 521–539, 1995.

Liu AK, Belliveau JW, Dale AM: Spatiotemporal imaging of human brain activity using functional MRI constrained magnetoencephalography data: Monte Carlo simulations. Proceedings of the National Academy of Sciences of the USA: 95; 8945–8950, 1998.

Llinás RR, Ribary U, Jeanmonod D, Kronberg E, Mitra PP: Thalamocortical dysrhythmia: A neurological and neuropsychiatric syndrome characterized by magnetoencephalography. Proceedings of the National Academy of Sciences of the USA: 96; 15222–15227, 1999.

Loo SK, Teale PD, Reite ML: EEG correlates of methylphenidate response among children with ADHD: a preliminary report. Biological Psychiatry: 45; 1657–1660, 1999.

Lovrich D, Novick B, Vaughan HG Jr: Topographic analysis of auditory event-related potentials associated with acoustic and semantic processing. Electroencephalography and Clinical Neurophysiology: 71; 40–54, 1988.

Luck SJ: Direct and indirect integration of event-related potentials, functional magnetic resonance images, and single-unit recordings. Human Brain Mapping; 8; 115–120, 1999.

Marosi E, Harmony T, Sánchez L, Becker J, Bernal J, Reyes A, Díaz de León AE, Rodrígues M, Fernández T: Maturation of the coherence of EEG activity in normal and learning-disabled children. Electroencephalography and Clinical Neurophysiology: 83; 350–357, 1992.

Martín-Loeches M, Hinojosa JA, Rubia FJ: Insights from event-related potentials into the temporal and hierarchical organization of the ventral and dorsal streams of the visual system in selective attention. Psychophysiology: 36; 721–736, 1999.

Mason JA, Hermann KR: Universal infant hearing screening by automated auditory brainstem response measurement. Pediatrics: 101; 221–228, 1998.

Mathiak K, Hertrich I, Lutzenberger W, Ackermann H: Preattentive processing of consonant vowel syllables at the level of the supratemporal plane: a whole-head magnetencephalography study. Cognitive Brain Research: 8; 251–257, 1999.

McAnally KI, Stein JF: Scalp potentials evoked by amplitude-modulated tones in dyslexia. Journal of Speech, Language, and Hearing Research: 40; 939–945, 1997.

McCallum WC: Potentials related to expectancy, preparation and motor activity. In Picton TW (Ed), Human Event-Related Potentials, EEG Handbook (revised series, Vol. 3). Amsterdam: Elsevier, pp. 427–534, 1988.

McCarthy G, Nobre AC, Bentin S, Spencer DD: Language-related field potentials in the anterior–medial temporal lobe: I. Intracranial distribution and neural generators. Journal of Neuroscience: 15; 1080–1089, 1995.

McCarthy G, Puce A, Belger A, Allison T: Electrophysiological studies of human face perception. II: Response properties of face-specific potentials generated in occipitotemporal cortex. Cerebral Cortex: 9; 431–444, 1999.

McClelland RJ, Eyre DG, Watson D, Calvert GJ, Sherrard E: Central conduction time in childhood autism. British Journal of Psychiatry: 60; 659–663, 1992.

McEvoy LK, Smith ME, Gevins A: Test–retest reliability of cognitive EEG. Clinical Neurophysiology: 111; 457–463, 2000.

McGee T, Kraus N, Killion M, Rosenberg R, King C: Improving the reliability of the auditory middle latency response by monitoring the EEG delta activity. Ear and Hearing: 14; 76–84, 1993.

McGee T, Kraus N, King C, Nicol T: Acoustic elements of speech-like stimuli are reflected in surface recorded responses over the guinea pig temporal lobe. Journal of the Acoustical Society of America: 99; 3606–3614, 1996.

McPherson WB, Ackerman PT, Holcomb PJ, Dykma RA: Event-related brain potentials elicited during phonological processing differentiate subgroups of reading disabled adolescents. Brain and Language: 62; 163–185, 1998.

Mehta AD, Ulbert I, Schroeder CE: Intermodal selective attention in monkeys. I. distribution and timing of effects across visual areas. Cerebral Cortex: 10; 343–358, 2000a.

Mehta AD, Ulbert I, Schroeder CE: Intermodal selective attention in monkeys. II. Physiological mechanisms of modulation. Cerebral Cortex: 10; 359–370, 2000b.

Merzenich MM, Jenkins WM, Johnson P, Schreiner C, Miller SL, Tallal P: Temporal processing deficits of language-learning impaired children ameliorated by training. Science: 271; 77–81, 1996.

Metcalfe K: Williams syndrome: an update on clinical and molecular aspects. Archives of Disease in Childhood: 81; 198–200, 1999.

Metherate R, Cox CL, Ashe JH: Cellular bases of neocortical activation: modulation of neural oscillations by the nucleus basalis and endogenous acetylcholine. Journal of Neuroscience: 12; 4701–4711, 1992.

Michie PT, Karayanides F, Smith GL, Barrett NA, Large MM, O'Sullivan BT, Kavanagh DJ: An exploration of varieties of visual attention: ERP findings. Cognitive Brain Research: 7; 419–450, 1999.

Miltner W, Braun C, Johnson R, Simson GV, Rushkin DS: A test of brain electrical source analysis (BESA): a simulation study. Electroencephalography and Clinical Neurophysiology: 91; 295–310, 1994.

Miyazaki M, Shibasaki H, Suwazono S, Honda M, Ikeda A, Nagamine T, Nishida S, Nakamura M, Hayakawa T, Mutoh K, Mikawa H: Characteristics of auditory P300 in children: application of single trial analysis. Brain and Development: 16; 374–381, 1994.

Molfese DL: Neuroelectric correlates of categorical speech perception in adults. Brain and Language: 5; 25–35, 1978.

Molfese DL: Hemispheric specialization for temporal information: implications for the perception of voicing cues during speech perception. Brain and Language: 11; 285–299, 1980.

Molfese DL: Predicting dyslexia at 8 years of age using neonatal brain responses. Brain and Language: 72; 238–245, 2000.

Molfese DL, Hess TM: Hemispheric specialization for VOT perception in the preschool child. Journal of Experimental Child Psychology: 26; 71–84, 1978.

Molfese DL, Molfese VJ: Right-hemisphere responses from preschool children to temporal cues to speech and nonspeech materials: electrophysiological evidence. Brain and Language: 33; 245–259, 1988.

Munk MHJ, Roelfsema PR, König P, Engel AK, Singer W: Role of reticular activation in the modulation of intracortical synchronization. Science: 272; 271–274, 1996.

Näätänen R: The role of attention in auditory information processing as revealed by event-related potentials and other brain measures of cognitive function. Behavioral Brain Science: 13; 201–288, 1990.

Näätänen R, Lehtokoski A, Lennes M, Cheour M, Houtilainen M, Iivonen A, Vainio M, Alkus P, Iimoniemi RJ, Luuk A, Allik J, Sinkkonen J: Language-specific phoneme representations revealed by electric and magnetic brain responses. Nature: 385; 432–434, 1997.

Näätänen R, Picton T: The N1 wave of the human electric and magnetic response to sound: a review and an analysis of the component structure. Psychophysiology: 24; 375–425, 1987.

Nagarajan S, Mahncke H, Salz T, Tallal P, Roberts T, Merzenich MM: Cortical auditory signal processing in poor readers. Proceedings of the National Academy of Sciences of the USA: 96; 6483–6488, 1999.

Narita T, Koga Y: Neuropsychological assessment of childhood autism. Advances in Biological Psychiatry: 16; 156–170, 1987.

Nicholson C, Freeman JA: Theory of current source–density analysis and determination of conductivity tensor for anuran cerebellum. Journal of Neurophysiology: 38; 356–368, 1975.

Nobre AC, McCarthy G: Language-related field potentials in the anterior–medial temporal lobe: II. Effects of word type and semantic priming. Journal of Neuroscience: 15; 1090–1098, 1995.

Novak GP, Kurtzberg D, Kreuzer JA, Vaughan HG Jr: Cortical responses to speech sounds and their formants in normal infants: maturational sequence and spatiotemporal analysis. Electroencephalography and Clinical Neurophysiology: 73; 295–305, 1989.

Novick B, Lovrich D, Vaughan HG Jr: Event-related potentials associated with the discrimination of acoustic and semantic aspects of speech. Neuropsychologia: 23; 87–101, 1985.

Novick B, Vaughan HG Jr, Kurtzberg D, Simson R: An electrophysiological indication of auditory processing defects in autism. Psychiatry Research: 3; 107–114, 1980.

Oades RD, Dittmann-Balcar A, Schepker R, Eggers C, Zerbin D: Auditory event-related potentials (ERPs) and mismatch negativity (MMN) in healthy children and those with attention-deficit or Tourette/tic symptoms. Biological Psychology: 43; 163–185, 1996.

Oades RD, Dittmann-Balcar A, Zerbin D: Development and topography of auditory event-related potentials (ERPs): Mismatch and processing negativity in individuals 8–22 years of age. Psychophysiology: 34; 677–693, 1997.

Oades RD, Walker MK, Geffen LB, Stern LM: Event related potentials in autistic and healthy children on an auditory choice reaction time task. International Journal of Psychophysiology: 6; 25–37, 1988.

Oades RD: Frontal, temporal and lateralized brain function in children with attention-deficit hyperactivity disorder: a psychophysiological and neurophysiological viewpoint on development. Behavioural Brain Research: 94; 83–95, 1998.

O'Craven KM, Downing PE, Kanwisher N: fMRI evidence for objects as the units of attentional selection. Nature: 401; 584–587, 1999.

Ohala JJ: Speech perception is hearing sounds, not tongues. Journal of the Acoustical Society of America: 99; 1718–1725, 1996.

Onitsuka T, Ninomiya H, Sato E, Yamamoto T, Tashiro N: The effect of interstimulus intervals and between-block rests on the auditory evoked potential and magnetic field: is the auditory P50 in humans an overlapping potential? Clinical Neurophysiology: 111; 237–245, 2000.

Overtoom CCE, Verbaten MN, Kemner C, Kenemans JL, Van Engeland H, Buitelaar JK, Camfferman G, Koelega HS: Associations between event-related potentials and measures of attention and inhibition in the continuous performance task in children with ADHD and normal controls. Journal of the American Academy of Child and Adolescent Psychiatry: 37; 977–985, 1998.

Pang EW, Edmonds GE, Desjardins R, Khan SC, Trainor LJ, Taylor MJ: Mismatch negativity to speech stimuli in 8-month-old infants and adults. International Journal of Psychophysiology: 29; 227–236, 1998.

Pang EW, Taylor MJ: Tracking the development of the N1 from age 3 to adulthood: an examination of speech and non-speech stimuli. Clinical Neurophysiology: 111; 388–397, 2000.

Pantev C, Bertrand O, Eulitz C, Verkindt C, Hampson S, Schuierer G, Elbert T: Specific tonotopic organizations of different areas of the human auditory cortex revealed by simultaneous magnetic and electric recordings. Electroencephalography and Clinical Neurophysiology: 94; 26–40, 1995.

Pantev C, Elbert T, Ross B, Eulitz C, Terhardt E: Binaural fusion and the representation of virtual pitch in the human auditory cortex. Hearing Research: 100; 164–170, 1996.

Paterson SJ, Brown JH, Gsödl MK, Johnson MH, Karmiloff-Smith A: Cognitive modularity and genetic disorders. Science: 286; 2355–2358, 1999.

Pegg JE, Werker JF: Adult and infant perception of two English phones. Journal of the Acoustical Society of America: 102; 3742–3753, 1997.

Pekkonen E, Rinne T, Näätänen R: Variability and replicability of the mismatch negativity. Electroencephalography and Clinical Neurophysiology: 96; 546–554, 1995.

Perrin F, Bertrand O, Pernier J: Scalp current density mapping: value and estimation from potential data. IEEE Transactions on Biomedical Engineering: 34; 283–288, 1987.

Pfurtscheller G: Event-related synchronization (ERS): an electrophysiological correlate of cortical areas at rest. Electroencephalography and Clinical Neurophysiology: 83; 62–69, 1992.

Pfurtscheller G, Lopes da Silva FH: Event-related EEG/MEG synchronization and desynchronization: basic principles. Clinical Neurophysiology: 110; 1842–1857, 1999.

Phillips DP, Taylor TL, Hall SE, Carr MM, Mossop JE: Detection of silent intervals between noises activating different perceptual channels: some properties of 'central' auditory gap detection. Journal of the Acoustical Society of America: 101; 3694–3705, 1997.

Picton TW, Hillyard SA: Endogenous event-related potentials. In Picton TW (Ed), Handbook of Electroencephalography and Clinical Neurophysiology, Vol. 3, Human Event-Related Potentials. Amsterdam: Elsevier, pp. 361–426, 1988.

Pike AA, Marlow N, Reber C: Maturation of the flash visual evoked potential in preterm infants. Early Human Development: 54; 215–222, 1999.

Pisoni DP: Identification and discrimination of the relative onset time of two component tones: implications for voicing perception in stops. Journal of the Acoustical Society of America: 61; 1352–1361, 1977.

Poeppel D, Phillips C, Yellin E, Rowley HA, Roberts TPL, Marantz A: Processing of vowels in supratemporal auditory cortex. Neuroscience Letters: 221; 145–148, 1997.

Polich J: P300 in clinical applications. In Niedermeyer E, Lopes Da Silva F (Eds), Electroencephalography: Basic Principles, Clinical Applications, and Related Fields. Philadelphia, PA: Lippincott Williams and Wilkins, pp. 1073–1091, 1999.

Ponton CW, Eggermont JJ, Kwong B, Don M: Maturation of human central auditory system activity: evidence from multichannel evoked potentials. Clinical Neurophysiology: 111; 220–236, 2000.

Puce A, Allison T, Asgari M, Gore JC, McCarthy G: Differential sensitivity of human visual cortex to faces, letterstrings, and textures: A functional magnetic resonance imaging study. Journal of Neuroscience: 16; 5205–5215, 1996.

Puce A, Allison T, Bentin S, Gore JC, McCarthy G: Temporal cortex activation in humans viewing eye and mouth movements. Journal of Neuroscience: 18; 2188–2199, 1998.

Puce A, Allison T, McCarthy G: Electrophysiological studies of human face perception. III: Effects of top-down processing on face-specific potentials. Cerebral Cortex: 9; 445–458, 1999.

Rapin I: Autism. New England Journal of Medicine: 337; 97–104, 1997.

Recanzone GH, Schreiner CE, Merzenich MM: Plasticity in the frequency representation of primary auditory cortex following discriminative training in adult owl monkeys. Journal of Neuroscience: 13; 87–103, 1993.

Reite M, Teale P, Rojas DC: Magnetoencephalography: applications in psychiatry. Biological Psychiatry: 45; 1553–1563, 1999.

Reite M, Teale P, Zimmerman J, Davis K, Whalen J: Source location of a 50 msec latency auditory evoked field component. Electroencephalography and Clinical Neurophysiology: 70; 490–498, 1988.

Reser DH, Fishman YI, Arezzo JC, Steinschneider M: Binaural interactions in primary auditory cortex of the awake monkey. Cerebral Cortex: 10; 574–584, 2000.

Ring HA, Baron-Cohen S, Wheelwright S, Williams SCR, Brammer M, Andrew C, Bullmore ET: Cerebral correlates of preserved cognitive skills in autism: a functional MRI study of Embedded Figures Task performance. Brain: 122; 1305–1315, 1999.

Ritter W, Simson R, Vaughan HG Jr, Friedman D: A brain event related to the making of a sensory discrimination. Science: 203; 1358–1361, 1979.

Riva D, Giorgi C: The cerebellum contributes to higher functions during development: evidence from a series of children surgically treated for posterior fossa tumors. Brain: 123; 1051–1061, 2000.

Robaey P, Cansino S, Dugas M, Renault B: A comparative study of ERP correlates of psychometric and Piagetian intelligence measures in normal and hyperactive children. Electroencephalography and Clinical Neurophysiology: 96; 56–75, 1995.

Rogers RL, Basile LFH, Papanicolaou AC, Eisenberg HM: Magnetoencephalography reveals two distinct sources associated with late positive evoked potentials during visual oddball task. Cerebral Cortex: 3; 163–169, 1993.

Rosen S: Language disorders: a problem with auditory processing? Current Biology: 9; R698–R700, 1999.

Rosenhall U, Johansson E, Gillberg C: Oculomotor finding in autistic children. Journal of Laryngology and Otology: 102; 435–439, 1988.

Rossion B, Campanella S, Gomez CM, Delinte A, Debatisse D, Liard L, Dubois S, Bruyer R, Crommelinck M, Guerit: Task modulation of brain activity related to familiar and unfamiliar face processing: an ERP study. Clinical Neurophysiology: 110; 449–462, 1999.

Rumsey JM, Grimes AM, Pikus AM, Duara R, Ismond DR: Auditory brainstem responses in pervasive developmental disorders. Biological Psychiatry: 19; 1403–1418, 1984.

Rutter M: Genetic studies of autism: from the 1970s into the millennium. Journal of Abnormal Child Psychology: 28; 3–14, 2000.

Salamy A: Maturation of the auditory brainstem response from birth through early childhood. Journal of Clinical Neurophysiology: 1; 293–329, 1984.

Sams M, Hietanen JK, Hari R, Ilmoniemi RJ, Lounasmaa OV: Face-specific responses from the human inferior occipitotemporal cortex. Neuroscience: 77; 49–55, 1997.

Sannita WG: Stimulus-specific oscillatory responses of the brain: a time/frequency-related coding process. Clinical Neurophysiology: 111; 565–583, 2000.

Sasama R: Hearing threshold investigations in infants and children. Audiology: 29; 76–84, 1990.

Satterfield JH, Schell AM, Nicholas T: Preferential neural processing of attended stimuli in attention-deficit hyperactivity disorder and normal boys. Psychophysiology: 31; 1–10, 1994.

Scherg M, Vajsar J, Picton TW: A source analysis of the late human auditory evoked potentials. Journal of Cognitive Neuroscience: 1; 336–355, 1989.

Scherg M, Von Cramon D: Evoked dipole source potentials of the human auditory cortex. Electroencephalography and Clinical Neurophysiology: 65; 344–360, 1986.

Schreiner CE: Spatial distribution of responses to simple and complex sounds in the primary auditory cortex. Audiology and Neuro-otology: 3; 104–122, 1998.

Schroeder CE, Seto S, Garraghty PE: Emergence of radial nerve dominance in median nerve cortex after median nerve transection in an adult squirrel monkey. Journal of Neurophysiology: 77; 522–526, 1997.

Schroeder CE, Steinschneider M, Javitt DC, Tenke CE, Givre SJ, Mehta AD, Simpson GV, Arezzo JC, Vaughan HG Jr: Localization of ERP generators and identification of underlying neural processes. In Karmos G, Molnár M, Csépe V, Czigler I, Desmedt JE (Eds), Perspectives of Event-Related Potentials Research (EEG Suppl 44). Elsevier: Amsterdam, pp. 55–75, 1995.

Schroeder CE, Tenke CE, Givre SJ, Arezzo JC, Vaughan HG Jr: Striate cortical contribution to the surface-recorded pattern-reversal VEP in the alert monkey. Vision Research: 31; 1143–1157, 1991.

Schröger E: Human brain potential signs of selection by location and frequency in an auditory transient attention situation. Neuroscience Letters: 173; 163–166, 1994.

Schulte-Körne G, Deimel W, Bartling J, Remschmidt H: Auditory processing and dyslexia: evidence for a specific speech processing deficit. NeuroReport: 9; 337–340, 1998.

Schulte-Körne G, Deimel W, Bartling J, Remschmidt H: Preattentive processing of auditory patterns in dyslexic human subjects. Neuroscience Letters: 276; 41–44, 1999.

Schulz KP, Himelstein J, Halperin JM, Newcorn JH: Neurobiological models of attention-deficit/hyperactivity disorder: a brief review of the empirical evidence. CNS Spectrums: 5; 34–44, 2000.

Shafer VL, Morr ML, Kreuzer JA, Kurtzberg D: Maturation of mismatch negativity in school-age children. Ear and Hearing: 21; 242–251, 2000.

Sharma A, Dorman MF: Cortical auditory evoked potential correlates of categorical perception of voice-onset time. Journal of the Acoustical Society of America: 106; 1078–1083, 1999.

Sharma A, Kraus N, McGee T, Carrell T, Nicol T: Acoustic versus phonetic representation of speech as reflected by the mismatch negativity event-related potential. Electroencephalography and Clinical Neurophysiology: 88; 64–71, 1993.

Sharma A, Kraus N, McGee TJ, Nicol TG: Developmental changes in P1 and N1 central auditory responses elicited by consonant–vowel syllables. Electroencephalography and Clinical Neurophysiology: 104; 540–545, 1997.

Shepherd AJ, Saunders KJ, McCulloch DL, Dutton GN: Prognostic value of flash visual evoked potentials in preterm infants. Developmental Medicine Child Neurology: 41; 9–15, 1999.

Simmons JQ, Baltaxe C: Language patterns of adolescent autistics. Journal of Autism and Childhood Schizophrenia: 5; 333–351, 1975.

Simos PG, Breier JI, Zouridakis G, Papanicolaou AC: Magnetic fields elicited by a tone onset time continuum in humans. Cognitive Brain Research: 6; 285–294, 1998a.

Simos PG, Breier JI, Zouridakis G, Papanicolaou AC: MEG correlates of categorical-like temporal cue perception in humans. NeuroReport: 9; 2475–2479, 1998c.

Simos PG, Diehl RL, Breier JI, Molis MR, Zouridakis G, Papanicolaou AC: MEG correlates of categorical perception of a voice onset time continuum in humans. Cognitive Brain Research: 7; 215–219, 1998b.

Simos PG, Molfese DL: Electrophysiological responses from a temporal order continuum in the newborn infant. Neuropsychologia: 35; 89–98, 1997.

Simos PG, Molfese DL, Brenden RA: Behavioral and electrophysiological indices of voicing-cue discrimination: laterality patterns and development. Brain and Language: 57; 122–150, 1997.

Singer W: Response synchronization: a universal coding strategy for the definition of relations. In Gazzaniga MS (Ed-in-Chief), The New Cognitive Neurosciences, 2nd ed. Cambridge, MA: MIT Press, pp. 325–338, 2000.

Smith AT, Singh KD, Greenlee MW: Attentional suppression of activity in the human visual cortex. NeuroReport: 11; 271–277, 2000.

Solanto MV: Neuropsychopharmacological mechanisms of stimulant drug action in attention-deficit hyperactivity disorder: a review and integration. Behavioral Brain Research: 94; 127–152, 1998.

Spillmann L, Werner JS: Long-range interactions in visual perception. Trends in Neuroscience: 19; 428–434, 1996.

Stapells DR: Auditory brainstem response assessment of infants and children. Seminars in Hearing: 10; 229–251, 1989.

Stapells DR, Galambos R, Costello JA, Makeig S: Inconsistency of auditory middle latency and steady-state responses in infants. Electroencephalography and Clinical Neurophysiology: 71; 289–295, 1988.

Stapells DR, Gravel JS, Martin BA: Thresholds for auditory brain stem responses to tones in notched noise from infants and young children with normal hearing or sensorineural hearing loss. Ear and Hearing: 16; 361–371, 1995.

Stapells DR, Kurtzberg D: Evoked potential assessment of auditory system integrity in infants. Clinics in Perinatology: 18; 497–518, 1991.

Stapells DR, Ruben RJ: Auditory brain stem responses to bone-conducted tones in infants. Annals of Otology, Rhinology and Laryngology: 98; 941–949, 1989.

Starr A, Sandroni P, Michalewski HJ: Readiness to respond in a target detection task: pre- and post-stimulus event-related potentials in normal subjects. Electroencephalography and Clinical Neurophysiology: 96; 76–92, 1995.

State MW, Lombroso PJ, Pauls DL, Leckman JF: The genetics of childhood psychiatric disorders: a decade of progress. Journal of the American Academy of Child and Adolescent Psychiatry: 39; 946–962, 2000.

Stefanatos GA, Green GGR, Ratcliff GG: Neurophysiological evidence of auditory channel anomalies in developmental dysphasia. Archives of Neurology: 46; 871–875, 1989.

Steinschneider M, Reser D, Schroeder CE, Arezzo JC: Tonotopic organization of responses reflecting stop consonant place of articulation in primary auditory cortex (A1) of the monkey. Brain Research: 674; 147–152, 1995b.

Steinschneider M, Schroeder CE, Arezzo JC, Vaughan HG Jr: Speech-evoked activity in primary auditory cortex: effects of voice onset time. Electroencephalography and Clinical Neurophysiology: 92; 30–43, 1994.

Steinschneider M, Schroeder CE, Arezzo JC, Vaughan HG Jr: Physiological correlates of the voice onset time boundary in primary auditory cortex (A1) of the awake monkey: temporal response patterns. Brain and Language: 48; 326–340, 1995a.

Steinschneider M, Tenke CE, Schroeder CE, Javitt DC, Simpson GV, Arezzo JC, Vaughan HG Jr: Cellular generators of the cortical auditory evoked potential initial component. Electroencephalography and Clinical Neurophysiology: 84; 196–200, 1992.

Steinschneider M, Volkov IO, Noh MD, Garell PC, Howard MA III: Temporal encoding of the voice onset time phonetic parameter by field potentials recorded directly from human auditory cortex. Journal of Neurophysiology: 82; 2346–2357, 1999.

Steriade M: Synchronized activities of coupled oscillators in the cerebral cortex and thalamus at different levels of vigilance. Cerebral Cortex: 7; 583–604, 1997.

Studdert-Kennedy M, Mody M: Auditory temporal perception deficits in the reading-impaired: a critical review of the evidence. Psychonomic Bulletin and Review: 2; 508–514, 1995.

Swanson J, Castellanos FX, Murias M, LeHoste G, Kennedy J: Cognitive neuroscience of attention deficit hyperactivity disorder and hyperkinetic disorder. Current Opinion in Neurobiology: 8; 263–271, 1998.

Szymanski MD, Yund EW, Woods DL: Phonemes, intensity and attention: differential effects on the mismatch negativity (MMN). Journal of the Acoustical Society of America: 106; 3492–3505, 1999.

Tager-Flusberg H: The conceptual basis for referential word meaning in children with autism. Child Development: 56; 1167–1178, 1985.

Tager-Flusberg H: A psycholinguistic perspective on language development in the autistic child. In Dawson G (Ed), Autism: Nature, Diagnosis, and Treatment. New York, Guilford, pp. 92–109, 1989.

Tallal P: Children with language impairment can be accurately identified using temporal processing measures: a response to Zhang and Tomblin, Brain and Language, 65, 395–403 (1998). Brain and Language: 69; 222–229, 1999.

Tallal P, Merzenich MM, Miller S, Jenkins W: Language learning impairments: integrated basic science, technology, and remediation. Experimental Brain Research: 123; 210–219, 1998.

Tallal P, Miller S, Bedi G, Byma G, Wang X, Nagarajan SS, Schreiner C, Jenkins WM, Merzenich MM: Language comprehension in language-learning impaired children improved with acoustically modified speech. Science: 271; 81–84, 1996.

Tallal P, Miller S, Fitch RH: Neurobiological basis of speech: a case for the preeminence of temporal processing. In Tallal P, Galaburda AM, Llinás RR, von Euler C (Eds), Temporal Information Processing in The Nervous System: Special Reference To Dyslexia And Dysphasia. Annals of the New York Academy of Sciences, 682; 27–47, 1993.

Taylor MJ: Maturational changes in ERPs to orthographic and phonological tasks. Electroencephalography and Clinical Neurophysiology: 88; 494–507, 1993.

Taylor MJ, Edmonds GE, McCarthy G, Allison T: Eyes first! Eye processing develops before face processing in children. NeuroReport: 12; 1671–1676, 2001.

Taylor MJ, McCarthy G, Saliba E, Degiovanni E: ERP evidence of developmental changes in processing of faces. Clinical Neurophysiology: 110; 910–915, 1999.

Taylor MJ, Menzies R, MacMillan LJ, Whyte HE: VEPs in normal full-term and premature neonates: longitudinal versus cross-sectional data. Electroencephalography and Clinical Neurophysiology: 68; 20–27, 1987.

Taylor MJ, Voros JG, Logan WJ, Malone MA: Changes in event-related potentials with stimulant medication in children with attention deficit hyperactivity disorder. Biological Psychology: 36; 139–156, 1993.

Temple CM: Cognitive neuropsychology and its application to children. Journal of Child Psychology and Psychiatry: 38; 27–52, 1997.

Temple E, Posner MI: Brain mechanisms of quantity are similar in 5-year-old children and adults. Proceedings of the National Academy of Sciences of the USA: 95; 7836–7841, 1998.

Thivierge J, Bedard C, Cole R, Maziade M: Brainstem auditory evoked response and subcortical abnormalities in autism. Amereican Journal of Psychiatry: 147; 1609–1613, 1990.

Tiitinen H, Alho K, Huotilainen M, Ilmoniemi RJ, Simola J, Näätänen R: Tonotopic auditory cortex and the magnetoencephalographic (MEG) equivalent of the mismatch negativity. Psychophysiology: 30; 537–540, 1993.

Tomoda Y, Tobimatsu S, Mitsudome A: Visual evoked potentials in school children: A comparative study of transient and steady-state methods with pattern reversal and flash stimulation. Clinical Neurophysiology: 110; 97–102, 1999.

Tonnquist-Uhlén I, Borg E, Persson HE, Spens KE: Topography of auditory evoked cortical potentials in children with severe language impairment: the N1 component. Electroencephalography and Clinical Neurophysiology: 100; 250–260, 1996.

Tonnquist-Uhlén I, Borg E, Spens KE: Topography of auditory evoked long-latency potentials in normal children, with particular reference to the N1 component. Electroencephalography and Clinical Neurophysiology: 95; 34–41, 1995.

Tootell RBH, Dale AM, Sereno MI, Malach R: New images from human visual cortex. Trends in Neuroscience: 19; 481–489, 1996.

Traub RD, Spruston N, Soltesz I, Konnerth A, Whittington MA, Jefferys JGR: Gamma-frequency oscillations: a neuronal population phenomenon, regulated by synaptic and intrinsic cellular processes, and inducing synaptic plasticity. Progress in Neurobiology: 55; 563–575, 1998.

Trejo LJ, Ryan-Jones DL, Kramer AF: Attentional modulation of the mismatch negativity elicited by frequency differences between binaurally presented tone bursts. Psychophysiology: 32; 319–328, 1995.

Ungerleider LG, Courtney SM, Haxby JV: A neural system for human visual working memory. Proceedings of the National Academy of Sciences of the USA: 95; 883–890, 1998.

Uwer R, von Suchodoletz W: Stability of mismatch negativities in children. Clinical Neurophysiology: 111; 45–52, 2000.

Van der Stelt O, Kok A, Smulders FTY, Snel J, Gunning WB: Cerebral event-related potentials associated with selective attention to color: developmental changes from childhood to adulthood. Psychophysiology: 35; 227–239, 1998.

Vaughan HG Jr, Arezzo JC: The neural basis of event-related potentials. In Picton TW (Ed), Handbook of Electroencephalography and Clinical Neurophysiology, Vol. 3, Human Event-Related Potentials. Amsterdam: Elsevier, pp. 45–96, 1988.

Vaughan HG Jr, Kurtzberg D: Electrophysiologic indices of human brain maturation and cognitive development. In Gunnar MR, Nelson C (Eds), Minnesota Symposia On Child Psychology, Vol. 24. Hillsdale, NJ: Larwrence Erlbaum, pp. 1–36, 1992.

Vaz Pato M, Jones SJ: Cortical processing of complex tone stimuli: mismatch negativity at the end of a period of rapid pitch modulation. Cognitive Brain Research: 7; 295–306, 1999.

Volkmar F, Cook EH, Pomeroy J, Realmuto G, Tanguay P: Practice parameters for the assessment and treatment of children, adolescents, and adults with autism and other pervasive developmental disorders. Journal of the American Academy of Child and Adolescent Psychiatry: 38(Suppl 12); S32–S54, 1999.

Wackermann J, Matoušek M: From the 'EEG age' to a rational scale of brain electric maturation. Electroencephalography and Clinical Neurophysiology: 107; 415–421, 1998.

Wang J, Zhou T, Qui M, Du A, Cai K, Wang Z, Zhou C, Meng M, Zhuo Y, Fan S, Chen L: Relationship between ventral stream for object vision and dorsal stream for spatial vision: an fMRI + ERP study. Human Brain Mapping: 8; 170–181, 1999a.

Weinberger NM: Learning-induced receptive field plasticity in the primary auditory cortex. Seminars in Neuroscience: 9; 59–67, 1997.

Werker JF, Tees RC: Influences on infant speech processing: toward a new synthesis. Annual Review of Psychology: 50; 509–535, 1999.

Werner LA, Folsom RC, Mancl LR: The relationship between auditory brainstem response latencies and behavioral thresholds in normal hearing infants and adults. Hearing Research: 15; 88–98, 1994.

Whyte HE: Visual-evoked potentials in neonates following asphyxia. Clinics in Perinatology: 20; 451–461, 1993.

Winkler I, Lehtokoski A, Alku P, Vainio M, Czigler I, Csépe V, Aaltonen O, Raimo I, Alho K, Lang H, Iivonen A, Näätänen R: Pre-attentive detection of vowel contrasts utilizes both phonetic and auditory memory representations. Cognitive Brain Research: 7; 357–369, 1999.

Woldorff MG, Gallen CC, Hampson SR, Hillyard SA, Pantev C, Sobel D, Bloom FE: Modulation of early sensory processing in human auditory cortex during auditory selective attention. Proceedings of the National Academy of Sciences of the USA: 90; 8722–8726, 1993.

Woldorff MG, Hillyard SA, Gallen CC, Hampson SR, Bloom FE: Magnetoencephalographic recordings demonstrate attentional modulation of mismatch-related neural activity in human auditory cortex. Psychophysiology: 35; 283–292, 1998.

Wolff S, Barlow A: Schizoid personality in childhood: a comparative study of schizoid, autistic and normal children. Journal of Child Psychology and Psychiatry: 20; 29–46, 1979.

Wong V, Wong SN: Brainstem auditory evoked potential study in children with autistic disorder. Journal of Autism and Developmental Disorders: 21; 329–340, 1991.

Wood CC, Wolpaw JR: Scalp distribution of human auditory evoked potentials. II. Evidence for overlapping sources and involvement of auditory cortex. Electroencephalography and Clinical Neurophysiology: 54; 25–38, 1982.

Woods DL, Alho K, Algazi A: Stages of auditory feature conjunction: an event-related brain potential study. Journal of Experimental Psychology: 20; 81–94, 1994.

Wright BA, Lombardino LJ, King WM, Puranik CS, Leonard CM, Merzenich MM: Deficits in auditory temporal and spectral resolution in language-impaired children. Nature: 387; 176–178, 1997.

Yordanova J, Banaschewski T, Kolev V, Woerner W, Rothenberger A: Abnormal early stages of task stimulus processing in children with attention-deficit hyperactivity disorder — evidence from event-related gamma oscillations. Clinical Neurophysiology: 112; 1096–1108, 2001.

Yordanova J, Kolev V: Developmental changes in the event-related EEG theta response and P300. Electroencephalography and Clinical Neurophysiology: 104; 418–430, 1997.

Yvert B, Bertrand O, Thévenet M, Echallier JF, Pernier J: A systematic evaluation of the spherical model accuracy in EEG dipole localization. Electroencephalography and Clinical Neurophysiology: 102; 452–459, 1997.

CHAPTER 6

# The neuropsychology of childhood seizure disorders

Michael T. Stowe [a,c,*], David M. Masur [a,c] and Shlomo Shinnar [a,b,c]

[a] *Department of Neurology, Montefiore Medical Center and the Albert Einstein College of Medicine, Bainbridge Avenue and
210th Street, Bronx, NY 10476, USA*
[b] *Department of Pediatrics, Montefiore Medical Center and the Albert Einstein College of Medicine, Bainbridge Avenue and
210th Street, Bronx, NY 10476, USA*
[c] *Comprehensive Epilepsy Management Center, Montefiore Medical Center and the Albert Einstein College of Medicine,
Bainbridge Avenue and 210th Street, Bronx, NY 10476, USA*

## Introduction

Seizures are paroxysmal events characterized by abnormal electrical activity in the brain, which produces a sudden disruption of ongoing behavior and cognition. Depending upon the localization, duration, and spread of the abnormal activity in the brain, seizures are capable of causing disturbances in movement, consciousness, sensation, and perception. Epilepsy is defined as two or more unprovoked seizures more than 24 hours apart (Commission on Epidemiology and Prognosis, 1993). Epilepsy affects approximately 0.5 to 1% of all children through the age of 16 (Berg, 1995; Camfield et al., 1996; Hauser, Annegers and Kurland, 1993; Hauser and Hesdorffer, 1990; Sillanpaa, Jalava, Kaleva and Shinnar, 1998). Each year, 120 out of every 100,000 persons in the United States seek medical attention for a newly recognized seizure. Of these 300,000 patients, 40% (120,000) are children under 18 years (Hauser and Hesdorffer, 1990). The most common seizure type in children is febrile seizures which accounts for the majority (75,000–100,000) of cases. However,

20,000–45,000 children will be diagnosed as having epilepsy annually (Berg, 1995; Hauser and Hesdorffer, 1990). The highest risk of developing epilepsy in children is in the first year of life. However, the median age of seizure onset is 5 to 6 years of age (Berg, Levy, Testa and Shinnar, 1999a; Berg, Shinnar, Levy and Testa, 1999b; Berg, Testa, Levy and Shinnar, 1996; Camfield et al., 1996; Sillanpaa et al., 1998). There is some suggestion that the incidence of epilepsy may have declined in the last few decades (Berg et al., 1996, 1999a,b; Camfield et al., 1996; Hauser et al., 1993; Sillanpaa et al., 1998). The reasons for this are not fully clear but may include factors that decrease the risk such as vaccines for meningitis and improved diagnosis which will exclude cases that in the past may have been included (Berg et al., 1996).

While many cases of childhood onset epilepsy attain remission (Annegers, Hauser and Elveback, 1999; Berg, 1995; Berg, Hauser and Shinnar, 1995; Berg et al., 1996; Camfield, Camfield, Gordon et al., 1993; Casetta, Granieri, Monetti, et al., 1997; Hauser and Hesdorffer, 1990; Sillanpaa et al., 1998), many continue to have active epilepsy. Overall, 1.5 million Americans, including as many as 325,000 children between the ages of 5 and 14 years, have active epilepsy (Berg, 1995; Hauser and Hesdorffer, 1990). While there is a secondary peak age of incidence in the elderly (Hauser et al., 1993; Hauser and Hesdorf-

---

* Corresponding author. Comprehensive Epilepsy Management Center, Montefiore Medical Center and the Albert Einstein College of Medicine, Bainbridge Avenue and 210th Street, Bronx, NY 10476, USA. Tel.: +1 (718) 920-7757;
E-mail: retroviseur@aol.com

fer, 1990), the majority of active cases even in adults are of childhood onset. Epilepsy is the third most common serious neurological disorder in childhood with mental retardation and cerebral palsy being the most common (D'Amelio, Shinnar and Hauser, 2002) and the most common treatable serious neurological disorder in children and young adults.

Epilepsy is a complicated disorder in that the observed cognitive and behavioral deficits are the result of interactions between biological and psychosocial factors in combination with the particular effects of the medications used to treat seizure activity (Hermann and Whitman, 1986). In this chapter we will try to describe the various epileptic syndromes, the medications used to treat them, and the variety of associated cognitive deficits. We will touch upon the use of surgery as an increasingly prevalent method for the treatment of intractable seizures. In addition, an approach to the neuropsychological evaluation of the child with epilepsy is outlined.

## Classification of seizures and epilepsies

A new internationally accepted classification of seizures has been adopted, replacing the often confusing older descriptive classification (Commission on Classification and Terminology of the International League Against Epilepsy, 1981). A simplified summary of the classification is shown in Table 1.

In the new classification, the basic distinction is between those seizures with focal onset, whether or not they generalize (partial), and seizures without focal onset (generalized) which are generalized from the onset. Both absence ('petit mal') and tonic–

TABLE 1

Classification of seizures

| Generalized | Partial |
| --- | --- |
| Absence | |
|   Typical absence | Simple partial |
|   Atypical absence | Complex partial |
| Myoclonic | Partial with secondary generalization |
| Tonic | |
| Tonic–clonic | |
| Atonic | |

[a] Modified from Commission on Classification and Terminology of the International League Against Epilepsy (1981).

clonic ('grand mal') are classified under generalized seizure disorders. The old 'psychomotor seizure' is included in the spectrum of a complex partial seizure, which is defined as a partial seizure with impaired consciousness. The new classification has a rational basis in terms of both common electrophysiologic features of the seizure types and the spectrum of drugs that are effective in their treatment.

Note that this is a classification of seizures and not of epilepsy. A person with juvenile myoclonic epilepsy may have absence, myoclonic, and tonic–clonic seizures. Similarly, a patient with a left posterior temporal spike focus still has temporal lobe epilepsy. His or her seizures, however, are complex partial or partial with secondary generalization. The current classification of epilepsies is summarized in several comprehensive reviews (Commission on Classification and Terminology of the International League Against Epilepsy, 1989; Roger, Dravet, Bureau et al., 1992). A simplified summary of some of the more common epileptic syndromes of childhood is shown in Table 2.

## Neuropsychological deficits associated with epilepsy

Epilepsy is a condition in which at least a small area of brain tissue is dysfunctional. Seizures themselves interrupt cognitive function, but neuropsychological dysfunction associated with an area of anomalous tissue, i.e., the epileptic focus, is also likely. While neural reorganization and plasticity may play roles in the resulting functional capabilities of epileptic children, there are likely to be some minor or greater deficits. Although the nature and extent of fixed cognitive deficits, or cognitive decline continue to be unclear, impairments of memory, abstraction, speed of performance, and general intellectual ability have been identified. The severity of these deficits has been related to the type of seizure (Farwell, Dodrill and Batzel, 1985; O'Leary, Seidenberg, Berent and Boll, 1981), seizure frequency (Farwell et al., 1985) as well as age of onset (O'Leary, Lovell, Sackellares et al., 1983). Studies of the precise relationship between epilepsy and cognitive impairment are affected by a number of methodological issues. A prominent one is the distinction between deficits related to seizure activity and the effects of the

TABLE 2

Classification of epilepsy syndromes [a]

Localization-related (partial) epilepsies:
*Idiopathic partial epilepsies*
   Benign childhood epilepsy with centro-temporal spikes
   Childhood epilepsy with occipital paroxysms
   Primary reading epilepsy

*Symptomatic partial epilepsies*
   Chronic progressive epilepsia partialis continua
   Seizures characterized by modes of precipitation
   Other based on localization (temporal lobe, frontal lobe etc)
   or etiology

*Cryptogenic partial epilepsy*

Generalized epilepsies:
*Idiopathic generalized epilepsies*
   Childhood absence epilepsy
   Juvenile absence epilepsy
   Juvenile myoclonic epilepsy
   Epilepsy with generalized tonic–clonic seizures on awakening
   Photo-convulsive epilepsy

*Cryptogenic and/or symptomatic generalized epilepsies*
   West syndrome/infantile spasms
   Lennox–Gastaut syndrome
   Epilepsy with myoclonic–astatic seizures

*Symptomatic generalized epilepsies*
   Generalized symptomatic epilepsies — nonspecific etiology
      Early myoclonic encephalopathy
      Early infantile epileptic encephalopathy with suppression
      bursts
   Generalized symptomatic epilepsies-specific
   syndromes/etiologies

Other epilepsies not determined whether partial or generalized:
*Epilepsies with both generalized and focal features*
   Neonatal seizures
   Severe myoclonic epilepsy in infancy
   Epilepsy with continuous spike and wave during slow wave
      sleep
   Landau–Kleffner (acquired epileptic aphasia)

*Epilepsies without unequivocal generalized or focal features*

Special syndromes (not clearly epilepsy):
*Situation-related seizures*
   Febrile seizures
   Seizures occurring only in the context of acute metabolic or
      toxic events

*Isolated events*
   Isolated seizure (or cluster of seizures in a single day)
   Isolated status epilepticus

[a] Adapted from the Commission on Classification and Terminology of the International League Against Epilepsy (1989), Roger et al. (1992) and Berg et al. (1999a).

medications used to treat the seizures. Anti-epileptic medications have potentially significant effects upon cognitive function. As neuropsychological evaluation has rarely been obtained prior to the start of treatment, the relative contribution of seizures or medication to the overall cognitive picture is difficult to ascertain. Other potentially confounding factors are the severity of the seizure disorder, the underlying brain pathology responsible for the seizures, as well as measurement issues. Meanwhile, the majority of children with epilepsy are essentially neuropsychologically normal. In the following sections a number of issues dealing with epilepsy's impact upon neuropsychological functioning are covered. These include the impact of seizure (ictal) events and inter-ictal spikes on cognitive processing, the question of epilepsy's impact on IQ, the cumulative effect of seizures on IQ, status epilepticus, seizure effects in children vs. adults, severe childhood epileptic encephalopathies, and finally modality-specific neuropsychological deficits associated with epilepsy.

## Ictal and inter-ictal spike effects

Except for simple partial seizure, clinical seizures affect consciousness. The severity of the loss of consciousness in complex partial seizure is variable. Ictal attention variation affects the acquisition of information for processing, and therefore gives rise to cognitive impairment during the seizure. This alteration of information processing can cause amnesia for the seizure episode (Rowan and Rosenbaum, 1991). Seizures involving language cortex result in a variety of language deficits, such as speech arrest, paraphasias, and impairments of comprehension and word retrieval. Seizures involving the non-dominant hemisphere may produce disturbances of spatial perception and cognition. Deficits may be limited to the ictal event, there being no fixed deficits between seizures. Yet, there are children who have fixed deficits related to their seizures. For example, a patient with a left hemisphere complex partial seizure may experience speech arrest as well as other ictal deficits. If this patient's focus involves language-related cortex, the seizures may be associated with mild, fixed deficits of language.

With the exception of myoclonic seizures, all generalized seizures involve impairment of consciousness. In the case of generalized tonic–clonic seizures, the loss of consciousness is complete. Children with absence seizures may experience ictal-related diminution of cognitive function. Absence (petit mal) seizures are generalized seizures characterized by lapses of consciousness that rarely last longer than 10 seconds. There is a sudden and complete cessation of ongoing activity and a brief motionless stare, and in many cases the child is unaware of the seizure and continues as if nothing had happened. The cognitive effect of these absence seizures is likely to be true of other seizure types associated with lapses of attention. On EEG, a typical absence seizure is characterized by generalized 3-Hz spike-and-wave discharges that begin suddenly and end abruptly (Engel, 1989). Even without noticeable loss of consciousness, discharges of this type have been associated with momentary impairments of scholastic skills such as reading and arithmetic (Kastelijn-Nolst Trenite, Bakker, Binnie et al., 1988), deficits in verbal learning (Siebelink, Bakker, Binnie and Kastelijn-Nolst Trenite, 1988) and impairment of spatial ability (Matsuoka, Okuma, Ueno and Saito, 1986). More recently, children with absence seizures were shown to have poorer visual–spatial skills, visual–spatial learning ability, and long-term visual and verbal memory ability than match controls (Pavone, Bianchini, Trifiletti et al., 2001). Verbal ability was comparable in both groups. Yet, as with many such studies, medication may have affected the results. The most severe deficits were in children with earlier onset of the disorder who were treated with more than one drug.

Inter-ictal spikes without clinical epileptiform activity may also be responsible for attention disruption in children with epilepsy. Simultaneous monitoring of EEG and neuropsychological test performance has elucidated the relationship between subclinical seizure activity evident on EEG and attentional disruption. This transient cognitive impairment represents a subtle cognitive change associated with subclinical epileptiform discharges (Aldenkamp, Gutter and Beun, 1992). They are epileptic events that are not observed by the individual nor by the casual observation of parents, teachers, physicians, or others (Aldenkamp, 1997). Cognitive function may be disturbed in both child and adult patients, because fleeting disruptions of awareness affect on-going cognitive activity. These gaps in processing have been shown to be associated with spike and spike–wave discharges on EEG. These in turn have been related to impairments on tests of verbal and non-verbal memory (Aarts, Binnie, Smith and Wilkins, 1984), and with continuous attention performance on computerized assessments (Rugland, 1990). The clinical significance of this phenomenon and its frequency among individuals with epilepsy remains controversial (Aldenkamp et al., 1992).

### The question of IQ decline

An association between epilepsy and declines in cognitive function has been observed clinically for more than three hundred years. Early onset of epilepsy and subsequent poor prognosis of cognitive functioning was described some one hundred years ago (Browne and Reynolds, 1981). However, prospective studies have failed to show clear evidence of IQ decline in children with epilepsy followed over a 3-year period with serial psychological testing (Nelson and Ellenberg, 1986).

When addressing the question of whether childhood epilepsy is associated with lowered intellectual functioning one must be clear about which 'epilepsies' are being discussed. Progressive cognitive deterioration is a hallmark of several devastating epileptic syndromes of childhood as follows: Lennox–Gastaut syndrome, West syndrome, electrical status epilepticus in slow wave sleep (ESES), and Landau–Kleffner syndrome (these will be described in more detail later in the chapter). The Lennox–Gastaut syndrome occurs in fewer children, 0.26 per 1000 in a recent population-based study of children in metropolitan Atlanta (Trevathan, Murphy and Yeargin-Allsopp, 1997). The Landau–Kleffner syndrome, or acquired epileptic aphasia, and ESES occur at similarly low rates (Gordon, 1997; Seri, Cerquiglini and Pisani, 1998). Initially normal, the development of these children suffers dramatic neurological deterioration. A recent near-population-based study of newly diagnosed epilepsy was conducted in children, ages 0 to 15 years in the state of Connecticut (Berg et al., 1999b). High quality diagnostic identification by child neurologists indicated the following rates of the more severe epilepsy syndromes as follows: West syndrome 3.9%, Lennox–Gastaut 0.7%, and electrographic status epilepticus in sleep (ESES) 0.2%. Epilepsy syndromes not associated with progressive neurological impairment were much more frequent, such as the following: childhood absence epilepsy 12.1%, benign rolandic epilepsy 9.6%, juvenile absence epilepsy 2.4%, and juvenile myoclonic epilepsy 2.0%. The question of the potential cognitive burden of these more benign childhood epilepsies, as well as that of the more common simple and complex partial epilepsies remains an issue.

A number of studies indicate that children with epilepsy have lower mean IQ scores than control subjects (Bourgeois, Prensky, Palkes et al., 1983; Ellenberg, Hirtz and Nelson, 1986; Farwell et al., 1985). Other investigators have found that the distribution of cognitive test scores in epileptic children does not deviate significantly from that of the normal population (Rutter, Graham and Yule, 1970). Yet, there is a tendency for the lower ranges of IQ to be overrepresented in unselected groups of epileptic individuals (Trimble and Thompson, 1986). More severely neurologically affected children, such as those with malignant epilepsy syndromes just discussed, probably account for this lowering of IQ.

Recently, concern has been raised whether inter-ictal epileptiform activity may complicate performance on intellectual assessments. It is the general consensus that epilepsy per se does not result in intellectual deficiency in children (Holmes, 1991), yet prolonged post-ictal effects and inter-ictal epileptiform discharges may diminish information processing during testing. The resulting performance of these children may be notable for particular difficulty with assessments of attention or memory. For example, a European study using a Dutch general intelligence test disclosed that children with suspected or proven epilepsy and documented EEG discharges had mean IQ scores that were one standard deviation below the mean of the test (Siebelink et al., 1988). A markedly deviant score on a subtest of verbal memory was largely responsible for the lowered IQ scores, as the other subtests of the test battery did not deviate from the mean. Transitory cognitive impairment (Gibbs, Lennox and Gibbs, 1936) may be responsible for such results and interfere with school performance. The adverse effects of inter-ictal spikes

have been demonstrated during WISC performance in a study coupling testing with EEG recording and video monitoring (Aldenkamp, Overweg, Gutter et al., 1996). Children with subclinical seizure activity during testing obtained significantly lower IQ scores for the Full, Verbal, and Performance Scales in comparison with controls. The affected children in this study did not obtain significantly impaired IQ scores, but subclinical events and prolonged post-ictal states should be considered in the assessment (Aldenkamp, 1997). Seizures may have a prolonged behavioral effect because the post-ictal state may negatively impact cognitive test performance for up to two days (Halgren, Stapleton, Domalski et al., 1991). Better seizure control may improve the school functioning of these children.

While evidence suggests that post-ictal states and inter-ictal spikes disturb cognitive testing of epileptic children, this does not constitute evidence that epilepsy results in neuropsychological deterioration. Certain severe syndromes that cause seizures are regularly associated with a decline in neuropsychological integrity, but epilepsy itself is not.

*Cumulative seizure effects on IQ*

A related issue with is whether the cumulative effect of seizures results in neuropsychological deterioration. The question has been framed primarily with regard to IQ. Do children who have frequent seizures experience intellectual decline? Again, in the case of the severe childhood epileptic encephalopathies, there is clear progressive impairment. In each of these syndromes, the prognosis for recovery to premorbid levels of cognitive functioning is generally poor, even if treatment is successful in stopping the seizure activity and normalizing the EEG. However, the deterioration associated with these syndromes is not directly correlated with the frequency of seizures. Furthermore, other seizure disorders, such as childhood absence, juvenile myoclonic, and benign rolandic epilepsies are clearly *not* associated with progressive intellectual impairment. Complicating the research addressing this issue is that studies can be difficult to interpret due to the assumption that there may be pre-existing or co-existing brain damage which gives rise to the seizures and also exerts its own deleterious effect upon cognitive performance.

This fact is especially pertinent with regard to studies conducted in tertiary epilepsy centers, which are skewed towards bad outcome.

Rodin (1968) conducted a longitudinal study of epileptics in which declines in intellectual performance were observed regardless of either etiology or the presence of brain damage. More recently, Farwell et al. (1985) found a highly significant inverse correlation between performance on the WISC-R and the number of years of seizures, suggesting that the more seizures experienced by a child over his/her lifetime, the greater the likelihood of lowered intellectual functioning. Dodrill (1986) addressed this issue in a well-studied group of adults with tonic–clonic seizures. He divided the subjects into four groups as follows: those with lifelong histories of 2–10 generalized tonic–clonic seizures, those with 11–100 convulsive episodes, those with more than 100 such seizures, and those with a history of at least one episode of generalized tonic–clonic status epilepticus, regardless of the number of seizures experienced. Each subject received extensive testing that included the WAIS and other measures of neuropsychological, social, and emotional functioning. Histories of previous brain damage and medication regimens of each subject were analyzed. Dodrill found that higher numbers of tonic–clonic seizures over the subject's lifetime were associated with lower levels of functioning, regardless of the area of functioning that was tested. Current seizure frequency did not produce such an association. Differences between the groups in cognitive ability as a function of the age of onset of the seizures also emerged. Yet, when the number of tonic–clonic seizures was controlled for, this difference was eliminated. From these data, Dodrill concluded that the cumulative frequency of convulsive episodes per se was related to increased cognitive impairment, and that individuals who had experienced more than 100 attacks were significantly impaired, regardless of the age of onset, a history of brain damage, or the particular medication regimen. However, individuals with more than 100 convulsive episodes represent a small proportion of the total, have refractory epilepsy, and are not representative all epileptics. In all but this most extreme group, there is little evidence of intellectual decline. The clinician should also remember that the determination of cognitive decline is best conducted on an individual basis with an appropriate battery of neuropsychological tests.

The above evidence correlating frequency of seizures with impairment of cognitive functioning comes almost exclusively from tertiary care centers which are skewed towards intractable seizure patients. Population-based studies have yielded far different results. Several studies based upon the National Collaborative Perinatal Project (NCPP) have failed to find an association between seizures and intellectual decline. Children with febrile seizures who were tested at age 7 years and compared with age-matched siblings showed no significant differences in test scores (Nelson and Ellenberg, 1978). This was true even for the group who experienced prolonged febrile seizures lasting for more than 30 minutes. More recently, Nelson and Ellenberg (1990) reported no decline in IQ scores in children with epilepsy from the NCPP cohort who were tested at ages 4 and 7 years. The children with epilepsy did not have lower scores than those without epilepsy, and there was no evidence of cognitive decline.

The majority of otherwise neurologically normal children who have experienced a convulsion have a self-limited disorder with excellent long-term prognosis. Many of these children may not even require therapy (Freeman, Tibbles, Camfield and Camfield, 1987; O'Dell and Shinnar, 2001; Shinnar, Berg, Moshe et al., 1990). There is no convincing evidence that infrequent brief seizure activity results in intellectual decline. Yet, the emerging issue of the effect of subclinical seizures upon the intelligence test performance and the school functioning of some children with epilepsy is an important one. This phenomenon may in fact lend explanation to the findings of some studies addressing the intelligence issue. When such silent 'seizures' are present, their stealthy interference in the functioning of these children may be studied with EEG and video technology. Most anti-epileptic drugs do not effectively suppress inter-ictal discharges.

*Status epilepticus*

More evidence that seizures per se are rarely responsible for intellectual decline comes from studies of status epilepticus in children. Status epilepticus is defined as a prolonged seizure lasting more than 30 minutes (Commission on Epidemiology and Prognosis, 1993). It is a life threatening neurological emergency. The duration of episodes varies considerably and can last for many hours. It occurs either in the context of seizure disorders or as a manifestation of an acute neurologic insult (e.g., trauma, encephalitis, stroke, neoplasm). Status can occur with various seizure types such as with convulsions, absence, or complex partial seizures.

Older studies in children (Aicardi and Chevrie, 1970, 1983) and adults (Hauser, 1983) reported a high rate of major neurological sequelae. Animal studies in adolescent and adult monkeys demonstrated that if status epilepticus persisted beyond one hour, changes in the brain would occur reflecting probable neurological damage even if the animal was adequately ventilated (Meldrum and Brierly, 1973; Meldrum and Horton, 1973; Meldrum, Horton and Brierly, 1974). These older studies provided the strongest evidence for permanent brain damage caused by seizures. However, in humans the cognitive sequelae of status epilepticus appear to be associated with the precipitating acute neurologic insult, rather than being the direct consequence of status epilepticus (Maytal, Shinnar, Moshe and Alvarez, 1989; Shinnar and Babb, 1997).

Prospective data from adults with epilepsy collected by Dodrill and Wilensky (1990) suggest that status epilepticus is associated with only slight adverse cognitive effects. In many individuals in their study they suggested that no discernable effects were evident. Their project followed 143 adults over a 5-year period with pre- and post-comprehensive neuropsychological testing. Nine individuals had an episode of status epilepticus in the intervening period, giving rise to the opportunity to study these cases in comparison with matched controls with epilepsy from the cohort. The patients with status episodes were seen to have lower IQ, along with other more frequent cognitive deficits in comparison to the control subjects. Yet, these neuropsychological findings were also for the most part seen at baseline. The findings are consistent with epidemiologic data indicating that status epilepticus occurs more commonly among those individuals who are already neurologically abnormal.

Ellenberg et al. (1986) provide prospective data in children to address the question. As part of the National Collaborative Perinatal Project, they examined cognitive test data in children at ages 4 years and 7 years. Eight children in the cohort experienced status epilepticus in the intervening years. The results indicated that there was no evidence of cognitive decline in these children from age 4 years to age 7 years.

At present, the accumulated evidence from animal studies suggests that the immature CNS is more susceptible to the development of episodes of status epilepticus. Yet, the developing brain also appears to be more resistant to the adverse sequelae of status (Holmes and Moshe, 1990; Shinnar and Babb, 1997).

Although good prospective research addressing the question of the cognitive effects stemming from status epilepticus is limited, the results are quite optimistic. These episodes, although serious neurologic events do not appear to be associated with more than minimal cognitive adverse effects if any at all. The findings also lend further evidence that seizures themselves do not appear to cause cognitive impairment.

*Seizure effects in children vs. adults*

A discussion of the effects of seizures on neuropsychological function would be incomplete without a discussion of the difference between children and adults. Clinical studies have all demonstrated that while children are more likely to develop seizures in general and status epilepticus in particular, they tend to have fewer sequelae. This is true even for more recent studies (Hauser, 1990). Studies in developing animals provide further evidence that the immature brain, while more susceptible to the development of seizures, is more resistant to any brain damage (Albala, Moshe and Okada, 1984; Holmes, 1997; Moshe and Albala, 1983). Young rats given convulsants are more prone than adult rats to develop seizures and status epilepticus. However, surviving young rats do not demonstrate the neuronal loss in Ammon's horn which is seen in older rats (Albala et al., 1984) and in adult primates (Meldrum and Brierly, 1973; Meldrum and Horton, 1973; Meldrum et al., 1974). In addition, these young rats do not demonstrate increased seizure susceptibility as adults (Moshe and Albala, 1983; Okada, Moshe and Albala, 1984). Thus, it appears that the immature brain is more resistant to damage from seizures. In summary, the available evidence suggests that while cognitive dysfunction does occur in the context of certain epileptic syndromes, seizures themselves, even prolonged ones, are rarely associated with any cognitive deterioration. Children with evidence of deteriorating cognitive function require an investigation into other possible causes such as an underlying progressive encephalopathy or drug toxicity.

### Malignant childhood epileptic encephalopathies

Several childhood epileptic encephalopathies lead to severe neuropsychological deficits with variable long-term prognoses.

### West syndrome or infantile spasms

The diagnosis of West syndrome is based on a triad of findings as follows: seizures associated with infantile spasms, an EEG pattern of hypsarrhythmia, and developmental arrest or regression (Arnold and Dodson, 1996). The syndrome always begins in infancy and a majority of these children end up cognitively impaired. Many cases are associated with an identifiable brain disorder, with tuberous sclerosis being the most common. Prognosis for these children is clearly poor for most cases. Yet, in those with some prior normal development, no clear underlying disorder, and appropriate therapy, the prognosis is more optimistic. Treatment is aimed not just at suppression of the clinical seizures but at reversal of the underlying hypsarrhythmic EEG. Standard anticonvulsants are ineffective on the syndrome but many children respond to high dose ACTH (adrenocorticotropic hormone) (Baram, Mitchell, Tournay et al., 1996). Other treatments have included steroid therapies, such as prednisone and hydrocortisone. A recent review of the literature (Hancock, Osborne and Milner, 2001) revealed preliminary evidence for vigabatrin as an effective non-standard anti-epileptic drug therapy for reducing the spasms associated with West syndrome. Another review article (Curatolo, Verdecchia and Bombardieri, 2001) suggested that vigabatrin is particularly effective for reducing spasms when West syndrome is associated with tuberous sclerosis. The non-standard anti-epileptic drug, zonisamide has shown some evidence as a possible treatment (Suzuki, 2001), as has vitamin B-6 (Toribe, 2001). Recent improvements in MRI

and PET scanning techniques have shown focal and multifocal cortical lesions in the majority of these children and allowed improvements in surgical interventions to be made (Asano, Chugani, Juhasz et al., 2001). Although early therapy can improve outcome, the majority of these children show below average intelligence (Jeavons, 1985).

### Lennox–Gastaut syndrome

The Lennox–Gastaut syndrome occurs primarily in infancy and childhood though there are cases of adolescent onset (Roger et al., 1992). Typically, there are multiple seizure types including myoclonic, atonic and atypical absence. The hallmark seizure type are tonic seizures in sleep. The characteristic EEG pattern is of inter-ictal slow spike and wave (<3 Hz). The majority of patients are mentally retarded though this is no longer felt to be necessary for the diagnosis. Ninety-one percent of the children with Lennox–Gastaut syndrome have IQ scores at or below 70 (Trevathan et al., 1997). Neuropsychological development is variable but may arrest or even regress. An identifiable brain disorder or lesion is seen in approximately half of these cases. Frequently associated disorders in the Metropolitan Atlanta study included tuberous sclerosis, brain malformations, perinatal asphyxia, stroke, and CNS infections. The child's prognosis is better if the syndrome is not associated with an underlying brain lesion. If the seizures stop, neuropsychological functioning usually improves. Many treatments have been tried with limited effectiveness. Valproic acid is the drug of choice and other anti-epileptic drugs are frequently tried, as well as the ketogenic diet if the drugs to not prove beneficial.

### Landau–Kleffner syndrome (LKS) and electrographic status epilepticus in sleep (ESES)

The Landau–Kleffner syndrome (or acquired epileptic aphasia) and ESES are typically discussed together in the literature. With clinical and EEG features in common, they are conditions that lead to deteriorating neuropsychological status. They are considered by many authorities to be different manifestations of a common brain disorder (Arnold and Dodson, 1996; Beaumanoir, 1992; Tassinari, Bureau, Dravet et al., 1992). Unlike the West and Lennox–Gastaut syndromes, these disorders occur in children at later, more variable ages. They arise abruptly over the course of days or months and result in cognitive decline in previously normally developing children. The neuropsychological decline in LKS is specifically language. Receptive and expressive language functioning become severely affected. In ESES, the deterioration is more global with respect to cognitive functioning. In the Landau–Kleffner syndrome, the epileptic discharges have a focal origin in the posterior temporal leads. The language impairment is severe. Seizures are less prominent than the neuropsychological symptoms. Clinical seizures are inconsistently present in the course, and 30% of the children do not have seizures but by definition must have an epileptiform EEG. The language deficit has been characterized as a severe inability to recognize and comprehend language, a verbal auditory agnosia (Gascon, Victor, Lombroso and Goodglass, 1973; Rapin, Mattis, Rowan and Golden, 1977). Indeed, evidence suggests that all auditory processing is disrupted, both verbal and non-verbal (Appleton, 1995). It is postulated that inter-ictal EEG activity impairs auditory processing thus leading to the language impairment (Seri et al., 1998). Gordon (1997) and others speculate that the epileptiform activity disrupts the development of language and cognitive function at a critical stage. Prognosis is variable. The course of the language impairment is unpredictable. Some children affected with the syndrome improve suddenly and recover well. Others are affected with lasting language deficits. Standard anti-epileptic medications are useful in controlling the seizures, but not the condition per se. As was the case with infantile spasms, treatment is directed at trying to abolish the underlying epileptiform EEG abnormalities. Steroids have been used with some success (Lerman, Lerman-Sagie and Kivity, 1991; Marescaux, Hirsch, Finck et al., 1990). Surgery using subpial transection of language cortex in attempt to abolish the epileptiform activity without resecting eloquent cortex has also been reported (Morrell, Whisler, Smith et al., 1995) but its use at this time remains experimental.

Although they may not experience clinical seizures, children affected with ESES evidence 85% or more of spike and wave activity in their EEGs during slow wave sleep (Tassinari et al., 1992). In contrast to the Landau–Kleffner syndrome, ESES typically results in a global deterioration of cognitive ability

from the premorbid normal development. The severity of the cognitive decline is greater in this condition than in Landau–Kleffner. The prognosis is also less positive, and the cognitive deficits are more lasting than in Landau–Kleffner. Seizures are usually nocturnal, yet can occur during wakefulness. They are of variable types, and usually respond to anti-epileptic drug therapy. As with Landau–Kleffner, treatment modalities for ESES include steroids and subpial resection of the cortex (Arnold and Dodson, 1996).

## Modality-specific neuropsychological deficits

Formal neuropsychological studies of individuals with epilepsy have not found a specific pattern of impairment. Nonetheless, deficits in memory, attention, language, and spatial abilities have been observed in samples of children with epilepsy. The presence and the severity of these deficits vary greatly as a function of the etiology and type of seizure, the duration of the seizure disorder, the presence and location of a seizure focus, and the use of anticonvulsant medication. As epilepsy is clearly a heterogeneous collection of disorders with varying neurophysiological abnormalities, it would follow that cognitive deficits would be disparate. Yet, this fact notwithstanding, a recent study of neuropsychological patterns of deficit (Williams, Griebel, Dykman and Roscoe, 1998) suggests that epilepsy in children often has a rather diffuse effect upon development and may be associated with decreased attention skills. In a sample of 79 children (ages 6 to 15 years), these investigators found that specific functions, such as memory, language, academics, executive, visual–motor, and fine motor ability, were commensurate with overall intellectual level. Still, as the following sections reveal, there is a body of evidence supporting the presence of specific deficits, most notably in the function of memory in children with epilepsy.

### Memory

Impairments of both verbal and non-verbal memory have been associated with both generalized and focal seizures. Loiseau, Strube, Broustet et al. (1980) found impairment of both verbal and non-verbal memory in a large group of epileptics with generalized seizures when compared to a control group matched for age, education, sex, and social status. Deficits were noted in the recall of word lists and simple geometric patterns. A number of investigators have found that partial epilepsy causes more substantial memory impairment than that associated with generalized epilepsy, particularly in individuals with complex partial seizures emanating from the temporal lobe. It was in fact the study of temporal lobe epilepsy patients, particularly those with intractable seizures, which confirmed the role of the hippocampal formation and temporal lobe structures in memory processes in humans (Novelly, 1992). Studies of adults with epilepsy using the Wechsler Memory Scale demonstrated greater impairment of verbal memory, learning, and attention (Bornstein, Pakalnis and Drake, 1988b; Glowinski, 1973; Quadfasel and Pruyser, 1955) than in control subjects. Research has demonstrated that memory impairment can present as the initial and major symptom in what eventually becomes a diagnosis of temporal lobe epilepsy, with claims of improvement in memory observed after introduction of anti-epileptic medication (Gallassi, Morreale, Lorusso et al., 1988).

Studies of the effect of laterality of partial epilepsy in non-surgical patients have been conducted in both children and adults. Children with left temporal lobe foci have relatively greater verbal memory deficits than children with right temporal seizures, who tend to have greater impairment of visual–spatial memory (Fedio and Mirsky, 1969). Although some earlier studies of adults with epilepsy failed to find differential impairment of verbal and non-verbal memory relative to the side of the seizure focus (Agnetti, Ganga, Murrigaile et al., 1979; Berent, Boll and Giordani, 1980; Glowinski, 1973), later well-controlled studies have found them (Bornstein, Pakalnis and Drake, 1988c; Hermann, Wyler and Richey, 1988a). In addition, when the difference between verbal and non-verbal memory test findings is great, the prediction of the location of seizure onset is more accurate (Loring, Lee and Martin, 1988). The sensitivity of neuropsychological testing for detecting site-specific memory deficits has been a major asset for predicting memory status following the surgical treatment of temporal lobe epilepsy (Dodrill, 1986; Rausch, 1987). Memory tests are also useful for distinguishing between patients with temporal versus extratemporal lobe epilepsy, especially for surgical decision-making of patients with intractable seizures (e.g., Breier, Plenger, Wheless et al., 1996).

*Attention*

Impairments of attention and overall slowing of mental processing are frequent, even in the absence of overt clinical seizure activity. Stores, Hart and Piran (1978) administered a battery of tests designed to measure attention in a group of children with epilepsy and controls without epilepsy. Boys with epilepsy had significantly greater difficulties with attention than controls. Surprisingly, these investigators did not find comparable attentional impairments in the girls with epilepsy. Loiseau, Signoret and Strube (1984) administered tests of learning and attention to adolescents and young adults with either partial or generalized seizures. They concluded that the generalized seizure group was significantly impaired in both areas relative to controls. In contrast, the partial seizure group did not have attentional deficits. The comprehensive neuropsychological study by Williams et al. (1998) cited earlier suggests that deficient verbal and visual attention skills complicate testing results by interfering with efficient performance on cognitive tests, such as memory. Thus attention is an important area for investigation of epilepsy-related deficits in children. This area of impairment may complicate the conclusions reached regarding other potential deficits for children with epilepsy.

A factor analytic study of the WAIS-R subtests in a sample of patients with a variety of seizure disorders (Bornstein, Drake and Pakalnis, 1988a) brought out the Freedom from Distractibility factor (i.e., attention) as prominent. Others have reported similar findings (Aldenkamp, Alpherts, De Bruine and Dekker, 1990; Dodrill, 1986; Rodin, Schmaltz and Twitty, 1986). This factor consists of the subtests, Digit Span and Arithmetic, which place the greatest demand upon sustained attention and concentration. The investigators interpreted their findings as suggesting that attentional factors have a more important influence on performance in this population than in other patient groups. A recent study of differential attention deficits in epileptic patients suggests that generalized seizure patients differ from temporal lobe epilepsy patients in the type of their attentional deficit (Goldstein, Rosenbaum and Taylor, 1997). Reaction time studies and continuous performance tests suggested that vigilance was deficient in both patient groups, with the generalized seizure patients most severely affected, in contrast to those with temporal lobe epilepsy whose deficit was limited to cognitive expectancy. They suggested that the primary deficit in patients with pure generalized seizure disorders stems from a subcortical reticular activating system dysfunction, while in temporal lobe epilepsy patients it is the limbic system and its projections to frontal cortical areas that is dysfunctional.

Other research paradigms support this finding. Lokeit, Seitz, Markowitsch et al. (1997) described hypometabolism of prefrontal cortex on PET scans of patients with temporal lobe epilepsy while they performed neuropsychological tests sensitive to frontal lobe function. Earlier research by Hermann et al. (1988a), replicated by Horner, Flashman, Freides and Epstein (1996), had suggested that patients with temporal lobe seizures demonstrate a disproportionate amount of frontal lobe pathology when compared with other epilepsy controls. This conclusion was based on their poor performance on the Wisconsin Card Sorting Test, a test of problem solving efficiency and mental flexibility. These findings suggest that frontal lobe inefficiency may be an integral part of the clinical picture of epilepsy with temporal lobe foci. Deficits of this type have been shown to predict occupational status, in that impairments of alertness, flexibility, and memory characterize many individuals with this type of seizure who were either unemployed or who held low level jobs (Dikmen, 1980).

*Language*

Deficits in specific aspects of language associated with epilepsy have been less well studied than memory. Shih and Peng (1998) attribute this lack of focus to neuroscientists' expectation of classic language disorder syndromes. The exception is the Landau–Kleffner syndrome (Landau and Kleffner, 1957) which, typically, is associated with complete or near-complete loss of language, generally because of a verbal auditory agnosia. More subtle language deficits are likely to arise in some epileptic children with foci that affect cortical language areas. Ballaban-Gil (1995) points out that it remains to be seen whether the epileptic activity is responsible for the language disorder or whether the language disorder and the epilepsy may be separate manifestations of some common underlying brain disorder. Abou-Khalil (1995) emphasizes that epilepsy has contributed information regarding language localization, notably through Wilder Penfield's mapping of cortical areas for language with cortical stimulation in patients undergoing surgical resections for epilepsy. Presurgical cortical mapping demonstrates that cortical language representation might be atypical in epileptics with seizure foci localized to the dominant hemisphere. Indeed, expressive and receptive language functions may be dissociated in some epileptics in whom receptive abilities may be localized in the left hemisphere, for example, and expressive abilities in the right (Kurthen, Helmstaedter, Linke and Solymosi et al., 1993).

Patients with left temporal epilepsy suffer from greater language deficits than those with right temporal lobe epilepsy (Hermann, Seidenberg, Haltiner and Wyler, 1993). Impairment of naming ability and word usage is a prominent symptom of partial complex seizures of left temporal origin, but these deficits are likely to be misinterpreted as memory impairment (Mayeux, Brandt, Rosen and Benson, 1980). Howell, Saling, Bradley and Berkovic (1994) indicated that epileptics with left temporal foci had significantly more naming deficits and pauses in speech than those with right temporal lobe foci. Hermann, Wyler and Steenman (1988b) reported that measures of language comprehension, naming, and verbal fluency were the most robust predictors of performance on tests of learning and memory in patients with complex partial seizures.

A neuropsychological study of children with epilepsy (Gaggero, Cirrincione, Zannoto and de Negri, 1993) showed that those affected by dominant hemisphere focal paroxysmal EEG abnormalities had language deficits. The longitudinal study by Cohen and LeNormand (1998) of six children with partial epilepsy is illustrative of the course of their language deficits. The six children were followed for five years beginning at about age three years, and were compared to a larger cohort. When first studied, the epileptic children had marked deficits in both receptive and expressive language functions. Over the course of the study, they improved to normal or near-normal levels in language comprehension, whereas expressive language failed to show comparable improvement. The subtle nature of language deficits in many epileptic children may, according to Galaburda (1993), stem from the effect of early brain dysfunction on a plastic and developing brain.

Studies of school achievement uncover mild language dysfunction in children who otherwise present with adequate speech. A number of studies have reported that these children average about a 12-month lag in reading ability by chronological age (Rutter et al., 1970) or grade placement (Green and Hartlage, 1971). Dodrill and Clemmons (1984) found that high school tests of language ability were the best predictors of vocational adjustment and independent living in young adult epileptics. Subclinical epileptiform EEG activity that disrupts reading efficiency (Kastelijn-Nolst Trenite et al., 1988) might explain the difficulty some of these children encounter in achieving a consistent level of academic performance.

*Spatial ability*

It is currently unclear to what extent epilepsy affects visuo-spatial functions, since the few studies in this area have utilized tests that require a number of different cognitive abilities. Children with seizures were found to perform more poorly than controls on the Bender Gestalt Test (Schwartz and Dennerll, 1970; Tymchuk, 1974), although it was uncertain whether graphomotor dysfunction rather than impairment of spatial organization was responsible. The neuropsychological study by Gaggero et al. (1993) of 67 children with partial and generalized epilepsies revealed deficits in memory, attention, and spatial organization. The previously mentioned comprehensive neuropsychological study of Williams et al. (1998) suggested overall performance lowering which was attributable to reduced attention, as scores were commensurate with the overall IQ. Shewmon and Erwin (1988) found that focal posterior interictal spikes were associated with prolonged reaction times as well as misperception of stimuli. Thus, it appears that transient, localized epileptiform electrical activity may impair spatially mediated functions.

Whether these are stable cognitive deficits or reversible disturbances related to the spikes remains unclear.

## Cognitive effects of anti-epileptic medications

Anti-epileptic drugs (AEDs) are potent medications that work by altering the function of synapses that are also involved in normal neuronal transmission. As such they all have adverse effects on cognition and behavior (Committee on Drugs, 1995; O'Dell and Shinnar, 2001). The choice of a particular drug is made based upon its pharmacologic properties as well as seizure type. These properties include the therapeutic window (ratio of the therapeutic drug dose to the toxic drug dose) and the half-life of the drug, which allows for the calculation of the loading dose, the dosage interval, and the maintenance dose to be employed (Dreifuss, 1983). The nature and extent of the cognitive deficits vary with the particular drug or combination of drugs used (monotherapy vs. polytherapy) as well as with the serum concentration of the drug (Shinnar, 1987; Trimble and Thompson, 1986). There is no drug that suppresses abnormal cerebral activity without having the potential of affecting normal cognitive functioning (Committee on Drugs, 1995; O'Dell and Shinnar, 2001). The question then is what are the cognitive side effects obtained from the use of anti-epileptic medications at their therapeutic dosage levels.

Distinguishing between the deficits produced by these medications and the deficits associated with the seizures themselves is a major issue in the neuropsychological study of epilepsy. Indeed there are many important methodological issues that complicate the validity of conclusions drawn from this area of research. Included among these issues are the non-randomized nature of much of the research, the necessity of clinical considerations in subject assignment, often small sample sizes and the validity of negative findings in studies lacking statistical power, the variety of seizure disorders themselves, individual differences in drug metabolism, polytherapy, tolerance, other drug use, age of onset of epilepsy, duration of epilepsy, the effect of individual medication histories and possible long-term effects of past medication use, individual differences in cognitive abilities, and seizure-related traumatic brain injury (i.e., from seizure precipitated falls). In addition to these various issues which can complicate detecting consistent adverse effects of the drugs in the treatment of epileptics is the fact that the drugs also appear to have cognitive benefit. For example, a review of the literature comparing cognitive effects of anti-epileptic drugs upon epileptic patients vs. healthy controls (Smith, 1991) suggests that non-epileptics experience negative cognitive effects to a greater degree than do their patient counterparts. This is presumably due to the beneficial effect of controlling epileptic activity in the patients, both seizure activity and inter-ictal epileptiform activity as well.

Determining the contribution of the medication effects to the overall neuropsychological picture is essential, because the majority of seizure patients will be maintained on some form of anticonvulsant drug for many years. The lack of baseline evaluations of children prior to the start of therapy has made it difficult to make this distinction accurately enough for sound clinical decision-making. Indeed, an extensive and rigorous review of the literature by Vermeulen and Aldenkamp (1995) revealed the lack of studies that followed basic standards of methodology, design, and analysis, thus limiting the clinician's ability to draw sound conclusions for therapeutic decision-making. Their review concluded, however, that "the tentative overall picture emerging from the creme de la creme of research on cognitive anti-epileptic drug effects is that differences in cognitive profiles may not be very large". As a result of their extensive review and critique of this area, Vermeulen and Aldenkamp provide a list of recommendations for anti-epileptic drug research as follows: examine monotherapy only; employ seizure-free subjects; employ a repeated measures design (parallel groups or crossover); use random treatment allocation when comparing anti-epileptic drugs; employ a no-treatment control group to assess absolute effects; interpret designs with a non-randomly assigned element (e.g., controls) with caution; discuss the rationale for the choice of anticipated treatment effects; use a sample size that results in adequate power (e.g., 0.80); exercise economy in the number of outcome measures; follow commonly accepted guidelines for reporting data.

The importance of methodological factors in study results is illustrated by past research findings of cognitive deficits associated with phenytoin. Dodrill (1989), for example, has made the argument that such cognitive side effects ascribed to phenytoin as vigilance, psychomotor function, memory, and general intellectual functioning may all be due to this drug's effect upon motor speed and accuracy because of its cerebellar effects. Since the delineation of various cognitive functions is complicated by their interrelationships, such caution in deficit determination is of extreme importance for drawing out conclusions of these drugs' true adverse effects.

Of special relevance to anti-epileptic drug use with children is Holmes (1997) review of animal research findings that indicate these drugs may have greater detrimental effects on the developing brain. He therefore questions the appropriateness of current treatment approaches of childhood seizure disorders.

*Phenobarbital*

Phenobarbital is used for the treatment of young children with both febrile and afebrile seizures. Farwell, Lee, Hirtz et al. (1990) found significantly lower IQ scores, as measured by the Bayley scales of infant development and the Stanford–Binet, in children with febrile seizures treated with phenobarbital, as compared to a placebo treated group, in a randomized, placebo-controlled double-blind study. However, the methodology of this two-year follow-up study is questionable. A further examination of IQ and other neuropsychological variables in children (Willis, Nelson, Black et al., 1997) treated with phenobarbital (or with mephobarbital) showed no difference in IQ with the WISC-R, yet the very small sample size of their case control study procedure leaves interpretation of this finding in question. As with many studies with children and adults on this issue, sample sizes are small, suggesting authors believe that only large side effects are worth detecting.

Chronic phenobarbital administration in children at therapeutic levels has been suggested to produce psychomotor slowing (Reynolds and Travers, 1974) and impaired fine motor coordination (Hellstrom and Barlach-Christoffersen, 1980). A significant negative correlation has been obtained between the WISC-R Performance IQ and children maintained for over one year on a constant dose of phenobarbital (Corbett, Trimble and Nichol, 1985), suggesting a decline in the ability to perform timed tasks of spatial functioning. Impairment of attention in children with administration of phenobarbital has also been observed. Studies correlating serum anticonvulsant levels of phenobarbital and performance on given neuropsychological tests revealed that measures of attention such as WISC-R Digit Span and Coding were the tests most sensitive to high serum levels (Hartlage, 1981). The consistent appearance of a visual–motor component in these studies is relevant to the hypothesis Dodrill tested with respect to phenytoin. If specific cognitive side effects are in fact associated with phenobarbital use at therapeutic doses, a motor speed effect may possibly underlie some of the positive findings to date. Yet findings of cognitive test performance that did not require a visual–motor response have been suggested as well. A double-blind crossover study comparing the cognitive side effects of phenobarbital with valproic acid in children (Vining, Mellits, Cataldo et al., 1983) demonstrated significantly poorer performance on tests of vocabulary, auditory attention, and spatial ability during administration of phenobarbital. A double-blind crossover study in adults with partial complex seizures found only subtle differences in overall neuropsychological performance during administration of either phenobarbital, phenytoin, or carbamazepine (Meador, Loring, Huh et al., 1990). However, significantly lower scores on Digit Symbol were observed during phenobarbital ingestion, corroborating previous findings of impaired attention and deficient complex motor performance.

*Phenytoin*

While adequately designed studies of the possible side effects of this drug in children are lacking, there is cautionary evidence for long-term use of the drug from a study of mentally retarded children at therapeutic dose levels. Vallarta, Bell and Reichert (1974) reported on ten children referred for progressive neurological and intellectual deterioration related to long-term phenytoin use. Symptoms of this chronic drug effect were insidious, and although the therapy was stopped, the effects were not reversed. While the concern for such potential encephalopathy is echoed by others (Hirtz and Nelson, 1985; Trimble, 1981), there remains little evidence to draw firm conclu-

sions that phenytoin directly causes intellectual decline. Indeed the results of Dodrill and Wilensky (1992) with adults argue otherwise. Their longitudinal study of stable, five-year therapy with phenytoin in monotherapy, phenytoin in polytherapy, or other anti-epileptic drug use (such as barbiturate medications, carbamazepine, or valproic acid) showed no significant cognitive changes on a comprehensive battery of neuropsychological variables.

The majority of research on the issue of cognitive side effects of phenytoin has been with adults. Phenytoin at high serum levels has been shown to be negatively correlated with Performance IQ (Corbett et al., 1985) and to be related to deficits in intelligence and visuomotor tracking in a group of seizure-free patients on monotherapy relative to controls (Gallassi, Morreale, Lorusso et al., 1987). These findings suggest that the deficits and their reversal were drug-related. In this study, unlike the results of Vallarta et al. (1974), the intellectual and tracking deficits disappeared one year after discontinuation of the therapy. Dodrill and Troupin (1977) found similar results in a comparison of phenytoin and carbamazepine therapy, in patients matched for IQ and seizure characteristics. The phenytoin patients evidenced lower scores on tests of memory and visuomotor tracking. A study of normal volunteers administered either phenytoin or placebo in a double-blind crossover design over a 2-week period demonstrated decreased memory and slower verbal and perceptual information processing (Thompson, Huppert and Trimble, 1980, 1981).

Important in the interpretation of these studies, however, is the finding by Dodrill (1989) that motor speed is a contaminating factor in studies of the cognitive side effects of phenytoin. Healthy controls randomized to either high or low serum phenytoin monotherapy showed deficits associated with high drug level in WAIS Performance IQ and a variety of problem-solving, perceptual, and attention and concentration tests, all of which statistical significance disappeared when motor speed was factored in as a covariate. This demonstration aids in the interpretation of more recent studies. For example, a discontinuation study of phenytoin, carbamazepine, and valproate (Duncan, Shorvon and Trimble, 1990) with patients on polytherapy revealed benefits associated with phenytoin discontinuation on specific tasks of attention and concentration. These tasks, however, were visual–motor. Similarly, a well designed crossover study of the effects of phenytoin, as well as phenobarbital and valproate in healthy volunteers (Meador, Loring, Moore et al., 1995) demonstrated statistically significant deficits ascribed to phenytoin on four of fifteen test variables. Three of the four involved a visual–motor component, while the fourth was a delayed verbal memory test. Interestingly, the latter study showed no deficit for verbal learning or for complex visual learning and delayed memory. The mean performance of these subjects on the delayed verbal memory test was only slightly below that of the control condition, seemingly a small, not clinically meaningful difference.

In summary, the majority of the research (in adults) suggests that phenytoin has primarily a negative visual–motor effect, and other potential side effects are uncertain.

### Carbamazepine

Carbamazepine, like phenytoin, also works by blocking repetitive firing by its action on the voltage-dependent sodium–potassium channel. It is the most commonly used anti-epileptic drug in children. Schain, Ward and Guthrie (1977) studied the effects of treating children who had major motor or partial complex seizures with carbamazepine as replacement for either phenobarbital or primidone. They were able to achieve the same degree of seizure control, and the children demonstrated improvement in attention, problem-solving ability, and in general intelligence as measured with the WISC. In children with newly diagnosed complex partial epilepsy who were assessed before and after institution of carbamazepine monotherapy (O'Dougherty, Wright, Cox and Walson, 1987), slight improvements of speeded eye–hand coordination and information processing were observed at low therapeutic levels. Higher carbamazepine plasma concentrations were associated with significantly poorer performance in these areas.

While carbamazepine monotherapy appeared to have little effect on overall psychometric performance in a group of adult epileptics, the use of carbamazepine in conjunction with another anticonvulsants did produce significant declines in Performance IQ and in Digit Span scores (Gillham, Williams,

Wiedman et al., 1988). Removal of carbamazepine in adult patients in a study of several neuropsychological variables showed only a small negative effect upon motor speed and coordination skills (Duncan et al., 1990). A revealing effect of acute versus chronic drug effects was recently demonstrated by Gigli, Maschio, Diomedi et al. (1996). They administered tests of attention and memory in newly diagnosed epileptics at baseline, acute (same-day) dosing, and one month after chronic use of controlled-release carbamazepine therapy. The results revealed that the patients experienced impaired verbal learning and memory performance in association with acute dosing, but that this effect disappeared at the one-month assessment. Thus, at moderate therapeutic dose levels and after an initial adjustment period, carbamazepine monotherapy appears to have little in the way of deleterious cognitive side effects.

### Valproic acid

Valproic acid is a potent broad-spectrum antiepileptic drug that is widely used in the treatment of generalized seizure disorders of all types. There remains a paucity of systematic research that has investigated the cognitive effects of valproic acid. The existing studies have been primarily with adults. Valproate appears to have minimal effect on the performance of cognitive tests by healthy volunteers (Trimble and Thompson, 1986), and there is some evidence that it has beneficial effects on attention and concentration at low therapeutic levels (Barnes and Bower, 1978; Trimble and Thompson, 1986). In a double-blind comparison with phenobarbital, valproic acid had significantly less effect on vocabulary, attention, and on spatial skills (Vining et al., 1983). Valproate removal showed little effect on attention–concentration tasks and only a small effect on motor speed performance (Duncan et al., 1990). Yet, in spite of the popularity of valproic acid in the treatment of epilepsy syndromes in children, little evidence of its cognitive effects in children specifically is available. A recent call for such work was made (Lagarda, Booth, Fennell and Maria, 1996) with guidelines suggested. A small case control study demonstrated no significant effect of valproate monotherapy discontinuation in children (Aldenkamp, Alpherts and Blennow, 1993). Yet more studies are needed to guide the use of this drug in children, particularly in light of a recent published finding of reversible parkinsonian symptoms and a suggestion of cognitive impairment in a study of discontinuing valproate in a clinic sample of patients (Armon, Shin, Miller et al., 1996). These patients were on long-term valproic acid treatment (at least twelve months) and were studied due to concerns about symptoms related to the drug. The parkinsonian symptoms improved after the drug was stopped, although whether or not significant cognitive improvement took place with discontinuation was difficult to determine from this report. Nevertheless, further study of the potential cognitive effects of this drug with chronic use is necessary.

**Newer anti-epileptic drugs**

Several newer anti-epileptic drugs have come into use, and these include the following: gabapentin, lamotrigine, tiagabine, topiramate, vigabatrin, felbamate, zonisamide, oxcarbamazepine, and levetarecetam. The possible cognitive side effects of these medications have received some recent attention, although all studies noted have been with adults. Thus far, these drugs, with the exception of topiramate, have demonstrated little in the way of adverse cognitive effects.

*Topiramate*

Topiramate is a broad-spectrum potent anti-epileptic drug effective against a wide variety of seizure types. It has a variety of different mechanisms. Topiramate was studied, along with gabapentin and lamotrigine, in a randomized, parallel groups study of healthy volunteers tested after acute and longer (2 weeks and then 4 weeks) dosing (Martin, Kuzniecky, Ho et al., 1999). Gabapentin and lamotrigine showed no significant effects on tests of word naming, verbal memory, reaction time, and other attention–concentration tests. The topiramate group, however, showed lower performances in attention and word naming at the 2-week testing and in memory and attention at the 4-week testing. A retrospective case control study of neuropsychological assessment results prior to and after the introduction of topiramate therapy similarly showed cognitive deficits (Thompson, Baxendale,

Duncan and Sander, 2000) for verbal IQ, verbal fluency, and verbal learning. Reduction or withdrawal of topiramate therapy in some of these subjects resulted in improvements in test scores of verbal fluency, verbal learning, and digit span performance. Thus topiramate may be associated with cognitive side effects which should be further evaluated and considered in its use.

*Gabapentin*

Gabapentin is a narrow-spectrum agent effective for partial and generalized tonic–clonic seizures. In the Martin et al. (1999) study, gabapentin showed no significant effects on tests of word naming, verbal memory, reaction time, and other attention–concentration tests at either the 2-week testing or 4-week testing sessions. In a study of seizure patients, gabapentin (Leach, Girvan, Paul and Brodie, 1997), tested in a double-blind, dose ranging, randomized crossover design showed no adverse effects on psychomotor nor memory tests. Thus gabapentin does not appear to have significant cognitive side effects upon neuropsychological tests of attention and memory in the research to date. Of additional note, however, gabapentin has also been implicated in intensifying pre-existing attention-deficit and disruptive behavior disorders in children (Wolf, Shinnar, Kang et al., 1995).

*Lamotrigine*

Lamotrigine is another broad-spectrum anti-epileptic drug effective against both generalized and partial seizures. As with gabapentin, lamotrigine does not appear to produce significant adverse effects on tests of word naming, verbal memory, reaction time, and other attention–concentration tests in the study by Martin et al. (1999). The lamotrigine group did not show adverse effects upon memory and attention at either the 2-week or the 4-week testing periods. Lamotrigine was further demonstrated, in a pre–post within-subjects add-on to carbamazepine study, to show no effects on motor speed, reaction time, and memory tests (Aldenkamp, Mulder and Overweg, 1997). A double-blind, randomized, placebo-controlled, crossover design, in which lamotrigine was added to existing therapy of refractory patients, also showed no effect on visual–motor speed, attention–concentration, and reaction time tests (Smith, Baker and Davies, 1993).

*Tiagabine*

Tiagabine is a narrow-spectrum agent effective against partial seizures. It works by blocking re-uptake of GABA at the nerve terminals (Shinnar and Sommerville, 2001). Dodrill, Arnett, Sommerville and Shu (1997) and Dodrill, Arnett, Shu et al. (1998) have demonstrated no effects of tiagabine on a variety of neuropsychological measures, including tests of motor functions, attention–concentration, memory, language, and overall IQ. This lack of effect was found in randomized, double-blind, parallel group research designs. Tiagabine was added to existing therapy at varying dose ranges in one (Dodrill et al., 1997) study. The second study involved patients on existing therapy with other anticonvulsant medications who were successfully moved to tiagabine monotherapy (Dodrill et al., 1998). Finally, a direct comparison of tiagabine with the 'older, standard' drug, carbamazepine, indicated it to be superior (Meador, Loring, Ray et al., 2001). A double-blind crossover design with two 10-week treatment periods of the two drugs was employed. The healthy study subjects were assessed at pre-treatment baseline, at the ends of the two treatment periods, then at post-treatment. Forty neuropsychological variables were measured in a comprehensive battery. Subjects showed better performance on 48% of the variables when they were treated with lamotrigine as compared to carbamazepine. No variables yielded better results with carbamazepine. Lamotrigine therapy compared with non-drug use in the study was closely comparable. These studies indicate little concern for cognitive side effects of tiagabine to date.

*Vigabatrin*

Vigabatrin is a narrow-spectrum drug which works by irreversible binding to GABA transaminase thus blocking GABA degradation and raising whole-brain GABA levels. Dodrill, Arnett, Sommerville and Sussman (1995) also demonstrated vigabatrin to have little effect upon a variety of neuropsy-

chological measures in a randomized double-blind parallel groups design. Vigabatrin, at various doses, was added to the existing therapy of patients with refractory epilepsy. The same study design used by another team (Provinciali, Bartolini, Mari et al., 1996) showed no effect of vigabatrin add-on therapy on memory, visual–motor, and attention–concentration tests. Therefore, vigabatrin appears also to demonstrate little in the way of concern regarding side effects on cognitive test performance.

*Other new anti-epileptic drugs*

Several other additions to the growing list of anti-epileptic drugs are felbamate, levetiracetam, oxcarbazepine, and zonisamide. Oxcarbazepine is structurally similar to, but not pharmacologically identical to the older drug, carbamazepine. These drugs require appropriately designed, controlled studies upon which to base conclusions about cognitive effects.

In sum, with the exception of topiramate, the new line drugs show promise for controlling seizures with little effect upon cognitive functioning. Still, further study is required. Beginning studies are needed for the latter several mentioned agents.

**Monotherapy versus polytherapy**

Currently, one of the principles of pharmacological treatment of epilepsy is to attempt to control seizures with a single medication. Anti-epileptic drugs can interact so as to affect each other's serum levels, thus causing potentially serious side effects or actually reducing seizure control. For example, valproate added to phenobarbital can produce toxic levels of the latter, since valproate is an enzyme inhibitor which increases the level of other drugs (Engel, 1989). It is not surprising that reducing the number of anticonvulsant medications used in a patient has been shown to ameliorate cognitive deficits substantially. Thompson and Trimble (1982) demonstrated improvement in perceptual and decision-making speed in epileptics who had their medication regimen reduced during a hospital stay. Improvements in performance and full-scale IQ scores, as well as improvements in non-verbal memory were observed in epileptics who were successfully reduced to one medication over the course of a year (Ludgate, Keating, O'Dwyer and Callaghan, 1985). Even medications such as carbamazepine, which by itself has relatively few cognitive side effects, may produce impairment of attention and motor speed when another drug is added (Gillham et al., 1988). Thus, knowledge of both the pharmacology and the cognitive effects of each medication is essential in order to develop a medication regimen achieving maximum seizure control with minimum impact on mental abilities.

In summary, there is evidence that phenobarbital and phenytoin both have adverse effects upon cognitive functions independent of that resulting from seizure activity or underlying brain pathology. The nature of these adverse effects is somewhat unclear, however, as the studies establishing various cognitive side effects of these drugs have limitations, and the results may be explained in part by their effect upon one variable of performance, namely motor speed. Studies of carbamazepine and valproic acid show less of an adverse cognitive effect. The new line of anti-epileptic drugs, including gabapentin, lamotrigine, tiagabine, and vigabatrin, show very little effect upon cognitive function in the study efforts to date. Topiramate has been shown to have some negative effects in healthy volunteers. Other of the new line anti-epileptic drugs require beginning studies to explore the cognitive side effect issue. The use of multiple anticonvulsants often exacerbates cognitive deficits, possibly without any clear improvement in seizure control.

## Neuropsychological assessment for epilepsy surgery

When recurrent seizures of localized cerebral onset prove intractable to medication therapy, resective neurosurgery is a viable alternative treatment. The rationale for resective surgery in epilepsy is to remove the dysfunctional, abnormal tissue presumably causing the abnormal brain activity (Spencer, 1994). Temporal and extratemporal epileptogenic foci have been resected in adults for many years. The recommendation of this treatment for children is a relatively recent development in the medical management of epilepsy. The procedure is not without side effects (Berg, 1994), among them cognitive effects. A review by Dodrill (1992) suggests that the

most important cognitive risk is for memory to be affected post-surgery, particularly troublesome when the procedure involves the hemisphere dominant for speech. He concludes that other cognitive changes are of lesser severity and importance. Methods of focus definition and presurgical neuropsychological assessments are utilized to predict, prevent, and limit cognitive disruptions from surgery. Baseline assessment of memory and other cognitive functions can aid in the decision-making process about surgery. For example, individuals with a dominant hemisphere, temporal lobe focus and average to high average baseline memory skills are at special risk for verbal memory decline post-surgery (e.g., Chelune, 1991). In fact, dominant hemisphere resections are likely to produce more prominent cognitive deficits than non-dominant ones. This is probably true because of the ubiquitous importance of language in human experience.

In 1935, the famous patient HM suffered devastating anterograde amnesia following sizable bilateral resections of the mesial temporal lobes. This unfortunate case proved instructive in the importance of mesial temporal structures for memory function, particularly that of the hippocampi. Bilateral mesial temporal resections involving the hippocampi have since been understood to be contraindicated. The case also dramatically indicated the need for evaluating patients prior to surgery for the possible adverse effects of surgery upon memory function. This need is met by the Wada procedure. During this procedure one hemisphere is anesthetized with amytal and the contralateral hemisphere is tested for its ability to support memory function. If the hemisphere contralateral to the defined seizure focus does not support memory, surgery is contraindicated. The neuropsychologist's evaluation of memory during this procedure is obviously an important aspect of the presurgical evaluation.

The Wada procedure allows for the assessment of language laterality as well, information about which may also prove vital for surgical decision-making. Language functions are localized to the left hemisphere in most individuals. In a small minority of right handers and in a minority of left handers the right hemisphere may support language functions, or, there may be a sharing of language functions between the two lateral hemispheres. Non-left language representation is more common in individuals with neurological impairment than normals, particularly when it is associated with early-life lateralized hemispheric lesions.

When the side of planned epilepsy surgery involves language cortex, the potential for disruption of language functions must be weighed in the decision to go forward with surgery. A language cortical mapping procedure provides information addressing this need. The language cortical mapping procedure provides a functional map of language sites in the temporal lobe to distinguish eloquent from non-eloquent cortex. During the procedure, sets of surgically placed electrodes are selectively stimulated while a neuropsychologist simultaneously elicits a verbal response to a simple stimulus (e.g., a word on a card, a pictured object to name). The verbal response is evaluated to determine whether a particular electrode site is a language or non-language area. In doing so, the cortical map can be drawn, and a plan of avoiding language cortex can be carried out in the surgical resection of the (typically mesial temporal) epileptogenic focus.

The timing of such surgery for children is an issue for continued research. The interplay of maturational factors and the child's psychosocial development in relation to seizures and surgical intervention is a prime area for continued study. Typically, seizure surgery is done in children 12 years or older. It is undertaken in younger children when the situation warrants, such as when there is evidence of deteriorating development owing to the neurological condition. By age 12 years localization of neuropsychological functions is believed to be congruent with that of the mature adult. For younger children, the potential for side effects of surgical intervention for seizure control upon the rapidly developing brain, with changing EEG patterns and seizure morphology, is unclear (Duchowny, Levin and Jayakar, 1994). The effect of these factors upon the developing limbic system, a brain subsystem frequently involved in epilepsy, is unknown. A relatively better known phenomenon relating to surgery for children is the typically superior functional ability of their nervous systems to recover. Behavioral consequences of chronic seizures are significant and can have a major impact upon the psychological development of maturing children (Resnick, Duchowny and Jayakar, 1994). The ben-efit of curing or substantially controlling intractable epilepsy in a child patient may have important benefits for the child's behavioral and social developmental outcome, preventing his or her becoming a chronically ill patient, with the accompanying psychic handicaps this involves (Dam, 1996). Longitudinal neuropsychological outcome studies assessing the developmental effects of surgery, both benefits and adverse cognitive effects, will be of great utility in the future of surgical decision-making for such children.

## Neuropsychological testing of children with epilepsy

The comprehensive neuropsychological assessment of children with epilepsy has become an important part of their overall management. Neuropsychological testing can identify specific areas of cognitive deficit which may be associated with epilepsy and which interfere with educational achievement. Academic performance may suffer due to deficits in memory, attentional skills, language functions, or other cognitive impairments. Neuropsychological testing can similarly be used to address the changes in cognitive function resulting from medication. The results of the evaluation can also provide a basis for the remediation of these deficits. Thus, the neuropsychologist plays an important role in both the diagnosis and treatment of the cognitive consequences of this disorder.

There are a wide variety of tests commonly used by neuropsychologists to assess cognitive function. Some of these available measures lack adequate normative data and psychometric validation (Reynolds, 1989), although this has become less true as further test development has proceeded in recent years. Still, much of the utility of neuropsychological assessment procedures comes from the clinical experience of the user. Specific knowledge of and experience with epilepsy is important for appropriate neuropsychological work.

Dodrill (1978, 1986) has assembled the Neuropsychological Battery for Epilepsy with a variety of measures meant to provide a comprehensive assessment of functions, with good coverage of areas observed to show deficits in patients with epilepsy. The reliability and validity of the battery has been studied; it is sensitive to brain-related deficits in epilepsy, and has established normative data with epileptics. Although a similar level of standardization has not yet been accomplished for children with epilepsy, as Dodrill points out, any comprehensive neuropsychological assessment battery is appropriate as long as it addresses the issues of relevance to these patients. Aside from the child's academic development, the various other issues involved include the assessment's sensitivity to the effects of seizures, the effects of medications, EEG epileptiform discharges, and surgical intervention. A comprehensive neuropsychological evaluation will include assessments of the following: overall intellectual ability, academic achievement, language functions, memory, attention and executive functions, motor speed and coordination, laterality, sensory-perceptual abilities, and visual–motor integration ability. In addition, an assessment of personality issues and psychological adjustment are of importance both for the impact these can have upon cognitive performance and for the impact of epilepsy and seizures upon emotional development. A comprehensive listing of neuropsychological instruments can be obtained in Spreen and Strauss (1998), while Oxbury (1997) provides a listing of instruments common to epilepsy evaluations. A welcome addition to the neuropsychological assessment of children with epilepsy, and others, was the introduction of the jointly normed Wechsler Intelligence Scale for Children, 3rd edition and the Wechsler Individual Achievement Test (WIAT) (The Psychological Corporation, 1992; Wechsler, 1991). These provide intellectual and achievement assessments standardized on the same normative sample, allowing more reliable evaluation of academic strengths and weaknesses in relation to overall ability level. Along with the IQ indices, the WISC-III includes attention–concentration and processing speed indices and the WIAT includes subtests assessing language comprehension and expression. In addition to the continuing need for adequately standardized measures is the importance of care and judgement that come with clinical neuropsychological experience. Sociocultural factors impact significantly upon test outcomes. Some measures claim to be more or less culture-free. Yet, the experience and judgement of the neuropsychologist are vital to the appropriate assessment of children with epilepsy. Sociocultural

factors can result in test scores that reflect lower ability than the individual's 'true' score. In the final analysis the neuropsychologist analyzes the 'pattern' of scores using good clinical judgement to reach decisions of cognitive deficit determination (Jones-Gotman, Smith and Zatorre, 1993).

An issue of primary importance in the neuropsychology of childhood epilepsy concerns the accurate estimate of the child's premorbid level of cognitive ability. The decision regarding the degree of impairment is based upon the relationship between current performance and performance prior to the onset of the disorder. The development of valid and reliable indices of premorbid functioning has been somewhat successful in adults, but has been difficult in children due to the particular influence of maturational, social–cultural, and situational factors on children's intellectual levels (Klesges and Troster, 1987; Sattler, 1982). Scores from tests such as the WISC Information and Vocabulary, the Wide Range Achievement Test (reading portion), the Raven Progressive Matrices have all been used to estimate the child's premorbid cognitive ability level. If the nature of the cognitive deficit(s) affects these scores, the highest subtest score achieved on the WISC may provide at least a gross measure of ability (Lezak, 1983). Individual consideration of the performance of a child with epilepsy relative to premorbid functioning, rather than in terms of 'average' or 'low average', is particularly important in this disorder, since many of the deficits are often subtle and variable. Ideally, baseline neuropsychological testing should be completed at the onset of the disorder for the further assessment of changes in cognitive status and the effects of treatment upon cognition. In children younger than 12 years, serial cognitive testing can prove invaluable. If the underlying neurological condition leads to disruption of development as evidenced by declining cognitive test scores, surgery may be seen as more viable for these tender ages.

In summary, neuropsychological assessment can address a number of specific issues. This assessment is of great use in the lateralization and localization of cognitive dysfunction arising from focal disturbances (Milner, 1975; Rausch, 1987). This is of particular relevance in the surgical treatment of epilepsy. Preoperative neuropsychological methods are used to provide confirmation of the location and severity of the dysfunctional area, aid in the prediction of the amount of seizure control that may be obtained following resection, and to limit as well as to predict the amount of cognitive loss following surgery (Rausch, 1987). Serial neuropsychological assessment can provide documentation of improvement in cognitive function following surgery, and alert the physician to potential toxic drug effects. Serial neuropsychological assessments can also alert to the need to act aggressively in cases of neurological deterioration, for example with surgical intervention. In addition, the recent use of neuropsychological assessment coupled with simultaneous EEG recording and video monitoring may aid in the detection of the effect of subtle epileptic disturbances of attentional functioning and ongoing cognitive processing. In non-surgical as well as surgical seizure patients, neuropsychological data elucidates cognitive strengths and weaknesses providing a guide to adequate academic planning and strategies for cognitive remediation treatment.

## Summary and future directions

Epilepsy is a common and complex disorder that can affect both general intellectual performance as well as specific cognitive processes. The nature and severity of these deficits are often unclear since seizures themselves, the underlying brain pathology, and anticonvulsant medications all contribute to the presenting clinical picture. Although some forms of epilepsy that are accompanied by progressive neurological deterioration can affect intellectual ability, epilepsy itself does not appear to affect IQ test scores. Specific neuropsychological deficits are nevertheless detectable, which appear to be associated with the underlying brain pathology. The underlying pathology in turn gives rise to the epileptic condition and to the cognitive disturbances, which may be complicated by the effects of some anti-epileptic medication regimens as well as by inter-ictal epileptiform activity. Neuropsychological assessment is an invaluable tool for both the diagnosis and treatment of the cognitive sequelae of epilepsy. It can help to monitor the progress of epilepsy. Through assessment before and after the initiation of anticonvulsant treatment, it can provide a basis for decision-making about the choice of anti-epileptic drugs and their dosage levels. The recent, more frequent use of surgery for children with intractable seizures is a positive step. The contributions of neuropsychological testing to the presurgical diagnostic work-up and post-surgery follow-up are of great importance. In addition, longitudinal research addressing neurodevelopmental issues involved in the timing of childhood epilepsy surgery may provide further understanding of neurodevelopmental processes, as well as improve the surgical decision-making process itself. Finally, neuropsychological assessment is instrumental in devising specific remediation programs for overcoming cognitive deficits. The implementation of more rigorously controlled studies combined with better standardization of test instruments will lead to a more complete understanding of the relationship between epilepsy-related and treatment effects upon the cognitive performance of these children.

## References

Aarts JHP, Binnie CD, Smith AM, Wilkins AJ: Selective cognitive impairment during focal and generalized epileptiform activity. Brain: 107; 293–308, 1984.

Abou-Khalil B: Insights into language mechanisms derived from the evaluation of epilepsy. In Kirshner HS (Ed), Handbook of Speech and Language Disorders. Neurological Disease and Therapy, Vol. 33. New York: Marcel Dekker, 1995.

Agnetti V, Ganga M, Murrigaile M, Piras MR, Ticca A: A memory assessment in temporal lobe epilepsy. Presented at the XIth Epilepsy International Symposium, Florence, 1979.

Aicardi J, Chevrie JJ: Convulsive status epilepticus in infants and children: a study of 239 cases. Epilepsy: 11; 187–197, 1970.

Aicardi J, Chevrie JJ: Consequences of status epilepticus in infants and children. In Delgado-Escueta AV, Wasterlain CG, Treiman DM (Eds), Status Epilepticus, Advances in Neurology, Vol. 34. New York: Raven Press, pp. 115–125, 1983.

Albala BJ, Moshe SL, Okada R: Kainic-acid induced seizures: A developmental study. Developmental Brain Research: 13; 139–148, 1984.

Aldenkamp AP: Effect of seizures and epileptiform discharges on cognitive function. Epilepsia: 38 (Suppl 1); S52–S55, 1997.

Aldenkamp AP, Alpherts WCJ, Blennow G: Withdrawal of antiepileptic medication in children, B, effects on cognitive function. The multicenter Holmfrid study. Neurology: 43; 41–50, 1993.

Aldenkamp AP, Alpherts WCJ, De Bruine D, Dekker MJA: Test-retest variability in children with epilepsy B a comparison of WISC-R subtest profiles. Epilepsy Research: 7; 165–172, 1990.

Aldenkamp AP, Gutter TH, Beun AM: The effect of seizure activity and paroxysmal electroencephalographic discharges on cognition. Acta Neurologica Scandinavica: 86(Suppl 140); 111–121, 1992.

Aldenkamp AP, Mulder OG, Overweg J: Cognitive effects of lamotrigine as first-line add-on in patients with localization-related (partial) epilepsy. Journal of Epilepsy: 10; 117–121, 1997.

Aldenkamp AP, Overweg J, Gutter T, Beun AM, Diepman L, Mulder OG: Effect of epilepsy, seizures and epileptiform EEG discharges on cognitive function. Acta Neurologica Scandinavica: 93; 253–259, 1996.

Annegers JF, Hauser WA, Elveback LR. Remission of seizures and relapse in patients with epilepsy. Epilepsia 1999; 20:729-737.

Appleton RE: The Landau-Kleffner syndrome. Archives of Diseases in Children: 72; 386–387, 1995.

Armon C, Shin C, Miller P, Carwile S, Brown E, Edinger JD, Paul RG: Reversible parkinsonism and cognitive impairment with chronic valproate use. Neurology: 47; 626–635, 1996.

Arnold ST, Dodson WE: Epilepsy in children. Bailliere's Clinical Neurology: 5; 783–802, 1996.

Asano E, Chugani DC, Juhasz C, Muzik O, Chugani HT: Surgical treatment of west syndrome. Brain and Development: 23; 662–669, 2001.

Ballaban-Gil K: Language disorders and epilepsy. In Pedley A, Meldrum BS (Eds), Recent Advances in Epilepsy, No. 6. New York: Churchill Livingstone, 1995.

Baram TZ, Mitchell WG, Tournay A, Snead OC, Hanson RA, Horton EJ: High-dose corticotropin (ACTH) versus prednisone for infantile spasms: a prospective, randomized, blinded study. Pediatrics: 97; 375–379, 1996.

Barnes SE, Bower BD: Sodium valproate in the treatment of intractable childhood epilepsy. Developmental Medicine and Child Neurology: 17; 151–158, 1978.

Beaumanoir A: The Landau–Kleffner syndrome. In Roger J, Bureau M, Dravet C et al. (Eds), Epileptic Syndromes in Infancy, Childhood, and Adolescence. 2nd ed., London: John Libbey Eurotext, pp. 231–243, 1992.

Berent S, Boll TJ, Giordani B: Hemispheric site of epileptogenic focus: cognitive, perceptual and psychosocial implications for children and adults. In Canger R, Angeleri F, Penry JK (Eds), Advances in Epileptology. New York: Raven Press, pp. 163–181, 1980.

Berg AT: Evaluating the outcomes of epilepsy surgery. Clinical Neuroscience: 2; 10–16, 1994.

Berg AT: The epidemiology of seizures and epilepsy in children. In Shinnar S, Amir N, Branski D (Eds), Childhood Seizures: Basel: S Karger, pp. 93–99, 1995.

Berg AT, Hauser WA, Shinnar S: The prognosis of childhood-onset epilepsy. In Shinnar S, Amir N, Branski D (Eds), Childhood Seizures. Basel: S Karger, pp. 93–99, 1995.

Berg AT, Levy SR, Testa FM, Shinnar S: Classification of childhood epilepsy syndromes in newly diagnosed epilepsy: Inter-rater agreement and reasons for disagreement. Epilepsia: 40; 439–444, 1999a.

Berg AT, Shinnar S, Levy SR, Testa FM: Newly diagnosed epilepsy in children: presentation at diagnosis. Epilepsia: 40; 445–452, 1999b.

Berg AT, Testa FM, Levy SR, Shinnar S: The epidemiology of epilepsy: past, present, and future. Neurologic Clinics: 14; 383–398, 1996.

Binnie CD: Methods of detecting transient cognitive impairment during epileptiform discharges. In WE Dodson, M Kinsbourne, Hiltbrunner B (Eds), The Assessment of Cognitive Functions in Epilepsy. New York: Remos Publications, pp. 127–138, 1991.

Binnie CD: Cognitive impairment: Is it inevitable? Seizure: 3(Suppl A); 17–22, 1995.

Bishop DVM: Age of onset and outcome in acquired aphasia with convulsive disorder (Landau–Kleffner syndrome). Developmental Medicine and Child Neurology: 27(6); 705–712, 1985.

Bornstein RA, Drake ME, Pakalnis A: WAIS factor structure in epileptic patients. Epilepsia: 29(1); 203–208, 1988a.

Bornstein RA, Pakalnis A, Drake ME: Effects of seizure type and waveform abnormality on memory and attention. Archives of Neurology: 45; 884–887, 1988b.

Bornstein RA, Pakalnis A, Drake ME: Verbal and nonverbal memory and learning in patients with complex partial seizures of temporal lobe origin. Journal of Epilepsy: 1(4); 203–208, 1988c.

Bourgeois BF, Prensky AL, Palkes H, Talent BK, Busch SG: Intelligence in epilepsy: a prospective study in children. Annals of Neurology: 14(4); 438–444, 1983.

Breier JI, Plenger PM, Wheless JW, Thomas AB, Brookshire BL, Curtis VL, Papanicolaou A, Willmore LJ, Clifton GL: Memory tests distinguish between patients with focal temporal and extratemporal lobe epilepsy. Epilepsia: 37; 165–170, 1996.

Browne SW, Reynolds EH: Cognitive impairment in epileptic patients. In Reynolds EH, Trimble MR (Eds), Epilepsy and Psychiatry. Edinburgh: Churchill Livingstone, 1981.

Browne TR, Feldman, RG (Eds): Epilepsy: Diagnosis and Management. Boston, MA: Little Brown and Co., 1983.

Camfield C, Camfield P, Gordon K, Smith B, Dooley J: Outcome of childhood epilepsy: a population-based study with a simple predictive scoring system for those treated with medication. Journal of Pediatrics: 122; 861–868, 1993.

Camfield CS, Camfield PR, Gordon K, Wirrell E, Dooley JM: Incidence of epilepsy in childhood and adolescence: a population-based study in Nova Scotia from 1977–1985. Epilepsia: 37; 19–23, 1996.

Casetta I, Granieri E, Monetti, V.C. et al., 1997: Prognosis of childhood epilepsy: a community-based study in Copparo, Italy. Neuroepidemiology: 16; 22–28, 1997.

Chelune GJ: Using neuropsychological data to forecast postsurgical cognitive outcome. In Pellock JM, Dodson WE, Bourgeois BFD (Eds), Pediatric Epilepsy: Diagnosis and Therapy. 2nd ed., New York: Raven Press, 1991.

Cohen S, LeNormand M-T: Language acquisition in children with partial epilepsy. Brain and Cognition: 37; 182–186, 1998.

Cole AJ, Andermann F, Taylor L, Olivier A, Rasmussen T, Robitaille Y, Spire JP: The Landau–Kleffner syndrome of acquired epileptic aphasia: unusual clinical outcome, surgical experience, and absence of encephalitis. Neurology: 38; 31–38, 1988.

Commission on Classification and Terminology of the International League Against Epilepsy, 1981: Proposal for revised clinical and electroencephalographic classification of epileptic seizures. Epilepsia: 22; 489–501, 1981.

Commission on Classification and Terminology of the International League Against Epilepsy, 1989: Proposal for revised classification of epilepsies and epileptic syndromes. Epilepsia: 30; 389–399, 1989.

Commission on Epidemiology and Prognosis, 1993: International League Against Epilepsy: Guidelines for epidemiologic studies on epilepsy. Epilepsia: 34; 592–596, 1993.

Committee on Drugs, American Academy of Pediatrics: Behavioral and cognitive effects of anticonvulsant therapy. Pediatrics: 96; 538–540, 1995.

Corbett JA, Trimble MR, Nichol TC: Behavioral and cognitive impairments in children with epilepsy. American Academy of Child Psychiatry: 24(1); 17–23, 1985.

Curatolo P, Verdecchia M, Bombardieri R: Vigabatrin for tuberous sclerosis complex. Brain and Development: 23; 654–657, 2001.

Dam M: Epilepsy surgery. Acta Neurologica Scandinavica: 94; 81–87, 1996.

D'Amelio M, Shinnar S, Hauser WA: Epilepsy in children with mental retardation and cerebral palsy. In Devinsky O, Westbrook LE (Eds), Epilepsy and Developmental Disabilities. Boston, MA: Butterworth Heinemann, pp. 3–16, 2002.

Dikmen S: Neuropsychological aspects of epilepsy. In Hermann BP (Ed), A Multidisciplinary Handbook of Epilepsy. Springfield, IL: Charles C. Thomas, pp. 36–73, 1980.

Dodrill CB: A neuropsychological battery for epilepsy. Epilepsia: 19; 611–623, 1978.

Dodrill CB: Correlates of generalized tonic–clonic seizures with intellectual, neuropsychological, emotional, and social function in patients with epilepsy. Epilepsia: 27; 399–411, 1986.

Dodrill CB: Motor speed is a contaminating factor in evaluating the cognitive effects of phenytoin. Epilepsia: 30; 453–457, 1989.

Dodrill CB: The relationship of neuropsychological abilities to seizure factors and to surgery for epilepsy. Acta Neurologica Scandinavica: 86(Suppl 140); 106–110, 1992.

Dodrill CB, Arnett JL, Shu V, Pixton GC, Lenz GT, Sommerville KW: Effects of tiagabine monotherapy on abilities, adjustment, and mood. Epilepsia: 39; 33–42, 1998.

Dodrill CB, Arnett JL, Sommerville KW, Sussman NM: Effects of differing dosages of vigabatril (sabril) on cognitive abilities and quality of life in epilepsy. Epilepsia: 36; 164–173, 1995.

Dodrill CB, Arnett JL, Sommerville KW, Shu V: Cognitive and quality of life effects of differing dosages of tiagabine in epilepsy. Neurology: 48; 1025–1031, 1997.

Dodrill CB, Clemmons D: Use of neuropsychological tests to identify high school students with epilepsy who later demonstrate inadequate performance in life. Journal of Consulting and Clinical Psychology: 52(4); 520–527, 1984.

Dodrill CB, Matthews CG: The role of neuropsychology in the assessment and treatment of persons with epilepsy. American Psychologist: 47; 1139–1142, 1992.

Dodrill CB, Troupin AS: Psychotropic effects of carbamazepine in epilepsy: A double-blind comparison with phenytoin. Neurology: 27; 1023–1028, 1977.

Dodrill CB, Wilensky AJ: Intellectual impairment as an outcome of status epilepticus. Neurology: 40(Suppl 2); 23–27, 1990.

Dodrill CB, Wilensky AJ: Neuropsychological abilities before and after 5 years of stable antiepileptic drug therapy. Epilepsia: 33; 327–334, 1992.

Dreifuss FE: Pediatric Epileptology. Boston, MA: John Wright, 1983.

Duchowny M, Levin B, Jayakar P: Neurobiologic considerations in early surgery for epilepsy. Journal of Child Neurology: 9(Suppl 2) 2S42–2S49, 1994.

Duncan JS, Shorvon SD, Trimble MR: Effects of removal of phenytoin, carbamazepine, and valproate on cognitive function. Epilepsia: 31; 584–591, 1990.

Ellenberg JH, Hirtz DG, Nelson KB: Do seizures in children cause intellectual deterioration? New England Journal of Medicine: 314(17); 1085–1088, 1986.

Engel J Jr: Seizures and Epilepsy. Philadelphia, PA: F.A. Davis, 1989.

Farwell JR, Dodrill CB, Batzel LW: Neuropsychological abilities of children with epilepsy. Epilepsia: 26(5); 395–400, 1985.

Farwell JR, Lee YJ, Hirtz DG, Sulzbacher SI, Ellenberg JH, Nelson KB: Phenobarbital for febrile seizures–effects on intelligence and on seizure recurrence. New England Journal of Medicine: 322; 364–369, 1990.

Fedio P, Mirsky AF: Selective intellectual deficits in children with temporal lobe or centrencephalic epilepsy. Neuropsychologia: 7; 287–300, 1969.

Freeman JM, Tibbles J, Camfield C, Camfield P: Benign epilepsy of childhood: a speculation and its ramifications. Pediatrics: 79; 864–868, 1987.

Gaggero R, Cirrincione M, Zannoto E, de Negri M: Profile of the impairment in children with epilepsy. Approche Neuropsychologique des Apprentissages Chez L'Enfant: 4; 32–37, 1993.

Galaburda AM: Dyslexia and Development: Neurobiological Aspects of Extra-ordinary Brains. Cambridge, MA: Harvard University Press, 1993.

Gallassi R, Morreale A, Lorusso S, Ferrari M, Procaccianti G, Lugaresi E, Baruzzi A: Cognitive effects of phenytoin during monotherapy. Acta Neurologica Scandinavica: 75; 258–261, 1987.

Gallassi R, Morreale A, Lorusso S, Pazzaglia P, Lugaresi E: Epilepsy presenting as memory disturbances. Epilepsia: 29(5); 624–629, 1988.

Gascon G, Victor D, Lombroso S, Goodglass H: Language disorder, convulsive disorders, and electroencephalographic abnormalities. Archives of Neurology: 28; 156–162, 1973.

Gibbs FA, Lennox WG, Gibbs EL: The electroencephalogram in diagnosis and in localisation of epileptic seizures. Archives of Neurology and Psychiatry: 36; 1225–1235, 1936.

Gigli GL, Maschio M, Diomedi M, Placidi F, Silvestri G, Marciani MG: Cognitive performances in newly referred patients with temporal lobe epilepsy: Comparison with normal subjects in basal condition and after treatment with controlled-release carbamazepine. International Journal of Neuroscience: 88; 97–107, 1996.

Gillham RA, Williams N, Wiedman K, Butler E, Larkin JG, Brodie MJ: Concentration effect relationships with carbamazepine and its epoxide on psychomotor and cognitive function in epileptic patients. Journal of Neurology, Neurosurgery and Psychiatry: 51; 929–933, 1988.

Glowinski H: Cognitive deficits in temporal lobe epilepsy: an investigation of memory functioning. Journal of Nervous and Mental Disease: 157; 129–137, 1973.

Goldstein PC, Rosenbaum G, Taylor MJ: Assessment of differential attention mechanisms in seizure disorders and schizophrenia. Neuropsychology: 11; 309–317, 1997.

Gordon N: The Landau–Kleffner syndrome: Increased understanding. Brain and Development: 19; 311–316, 1997.

Green JB, Hartlage LG: Comparative performance of epileptic and non-epileptic children and adolescents. Diseases of the Nervous System: 32; 418–421, 1971.

Gumnit RJ: The Epilepsy Handbook: The Practical Management of Seizures. New York: Raven Press, 1983.

Halgren E, Stapleton J, Domalski P, Swartz BE, Delgado-Escueta AV, Walsh GO, Mandelkern M, Blahd W, Ropchan J: In Smith D, Trieman D, Trimble M (Eds), Advances in Neurology (Vol. 55). New York: Raven Press, pp. 385–410, 1991.

Hancock E, Osborne JP, Milner P: The treatment of west syndrome: a Cochrane review of the literature to December 2000. Brain and Development: 23; 624–634, 2001.

Hartlage LC: Neuropsychological assessment of anti-convulsant drug toxicity. Clinical Neuropsychology: 3; 20–22, 1981.

Hauser WA: Status epilepticus, frequency, etiology, and neurological sequelae. In Delgado-Escueta AV, Wasterlain CG, Treiman DM (Eds), Status Epilepticus: Advances in Neurology, Vol. 34. New York: Raven Press, pp. 3–14, 1983.

Hauser WA: Status epilepticus: epidemiologic considerations. Neurology: 40(Suppl 2); 9–13, 1990.

Hauser WA, Hesdorffer DC: Epilepsy: Frequency, Causes and Consequences. New York: Demos, 1990.

Hauser WA, Annegers J, Kurland L: Incidence of epilepsy and unprovoked seizures in Rochester, Minnesota: 1935–1984. Epilepsia 1993; 34: 453–468.

Hellstrom B, Barlach-Christoffersen M: Influence on phenobarbital on the psychomotor development and behavior in preschool children with convulsions. Neuropediatrie: 11; 151–160, 1980.

Hermann BP, Seidenberg M, Haltiner A, Wyler AR: Adequacy of language function and verbal memory performance in unilateral temporal lobe epilepsy. Cortex: 28; 423–433, 1993.

Hermann BP, Wyler AR, Richey ET: Wisconsin card sorting test performance in patients with complex partial seizures of temporal lobe origin. Journal of Clinical and Experimental Neuropsychology: 10(4); 467–476, 1988a.

Hermann BP, Wyler AR, Steenman H: The interrelationship between language function and verbal learning/memory performance in patients with complex partial seizures. Cortex: 24; 245–253, 1988b.

Hermann BP, Whitman S: Psychopathology in epilepsy: a multietiologic model. In Whitman S, Hermann BP (Eds), Psy-

chopathology in Epilepsy: Social Dimensions. New York: Oxford University Press, pp. 5–38, 1986.

Hirtz DG, Nelson KB: Cognitive effects of antiepileptic drugs. In Pedley TA, Meldum KS (Eds), Recent Advances in Epilepsy II. New York: Churchill Livingstone, 1985.

Holmes GL: Do seizures cause brain damage? Epilepsia: 32(Suppl. 5); S14–S28, 1991.

Holmes GL: Epilepsy in the developing brain: lessons from the laboratory and clinic. Epilepsia: 38; 12–30, 1997.

Holmes GL, McKeever M, Saunders Z: Epileptiform activity in aphasia of childhood an epiphenomenon? Epilepsia: 22; 631–639, 1981.

Holmes GL, Moshe SL: Consequences of seizures in the developing brain. Journal of Epilepsy: 3(Suppl); 1–13, 1990.

Horner MD, Flashman LA, Freides D, Epstein CM: Temporal lobe epilepsy and performance on the Wisconsin Card Sorting Test. Journal of Clinical Neuropsychology: 18; 310–313, 1996.

Howell RA, Saling MM, Bradley DC, Berkovic SF: Interictal language fluency in temporal lobe epilepsy. Cortex: 30; 469–478, 1994.

Jeavons PM: West Syndrome: Infantile spasms. In Roger J, Dravet C, Bureau M, Dreifuss FE, Wolf P (Eds), Epileptic Syndromes in Infancy, Childhood, and Adolescence. London: John Libbey, pp. 42–50, 1985.

Jones-Gotman M, Smith ML, Zatorre RJ: Neuropsychological testing for localising and lateralising the epileptogenic region. In Engel J Jr (Ed), Surgical Treatment of the Epilepsies. 2nd ed., New York: Raven Press, pp. 245–261, 1993.

Kastelijn-Nolst Trenite DGA, Bakker DJ, Binnie CD, Buerman A, Van Raaij MB: Psychological effect of subclinical epileptiform EEG discharges. I. Scholastic skills. Epilepsy Research: 2; 111–116, 1988.

Klesges RC, Troster AI: A review of premorbid indices of intellectual and neuropsychological functioning: what have we learned in the past five years? International Journal of Clinical Neuropsychology: 9(1); 1–11, 1987.

Kramer U, Nevo Y, Neufeld MY, Fatal A, Leitner Y, Harel S: Epidemiology of epilepsy in childhood: a cohort of 440 consecutive patients. Pediatric Neurology: 18; 46–50, 1998.

Kurthen M, Helmstaedter C, Linke DB, Solymosi L et al.: Interhemispheric dissociation of expressive and receptive language functions in patients with complex partial seizures: An amobarbital study. Brain and Language: 43; 694–712, 1993.

Lagarda SB, Booth MP, Fennell EB, Maria BL: Altered cognitive functioning in children with idiopathic epilepsy receiving valproate monotherapy. Journal of Child Neurology: 11; 321–330, 1996.

Landau WM, Kleffner F: Syndrome of acquired aphasia with convulsive disorder in children. Neurology: 7; 523–530, 1957.

Leach JP, Girvan J, Paul A, Brodie MJ: Gabapentin and cognition: A double blind, dose ranging, placebo controlled study in refractory epilepsy. Journal of Neurology, Neurosurgery, and Psychiatry: 62; 372–376, 1997.

Lennox WG: Epilepsy and Related Disorders, Vol. 1–2. Boston, MA; Little, Brown, and Co., 1960.

Lerman P, Lerman-Sagie T, Kivity S: Effect of early corticosteroid therapy for Landau–Kleffner syndrome. Developmental Medicine and Child Neurology: 33; 257–260, 1991.

Lezak MD: Neuropsychological Assessment. 2nd ed., New York: Oxford University Press, 1983.

Loiseau P, Signoret JL, Strube E: Attention problems in adult epileptic patients. Acta Neurologica Scandinavica: Suppl. 99; 31–34, 1984.

Loiseau P, Strube E, Broustet D, Battellochi S, Gomeni C, Morselli PL: Evaluation of memory function in a population of epileptics and matched controls. Acta Neurologica Scandinavica: Suppl. 80; 58–61, 1980.

Lokeit H, Seitz RJ, Markowitsch HJ, Neumann N, Witte OW, Ebner A: Prefrontal asymmetric interictal glucose hypometabolism and cognitive impairment in patients with temporal lobe epilepsy. Brain: 120; 2283–2294, 1997.

Loring DW, Lee GP, Martin RC: Material specific learning in patients with partial complex seizures of temporal lobe origin: convergent validation of memory constructs. Journal of Epilepsy: 1(2); 53–59, 1988.

Ludgate J, Keating J, O'Dwyer R, Callaghan N: An improvement in cognitive function following polypharmacy reduction in a group of epileptic patients. Acta Neurologica Scandinavica: 71; 448–452, 1985.

Marescaux C, Hirsch E, Finck S et al: Landau–Kleffner syndrome: a pharmacologic study of five cases. Epilepsia: 31; 768–777, 1990.

Martin R, Kuzniecky R, Ho S, Hetherington H, Pan J, Sinclair K, Gilliam F, Faught E: Cognitive effects of topiramate, gabapentin, and lamotrigine in healthy young adults. Neurology: 52; 321–327, 1999.

Matsuoka H, Okuma T, Ueno T, Saito H: Impairment of parietal cortical functions associated with episodic prolonged spike-and-wave discharges. Epilepsia: 27(4); 432–436, 1986.

Mayeux R, Brandt J, Rosen J, Benson DF: Interictal memory and language impairment in temporal lobe epilepsy. Neurology: 30; 120–125, 1980.

Maytal J, Shinnar S, Moshe SL, Alvarez LA: Low morbidity and mortality of status epilepticus in children. Pediatrics: 83(3); 323–331, 1989.

Meador KJ, Loring DW, Huh K, Gallager BB, King DW: Comparative cognitive effects of anticonvulsants. Neurology: 40; 391–394, 1990.

Meador KJ, Loring DW, Moore EE, Thompson WO, Nichols ME, Oberzan RE, Durkin MW, Gallagher BB, King DW: Comparative cognitive effects of phenobarbital, phenytoin, and valproate in healthy adults. Neurology: 45; 1494–1499, 1995.

Meador KJ, Loring DW, Ray PG, Murro AM, King DW, Perrine KR, Vazquez BR, Kiolbasa T: Differential cognitive and behavioral effects of carbamazepine and lamotrigine. Neurology: 56; 1177–1182, 2001.

Meldrum BS, Brierly JB: Prolonged epileptic seizure in primates: Ischemic cell change and its relation to ictal physiological events. Archives of Neurology: 28; 10–17, 1973.

Meldrum BS, Horton RW: Physiology of status epilepticus in primates. Archives of Neurology: 28; 1–9, 1973.

Meldrum BS, Horton RW, Brierly JB: Epileptic brain damage in adolescent baboon following seizures induced by allylglycine. Brain: 97; 407–418, 1974.

Milner B: Psychological aspects of focal epilepsy and its neurosurgical management. In Purpura D, Penry J, Walter R (Eds), Advances in Neurology. New York: Raven Press, pp. 299–321, 1975.

Morrell F, Whisler WW, Smith MC, Hoeppner TJ, De Toledo-Morrell L, Pierre-Louis SJC, Kanner AM, Buelow JM, Ristanovic R, Bergen D, Chez M, Hasegawa H: Landau–Kleffner syndrome. Treatment with multiple subpial transection. Brain: 118; 1529–1546, 1995.

Moshe SL, Albala BJ: Increased seizure susceptibility in the immature brain. Developmental Brain Research: 7; 81–85, 1983.

Nelson KB, Ellenberg JH: Prognosis in children with febrile seizures. Pediatrics: 61; 720–727, 1978.

Nelson KB, Ellenberg JH: Antecedents of seizure disorders in early childhood. American Journal of Diseases of Children: 140; 1053–1061, 1986.

Nelson KB, Ellenberg JH: Prenatal and perinatal antecedents of febrile seizures. Annals of Neurology: 27; 127–131, 1990.

Novelly RA: The debt of neuropsychology to the epilepsies. American Psychologist: 47; 1126–1129, 1992.

O'Dell C, Shinnar S: Initiation and discontinuation of antiepileptic drugs. Neurologic Clinics: 19; 289–311, 2001.

O'Dougherty M, Wright FS, Cox S, Walson P: Carbamazepine plasma concentration: Relationship to cognitive impairment. Archives of Neurology: 44; 863–867, 1987.

Okada R, Moshe SL, Albala BJ: Infantile status epilepticus and future seizure susceptibility in the rat. Developmental Brain Research: 15; 177–183, 1984.

O'Leary DS, Lovell MR, Sackellares JC, Berent S, Giordano B, Seidenberg M, Boll TJ: Effects of age of onset of partial and generalized seizures on neuropsychological performance in children. Journal of Nervous and Mental Disease: 171(10); 624–629, 1983.

O'Leary DS, Seidenberg M, Berent S, Boll TJ: Effects of age of onset of tonic–clonic seizures on neuropsychological performance in children. Epilepsia: 22; 197–204, 1981.

Oxbury S: Neuropsychological evaluation-Children: In Engel J, Pedley TA (Eds), Epilepsy: A Comprehensive Textbook. Philadelphia: Lippincott-Raven Publishers, 989–999, 1997.

Pavone P, Bianchini R, Trifiletti RR, Incorpora G, Pavone A, Parano E: Neuropsychological assessment in children with absence epilepsy. Neurology: 56; 1047–1051, 2001.

Provinciali L, Bartolini M, Mari F, Del Pesce M, Ceravolo MG: Influence of vigabatrin on cognitive performances and behaviour in patients with drug-resistant epilepsy. Acta Neurologica Scandinavica: 94; 12–18, 1996.

Quadfasel AF, Pruyser PW: Cognitive deficits in patients with psychomotor epilepsy. Epilepsia: 4; 80–90, 1955.

Rapin I, Mattis S, Rowan AJ, Golden GS: Verbal auditory agnosia in children. Developmental Medicine and Child Neurology: 19; 192–207, 1977.

Rausch R: Psychological Evaluation. In Engel J Jr (Ed), Surgical Treatment of the Epilepsies. New York: Raven Press, 1987.

Resnick TJ, Duchowny M, Jayakar P: Early surgery for epilepsy:

Redefining candidacy. Journal of Child Neurology: 9(Suppl 2) 2S36–2S41, 1994.

Reynolds CR: Measurement and statistical problems in neuropsychological assessment of children. In Reynolds CR, Fletcher-Janzen E (Eds), Handbook of Child Clinical Neuropsychology. New York; Plenum, pp. 145–166, 1989.

Reynolds EH, Travers RD: Serum anticonvulsant concentrations in epileptic patients with mental symptoms. British Journal of Psychiatry: 124; 440–445, 1974.

Rodin EA: The Prognosis of Patients with Epilepsy. Springfield, IL: Thomas, 1968.

Rodin EA, Schmaltz S, Twitty G: Intellectual functions of patients with childhood-onset epilepsy. Developmental Medicine and Child Neurology: 28; 25–33, 1986.

Roger J, Dravet C, Bureau M, Dreifuss FE, Wolf P (Eds): Epileptic Syndromes in Infancy, Childhood, and Adolescence. London: John Libbey, 1985.

Roger J, Dravet C, Bureau M, Dreifuss FE, Wolf P (Eds): Epileptic Syndromes in Infancy, Childhood, and Adolescence. 2nd ed., London: John Libbey Eurotext, 1992.

Rowan AJ, Rosenbaum DH: Ictal amnesia and fugue states. In Smith D, Treiman D, Trimble M (Eds), Advances in Neurology, Vol. 55. New York: Raven Press, pp. 357–367, 1991.

Rugland AL: "Subclinical" epileptogenic activity. In Sillanpaa M et al (Eds), Paediatric Epilepsy. Petersfield: Wrightson Biomedical Publishers, pp. 217–224, 1990.

Rutter M, Graham P, Yule W: A Neuropsychiatric Study in Childhood. Philadelphia, PA: Lippincott, 1970.

Sattler JM: Assessment of Children's Intelligence and Special Abilities. 2nd ed., Boston, MA: Allyn and Bacon, 1982.

Schain RJ, Ward JW, Guthrie D: Carbamazepine as an anticonvulsant in children. Neurology: 27; 476–480, 1977.

Schwartz ML, Dennerll RD: Neuropsychological assessment of children with and without questionable epileptogenic dysfunction. Perceptual and Motor Skills: 30; 111–121, 1970.

Seri S, Cerquiglini A, Pisani F: Spike-induced interference in auditory sensory processing in Landau–Kleffner syndrome. Electroencephalography and Clinical Neurophysiology: 108; 506–510, 1998.

Shewmon DA, Erwin RJ: Focal spike induced cerebral dysfunction is related to the after-coming slow wave. Annals of Neurology: 23; 131–137, 1988.

Shih Y-H, Peng FCC: An outline of the theoretical constructs of epilepsy and language disorders based on surgical treatment of epilepsies. Journal of Linguistics: 7; 11–21, 1998.

Shinnar S: Antiepileptic drugs in adolescents. Journal of Adolescent Health Care: 8; 105–112, 1987.

Shinnar S, Babb TL: Long-term sequelae of status epilepticus. In Engel J, Pedley TA (Eds), Epilepsy: A Comprehensive Textbook. Philadelphia, PA: Lippincott-Raven, 1997.

Shinnar S, Berg AT, Moshe SL, Petix M, Maytal J, Kang H, Goldensohn ES, Hausar WA: Risk of seizure recurrence following a first unprovoked seizure in childhood: a prospective study. Pediatrics: 85(6); 1076–1085, 1990.

Shinnar S, Sommerville KW: Tiagabine. In Pellock JM, Dodson WE, Bourgeois BF (Eds), Pediatric Epilepsy: Diagnosis and Therapy. 2nd ed., New York, NY: Demos, pp 489–498, 2001.

Siebelink BM, Bakker DJ, Binnie CD, Kastelijn-Nolst Trenite DGA: Psychological effects of subclinical epileptiform EEG discharges in children. II. General intelligence tests. Epilepsy Resarch: 2; 117–121, 1988.

Sillanpaa M, Jalava M, Kaleva O, Shinnar S: Long-term prognosis of seizures with onset in childhood. New England Journal of Medicine: 338; 1715–1722, 1998.

Smith DB: Cognitive effects of antiepileptic drugs. In Smith, D, Trieman D, Trimble M (Eds), Advances in Neurology, Vol. 55. New York: Raven Press, pp. 197–212, 1991.

Smith DB, Baker G, Davies G: Outcomes of add-on treatment with lamotrigine in partial epilepsy. Epilepsia: 34(Suppl 2); 312–322, 1993.

Smith DB, Craft BR, Collins J, Mattson RH, Cramer JA: Behavioral characteristics of epilepsy patients compared with normal controls. Epilepsia: 27(6); 123–131, 1986.

Spencer SS: Evolving indications and applications of epilepsy surgery. Clinical Neuroscience: 2; 3–9, 1994.

Spreen O, Strauss E: A Compendium of Neuropsychological Tests. 2nd ed., New York: Oxford University Press, 1998.

Stores G, Hart J, Piran N: Inattentiveness in school children with epilepsy. Epilepsia: 19; 169–175, 1978.

Suzuki Y: Zonisamide in West syndrome. Brain and Development: 23; 658–661, 2001.

Tassinari CA, Bureau M, Dravet C, Dalla Bernardina B, Roger J: Epilepsy with continuous spikes and waves during slow wave sleep–ESES. In Roger J, Dravet C, Bureau M, Dreifuss FE, Wolf P (Eds), Epileptic Syndromes in Infancy, Childhood, and Adolescence. 2nd ed., London: John Libbey Eurotext, pp. 245–246, 1992.

The Psychological Corporation: Wechsler Individual Achievement Test. San Antonia, TX: Author, 1992.

Thompson PJ, Baxendale SA, Duncan JS, Sander JWAS: Effects of topiramate on cognitive function. Journal of Neurology, Neurosurgery and Psychiatry: 69; 636–641, 2000.

Thompson PJ, Huppert FA, Trimble MR: Anticonvulsant drugs, cognitive function, and memory. Acta Neurologica Scandinavica: 80(Suppl); 75–81, 1980.

Thompson PJ, Huppert FA, Trimble MR: Phenytoin and cognitive functions: effects on normal volunteers and implications for epilepsy. British Journal of Clinical Psychology: 20; 155–162, 1981.

Thompson PJ, Trimble MR: Comparative effects of anticonvulsant drugs on cognitive functioning. British Journal of Clinical Practice: Suppl 18; 154–156, 1982.

Toribe Y: High-dose vitamin B-6 treatment in west syndrome. Brain and Development: 23; 654–657, 2001.

Trevathan E, Murphy CC, Yeargin-Allsopp M: Prevalence and descriptive epidemiology of Lennox–Gastaut syndrome among Atlanta children. Epilepsia: 38; 1283–1288, 1997.

Trimble MR: Anticonvulsant drugs, behavior, and cognitive abilities. Current Developments in Psychopharmacology: 6; 65–91, 1981.

Trimble MR, Thompson PJ: Neuropsychological aspects of epilepsy. In Grant I, Adams KM (Eds), Neuropsychologic Assessment of Neuropsychiatric Disorders. New York: Oxford University Press, pp. 321–346, 1986.

Tymchuk AJ: Comparison of Bender error and time scores for groups of epileptic, retarded, and behavior problem children. Perceptual and Motor Skills: 38; 71–74, 1974.

Vallarta JM, Bell DB, Reichert A: A progressive encephalopathy due to chronic hydrantoin intoxication. American Journal of Diseases of Children: 128; 27–34, 1974.

Vermeulen J, Aldenkamp AP: Cognitive side-effects of chronic antiepileptic drug treatment: A review of 25 years of research. Epilepsy Research: 22, 65–95, 1995.

Vining EPG, Mellits ED, Cataldo MF, Dorsen MM, Speilberg SP, Freeman JA: Effects of phenobarbital and sodium valproate on neuropsychological function and behavior. Annals of Neurology: 14; 360, 1983.

Wechsler D: Manual for the Wechsler Intelligence Scale for Children. 3rd ed., San Antonio, TX: The Psychological Corporation, 1991.

Wheless JW, Constantinou JE: Lennox–Gastaut syndrome. Pediatric Neurology: 17; 203–211, 1997.

Williams J, Griebel ML, Dykman A, Roscoe A: Neuropsychological patterns in pediatric epilepsy. Seizure: 3; 223–228, 1998.

Willis J, Nelson A, Black W, Borges A, An A, Rice J: Barbiturate anticonvulsants: A neuropsychological and quantitative electroencephalographic study. Journal of Child Neurology: 12; 169–171, 1997.

Wolf SM, Shinnar S, Kang H, Gil KB, Moshe SL: Gabapentin toxicity in children manifesting as behavioral changes. Epilepsia: 37; 87–90, 1995.

CHAPTER 7

# Neuroimaging in the developmental disorders

Jenifer Juranek [a],[*] and Pauline A. Filipek [a],[b]

[a] *Department of Pediatrics, University of California, Irvine, College of Medicine, UC Irvine Medical Center, Route 81-4482,
101 City Drive South, Orange, CA 92868-3298, USA*
[b] *Department of Neurology, University of California, Irvine, College of Medicine, UC Irvine Medical Center, Route 81-4482,
101 City Drive South, Orange, CA 92868-3298, USA*

## Introduction

Over the past decade, a tremendous surge in research activity has significantly expanded our current understanding of brain–behavior relationships in human subjects. Vast advances in MRI technology have dramatically improved the quality and resolution of 3-D whole-brain images acquired for neuroanatomical localization studies. Parallel advances in computer technology and software development have greatly facilitated quantitative analyses of large contiguous image sets containing essentially isotropic data. Additionally, computerized administration and scoring of standardized neuropsychological assessments have been developed and are currently available as an alternative to pencil and paper versions. This move toward computerized test administration and response evaluation significantly improves efficiency and accuracy of professional assessments of subjects' performance within the traditional behavior domains of cognition, language, visual–spatial function, and socialization. The purpose of the present review is to address the following issues: (1) review investigative approaches to understanding brain–behavior relationships; (2) discuss state-of-the-art neuroimaging techniques utilized for quanti-

tative neuroanatomical analyses; (3) summarize current knowledge of structural–functional relationships underlying cognitive function and behavior in normal and developmentally disordered children.

Cognitive neuroscientists share a common goal: to elucidate the neural substrates underlying various cognitive functions. In order to address this issue, several divergent approaches have emerged: (1) determine neurological bases of impaired cognitive function resultant from head trauma or disease; (2) identify anomalous patterns of neural development among cohorts representative of various developmental disorders; (3) characterize progressive neurological changes underlying normal brain development from infancy through adulthood. Attempts to identify anatomically based relationships between neural networks and human behavior have been diverse in methodology, often yielding discordant results and conclusions. Such conflicting evidence can be directly attributed to a lack of common standards for subject recruitment, exclusionary criteria, scanning protocols, image analysis methodologies, anatomical definitions, and uniform matching of control subjects (Filipek, 1995b, 1996; Filipek, Kennedy and Caviness, 1992a).

Given the current state of the science, standardized study protocols should be implemented across research centers, thereby making comparisons possible and eliminating some of the confusion in the field.

---
[*] Corresponding author: Tel. +1 (714) 456-8622; Fax: +1 (714) 456-8883; E-mail: jjuranek@uci.edu

**Case studies: lesions**

*Adults*

Cognitive neuroscientists have traditionally posed experimentally challenging questions as we investigate relationships between brain organization and behavior. Retrospective chart reviews of impaired cognitive or behavioral performance correlated with discrete focal lesions in the adult population have contributed to the formulation of hypotheses regarding brain–behavior relationships. Thus, cognitive and behavioral deficits are typically evaluated within the context of lesion size, location, extent, and age of onset as a means to localize the underlying neural systems mediating various functions (Damasio and Damasio, 1989; Heilman and Valenstein, 1985; Mesulam, 1985). This classic bottom-up approach from lesion to behavior assumes that brain organization is modular in design with minimal variability across individuals. However, information streams are often processed in a distributed fashion, generally recruiting complex interactions between numerous neural networks (Ishai, Ungerleider, Martin et al., 1999). Additionally, self-reports of premorbid normal performance may represent a 'mixed bag' whereby abnormalities or symptomatologies may simply lack robustness, and therefore they are not explicitly reported by the individual during the course of an interview. Although these types of criticisms limit the conclusions that can be drawn from lesion case studies, when combined with additional lines of evidence, results from these studies add considerable depth to our current understanding of brain–behavior relationships.

*Children*

Since discrete focal lesions are rare in children, relatively little information is available about lesion-based brain–behavior correlations along the developmental trajectory (Filipek, 1995b, 1996; Filipek et al., 1992a). The inherently dynamic nature of human brain growth, development, and plasticity throughout childhood and adolescence complicates attempts to characterize relationships between neuroanatomical structures and cognitive functions. Furthermore, results from lesion-based studies in the adult brain cannot be readily extrapolated to the developing brain in children. While both large and small lesions in adults can produce large behavioral deficits, large lesions in children frequently result in relatively small behavioral deficits, presumably due to the greater capacity for neural plasticity in children (Johnson, 1997; Kolb, 1995; Nass and Gazzaniga, 1987).

**Neuroimaging studies**

*Image acquisition: aMRI*

Rapid technological advances in anatomical magnetic resonance imaging methods (aMRI) have significantly improved the quality and resolution of whole-brain image sets acquired for quantitative neuroanatomical analyses. Pulse sequence protocols currently implemented across most research centers have been specifically developed to acquire 3-D whole-brain image sets of 1 mm contiguous sections of essentially isotropic data with less than 30 min of imaging time. This development has greatly facilitated our ability to conduct neuroimaging studies in small children. Quantitative analyses of neuroanatomical structures performed in earlier MR imaging studies were substantially limited by thick, non-contiguous slice acquisition protocols. Such limitations precluded quantitative measurements of tissue located between slices, since they were skipped and not directly imaged. Similarly, volume-averaging effects associated with large slice thickness acquisitions significantly limited the resolving power of quantitative analyses. Since voxel intensity values are integrated over slice thickness, structural boundary changes occurring throughout the depth of an individual slice are simply averaged. Thus, large slice thickness values are generally associated with greater margin of error values for volumetric measurements. However, many of these issues have been resolved over the last decade as nearly all research centers are currently capable of utilizing volumetric pulse sequences to acquire thin (1 mm) contiguous sections of nearly isotropic data for their brain neuroimaging studies. Specifically, the spoiled gradient recalled (SPGR) and magnetization prepared gradient echo (MPRAGE) sequences provide outstanding spatial resolution and contrast for T1-weighted images within an acceptable total imaging time (less than 30 min) for adults as well as small children.

*Image processing*

Software algorithms have been successfully developed to digitally reformat isotropic 3-D anatomical MRI data into any plane. Since the plane of image acquisition (i.e. sagittal, axial, coronal) may not necessarily be identical to the plane of image analysis, constructing digitally reformatted image sets serves a crucial role in the image analysis pipeline. For instance, the sagittal plane may be selected as the acquisition plane for MR images in order to minimize the total amount of imaging time. Consequently, digital reconstructions are required to reliably and accurately transform isotropic image sets into a coronal or axial plane, as appropriate for image analysis. Additionally, semi- and fully-automated software algorithms have been specifically developed to positionally normalize intra- and inter-subject MR image sets. Although nearly all MR scanners currently use a laser crossbeam for positional alignment of human subjects within the head coil, some positional variability is inevitably introduced across subjects over the course of a research project. Positional normalization of each subject's volumetric image set into a standardized 3-D coordinate system (Talairach or stereotaxic space) produces essentially identical image planes across subjects, independent of size, position, or orientation of each subject's head within the scanner (Alpert, Bradshaw, Kennedy and Correia, 1990; Collins, Neelin, Peters and Evans, 1994; Filipek et al., 1992a).

Intra-subject registration methods for aligning MR image sets acquired from the same individual across successive scanning sessions have facilitated longitudinal neuroimaging studies designed to assess normal patterns of structural development in children's brains (Thompson, Giedd, Woods et al., 2000). Naturally, as children progress through typical developmental stages and expand their behavioral repertoire, accompanying changes in brain structure and function should be evident. Thus, dynamic patterns of tissue growth and recession can be imaged and correlated with age-appropriate cognitive development. Such information will provide valuable insight into the degree of variability typ-

ically expressed in brains of normally developing children. These longitudinal neuroimaging studies have already begun to identify neural developmental patterns underlying normal and abnormal cognitive development throughout childhood and adolescence (Giedd, Blumenthal, Jeffries et al., 1999; Thompson et al., 2000).

Intra-subject registration methods have also been utilized for cross-modality MR imaging studies (i.e. anatomical and functional MRI). Thus, aMRI and fMRI image sets are co-registered into the same stereotaxic space, enabling direct voxel-to-voxel comparisons of anatomical and functional layers. Such comparisons provide the investigator with outstanding spatial and temporal resolution, respectively. Thus, pediatric neuroimaging studies have the potential to track not only maturational changes in brain structure and function in normally developing children, but also to track efficacy of pharmacological or behavioral intervention treatment strategies on shaping the course of those developmental patterns in developmentally disordered children (Giedd, Rapoport, Leonard et al., 1996; Vaidya, Austin, Kirkorian et al., 1998).

*Image analyses*

The analytical power of neuroimaging studies has significantly improved as morphometric methodologies have progressed from measurements of global and regional boundaries to measurements of individual gyri defined by delimiting sulci. Such cortical parcellation techniques (Rademacher, Galaburda, Kennedy et al., 1992) have dramatically increased our ability to precisely localize neural correlates of cognitive function using traditional brain–behavior nomenclature (Damasio and Damasio, 1989; Damasio and Frank, 1992; Heilman and Valenstein, 1985; Mesulam, 1985). The significance of this increased resolving power is readily appreciated as one compares conclusions drawn by researchers reporting morphometric or functional differences in 'primary auditory and auditory association cortices' vs. 'posterior temporal region'. The application of these morphometric methods to investigations of normally developing and developmentally disordered children's brains provides exceptional specificity for identifying age-related structural parameters underlying normal and anomalous cognitive development. This top-down approach from behavior to neural substrates is ideally suited for identifying correlative associations between brain organization and behavior in the developmental disorders. The state of the science is indeed ready to address such challenging questions posed by developmental cognitive neuroscientists.

## Autistic spectrum disorders

Autism is a lifelong developmental disorder characterized by a broad spectrum of deficits in behavioral, social, and communication domains. As specified in the fourth edition of the *Diagnostic and Statistical Manual of Mental Disorders* (American Psychological Association, 1994), autistic disorder falls under the umbrella diagnosis of pervasive developmental disorders which includes: autistic disorder, Asperger's disorder, childhood disintegrative disorder, Rett's disorder, and pervasive developmental disorder — not otherwise specified. Although a growing trend among clinicians is to group these five diagnostic entities together on an autistic spectrum continuum, the present review will limit its discussions to autistic disorder (AD) unless otherwise noted.

Definitive diagnostic criteria for AD include deficits in social interaction, verbal and non-verbal communication, restrictive interests, and repetitive movements. Although these diagnostic criteria appear fairly simple and straightforward, the heterogeneity of AD behavioral phenotypes expressed across affected individuals is indicative of the complexity of neural interactions hypothesized to underlie AD symptomatology. Although numerous attempts to identify anatomical correlates of AD have not yet yielded unequivocal structural anomalies that are AD-specific, the varied experimental designs and methodologies employed in these studies limit the validity of cross-study comparisons. However, several key findings have proven to be replicable and serve as a useful reference point for discussion in the following review of physical, histological, and structural data pertaining to AD cohorts.

### Physical examination in AD

As reported in the literature, mean head circumference measurements are consistently larger in both children and adults diagnosed with AD relative to controls (Bailey, LeCouteur, Gottesman et al., 1995; Bailey, Luthert, Dean et al., 1998; Bolton, MacDonald, Pickles et al., 1994; Davidovitch, Patterson and Gartside, 1996; Lainhart, Piven, Wzorek et al., 1997; Miles, Hadden, Takahashi and Hillman, 2000; Skjeldal, Sponheim, Ganes et al., 1998; Woodhouse, Bailey, Rutter et al., 1996). Although relatively few cases exhibit frank macrocephaly (i.e. head circumference > 97th percentile), the distribution of head circumference measurements among AD cohorts are positively skewed with the majority of individuals placing above the 50th percentile of the normal range (Bailey et al., 1995; Bailey et al., 1998; Bolton et al., 1994; Davidovitch et al., 1996; Lainhart et al., 1997; Rapin, 1996; Woodhouse et al., 1996). However, current estimates, pooled across several studies, indicate that approximately 20% of autistic individuals are macrocephalic (Fombonne, Roge, Claverie et al., 1999). Furthermore, recent reports have indicated that rates of macrocephaly among AD cohorts as well as their first-degree relatives are significantly higher than rates of macrocephaly observed in normative samples (Fidler, Bailey and Smalley, 2000; Miles et al., 2000). These findings of enlarged head circumference values among AD cohorts are corroborated by independent reports of larger than average cerebral volume measurements in approximately 25% of AD individuals studied using aMRI neuroimaging methods (Filipek, Richelme, Kennedy and Caviness, 1992b; Piven, Arndt, Bailey et al., 1995; Piven, Arndt, Bailey and Andreasen, 1996). While the enlarged head circumference may not necessarily be present at birth, the trend does appear in early to mid-childhood (ages 1–12 years) among AD cohorts (Lainhart et al., 1997; Mason-Brothers, Ritvo, Guze et al., 1987; Mason-Brothers, Ritvo, Pingree et al., 1990). Thus, an interesting aim of future studies would be to investigate patterns of head growth in autistic populations from a longitudinal perspective. Such information should provide valuable insight into age(s) of onset of macrocephaly and indicate rates of growth as a function of age.

### Neurohistological findings in AD

Although relatively few comprehensive neuropathological studies have been completed on autistic brains, gross pathology does not appear to be a characteristic feature of the autistic brain. However, consistent with reports of enlarged head circumference measurements among AD cohorts detailed above, Bailey, Luthert, Bolton et al. (1993) and Bailey et al. (1998) described heavier-than-average brain weights in three out of five autistic adults and normal weights in the remaining two specimens. Similarly, Bauman and Kemper (1997) reported heavier-than-average brain weights (e.g. 100–200 g) in 11 specimens obtained from autistic children, aged 5–12 years. Further microscopic analyses of these same 11 specimens revealed enlarged neuronal cell size in the septum, deep cerebellar nuclei, and the inferior olive. Interestingly, Bauman and Kemper (1997) noted slightly less than average brain weights (e.g. 100–300 g) in specimens obtained from 8 autistic adults, aged 18 to 54 years. Upon further microscopic examination of these adult specimens, the authors reported decreased neuronal size and number in the same areas observed to have enlarged neurons in the children's specimens (i.e. septum, deep cerebellar nuclei, and inferior olive). Since a multitude of factors can contribute to the types of neurohistological changes described above, more neuropathological specimens from autistic individuals, both children and adults, are required for continued study.

Cytoarchitectural analyses of cerebral cortex in autistic brains have revealed limited mild abnormalities, principally confined to the anterior cingulate gyrus, without evidence for microscopic abnormalities in the basal forebrain, thalamus, hypothalamus, or basal ganglia (Bauman and Kemper, 1994). Similar analyses of limbic structures in autistic specimens have indicated a reduction in neuronal size and an increase in cell-packing density of neurons in the hippocampus, subiculum, entorhinal cortex, and amygdala (Bauman and Kemper, 1985). Additionally, Golgi analysis of CA4 and CA1 regions of the hippocampus in two childhood cases of AD revealed smaller area measurements of perikarya in CA4 neurons and decreased dendritic branching of both CA4 and CA1 neurons relative to age-matched controls (Raymond, Bauman and Kemper, 1996). Collectively, this line of neuropathological evidence for cellular morphological abnormalities in limbic structures of autis-

tic individuals highlights the need for additional studies. (See DeLong, 2003, in this volume for further discussion on hippocampal insufficiency in autism.)

Neurohistological analyses of cerebellar tissue from autistic brains have identified microscopic abnormalities in the cerebellar hemispheres. Specifically, the posterior inferior hemispheres were found to display a marked reduction (50–60%) in the number of Purkinje and granule cells that was not accompanied by any evidence of increased gliosis typically indicative of degenerative processes (Arin, Bauman and Kemper, 1991; Bauman and Kemper, 1985, 1986, 1988, 1994; Ritvo, Freeman, Scheibel et al., 1986; Williams, Hauser, Purpura et al., 1980). In the posterior vermis, a mild reduction (~25%) in counts of Purkinje cells has been reported without evidence for gross hypoplasia (Bauman and Kemper, 1994; Ritvo et al., 1986). Furthermore, no evidence of retrograde cell loss in the inferior olivary nuclei, which are typically associated with Purkinje cell loss, was observed (Bauman and Kemper, 1985, 1994). Yet, differences in cell morphology were noted in inferior olivary neurons of autistic samples relative to control samples, including small and pale appearance in the adult cases and slightly enlarged size in the child cases (Bauman and Kemper, 1985, 1994). Clearly, additional specimens for postmortem analyses are required to identify trends in neuropathology that appear to be AD-specific from those that are non-specific and unrelated to AD.

A particularly exciting direction for future neuropathological investigations that has not yet been pursued involves the application of immunohistochemical techniques to assess expression of various substances in autistic brains, including nerve growth factor and glial fibrillary acidic protein. Assays of these biochemical markers would enable investigators to characterize neuronal–glial interactions in autistic brains and evaluate whether they differ relative to normal controls. Given the rapidly accumulating evidence supporting a dynamically active relationship between neurons and glia, especially within the context of neural plasticity within the central nervous system, this line of research would add considerable depth to our current knowledge cultivated from neuropathological studies of autistic brains.

*Anatomical magnetic resonance imaging (aMRI) studies in AD*

*Cerebral volume*
Consistent with evidence from physical measurements of head circumference and neuropathological findings of increased brain weights, structural imaging studies have reported larger than average cerebral volumes using quantitative MRI-based morphometric methods (Filipek et al., 1992b; Piven et al., 1995, 1996). Additionally, these authors reported that the enlarged cerebral volumes in their AD cohorts were localized to temporal, parietal, and occipital regions. More specifically, as first reported by Filipek et al. (1992b), enlarged cerebral volumes were found to be principally due to increased white matter volumes in these areas since gray matter volumes were not significantly different relative to controls. Despite the generally accepted association between posterior temporal–parietal regions and the traditional language regions based on the adult model (Damasio and Damasio, 1989; Damasio and Frank, 1992; Heilman and Valenstein, 1985; Mesulam, 1985), the relationship between language deficits among AD cohorts and increased brain volumes in typical language areas is not so readily apparent. Indeed, it is difficult to sort direct from compensatory effects of neural developmental patterns in children with AD. While it is plausible for increased regional volumes to result from abnormal progressive or regressive histogenic mechanisms early in pre- or postnatal development (Filipek et al., 1992b), these effects may only be secondary to more central, and subtle, neurobiological mechanisms underlying AD symptomatology (Bailey et al., 1993). Clearly, additional neuroimaging studies are needed to capture patterns of structural development in early childhood of autistic and normal children. Thus, diffusion tensor imaging (DTI) studies designed to assess myelination patterns in small children (Bihan, Mangin, Poupon et al., 2001) may be appropriate at this time to identify age of onset and location(s) of aberrant development of white matter tracts within the autistic population. MRI-based DTI protocols consist of echoplanar imaging (EPI) pulse sequences to non-invasively provide microstructural information about white matter tracts that cannot be obtained using conventional T1- or T2-weighted imaging techniques.

Whereas T1- or T2-weighted images provide sufficient contrast for differentiating between gray and white matter, DTI has the powerful potential to ascertain the orientation and trajectory of white matter tracts. Thus, combined with functional imaging techniques, DTI is expected to significantly contribute to the development of a functional neuroanatomical atlas whereby the issue of connectivity is finally approachable using non-invasive techniques (Stieltjes, Kaufmann, van Zijl et al., 2001).

*Limbic structural volumes*
Subsequent to the first published reports of microscopic neuroanatomical differences in the limbic system of autistic individuals (Bauman, 1991; Bauman and Kemper, 1985, 1990, 1994), several neuroimaging studies have attempted to identify corroborating macroscopic differences in limbic structures of autistic individuals in vivo. However, quantitative cross-sectional area measurements of the posterior hippocampus, including the subiculum and the dentate gyrus, revealed similar values for AD subjects and controls (Saitoh, Courchesne, Egaas et al., 1995). Quantitative volumetric measurements of the amygdala and hippocampus also failed to identify significant differences between AD and control subjects (Filipek et al., 1992b; Piven, Bailey, Ranson and Arndt, 1998). Yet, a more recent aMRI volumetric study did report significantly smaller amygdala and hippocampal volumes in non-mentally retarded autistic adolescents and adults (Aylward, Minshew, Goldstein et al., 1999). As reported by these authors, the decreased volume of the amygdala in AD subjects was rather robust since the effect was evident irrespective of application of correction factors to adjust for inter-subject differences in total brain size. However, the volume reduction observed in the hippocampus of AD subjects was less pronounced since the effect was only observed after hippocampal volume had been corrected for total brain volume within each subject. Curiously, these authors failed to observe a significant difference in brain volume between autistic and control subjects.

Quantitative measurements of the corpus callosum among AD cohorts have yielded reasonably consistent results across research centers, despite different methodological approaches (see Fig. 1). Using a 5-segment division method for the corpus

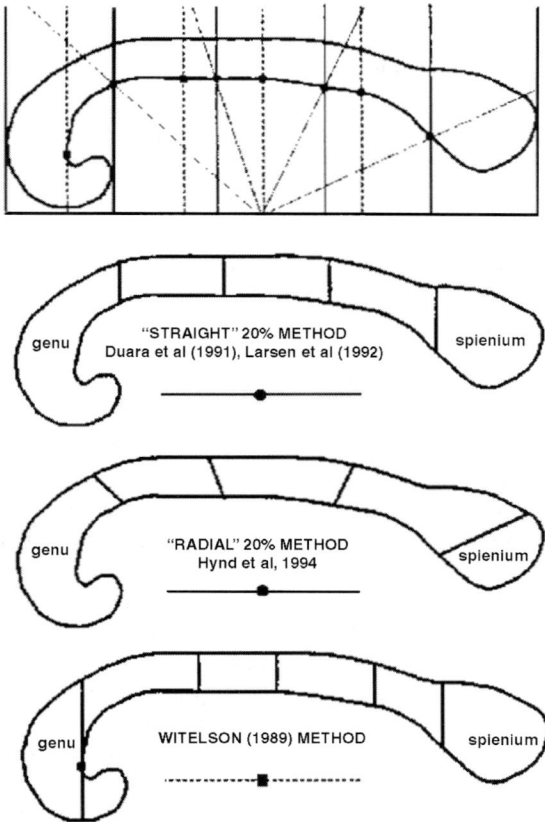

Fig. 1. Author's reconstruction of the three conventional methods used to subdivide the corpus callosum for morphometric analysis. Note the variable regional definitions leading to variable area measurements. The MRI studies in dyslexia that utilized theses methods are referenced within the figure. The method of Witelson (1989) generated the majority of the existing postmortem data in normal subjects.

callosum, Egaas et al. (1995) reported a significant reduction in cross-sectional areas of the posterior subregions 4 and 5. Their measurements were not corrected for inter-individual variations in total brain size. Using a 3-segment division method for quantifying area measurements of the corpus callosum, Piven, Bailey, Ranson and Arndt (1997a) reported a reduced size of the body and posterior subregions of the corpus callosum in their AD cohort relative to their control subjects. In this study, as well as in an earlier investigation by Filipek et al. (1992b), the decreased area measurements of posterior regions of the corpus callosum were evident

after the area measurements had been corrected for total brain size. Yet, a more recent study reported a significant reduction in the area of *anterior* regions of the corpus callosum as opposed to the posterior regions (Hardan, Minshew and Keshavan, 2000). Although these authors used a 7-segment division method for measurements of the corpus callosum, this difference would not be expected to account for the contradictory results. However, the authors themselves suggest that the severity of autism may not be comparable between subjects included in their study and the previous studies. Consequently, methodological differences in subject selection criteria may have contributed to these distinctly different findings. Despite these differences across studies, a featured result common to these studies is a reduction in area measurements of the corpus callosum in AD subjects (see Table 1). Thus, fewer interhemispheric myelinated fibers appear to be available for mediating interhemispheric communication between neural structures in the autistic population. Alternatively, the number of myelinated fibers may not be significantly reduced, but rather the fibers are more densely packed, thereby occupying less area.

*Basal ganglia volumes*

Relatively few MRI-based morphometric analyses of the basal ganglia in AD brains have been reported in the literature. While Filipek et al. (1992b) found lenticulate volumes to be significantly larger in autistic cohorts relative to control subjects, a subsequent study failed to observe any significant differences in lenticulate volumes between autistic and control subjects (Sears, Vest, Mohamed et al., 1999). However, this second study did report a significant increase in caudate volume in AD cohorts relative to control subjects. Thus, additional neuroimaging studies are required to determine whether changes in component structures of the basal ganglia are associated with AD. This line of research should prove to be particularly interesting given the behavioral overlap of symptoms associated with autism, obsessive–compulsive disorder, and Tourette syndrome (i.e. stereotyped, ritualistic, and repetitive behaviors).

*Cerebellar volume*

Dominating the scientific literature are hotly contested quantitative area measurements of the cerebel-

TABLE 1

Area measurements of the corpus callosum in autism

| Authors | Finding | Method |
|---|---|---|
| Egaas et al. (1995) | decreased posterior regions in autistics | 5 division |
| Piven et al. (1997a); Piven, Saliba, Bailey and Arndt (1997b) | decreased body and posterior regions in autistics | 3 division |
| Filipek et al. (1992a) | decreased posterior regions in autistics | 7 division |
| Hardan et al. (2000) | decreased anterior regions in autistics | 7 division |

lar vermis in AD cohorts. One group of investigators has reported a significant reduction in vermal lobules VI–VII in their autistic relative to nonautistic subjects (Courchesne, Hesselink, Jernigan and Yeung-Courchesne, 1987; Courchesne, Saitoh, Yeung-Courchesne et al., 1994; Courchesne, Yeung-Courchesne, Press et al., 1988). However, additional studies performed by other investigators have specifically reported no significant differences in measurements of vermal lobules VI–VII between AD and control subjects (Filipek et al., 1992b; Garber and Ritvo, 1992; Holttum, Minshew, Sanders and Phillips, 1992; Kleiman, Neff and Rosman, 1992; Levitt, Blanton, Capetillo-Cunliffe et al., 1999; Piven, Nehme, Simon et al., 1992; Piven et al., 1997b). Central to these controversial findings are methodological issues pertaining to study design (i.e. selection strategies of normal control groups for comparison with autistic groups) and data analysis (i.e. failure to account for confounding variables such as differences in IQ and gender between subject groups). Investigations that have adequately controlled for these variables have not been able to replicate the initial findings of AD-specific cerebellar hypoplasia by Courchesne and colleagues (for further review, see Filipek, 1999). In fact, area measurements of the cerebellar vermis in a patient population representative of a broad range of unrelated neurogenetic abnormalities revealed that hypoplasia of vermal lobules VI–VII frequently occurred in a variety of disorders (Schaefer, Thompson, Bodensteiner et al., 1996). Thus, the issue of whether cerebellar dysgenesis underlies the behavioral deficits associated with AD remains controversial. Future neuroimaging studies should recognize the need for IQ-matched autistic and control subjects for quantitative measurements of the cerebellar vermis.

## Developmental dyslexia

Along the continuum of language disorders, developmental dyslexia has received considerable attention in the scientific community. Specifically, developmental dyslexia is a reading disorder that affects approximately 5–10% of America's school-aged population (American Psychological Association, 1994; Eliez, Rumsey, Giedd et al., 2000; Shaywitz, Shaywitz, Fletcher and Escobar, 1990; Wadsworth, DeFries, Stevenson et al., 1992). Developmental dyslexia impacts both genders nearly equally, with some reports indicating a slightly male-biased ratio between 1.25 and 1.52 (Habib, 2000; Wadsworth et al., 1992). Although a spectrum of cognitive phenotypes constitutes a heterogeneous population of dyslexics, a commonly accepted definition for the disorder specifies a significant impairment in reading abilities, particularly single words, unexplainable by intelligence, sensory, or attentional deficits (Critchley, 1970; Grigorenko, 2001; Habib, 2000; World Health Organization, 1993). Central to the theoretical framework currently guiding empirical studies of developmental dyslexia are measurable deficits in phonological skills (Coltheart, Curtis, Atkins and Haller, 1993; Jorm, 1983; Shaywitz, 1998; Shaywitz, Shaywitz, Pugh et al., 1998; Torgesen, Wagner and Rashotte, 1994). However, the prevalence of co-morbid psychopathology, reportedly observed in approximately 20–30% of the dyslexic population (Hiemenz and Hynd, 2000; Hynd, Hall, Novey et al., 1995), complicates attempts to identify the underlying etiological factors that are specific to dyslexia and to determine the relative weight contributed by each factor to the expression of the disorder (for recent reviews, see Grigorenko, 2001; Habib, 2000). Based on results obtained from neuropathological investigations and in vivo neuroimaging studies completed over the last decade, the conceptualization of developmental dyslexia as a neurodevelopmental disorder is supported (Galaburda, 1993a; Hynd and Semrud-Clikeman, 1989). Furthermore, accumulating evidence indicates a contributory role for genetic influences in the etiology of dyslexia (Pennington, 1995; Pennington, Filipek, Lefly et al., 2000). As reviewed by Grigorenko (2001), three converging lines of evidence support the hypothesis that developmental dyslexia is heritable: (1) monozygotic and dizygotic twin studies (Bakwin, 1973; Cardon, Smith, Fulker et al., 1994; DeFries, Fulker and LaBuda, 1987; Pennington et al., 2000); (2) familial studies (Pennington, Gilger, Pauls et al., 1991; Smith, Pennington, Kimberling and Ing, 1990; Wolff and Melngailis, 1994); and (3) molecular–genetic studies (Cardon et al., 1994; Grigorenko, Wood, Meyer et al., 1997; Smith, Kimberling, Pennington and Lubs, 1983). Thus, substantial progress is being made toward determining the neurobiological bases of developmental dyslexia utilizing a multidisciplinary approach.

## Neuropathology in dyslexia

Remarkably few comprehensive postmortem studies of dyslexic brains have been completed in adults, let alone children. Overall, these studies have generated heightened interest in the planum temporale. The planum temporale is a triangular-shaped area located on the posterior aspect of the superior surface of the temporal lobes, just posterior to Heschl's gyrus, and is thus thought to serve a role in mediating receptive language function. The first postmortem analyses of plana in a normal population of adult brains indicated hemispheric asymmetry with a leftward bias (left > right) in approximately 65% of the normal subjects studied (Geschwind and Levitsky, 1968). Interestingly, such hemispheric asymmetry in plana size was conspicuously absent in postmortem analyses of dyslexic brains (Galaburda, Sherman, Rosen et al., 1985; Humphreys, Kaufman and Galaburda, 1990). In fact, 100% of dyslexic specimens studied by Galaburda et al. (1985) and Humphreys et al. (1990) reportedly exhibited symmetrical plana whereas only 24% of normal specimens were found by Geschwind and Levitsky (1968) to display symmetrical plana. However, subsequent studies have identified handedness to be a confounding variable that influences

symmetrical distribution of the planum temporale in adults (Foundas, Leonard and Heilman, 1995; Steinmetz, Volkmann, Jancke and Freund, 1991). These authors reported that left-handedness is associated with symmetrical plana or asymmetrical plana with a reversed bias (i.e. rightward; right > left). As discussed by Eliez et al. (2000), the dyslexic sample studied by Galaburda et al. (1985) and Humphreys et al. (1990) consisted of several left-handed individuals, thereby limiting the conclusions drawn from those studies since symmetrical plana might be related to handedness rather than diagnosis of dyslexia. Thus, given the constraints imposed by autopsy investigations, mainly rarity of specimens available for study, in vivo neuroimaging studies have engendered great enthusiasm, providing researchers with opportunities to evaluate fine structural details in well-defined subject populations.

## aMRI in dyslexia

Since the planum temporale is not readily defined by distinct anatomical boundaries, numerous constructs have emerged across research groups for defining this region in their quantitative neuroimaging studies (Filipek, 1995a; Filipek et al., 1992a; Galaburda, 1988, 1993b; Green, Hutsler, Loftus et al., 1999; Westbury, Zatorre and Evans, 1999). Additionally, some groups have used surface area (Galaburda, 1993a; Green et al., 1999; Larsen, Hoien, Lundberg and Odegaard, 1990; Rumsey, Donohue, Brady et al., 1997; Schultz, Cho, Staib et al., 1994), while others have used units of length for their measurements (Hynd, Semrud-Clikeman, Lorys et al., 1990; Leonard, Voeller, Lombardion et al., 1993). Furthermore, similar to the neuropathological investigations described above, not all neuroimaging experimental designs have included strict controls for handedness in their subject populations. Consequently, cross-study comparisons have limited interpretive value given the heterogeneity of definitions, methods of measurement, and subject selection criteria. Thus, the literature is split between reports on the planum temporale in dyslexics; some reports supporting the initial neuropathological findings relating atypical symmetry (Galaburda, 1993a; Larsen et al., 1990) or reversed asymmetry (Hynd et al., 1990), while others report no such significant differences in planum measurements between their dyslexic and normal control subjects (Rumsey et al., 1997; Schultz et al., 1994). Furthermore, Hiemenz and Hynd (2000) recently reported a lack of an association between sulcal morphology and developmental dyslexia in their evaluation of the caudal perisylvian region in dyslexic, ADHD, and control children between 8 and 12 years of age.

Another structure that has received considerable attention is the corpus callosum, mainly because of its role in mediating interhemispheric communication. This interest in the corpus callosum has emerged from numerous studies in which impaired interhemispheric transfer of sensory or motor information has been observed in dyslexic relative to control subjects (Best, 1985; Gladstone, Best and Davidson, 1989; Gross-Glenn and Rothenberg, 1984; Markee, Brown and Moore, 1996; Moore, Brown, Markee et al., 1995). However, quantitative measurements of midsagittal area of the corpus callosum in neuroimaging studies have yielded inconsistent results (see Table 2). While total callosal area was reportedly larger only in female adult dyslexics relative to age-matched controls, the posterior (splenial) region was found to be larger in both male and female adult dyslexics, many of whom were co-diagnosed with ADHD (Duara, Kushch, Gross-Glenn et al., 1991). Similarly, Rumsey, Casanova, Mannheim et al. (1996) reported a significantly larger posterior region of the corpus callosum, including the isthmus and splenium, in adult male dyslexics relative to control subjects matched for gender, age, handedness, socioeconomic status, and IQ. However, Hynd et al. (1995) failed to observe a group difference between dyslexic and age-matched controls in the posterior region of the corpus callosum in young children. Instead, these authors reported significantly smaller area measurements of the anterior region of the corpus callosum, the genu, in dyslexic relative to control subjects. Conversely, Larsen, Hoien and Odegaard (1992) reported no significant differences in their area measurements of the corpus callosum in dyslexic relative to control adolescents. Thus, these authors reported that total area and regional areas (genu or splenium) were similar in both dyslexic and control adolescents. More recently, using a twin-pair design, Pennington, Filipek, Lefly et al. (1999) also reported no significant group differences in mid-sagittal area measurements of the corpus callosum in dyslexic and control adolescents.

These highly varied results across research groups are indicative of the equally varied methodologies employed. Each of the studies summarized above are composed of subjects differing in age ranges, from adults to adolescents to children. Each study utilized different methodologies for delineating subregional boundaries of the corpus callosum in their midsagittal area measurements (see Fig. 1), ranging from an equal linear thirds method (Rumsey et al., 1996) to a 'straight' 20% method (Duara et al., 1991; Larsen et al., 1992) to a 'radial' 20% method (Hynd et al., 1995) to the Witelson method (Pennington et al., 1999). Since these methodologies yield non-equivalent subdivisions of the corpus callosum across research groups, cross-study comparisons are severely limited in their interpretive value. The interested reader is referred to reviews by Filipek (1995a) and Hynd and Semrud-Clikeman (1989) for more comprehensive discussions of this issue.

Morphometric analyses of neocortical regions and subcortical structures in adolescent twin pairs with and without developmental dyslexia (Pennington et al., 1999) revealed a significant interaction between diagnosis for dyslexia and neocortical regions, but not for subcortical structures. Specifically, volumetric measurements of the insula and anterior superior neocortex were significantly smaller in the dyslexic cohort while the retrocallosal cortex was larger relative to control subjects without dyslexia. The notable strengths of this study by Pennington et al. (1999) include twin-pair design, large sample size ($n = 75$ dyslexic and $n = 22$ control individuals), large number of structures quantified ($n = 13$), and appropriate control of confounds such as age, gender, handedness, and IQ. A decreased insula length (bilaterally) in dyslexic cohorts has also been observed by Hynd et al. (1990). Additionally, Eliez et al. (2000) recently reported a significant reduction in tissue volume localized to the temporal lobes, with an especially prominent decrease in gray matter on the left side, in dyslexic male adults relative to controls matched for age, gender, handedness, IQ, educational level, and socioeconomic status. Collectively, these results suggest neocortical development is altered subtly, yet to a measurable degree, and observable in dyslexic adults and adolescents.

TABLE 2

Area measurements of the corpus callosum in dyslexia

| Authors | Finding | Method |
|---------|---------|--------|
| Duara et al. (1991) | increased posterior region in dyslexics | 5 division |
| Rumsey et al. (1996) | increased posterior region in dyslexics | 3 division |
| Hynd et al. (1995) | decreased anterior region in dyslexics | 5 division |
| Larsen et al. (1992) | no significant difference | 5 division |
| Pennington et al. (1999) | no significant difference | 7 division |

## Attention deficit–hyperactivity disorder (ADHD)

ADHD is a childhood developmental disorder characterized by behavioral symptoms indicative of disruptions in attention, impulsivity, and activity level. Although prevalence estimates have been difficult to ascertain, epidemiological studies have reported that approximately 3–5% of school-aged children in the United States are affected with ADHD (American Psychological Association, 1994; Swanson, Sergeant, Taylor et al., 1998). More recently published estimates suggest that the prevalence of ADHD may actually fall between two and three times this commonly reported 3–5% prevalence estimate (Paule, Rowland, Ferguson et al., 2000). At least part of the difficulty in capturing this information can be attributed to problems with applying diagnostic criteria, as outlined in American Psychological Association (1994), in a clinical setting (Cantwell, 1996). For instance, expression of ADHD behavior is unpredictable, often context-sensitive, and frequently associated with other disorders. Furthermore, behavioral symptoms of ADHD are commonly dismissed or tolerated without seeking a professional's assessment, as parents believe their children will simply 'grow out of it'. Consequently, many cases of ADHD in children are never diagnosed (Cantwell, 1996; Swanson et al., 1998).

Investigative attempts to determine the neurobiological bases of ADHD are currently driven by neural network theories of attention that encompass the following perspectives: biochemical, neuroanatomical, and genetic. As postulated by Posner and Petersen (1990) and Posner and Raichle (1994), neural networks underlying attention can be described in terms of three major functions of attention: (1) orienting (selective) attention network for orienting to sensory stimuli, especially visual cues; (2) alerting (vigilance) attention network for maintaining an alert state for sustained attention; (3) executive network for control of goal-directed behavior. Within this context of formulating distinct functions of attention, localization of distinct neural networks subserving each function of attention has been a specific aim best addressed by neuroimaging, neuropharmacological, and lesion analysis studies. Thus, functional neuroimaging studies have indicated that the orienting network of attention is localized to posterior parietal lobules, thalamus, and midbrain (Corbetta, 1998; Posner and Dahaene, 1994). Pharmacological (Marrocco and Davidson, 1998) and lesion analysis studies (Robertson, Manly, Beschin et al., 1997) have suggested that the alerting network of attention is localized to the right lateral prefrontal lobe, right parietal lobe, and the locus coeruleus (Posner and Petersen, 1990; Posner and Raichle, 1994). Functional neuroimaging studies have indicated that the executive network of attention function is localized to the anterior cingulate gyrus, supplemental motor area, and portions of the basal ganglia (Bush, Frazier, Rauch et al., 1999; Posner and DiGirolamo, 1998). As reviewed in the following section, numerous aMRI studies on children with ADHD have revealed volumetric differences in various brain regions that may correlate with this diagnosis, especially those regions associated with fronto-striatal pathways, including prefrontal cortical–striatal–pallidal neural circuitry.

### aMRI in ADHD

#### Brain volume

Relative to normal controls, the volumes of the cerebral hemispheres have been reported to be approximately 5% smaller in subjects with ADHD (Castellanos, Giedd, Eckburg et al., 1994; Castellanos, Giedd, Marsh et al., 1996). An additional study by Berquin, Giedd, Jacobsen et al. (1998) found a significant reduction in total cerebral volume in the ADHD cohort relative to controls that no longer reached significance when scores from vocabulary IQ tests were factored into the analyses as a covariate. Since a positive correlation between IQ and brain volume has been reported (Reiss, Abrams, Singer et al., 1996), one must critically evaluate the experimental design and methodologies employed for each neuroimaging study when interpreting the results. In a subsequent study by Filipek, Semrud-Clikeman, Steingard et al. (1997), subject criteria carefully controlled for age, gender, handedness, and IQ of ADHD and control cohorts. Additionally, unlike the previous studies, these ADHD subjects were carefully screened and excluded from the study for co-morbid diagnoses. Although Filipek et al. (1997) did not observe a significant global reduction in cerebral hemispheric volume, a significant decrease in global white matter volume, predominately localized to the right frontal region, was observed in subjects with ADHD. This observation is particularly interesting given the proposed role for the right frontal region in the alerting network of attention and working memory (Posner and Petersen, 1990; Posner and Raichle, 1994; Smith and Jonides, 1999).

## Basal ganglia

### Caudate

Inconsistent findings have emerged across aMRI studies quantifying measurements of the caudate in ADHD and control cohorts. While some studies have reported the left caudate to be smaller than the right in ADHD subjects (Filipek et al., 1997; Hynd, Hern, Novey et al., 1993), other researchers have found a reversed asymmetry such that the right caudate was smaller than the left in ADHD subjects (Castellanos et al., 1994; Castellanos et al., 1996). While one study failed to observe any asymmetry in caudate volumes of children with ADHD (Aylward, Reiss, Reader et al., 1996), another study found larger right caudate areas in adolescent ADHD subjects relative to controls (Mataro, Garcia-Sanchez, Junque et al., 1997). Interestingly, in a sample of girls with ADHD,

Castellanos, Giedd, Berquin et al. (2001) recently reported symmetrical caudate volumes where the total caudate volume was found to be significantly smaller relative to controls, principally due to a smaller left caudate volume in the girls with ADHD. Collectively, these results fail to unambiguously identify a common structural variation specific to ADHD. However, despite the discrepancies, these results do implicate an etiological basis for the caudate in the expression of ADHD. Therefore, future volumetric studies are warranted in which age, gender, IQ, and co-morbid diagnoses are properly controlled in the experimental design. Furthermore, anatomical definition (i.e. head of the caudate vs. head and body and tail of the caudate) and quantitative methodology (i.e. area vs. 3-D volumetrics) should be operationalized and codified to yield comparable results across research centers.

### Pallidum

In aMRI studies, the globus pallidus is generally quantified as a single unit, including both lateral and medial segments without distinction between the two segments. Even so, measurements of the pallidum are not made without difficulty. Aylward et al. (1996) found male subjects with ADHD to have significantly smaller total volumes of the pallidum measured globally (i.e. bilaterally) with a predominate decrease in the left pallidum relative to control subjects. In contrast, Castellanos et al. (1996) reported smaller right pallidum volumes in ADHD subjects relative to controls. However, as noted by Castellanos et al. (1996), their measurements were limited to only a portion of the pallidum, thereby using an anatomical definition of the pallidum that differed from Aylward et al. (1996).

### Corpus callosum

Area measurements of the corpus callosum in aMRI studies have yielded inconsistent results (see Table 3). Although measures of total corpus callosum area have not significantly differed between ADHD and control subjects, area differences in regional subdivisions of the corpus callosum have been noted by several research groups (Baumgardner, Singer, Denckla et al., 1996; Castellanos et al., 1996; Giedd, Castellanos, Casey et al., 1994; Hynd, Semrud-Clikeman, Lorys et

TABLE 3

Area measurements of the corpus callosum in ADHD

| Authors | Finding | Method |
|---|---|---|
| Hynd et al. (1991) | decreased anterior and posterior regions in ADHD | 5 division |
| Semrud-Clikeman et al. (1994) | decreased posterior regions in ADHD | 7 division |
| Giedd et al. (1994) | decreased anterior regions in ADHD | 7 division |
| Baumgardner et al. (1996) | decreased anterior regions in ADHD | 5 division |
| Castellanos et al. (1996) | no significant difference | 7 division |

al., 1991; Semrud-Clikeman, Filipek, Biederman et al., 1994). Generally, reduced area measurements of corpus callosum subdivisions have been reported in ADHD subjects. However, the specific subregions of the corpus callosum that were significantly reduced between ADHD and control subjects in each of these studies varied from anterior segments (Baumgardner et al., 1996; Giedd et al., 1994) to posterior segments (Semrud-Clikeman et al., 1994) to both anterior and posterior segments (Hynd et al., 1991). Conversely, Castellanos et al. (1996) reported no significant differences in any subregional area of the corpus callosum between ADHD and control subjects. As discussed by Filipek (1995b), cross-study comparisons such as these have limited interpretive value given the diverse methodologies employed for performing quantitative measurements. Fundamentally, boundary delineations of subregional sections of the corpus callosum qualitatively differed across studies due to the implementation of a 5-division method (Baumgardner et al., 1996; Hynd et al., 1991) and a 7-division method (Castellanos et al., 1996; Giedd et al., 1994; Semrud-Clikeman et al., 1994). Additionally, inclusion or exclusion of ADHD subjects with co-morbid diagnoses, heterogeneity of ADHD severity, and non-uniformity of image acquisition protocols would all be expected to contribute to inter-study variability of results. Yet, interestingly, reductions in area measurements from the anterior segments of the corpus callosum in ADHD subjects noted above are consistent with reports of decreased right frontal volumes in ADHD subjects (Castellanos et al., 1996; Filipek et al., 1997). Taken together, these structural findings are consistent with the proposed role for the right frontal region in the attentional network hypothesis by Posner and Petersen (1990) and Posner and Raichle (1994).

*Functional magnetic resonance imaging (fMRI) in the developmental disorders*

Due to its non-invasive nature and lack of ionizing radiation, fMRI provides an unprecedented opportunity to investigate functional brain state changes in normal and developmentally disordered children. The fundamental principles of fMRI enable investigators to examine brain state changes based on blood oxygenation level dependent (BOLD) contrast. Due to inherent differences in paramagnetic properties of oxygenated and deoxygenated hemoglobin, changes in MR signal intensity can be captured and evaluated as a function of local blood flow changes associated with increased neural activity (Buxton and Frank, 1997). Whereas oxygenated blood yields greater MR signal intensity than deoxygenated blood, local changes in neural activity can be indirectly observed (Cohen and Bookheimer, 1994).

Although the application of fMRI to research investigations of developmental disorders is still in its infancy, combined with aMRI, this experimental approach promises to expand our current understanding of neurological changes underlying normal and abnormal brain development throughout childhood and adolescence. Whereas previous functional neuroimaging studies were necessarily limited to adult-based populations due to a requisite exposure to ionizing radiation, the advent of fMRI provides us with an opportunity to investigate developmental disorders in pediatric-aged cohorts. Thus, the number of pediatric studies utilizing fMRI is expected to rise over the next few years, especially in the areas of dyslexia and ADHD where school-aged children can be sufficiently cooperative (See Lovett and Barron, 2003, in this volume for further discussion of fMRI and dyslexia in children).

Currently, the application of fMRI to investigations of AD is hampered by methodological constraints associated with fMRI for acquiring adequate image quality. Such constraints include the need for the child to lie still while fully awake and follow directions as well as the ability to remain calm during the scanning procedure. Consequently, fMRI investigations of cognitive function in autism have been few and limited to high-functioning adolescents or adults (Baron-Cohen, Ring, Wheelwright et al., 1999; Ring, Baron-Cohen, Wheelwright et al., 1999; Schultz, Gauthier, Klin et al., 2000). Therefore, results from these studies should not be extrapolated to children or generalized to all autistic phenotypes. As reviewed by Rumsey and Ernst (2000), these initial reports should be viewed as exploratory as they clearly highlight the need for further study. Yet, these investigations have provided preliminary evidence supporting various hypotheses of anatomically distinct regions underlying behavioral symptoms associated with AD.

Given the characteristic social deficits exhibited by individuals diagnosed with AD, social information processing has been a key interest of the relatively few fMRI studies performed to date on AD subjects. Schultz et al. (2000) used fMRI to investigate patterns of brain activity during perceptual discrimination tasks between faces or objects in high-functioning adult subjects diagnosed with AD or Asperger's syndrome relative to control subjects matched for age, gender, IQ and handedness. Interestingly, increased activity in the inferior temporal gyrus was exhibited during perceptual processing of faces in the autistic group and during perceptual processing of objects in the controls. These results support other lines of evidence suggesting that autistic subjects perceptually evaluate faces as though they were objects by performing better than expected on recognition tasks with inverted faces (Tantam, Monaghan, Nicholson and Stirling, 1989). Whereas normal face perception is typically a holistic process, an inverted face perceptual task is predominately driven by feature-based object analysis (Hobson, Ouston and Lee, 1988; Langdell, 1978). A separate study by Baron-Cohen et al. (1999) reported adult subjects diagnosed with autism or Asperger's disorder demonstrated different patterns of relative brain activity compared to control subjects while performing

a Theory of Mind task requiring judgment of mental state from photographs of eyes. Specifically, the autistic group exhibited greater activity in the superior temporal gyrus, reduced activity in prefrontal regions, and a notable absence of activity in the amygdala. Ring et al. (1999) also reported differences in regional activation patterns in high-functioning adult autistic subjects during an Embedded Figures Task (EFT). Relative to control subjects, the autistic group exhibited more activity in the right ventral occipitotemporal region, an area implicated in object perception and visual imagery (Kosslyn, Thompson, Kim and Alpert, 1995; Ungerleider, Courtney and Haxby, 1998). Additionally, Ring et al. (1999) found their autistic group exhibited less activity relative to controls in parietal and dorsolateral prefrontal cortices, areas that have been implicated in spatial relations and working memory for objects (Smith and Jonides, 1995). Whether these phenomena characterize young children or individuals across the AD spectrum has yet to be investigated.

## Summary and future directions

As a progressive research field, neuroimaging in childhood developmental disorders continues to evolve as technological advances lead the way to more sophisticated levels of analyses. Such advances in technology have facilitated our ability to investigate normal patterns of brain growth and maturation of structural parameters in well-designed aMRI studies of developing children. These characterizations of normal child development provide an essential context for studies focused on determining the etiology of children's developmental disorders. As new neuroimaging techniques continue to emerge and gain momentum in their application to research investigations, especially fMRI and DTI, we collectively find ourselves gaining a more comprehensive and integrative understanding of brain anatomy and function in developing children. The development of consistent study protocols that can be implemented across research centers greatly facilitates this integrative process since results can be directly compared between studies. Such cooperative efforts significantly increase the power of our analyses since small sample sizes are frequently associated with any individual research center.

Over the next decade, exciting discoveries will undoubtedly transform the field as the science of pediatric neuroimaging in the developmental disorders continues to mature. Given the safe and non-invasive methodology of MRI studies that can be completed within a reasonable imaging time for small children, multiple scanning sessions can be used to follow individual children through the course of therapeutic intervention. Monitoring structural and functional cortical changes as an outcome measure of interventional treatment is an intriguing area for basic research that may eventually impact clinical practices in the developmental disorders (Casey, Thomas and McCandliss, 2001). The future is filled with many possibilities as we continue to experimentally address challenging questions about cortical development and behavior. While we seek to understand differences in brain structure and function as they relate to developmental disorders in children, we proceed with the expectation of discovering not only the neurobiological causes but also sound and effective interventional strategies.

# References

Alpert N, Bradshaw J, Kennedy D, Correia J: The principle axis transformation — A method for image registration. Journal of Nuclear Medicine: 31; 1717–1722, 1990.

Arin D, Bauman M, Kemper TL: The distribution of Purkinje cell loss in the cerebellum in autism. Neurology: 41; 307, 1991.

American Psychological Association: Diagnostic and Statistical Manual of Mental Disorders. 4th ed., Washington, D.C., 1994.

Aylward E, Minshew N, Goldstein G, Honeycutt N, Augustine A, Yates K, Barta P, Pearlson G: MRI volumes of amygdala and hippocampus in non-mentally retarded autistic adolescents and adults. Neurology: 53; 2145–2150, 1999.

Aylward E, Reiss AL, Reader M, Singer HS, Brown J, Denckla MB: Basal ganglia volumes in children with attention-deficit hyperactivity disorder. Journal of Child Neurology: 11; 112–115, 1996.

Bailey A, LeCouteur A, Gottesman I, Bolton P, Simonoff E, Yuzda E, Rutter M: Autism as a strongly genetic disorder: Evidence from a British twin study. Psychological Medicine: 25; 63–77, 1995.

Bailey A, Luthert P, Bolton P, LeCouteur A, Rutter M, Harding B: Autism and megalencephaly. Lancet: 341; 1225–1226, 1993.

Bailey A, Luthert P, Dean A, Harding B, Janota I, Montgomery M, Rutter M, Lantos P: A clinicopathological study of autism. Brain: 121; 899–905, 1998.

Bakwin H: Reading disability in twins. Developmental Medicine and Child Neurology: 15; 184–187, 1973.

Baron-Cohen S, Ring H, Wheelwright S, Bullmore E, Brammer M, Simmons A, Williams S: Social intelligence in the normal and autistic brain: an fMRI study. European Journal of Neuroscience: 11; 1891–1898, 1999.

Bauman M: Microscopic neuroanatomic abnormalities in autism. Pediatrics: 87; 791–796, 1991.

Bauman M, Kemper T: Histoanatomic observations of the brain in early infantile autism. Neurology: 35; 866–874, 1985.

Bauman M, Kemper TL: Developmental cerebellar abnormalities. A consistent finding in early infantile autism (Abstract). Neurology: 36; 190, 1986.

Bauman M, Kemper TL: Limbic and cerebellar abnormalities: Consistent findings in infantile autism (Abstract). Journal of Neuropathology and Experimental Neurology: 47; 369, 1988.

Bauman M, Kemper TL: Limbic and cerebellar abnormalities are also present in an autistic child of normal intelligence (Abstract). Neurology: 40; 359, 1990.

Bauman M, Kemper T: Neuroanatomic observations of the brain in autism. In Bauman M, Kemper T (Eds), The Neurobiology of Autism. Baltimore, MD: Johns Hopkins University Press, pp. 119–145, 1994.

Bauman M, Kemper T: Is autism a progressive process? (Abstract). Neurology Suppl: A285, 1997.

Baumgardner T, Singer HS, Denckla MB, Rubin M, Abrams M, Colli M, Reiss AL: Corpus callosum morphology in children with Tourette syndrome and attention deficit hyperactivity disorder. Neurology: 47; 477–482, 1996.

Berquin P, Giedd J, Jacobsen L, Hamburger S, Krain A, Rapoport J, Castellanos FX: Cerebellum in attention-deficit hyperactivity disorder: A morphometric MRI study. Neurology: 50; 1087–1093, 1998.

Best C: Hemispheric Function and Collaboration in the Child. Orlando, FL: Academic Press, 1985.

Bihan D, Mangin J, Poupon C, Clark C, Pappata S, Molko N, Chabriat H: Diffusion tensor imaging: concepts and applications. Journal of Magnetic Resonance Imaging: 13; 534–546, 2001.

Bolton P, MacDonald H, Pickles A, Rios P, Goode S, Crowson M, Bailey A, Rutter M: A case-control family history study of autism. Journal of Child Psychology and Psychiatry and Allied Disciplines: 35; 877–900, 1994.

Bush G, Frazier J, Rauch S, Seidman L, Whalen P, Jenike M, Rosen B, Biederman J: Anterior cingulate cortex dysfunction in attention/hyperactivity disorder revealed by fMRI and the counting stroop. Biological Psychiatry: 45; 1542–1552, 1999.

Buxton R, Frank L: A model for the coupling between cerebral blood flow and oxygen metabolism during neural stimulation. Journal of Cerebral Blood Flow and Metabolism: 17; 64–72, 1997.

Cantwell D: Attention deficit disorder: A review of the past 10 years. Journal of American Academy of Child Adolescent Psychiatry: 35; 978–987, 1996.

Cardon L, Smith S, Fulker D, Kimberling W, Pennington B, DeFries J: Quantitative trait locus for reading disability on chromosome 6. Science: 266; 276–279, 1994.

Casey B, Thomas K, McCandliss B: Applications of magnetic resonance imaging to the study of development. In: Handbook of Developmental Cognitive Neuroscience (Johnson M, Pennington B, eds), pp 137–147. Cambridge, MA: MIT Press, 2001.

Castellanos F, Giedd J, Berquin P, Walter J, Sharp W, Tran T, Vaituzis A, Blumenthal J, Nelson J, Bastain T, Zijdenbos A, Evans AC, Rapoport J: Quantitative brain magnetic resonance imaging in girls with attention-deficit/hyperactivity disorder. Archives of General Psychiatry: 58; 289–295, 2001.

Castellanos FX, Giedd JN, Eckburg P, Marsh W, Vaituzis A, Kaysen D, Hamburger S, Rapoport J: Quantitative morphology of the caudate nucleus in attention deficit hyperactivity disorder. Am J Psychiatry: 151; 1791–1796, 1994.

Castellanos FX, Giedd JN, Marsh W, Hamburger S, Vaituzis A, Dickstein D, Sarfatti S, Vauss Y, Snell J, Lange N, Kaysen D, Krain A, Ritchie G, Rajapaske J, Rapoport J: Quantitative brain magnetic resonance imaging in attention-deficit hyperactivity disorder. Archives of General Psychiatry: 53; 607–616, 1996.

Cohen M, Bookheimer S: Localization of brain function using Magnetic Resonance Imaging. Trends in Neurosciences: 17; 268–277, 1994.

Collins D, Neelin P, Peters T, Evans A: Automatic 3D intersubject registration of MR volumetric data in standardized talairach space. Journal of Computer Assisted Tomography: 18; 192–205, 1994.

Coltheart M, Curtis B, Atkins P, Haller M: Models of reading aloud: Dual-route and parallel- distributed-processing approaches. Psychological Review: 100; 580–608, 1993.

Corbetta M: Frontoparietal cortical networks for directing attention and the eye to visual locations: Identical, independent, or overlapping neural systems? Proceedings of the National Academy of Science, USA: 95; 831–838, 1998.

Courchesne E, Hesselink J, Jernigan T, Yeung-Courchesne R: Abnormal neuroanatomy in a non-retarded person with autism. Unusual findings with magnetic resonance imaging. Archives of Neurology: 44; 335–341, 1987.

Courchesne E, Saitoh O, Yeung-Courchesne R, Press G, Lincoln A, Haas R, Schreibman L: Abnormalities of cerebellar vermian lobules VI and VII in patients with infantile autism: Identification of hypoplastic and hyperplastic subgroups by MR imaging. American Journal of Roentgenology: 162; 123–130, 1994.

Courchesne E, Yeung-Courchesne R, Press G, Hesselink J, Jernigan T: Hypoplasia of cerebellar vermal lobules VI and VII in autism. New England Journal of Medicine: 318; 1349–1354, 1988.

Critchley M: The Dyslexic Child, 2nd Edition. London: Heinemann Medical, 1970.

Damasio H, Damasio A: Lesion Analysis in Neuropsychology. New York: Oxford University Press, 1989.

Damasio A, Frank R: Three-dimensional in vivo mapping of brain lesions in humans. Archives of Neurology: 49; 137–143, 1992.

Davidovitch M, Patterson B, Gartside P: Head circumference measurements in children with autism. Journal of Child Neurology: 11; 389–393, 1996.

DeFries J, Fulker D, LaBuda M: Evidence for a genetic aetiology in reading disability in twins. Nature: 329; 537–539, 1987.

DeLong GR: Disorders of memory in childhood with a focus on temporal lobe disease and autism. In Segalowitz SJ, Rapin I (Eds), Child Neuropsychology, Handbook of Neuropsychology, 2nd Edition, vol. 8, part II. Amsterdam: Elsevier, chapter 27, 2003.

Duara R, Kushch A, Gross-Glenn K, Barker W, Jallad B, Pascal S: Neuroanatomic differences between dyslexic and normal readers on magnetic resonance imaging scans. Archives of Neurology: 48; 410–416, 1991.

Egaas B, Courchesne E, Saitoh O: Reduced size of corpus callosum in autism. Archives of Neurology: 52; 794–801, 1995.

Eliez S, Rumsey J, Giedd J, Schmitt J, Patwardhan A, Reiss A: Morphological alteration of temporal lobe gray matter in dyslexia: An MRI study. Journal of Child Psychology and Psychiatry and Allied Disciplines: 41; 637–644, 2000.

Fidler D, Bailey J, Smalley S: Macrocephaly in autism and other pervasive developmental disorders. Developmental Medicine and Child Neurology: 42; 737–740, 2000.

Filipek PA: Neurobiological correlates of developmental dyslexia — What do we know about how the dyslexics' brains differ from those of normal readers? Journal of Child Neurology 10: S62–69, 1995a.

Filipek PA: Quantitative magnetic resonance imaging in autism: The cerebellar vermis. Current Opinion in Neurology: 8; 134–138, 1995b.

Filipek PA: Brief report: Neuroimaging in autism: The state of the science 1995. Journal of Autism and Developmental Disorders: 26; 211–215, 1996.

Filipek PA: Neuroimaging in the developmental disorders: The state of the science. Journal of Child Psychology and Psychiatry and Allied Disciplines: 40; 113–128, 1999.

Filipek PA, Kennedy DN, Caviness VS: Neuroimaging in child neuropsychology. In Rapin I, Segalowitz S (Eds), Handbook of Neuropsychology. Amsterdam: Elsevier Science Publishers, pp. 301–329, 1992a.

Filipek PA, Richelme C, Kennedy DN, Caviness VS: Morphometric analysis of the brain in developmental language disorders and autism (Abstract). Annals of Neurology: 32; 475, 1992b.

Filipek PA, Semrud-Clikeman M, Steingard RJ, Renshaw PF, Kennedy DN, Biederman J: Volumetric MRI analysis comparing subjects having attention-deficit hyperactivity disorder with normal controls. Neurology: 48; 589–601, 1997.

Fombonne E, Roge B, Claverie J, Courty S, Fremolle J: Microcephaly and macrocephaly in autism. Journal of Autism and Developmental Disorders: 29; 113–119, 1999.

Foundas A, Leonard C, Heilman KM: Morphological cerebral asymmetries and handedness. The pars triangularis and planum temporale. Archives of Neurology: 52; 501–508, 1995.

Galaburda A: The pathogenesis of childhood dyslexia. Association for Research in Nervous Mental Disorders: 66; 127–138, 1988.

Galaburda A: Neuroanatomic basis of developmental dyslexia. Neurologic Clinics: 11; 161–173, 1993a.

Galaburda A: The planum temporale. (Editorial). Archives of Neurology: 50; 457, 1993b.

Galaburda A, Sherman G, Rosen G, Aboitiz F, Geschwind N: Developmental dyslexia: Four consecutive patients with cortical anomalies. Annals of Neurology: 18; 222–233, 1985.

Garber H, Ritvo E: Magnetic resonance imaging of the posterior fossa in autistic adults. American Journal of Psychiatry: 149; 245–247, 1992.

Geschwind N, Levitsky W: Human brain: Left–right asymmetry in temporal speech region. Science: 161; 186–187, 1968.

Giedd JN, Blumenthal J, Jeffries NO, Castellanos FX, Liu H, Zijdenbos A, Paus T, Evans AC, Rapoport J: Brain development during childhood and adolescence: A longitudinal MRI study. Nature Neuroscience: 2; 861–863, 1999.

Giedd JN, Castellanos FX, Casey BJ, Kozuch P, King A, Hamburger S, Rapoport J: Quantitative morphology of the corpus callosum in attention deficit hyperactivity disorder. American Journal of Psychiatry: 151; 665–669, 1994.

Giedd JN, Rapoport J, Leonard HL, Richter D, Swedo SE: Case study: Acute basal ganglia enlargement and obsessive–compulsive symptoms in an adolescent boy. Journal of the American Academy of Child and Adolescent Psychiatry: 35; 913–915, 1996.

Gladstone M, Best C, Davidson R: Anomalous bimanual coordination among dyslexic boys. Developmental Psychology: 25; 236–246, 1989.

Green RL, Hutsler JJ, Loftus WC, Tramo MJ, Thomas CE, Silberfarb AW, Nordgren RE, Nordgren RA, Gazzaniga MS: The caudal infrasylvian surface in dyslexia: Novel magnetic resonance imaging-based findings. Neurology: 53; 974, 1999.

Grigorenko E: Developmental dyslexia: An update on genes, brains, and environments. Journal of Child Psychology and Psychiatry and Allied Disciplines: 42; 91–125, 2001.

Grigorenko E, Wood F, Meyer M, Hart L, Speed W, Shuster A, Pauls D: Susceptibility loci for distinct components of developmental dyslexia on chromosome 6 and 15. American Journal of Human Genetics: 60; 27–39, 1997.

Gross-Glenn K, Rothenberg S: Evidence for deficit in interhemispheric transfer of information in dyslexic boys. International Journal of Neuroscience: 24; 23–35, 1984.

Habib M: The neurological basis of developmental dyslexia: An overview and working hypothesis. Brain: 123; 2373–2399, 2000.

Hardan A, Minshew N, Keshavan M: Corpus callosum size in autism. Neurology: 55; 1033–1036, 2000.

Heilman KM, Valenstein E: Clinical Neuropsychology. New York: Oxford University Press, 1985.

Hiemenz J, Hynd G: Sulcal/gyral pattern morphology of the perisylvian language region in developmental dyslexia. Brain and Language: 74; 113–133, 2000.

Hobson R, Ouston J, Lee A: What's in a face? The case of autism. British Journal of Psychology: 79; 441–453, 1988.

Holttum J, Minshew N, Sanders R, Phillips N: Magnetic resonance imaging of the posterior fossa in autism. Biological Psychiatry: 32; 1091–1101, 1992.

Humphreys P, Kaufman W, Galaburda A: Developmental dyslexia in women: Neuropsychological findings in three patients. Annals of Neurology: 28; 727–738, 1990.

Hynd G, Hall J, Novey E, Eliopulos D, Black K, Gonzales J: Dyslexia and corpus callosum morphology. Archives of Neurology: 1995; 32–38, 1995.

Hynd G, Hern K, Novey E, Eliopulos D, Marshall R, Gonzalez J, Voeller K: Attention deficit–hyperactivity disorder and asymmetry of the caudate nucleus. Journal of Child Neurology: 8; 339–347, 1993.

Hynd G, Semrud-Clikeman M: Dyslexia and brain morphology. Psychological Bulletin: 106; 447–482, 1989.

Hynd G, Semrud-Clikeman M, Lorys A, Novey E, Eliopulos D: Brain morphology in developmental dyslexia and attention deficit disorder/hyperactivity. Archives of Neurology: 47; 919–926, 1990.

Hynd G, Semrud-Clikeman M, Lorys A, Novey E, Eliopulos D, Lyytinen H: Corpus callosum morphology in attention-deficit–hyperactivity disorder: Morphometric analysis of MRI. Journal of Learning Disabilities: 24; 141–146, 1991.

Ishai A, Ungerleider LG, Martin A, Schouten JL, Haxby JV: Distributed representation of objects in the human ventral visual pathway. Proceedings of the National Academy of Science, USA: 96; 9379–9384, 1999.

Johnson MH: Developmental Cognitive Neuroscience. Cambridge, MA: Blackwell Publishers, 1997.

Jorm A: Specific reading retardation and working memory: A review. British Journal of Psychology: 74; 311–342, 1983.

Kleiman M, Neff S, Rosman N: The brain in infantile autism: are posterior fossa structures abnormal? Neurology: 42; 753–760, 1992.

Kolb B: Brain Plasticity and Behavior. Mahwah, NJ: Lawrence Erlbaum, 1995.

Kosslyn S, Thompson W, Kim I, Alpert N: Topographical representations of mental images in primary visual cortex. Nature: 378; 496–498, 1995.

Lainhart JE, Piven J, Wzorek M, Landa R, Santangelo SL, Coon H, Folstein SE: Macrocephaly in children and adults with autism. Journal of the American Academy of Child and Adolescent Psychiatry: 36; 282–290, 1997.

Langdell T: Recognition of faces: An approach to the study of autism. Journal of Child Psychology and Psychiatry and Allied Disciplines: 19; 255–268, 1978.

Larsen J, Hoien T, Lundberg I, Odegaard H: MRI evaluation of the size and symmetry of the planum temporale in adolescents with developmental dyslexia. Brain and Language: 39; 289–301, 1990.

Larsen J, Hoien T, Odegaard H: Magnetic resonance imaging of the corpus callosum in developmental dyslexia. Cognitive Neuropsychology: 9; 123–134, 1992.

Leonard C, Voeller K, Lombardion L, Morris M, Hynd G, Alexander A, Andersen H, Garofalakis M, Honeyman J, Mao J, Agee O, Staab E: Anomalous cerebral structure in dyslexia revealed with magnetic resonance imaging. Archives of Neurology: 50; 461–469, 1993.

Levitt J, Blanton R, Capetillo-Cunliffe L, Guthrie D, Toga AW, McCracken J: Cerebellar vermis lobules VIII–X in autism.

Progress in Neuro-Psychopharmacology and Biological Psychiatry: 23; 625–633, 1999.

Lovett MW, Barron RW: Neuropsychological perspectives on reading development and developmental reading disorders. In Segalowitz SJ, Rapin I (Eds), Child Neuropsychology, Handbook of Neuropsychology, 2nd Edition, vol. 8, part II. Amsterdam: Elsevier, chapter 25, 2003.

Markee T, Brown W, Moore L: Callosal function in dyslexia: evoked potential interhemispheric transfer time and bilateral field advantage. Developmental Neuropsychology: 12; 409–428, 1996.

Marrocco RT, Davidson MC: Neurochemistry of attention. In Parasuraman R (Ed), The Attentive Brain. Cambridge, MA: MIT Press, pp. 35–50, 1998.

Mason-Brothers A, Ritvo ER, Guze B, Mo A, Freeman BJ, Funderburk SJ, Schroth PC: Pre-, peri-, and postnatal factors in 181 autistic patients from single and multiple incidence families. Journal of the American Academy of Child and Adolescent Psychiatry: 26; 39–42, 1987.

Mason-Brothers A, Ritvo ER, Pingree C, Petersen PB, Jenson WR, McMahon WM, Freeman BJ, Jorde LB, Spencer MJ, Mo A, Ritvo A: The UCLA-University of Utah epidemiologic survey of autism: Prenatal, perinatal, and postnatal factors. Pediatrics: 86; 514–519, 1990.

Mataro M, Garcia-Sanchez C, Junque C, Estevez-Gonzalez A, Pujol J: Magnetic resonance imaging measurement of the caudate nucleus in adolescents with attention-deficit hyperactivity disorder and its relationship with neuropsychological and behavioral measures. Archives of Neurology: 54; 963–968, 1997.

Mesulam MM: Patterns in behavioral neuroanatomy: Association areas, the limbic system, and hemispheric specialization. In Mesulam MM (Ed), Principles of Behavioral Neurology. Philadelphia, PA: F.A. Davis Company, pp. 1–70, 1985.

Miles JH, Hadden LL, Takahashi TN, Hillman RE: Head circumference is an independent clinical finding associated with autism. American Journal of Medical Genetics: 95; 339–350, 2000.

Moore L, Brown W, Markee T, Theberge D, Zvi J: Bimanual coordination in dyslexic adults. Neuropsychologia: 33; 781–793, 1995.

Nass RD, Gazzaniga MS: Cerebral lateralization and specialization in human central nervous system. In Mountcastle VB, Plum F, Geiger SR (Eds), Handbook of Physiology — The Nervous System: Higher Functions of the Brain. Baltimore, MD: Waverly Press, pp. 701–762, 1987.

World Health Organization: Classification of mental and behavioral disorders. In: ICD-10: The international classification of diseases. Geneva: World Health Organization, 1993.

Paule M, Rowland A, Ferguson S, Chelonis J, Tannock R, Swanson JM, Castellanos FX: Attention deficit/hyperactivity disorder: Characteristics, interventions, and models. Neurotoxicology and Teratology: 22; 631–651, 2000.

Pennington B: Genetics of learning disabilities. Journal of Child Neurology 10: S69–77, 1995.

Pennington B, Filipek P, Lefly D, Chhabildas N, Kennedy D, Simon J, Filley C, Galaburda A, DeFries J: A twin MRI study

of size variations in the human brain. Journal of Cognitive Neuroscience: 12; 223–232, 2000.

Pennington B, Filipek PA, Lefly D, Churchwell J, Kennedy DN, Simon J, Filley C, Galaburda A, Alarcon M, DeFries J: Brain morphometry in reading-disabled twins. Neurology: 53; 723–729, 1999.

Pennington B, Gilger L, Pauls D, Smith S, Smith S, DeFries J: Evidence for a major gene transmission of developmental dyslexia. Journal of the American Medical Association: 266; 1527–1534, 1991.

Piven J, Arndt S, Bailey J, Andreasen N: Regional brain enlargement in autism: A magnetic resonance imaging study. Journal of the American Academy of Child and Adolescent Psychiatry: 35; 530–536, 1996.

Piven J, Arndt S, Bailey J, Havercamp S, Andreasen N, Palmer P: An MRI study of brain size in autism. American Journal of Psychiatry: 152; 1145–1057, 1995.

Piven J, Bailey J, Ranson B, Arndt S: An MRI study of the corpus callosum in autism. American Journal of Psychiatry: 154; 1051–1056, 1997a.

Piven J, Bailey A, Ranson B, Arndt S: No difference in hippocampus volume detected on magnetic resonance imaging in autistic individuals. Journal of Autism and Developmental Disorders: 28; 105–110, 1998.

Piven J, Nehme E, Simon J, Barta P, Pearlson G, Folstein S: Magnetic resonance imaging in autism: Measurement of the cerebellum, pons, and fourth ventricle. Biological Psychiatry: 31; 491–504, 1992.

Piven J, Saliba K, Bailey J, Arndt S: An MRI study of autism: The cerebellum revisited. Neurology: 49; 546–551, 1997b.

Posner MI, Dahaene S: Attentional networks. Trends in Neurosciences: 7; 75–79, 1994.

Posner MI, DiGirolamo GJ: Executive attention: Conflict, target detection and cognitive control. In: Parasuraman R (Ed), The Attentive Brain. Cambridge, MA: MIT Press, pp. 401–423, 1998.

Posner MI, Petersen SE: The attention system of the human brain. Annual Review of Neuroscience: 13; 25–42, 1990.

Posner MI, Raichle ME: Neural networks of attention. In Posner MI, Raichle ME (Eds), Images of Mind. New York: Scientific American Library, pp. 153–179, 1994.

Rademacher J, Galaburda AM, Kennedy DN, Filipek PA, Caviness VSJ: Human cerebral cortex: Localization, parcellation, and morphometry with magnetic resonance imaging. Journal of Cognitive Neuroscience: 4; 352–374, 1992.

Rapin I: Neurological examination. In Rapin I (Ed), Preschool Children with Inadequate Communication: Developmental Language Disorder, Autism, Low IQ. London: MacKeith Press, 1996.

Raymond G, Bauman M, Kemper T: Hippocampus in autism: A Golgi analysis. Acta Neuropathologica (Berlin) 91: 117–119, 1996.

Reiss AL, Abrams MT, Singer HS, Ross JL, Denckla MB: Brain development, gender and IQ in children: A volumetric imaging study. Brain: 119; 1763–1774, 1996.

Ring H, Baron-Cohen S, Wheelwright S, Williams S, Brammer M, Andrew C, Bullmore E: Cerebral correlates of preserved cognitive skills in autism: A functional MRI study of Embedded Figures Task performance. Brain: 122; 1305–1315, 1999.

Ritvo E, Freeman B, Scheibel A, Duong T, Robinson H, Guthrie D, Ritvo A: Lower Purkinje cell counts in the cerebella of four autistic subjects: Initial findings of the UCLA–NSAC Autopsy Research Report. American Journal of Psychiatry: 143; 862–866, 1986.

Robertson IH, Manly T, Beschin N, Daini R, Haeske-Dewick H, Homberg V, Jehkonen M, Pizzamiglio G, Shiel A, Weber E: Auditory sustained attention is a marker of unilateral spatial neglect. Neuropsychologia: 35; 1527–1532, 1997.

Rumsey J, Casanova M, Mannheim G, Patronas N, DeVaughn N, Hamburger S, Aquino T: Corpus Callosum Morphology, as Measured with MRI, in Dyslexic Men. Biological Psychiatry: 39; 769–775, 1996.

Rumsey J, Donohue B, Brady D, Nace K, Giedd JN, Andreason P: A magnetic resonance imaging study of planum temporale asymmetry in men with developmental dyslexia. Archives of Neurology: 54; 1481–1489, 1997.

Rumsey JM, Ernst M: Functional neuroimaging of autistic disorders. Mental Retardation and Developmental Disabilities Research Reviews: 6; 171–179, 2000.

Saitoh O, Courchesne E, Egaas B, Lincoln A, Schreibman L: Cross-sectional area of the posterior hippocampus in autistic patients with cerebellar and corpus callosum abnormalities. Neurology: 45; 317–324, 1995.

Schaefer B, Thompson JJ, Bodensteiner J, McConnell J, Kimberling W, Gay C, Dutton W, Hutchings D, Gray S: Hypoplasia of the cerebellar vermis in neurogenetic syndromes. Annals of Neurology: 39; 382–385, 1996.

Schultz R, Cho N, Staib L, Kier L, Fletcher JM, Shaywitz S, Shankweiler D, Katz L, Gore J, Duncan J, Shaywitz B: Brain morphology in normal and dyslexic children: The influence of sex and age. Annals of Neurology: 35; 732–742, 1994.

Schultz R, Gauthier I, Klin A, Fulbright R, Anderson A, Volkmar F, Skudlarski P, Lacadie C, Cohen D, Gore J: Abnormal ventral temporal cortical activity during face discrimination among individuals with autism and Asperger syndrome. Archives of General Psychiatry: 57; 331–340, 2000.

Sears L, Vest C, Mohamed S, Bailey J, Ranson B, Piven J: An MRI study of the basal ganglia in autism. Progress in Neuro-Psychopharmacology and Biological Psychiatry: 23; 613–624, 1999.

Semrud-Clikeman M, Filipek PA, Biederman J, Steingard R, Kennedy DN, Renshaw P, Bekken K: Attention-deficit hyperactivity disorder: Magnetic resonance imaging morphometric analysis of the corpus callosum. Journal of American Academy of Child Adolescent Psychiatry: 33; 875–881, 1994.

Shaywitz S: Dyslexia. New England Journal of Medicine: 338; 307–312, 1998.

Shaywitz S, Shaywitz B, Fletcher JM, Escobar M: Prevalence of reading disability in boys and girls. Results of the Connecticut Longitudinal Study. Journal of the American Medical Association: 264; 998–1002, 1990.

Shaywitz SE, Shaywitz BA, Pugh KR, Fulbright RK, Constable RT, Mencl WE, Shankweiler DP, Liberman AM, Skudlarski P,

Fletcher JM, Katz L, Marchione KE, Lacadie C, Gatenby C, Gore JC: Functional disruption in the organization of the brain for reading in dyslexia. Proceedings of the National Academy of Science, USA: 95; 2636–2641, 1998.

Skjeldal OH, Sponheim E, Ganes T, Jellum E, Bakke S: Childhood autism: the need for physical investigations. Brain and Development: 20; 227–233, 1998.

Smith E, Jonides J: Working memory in humans: neuropsychological evidence. In Gazzaniga M (Ed), The Cognitive Neurosciences. Cambridge, MA: MIT Press, pp. 1009–1020, 1995.

Smith EE, Jonides J: Storage and executive processes in the frontal lobes. Science: 283; 1657–1661, 1999.

Smith S, Kimberling W, Pennington B, Lubs H: Specific reading disability: Identification of an inherited form through linkage analysis. Science: 219; 1345–1347, 1983.

Smith S, Pennington B, Kimberling W, Ing P: Familial dyslexia: Use of genetic linkage data to define subtypes. Journal of the American Academy of Child and Adolescent Psychiatry: 29; 204–213, 1990.

Steinmetz H, Volkmann J, Jancke L, Freund H: Anatomical left–right asymmetry of language-related temporal cortex is different in left- and right-handers. Annals of Neurology: 29; 315–319, 1991.

Stieltjes B, Kaufmann W, van Zijl P, Fredericksen K, Pearlson G, Solaiyappan M, Mori S: Diffusion tensor imaging and axonal tracking in the human brainstem. NeuroImage: 14; 723–735, 2001.

Swanson JM, Sergeant J, Taylor E, Sonuga-Barke E, Jensen P, Cantwell D: Attention-deficit hyperactivity disorder and hyperkinetic disorder. Lancet: 351; 429–433, 1998.

Tantam D, Monaghan L, Nicholson H, Stirling J: Autistic children's ability to interpret faces: a research note. Journal of Child Psychology and Psychiatry and Allied Disciplines: 30; 623–630, 1989.

Thompson PM, Giedd JN, Woods RP, MacDonald D, Evans AC, Toga AW: Growth patterns in the developing brain detected by using continuum mechanical tensor maps. Nature: 404; 190–193, 2000.

Torgesen J, Wagner R, Rashotte C: Longitudinal study of phonological processing in reading. Journal of Learning Disabilities: 27; 276–286, 1994.

Ungerleider LG, Courtney SM, Haxby JV: A neural system for human visual working memory. Proceedings of the National Academy of Science, USA: 95; 883–890, 1998.

Vaidya CJ, Austin G, Kirkorian G, Ridlehuber HW, Desmond JE, Glover GH, Gabrieli JDE: Selective effects of methylphenidate in attention deficit hyperactivity disorder: A functional magnetic resonance study. Proceedings of the National Academy of Science, USA: 95; 14494–14499, 1998.

Wadsworth S, DeFries J, Stevenson J, Gilger J, Pennington B: Gender ratios among reading-disabled children and their siblings as a function of parental impairment. Journal of Child Psychology and Psychiatry and Allied Disciplines: 33; 1229–1239, 1992.

Westbury C, Zatorre R, Evans A: Quantifying variability in the planum temporale: A probability map. Cerebral Cortex: 9; 392–405, 1999.

Williams R, Hauser S, Purpura D, DeLong G, Swisher C: Autism and mental retardation: Neuropathologic studies performed in four retarded persons with autistic behavior. Archives of Neurology: 37; 749–753, 1980.

Witelson SF: Hand and sex differences in the isthmus and genu of the human corpus callosum: A postmortem morphological study. Brain: 112; 799–835, 1989.

Wolff P, Melngailis I: Family patterns of developmental dyslexia. American Journal of Medical Genetics: 54; 122–131, 1994.

Woodhouse W, Bailey A, Rutter M, Bolton P, Baird G, LeCouteur A: Head circumference in autism and other pervasive developmental disorders. Journal of Child Psychology and Psychiatry and Allied Disciplines: 37; 665–671, 1996.

CHAPTER 8

# Positron emission tomography (PET) and single photon emission computed tomography (SPECT) in developmental disorders

Diane C. Chugani [a,b,*] and Harry T. Chugani [a,b,c]

[a] *Department of Pediatrics, Children's Hospital of Michigan, Wayne State University School of Medicine, Detroit, MI 48201, USA*
[b] *Department of Radiology, Children's Hospital of Michigan, Wayne State University School of Medicine, Detroit, MI 48201, USA*
[c] *Department of Neurology, Children's Hospital of Michigan, Wayne State University School of Medicine, Detroit, MI 48201, USA*

## Introduction

In 1957, Kennedy and Sokoloff demonstrated that the average *global* cerebral blood flow in children was 1.8 times that of normal young adults, and average cerebral oxygen utilization was 1.3 times higher than in adults. These findings extended to humans the prior observation in rats that both oxygen and glucose consumption of excised brain regions (cerebral cortex, striatum, cerebellum and brainstem) were higher between postnatal weeks four and seven, compared to adult values (Tyler and van Harreveld, 1942). Advances in neuroimaging have made it possible to study non-invasively regional cerebral glucose utilization and blood flow in the human brain during development, as well as many other physiological and biochemical processes, including neuroreceptor binding, neurotransmitter synthesis and transport, amino acid transport and protein synthesis. These methods are being used increasingly to demonstrate biochemical changes characteristic of developmental disorders at various ages, in an at-

tempt to better understand the underlying pathophysiology of disorders which disrupt cognitive development in children.

Due to the wide application of these techniques to developmental disorders in recent years, an in-depth coverage of all developmental disorders is beyond the scope of this chapter. We have therefore focussed on autism, and touched upon several other disorders including attention deficit and hyperactivity disorder and Tourette syndrome. Functional MRI is also being increasingly applied in children and in developmental disorders, but this is also beyond the scope of this chapter. The reader is referred to recent reviews of this topic (Boddaert and Zilbovicius, 2002; Bookheimer, 2000; Poldrack, Pare-Blagoev and Grant, 2002).

## PET and SPECT methodology

Positron emission tomography (PET) and single photon emission computed tomography (SPECT) are both relatively non-invasive methods which can be used to image physiological and biochemical processes within the brain and other organs through the use of radiolabeled tracers which are injected into the patient. These functional imaging techniques are now used in the clinical setting as well as in research applications.

* Corresponding author. Dr. Diane C. Chugani, PET Center, Children's Hospital of Michigan, 3901 Beaubien Boulevard, Detroit, MI 48201, USA. Tel.: +1 (313) 993-3847; Fax: +1 (313) 993-3845; E-mail: dchugani@pet.wayne.edu

With PET, the tracers are labeled with short-lived isotopes which emit positrons that in turn collide with surrounding electrons resulting in annihilation of both particles and the release of two high-energy (511 keV) gamma rays. The *two gamma rays generated by a single event travel in opposite directions* and can be recorded by multiple pairs of oppositely situated detectors that constitute the PET camera (Hoffman and Phelps, 1986; Ter-Pogossian, 1995). The [$^{14}$C]2-deoxyglucose autoradiography method for the measurements of the local brain metabolic rate for glucose in laboratory animals (Sokoloff, Reivich, Kennedy et al., 1977) has been adapted for human use with PET and 2-deoxy-2[$^{18}$F]fluoro-D-glucose (FDG) (Huang, Phelps, Hoffman et al., 1980; Phelps, Huang, Hoffman et al., 1979), allowing quantitative measurement of glucose metabolism in vivo in human brain. In addition to regional brain glucose utilization and blood flow, PET methods have been developed to image and measure many other processes, including neuroreceptor binding, neurotransmitter synthesis, amino acid transport and protein synthesis (for review see Langstrom and Dannals, 1995; Stocklin, 1995).

Similarly, SPECT makes use of gamma-emitting compounds for the imaging of many of the same physiological and biochemical processes. Since the isotopes used for SPECT release only a *single gamma ray* (or single photon) for detection by the SPECT camera, the spatial resolution is somewhat less for this method than for PET (5–7 mm for SPECT vs. 3–4 mm for PET state of the art cameras). The quality of SPECT scans is further limited by the inability to correct completely for attenuation (the absorption of some gamma rays within the tissue), and thus absolute quantification of metabolic rates is not possible with SPECT.

Functional brain imaging techniques linked to the performance of specific cognitive or sensorimotor tasks rely on task-related changes in regional cerebral blood flow (rCBF) which reflect increased neuronal and synaptic activity in corresponding brain areas (Ramsey, Kirkby, Van Gelderen et al., 1996). The most advanced rCBF imaging techniques are [$^{15}$O]water PET (Raichle, 1998) and functional magnetic resonance imaging (fMRI) (Rosen, Buckner and Dale, 1998). In [$^{15}$O]water PET, a radioisotope (oxygen-15) contained in saline is injected into

a subject's vein and regional differences in tracer uptake are detected while the subject engages in a specified task. Since oxygen-15 has a very short half-life (approximately 2 min), many scans for different task conditions can be acquired in a single session and resulting images can be compared by means of a subtraction technique (Fox, Mintun, Reiman et al., 1988). These techniques require significant subject cooperation (e.g., to lie still, to perform the task, not be distracted) and thus their application in children is limited to older and relatively high-functioning individuals.

## PET and SPECT studies in children: design issues

### Brain functional changes with development

Since functional neuroimaging has demonstrated striking changes in brain metabolism during maturation, there has been an attempt to determine whether regional values for various markers of brain function in developmental disorders are perturbed during maturation compared to age-matched normal children. In this regard, the study of young children soon after identification of a developmental disorder is more likely to yield important information relevant to the pathophysiology of the disorder than the study of older individuals who are likely to have undergone various interventions. Furthermore, functional brain abnormalities are also likely to change with age, even in disorders which are not progressive in nature.

Due to the dynamic processes which occur during brain development, neuroimaging studies in children need to take into account relatively large changes with age. While the use of age-matched control subjects will guard, to some extent, against drawing invalid conclusions which are artifacts of age differences between groups, this approach may decrease the sensitivity in detecting differences between groups due to the introduction of age-generated variability. Muzik, Ager, Janisse et al. (1999) have attempted to address this problem by devising a mathematical developmental algorithm with identifiable parameters representing different stages of development, such as the glucose metabolic rate value of the 'plateau phase' and the age at which glucose metabolic rates begin to decline, thus allowing for statistical comparisons of the various parameters compared among groups. In addition, longitudinal studies using large samples need to be undertaken to appreciate changes in functional brain activity with development.

*Control subjects or comparison groups*

A difficult problem in applying PET and SPECT imaging to disorders of childhood is to obtain an appropriate age-matched normal control group. The main potential risks of performing functional imaging studies with PET or SPECT include exposure to ionizing radiation and the use of sedation. Ernst, Freed and Zametkin (1998) reviewed studies of low-level radiation exposure with large sample sizes and long follow-up and concluded that health risks from low-level radiation could not be detected above those of adverse events of daily life. Furthermore, they found no evidence that low levels of radiation were more harmful to children than to adults. Nonetheless, current recommendations for radiation dosimetry in children for research purposes dictate a 10-fold lower dose limit for minors (less than 18 years of age) compared to adult doses (IRCP Publication 53, 1988). This restriction effectively eliminates the use of many SPECT tracers and some PET tracers from research use in children. Control studies of normal children younger than the age of 6–8 years are even more problematic. First, they are more difficult because of the need for cooperation, and in particular the need to stay still in a scanner for relatively long periods of time (for example, 30 min for an FDG scan and 90 min for a $[^{11}C]$AMT scan). Due to this requirement, sedation must be employed for many imaging procedures, adding to the overall risk. However, several large studies indicate that this is a small risk, and that sedation of children can be done in a safe and highly efficacious manner in a hospital radiology department using a structured sedation program modeled after the guidelines of the American Academy of Pediatrics (Egelhoff, Ball, Koch et al., 1997; Merola, Albarracin, Lebowitz et al., 1995). Secondly, very young children are not as capable of coping with the insertion of intravenous needles and the laboratory environment. Behavioral approaches have been developed to address

these issues for children. Acclimation techniques and strategies such as making the scanning environment more child-friendly (for example, using a facade to make the scanner look like a spaceship) have resulted in decreased stress to the children and increased cooperation, thus diminishing the need for sedation (Rosenberg, Sweeney, Gillen et al., 1997; Slifer, Bucholts and Cataldo, 1994; Slifer, Cataldo, Cataldo et al., 1993). Even in children who are able to cooperate for the studies, it is difficult to control for the possible effects of stress on the results of the study. A differential response to stress with age could produce misleading results regarding the normative maturational pattern. Furthermore, children with developmental disorders may show heightened stress to the imaging procedure, leading to potential artifactual differences between the disorder and age-matched controls.

Ethical guidelines permit the study of children for comparison groups if they also derive potential direct benefit from the study. Since there is considerable evidence that some developmental disorders are transmitted genetically through family members carrying a milder phenotype (for example as in autism; see Bailey, Le Couteur, Gottesman et al., 1995; Folstein and Rutter, 1977; Steffenburg, Gillberg, Hellgren et al., 1989), the normal siblings of autistic children have served as control subjects (Chugani, Muzik, Behen et al., 1999; Chugani, Muzik, Rothermel et al., 1997). Older children with an autistic sibling are capable of understanding the psychological, social and economic impact of this genetic disorder on their family, as well as the value of their participation in the study. As a precaution against parental coercion, the child should be interviewed in the absence of the parents to ascertain the child's motivation (or lack of motivation) for participation in the study before obtaining the child's written assent.

Another approach for obtaining a comparison group is to employ a group of children with a different disorder but with otherwise normal development who might benefit from the study. This type of control does not constitute an ideal comparison group since their imaging studies will show abnormalities related to their disorder. If the abnormalities are limited to a certain brain region, the remainder of the brain might be used for comparison to the autistic group. Children with epilepsy, for example, have been reported to show focal increases in uptake of the tracer $\alpha[^{11}C]$methyl-tryptophan associated with epileptogenic cortex. Values for whole-brain serotonin synthesis capacity have been calculated for children with epilepsy (excluding the epileptogenic region) for comparison of whole-brain values in autistic children (Chugani et al., 1999). It must be kept in mind when using this experimental approach, however, that adaptive changes can take place in areas of the brain outside the epileptic focus in response to the primary lesion.

Finally, in some circumstances, adults may be suitable as controls. The rationale for suggesting the employment an adult control group for studies of glucose metabolism was based upon previous studies showing that, although there are large changes in the quantitative values of regional brain glucose metabolism between one year of age and adulthood, the overall pattern of brain glucose metabolism at one year of age is similar to that seen in adults (Chugani and Phelps, 1986; Chugani, Phelps and Mazziotta, 1987). If the regional *pattern* of glucose utilization is indeed 'fixed' by one year of age, comparison of glucose metabolism PET scans from pediatric and adult groups might be made using statistical parametric mapping (SPM; Friston, Holmes, Worsley et al., 1995), a technique which compares data which are normalized to the global mean. However, SPM relies upon the accurate normalization and spatial registration of images to a standard template. In order to determine whether spatial normalization of PET image volumes to a PET image template could be successfully used in the pediatric population, we applied PET-derived transformation parameters to coregistered MRI image volumes (Muzik, Chugani, Juhasz et al., 2000). We then compared coronal, sagittal and transaxial contours of spatially normalized MRI image volumes obtained from epileptic children aged 2–14 years with those derived from adult controls. The epileptic children selected for this comparison all had focal epilepsy based on their EEGs and seizure semiology. In addition, they all had normal MRI scans. Our results indicated that the spatial normalization of pediatric brains to an adult template causes a higher level of artifacts in statistical parametric maps as compared to SPM analyses which involve only adult subjects. The error associated with this procedure in children less than 6

years of age precludes the application of SPM in this age group. However, although the error in the spatial normalization procedure for children ages 6 to 14 years was higher than in adults, the error did not result in artifacts in the SPM analysis. In addition, children over 6 years of age appeared to display the same pattern of glucose utilization as adults, with the exception of focal decreases due to epilepsy. Consequently, normal adult subjects appear to be adequate controls for studies of glucose utilization on pediatric study groups, but only if the children are over the age of 6 years. When interpreting results of an SPM analysis comparing children with adults, it must be kept firmly in mind that it is only the *pattern* that is being compared, and that there are large global changes in glucose metabolism with age in children (Chugani et al., 1987; see below).

## Functional maturation of the brain

### Brain glucose metabolism

Studies of regional cerebral glucose metabolism in human infants using PET with FDG have shown that the pattern of glucose utilization undergoes dramatic changes in the first postnatal year. A consistent pattern is seen in the newborn, with the highest glucose metabolic activity in primary sensorimotor cortex, thalamus, brainstem and cerebellar vermis (Chugani, 1994; Chugani and Phelps, 1986; Chugani et al., 1987; Kinnala, Suhonen-Polvi, Äärimaa et al., 1996). Intermediate levels of glucose metabolism are present in cingulate cortex, amygdala, hippocampus, and occasionally the basal ganglia (Chugani, 1996, 1998). The major portion of cerebral cortex shows the lowest glucose metabolism (Fig. 1). This neonatal pattern of glucose metabolism, largely confined to subcortical structures, is consistent with the less complex behavior of neonates compared to infants. For example, reflex behaviors, such as the Moro, root and grasp responses are prominent in newborns and are mediated by subcortical brain regions (Andre-Thomas and Saint-Anne Dargassies, 1960).

Subsequently, the ontogeny of regional brain glucose metabolism appears to follow a phylogenetic order, with functional maturation of older anatomical structures preceding that of newer areas (Chugani, 1994, 1996, 1998; Chugani and Phelps,

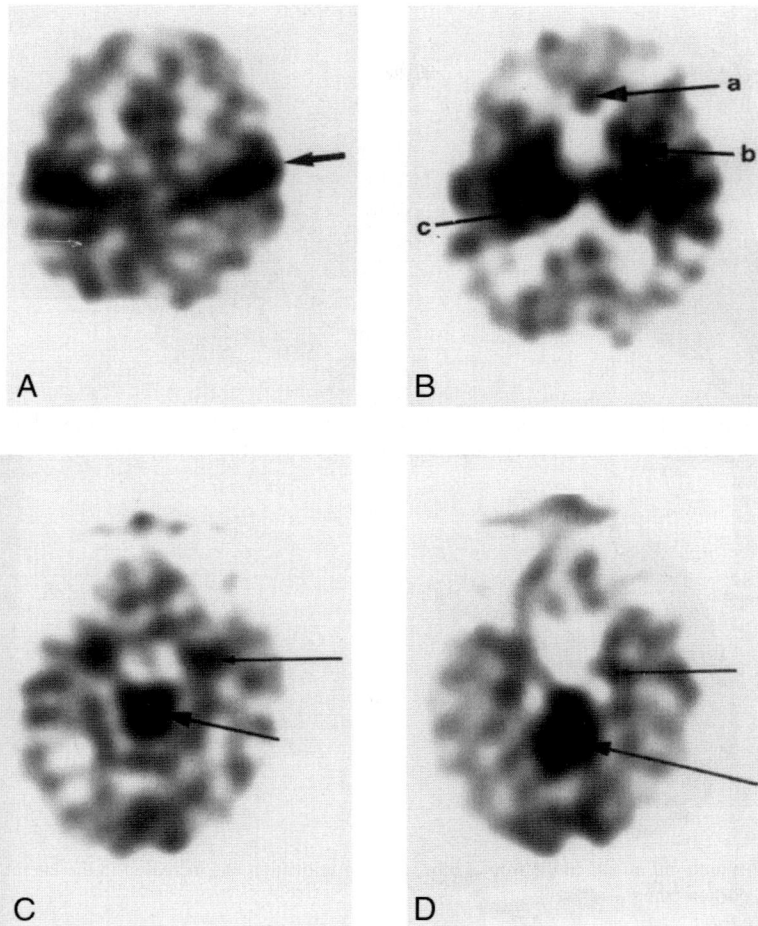

Fig. 1. Pattern of cerebral glucose utilization in human newborn shown on PET scan. (A) Sensorimotor cortex (arrow); (B) anterior cingulate cortex (a), basal ganglia (b), thalamus (c); (C) brainstem (thick arrow) and amygdala (thin arrow); (D) cerebellar vermis (thick arrow) and medial temporal (hippocampal) region. Note the relatively low glucose metabolic rate in most of the cerebral and cerebellar cortex.

1986; Chugani et al., 1987; Kinnala et al., 1996). Moreover, functional maturation of various brain regions as depicted by a rise in regional glucose metabolism correlates well with the maturation of behavioral, neurophysiological and neuroanatomical events in the infant. As visuo-spatial and visuo-sensorimotor integrative functions are acquired in the second and third months of life (Bronson, 1974), and primitive reflexes become reorganized (Andre-Thomas and Saint-Anne Dargassies, 1960; Parmelee and Sigman, 1983), increases in glucose metabolism are observed in parietal, temporal and primary visual cortical regions, frontal eye fields (Brodmann

area 8), basal ganglia, and cerebellar hemispheres (Fig. 2). Increasing glucose metabolism in cerebral cortex during the second and third months of life presumably reflects maturation of the cortex (Lipsitt, 1986), and is consistent with the dramatic maturation of the electroencephalogram seen during the same period (Kellaway, 1979). The observation that infants demonstrate a capacity to learn through exposure to language prior to their ability to speak (Kuhl, Williams, Lacerda et al., 1992) is consistent with the earlier functional maturation (glucose utilization) in receptive compared to expressive language areas.

199

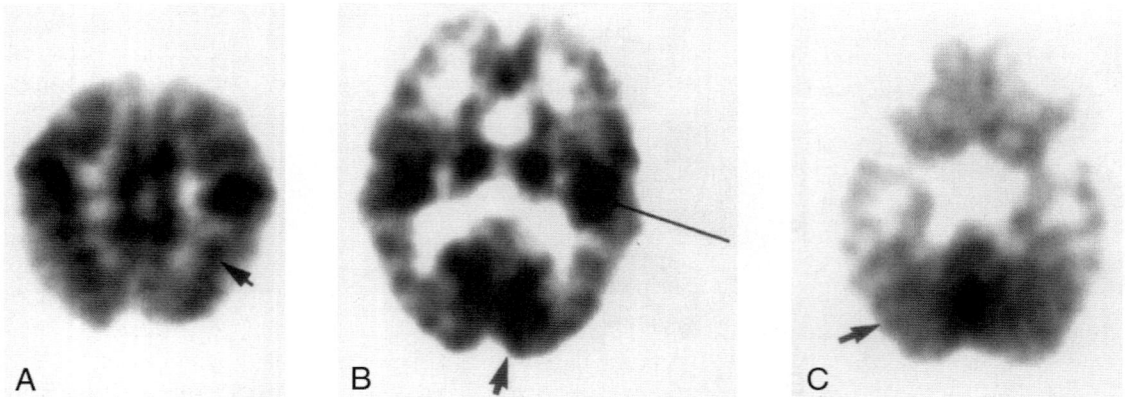

Fig. 2. Pattern of cerebral glucose utilization in a 3-month-old infant. Compared to newborns, there is now increased glucose utilization in: (A) parietal cortex (arrow); (B) temporal cortex (long arrow), occipital cortex (short arrow); and (C) cerebellar cortex (arrow).

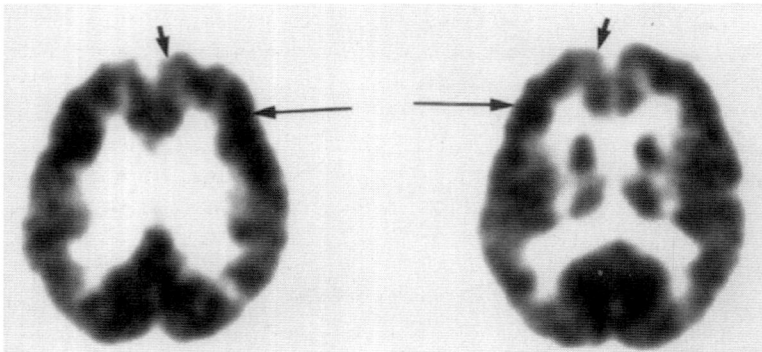

Fig. 3. Pattern of cerebral glucose utilization in an 8-month-old infant. In the frontal lobe, glucose utilization has increased in the lateral portion (long arrows) much more than in the medial portion (short arrows).

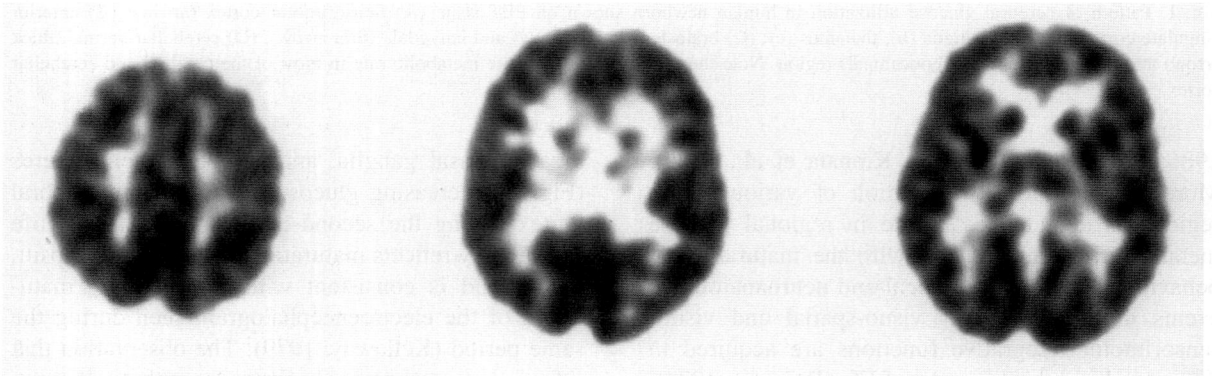

Fig. 4. Pattern of cerebral glucose utilization in a 1-year-old infant resembles that of an adult.

Between 6 and 8 months, the remaining frontal cortex begins to show a maturational rise in glucose metabolism, which continues until one year of age. Functional maturation of the frontal cortex begins in the lateral and inferior portions (Fig. 3), and later proceeds to include the mesial and lastly the dorsal prefrontal areas (Fig. 4). Functional maturation of these frontal cortical regions coincides with the emergence of higher cortical and cognitive abilities. For example, the infant now shows more sophisticated interaction with its surroundings and exhibits the phenomenon of stranger anxiety (Kagan, 1972). Performance on the delayed response task, which is a commonly used neuropsychological paradigm for evaluating prefrontal lobe integrity (Fuster, 1997; Goldman-Rakic, 1984) markedly improves during this period of frontal lobe metabolic maturation. Neuroanatomical studies in human infants have shown that there is an expansion of dendritic fields (Schade and van Groenigen, 1961) and an increase in capillary density (Diemer, 1968) in frontal cortex during this stage of development. By one year of age, the overall pattern of brain glucose metabolism is similar to that seen in adults. These findings demonstrate that the relationship between behavioral development and maturation of regional glucose metabolism is as predicted by Kennedy, Sakurada, Shinohara et al. (1982).

Measurement of the local cerebral metabolic rates of glucose utilization (LCMRglc) in children using PET have confirmed the findings of Kennedy and Sokoloff (1957) that children undergo a period during development when brain energy demand exceeds that of adults (Chugani et al., 1987). Unlike the study of Kennedy and Sokoloff (1957) which measured global cerebral blood flow and oxygen utilization, PET measurements of LCMRglc showed that the magnitude of increase over adult values is most marked for the neocortex, intermediate for basal ganglia and thalamus, and are probably not present in brainstem and cerebellum (Fig. 5). In other words, there appears to be a hierarchical ordering of structures in terms of the degree to which maturational increases in LCMRglc exceed adult values.

The typically low neonatal values of LCMRglc, which are about 30% lower than adult rates, rapidly increase from birth and reach adult values by about the second year. Thereafter, LCMRglc values continue to increase and begin to exceed adult values during the third postnatal year. By about 3 years, a plateau is reached which extends until about 9–10 years; following this, there is a gradual decline in LCMRGgc to reach adult values again by about 16–18 years (Chugani, 1994, 1998; Chugani et al.,

1987). The relative increase of LCMRglc over adult values, which is most pronounced in neocortical regions between 3 and 10 years, reaches a peak LCMRglc of over twice the LCMRglc levels seen in adults.

*Cerebral blood flow*

Similar developmental changes in children and adolescents have been reported for cerebral blood flow (Chiron, Raynaud, Maziere et al., 1992; Lou, Henriksen, Greisen et al., 1990). Chiron et al. (1992) studied regional cerebral blood flow (rCBF) with $^{133}$Xe SPECT in 42 neurologically normal children between the ages of 2 days and 19 years. Values for rCBF in cortex were lower in infants than in adults. Cortical rCBF increased with age so that at 5–6 years of age, values were 50%–85% higher than in adults. Thereafter, cortical rCBF values decreased gradually to reach adult values between the ages of 15 and 19 years. Chiron, Jambaque, Nabbout et al. (1997) have also reported hemispheric differences in their measurements of rCBF during development. Between 1 and 3 years of age, cerebral blood flow appeared to be higher in the right hemisphere compared to the left hemisphere. After 3 years of age in their sample, the left hemisphere showed higher cerebral blood flow. Based on these data, Chiron et al. (1997) have suggested that functional maturation of the right hemisphere might precede that of the left hemisphere. Future studies will be required to replicate the findings of Chiron et al. (1997), although their results are consistent with measures of electroencephalographic coherence data which also support the notion that the left and right hemispheres develop at different rates (Thatcher, Walker and Giudice, 1987).

*Serotonin synthesis capacity*

Similar to developmental changes shown for cerebral glucose metabolism and blood flow, ontogeny studies in nonhuman primates also demonstrate nonlinear changes in neurotransmitter content and receptor binding (Goldman-Rakic and Brown, 1982; Lidow, Goldman-Rakic and Pakic, 1991). For example, in the macaque, there is a steep rise in cortical serotonin content beginning before birth and reaching a

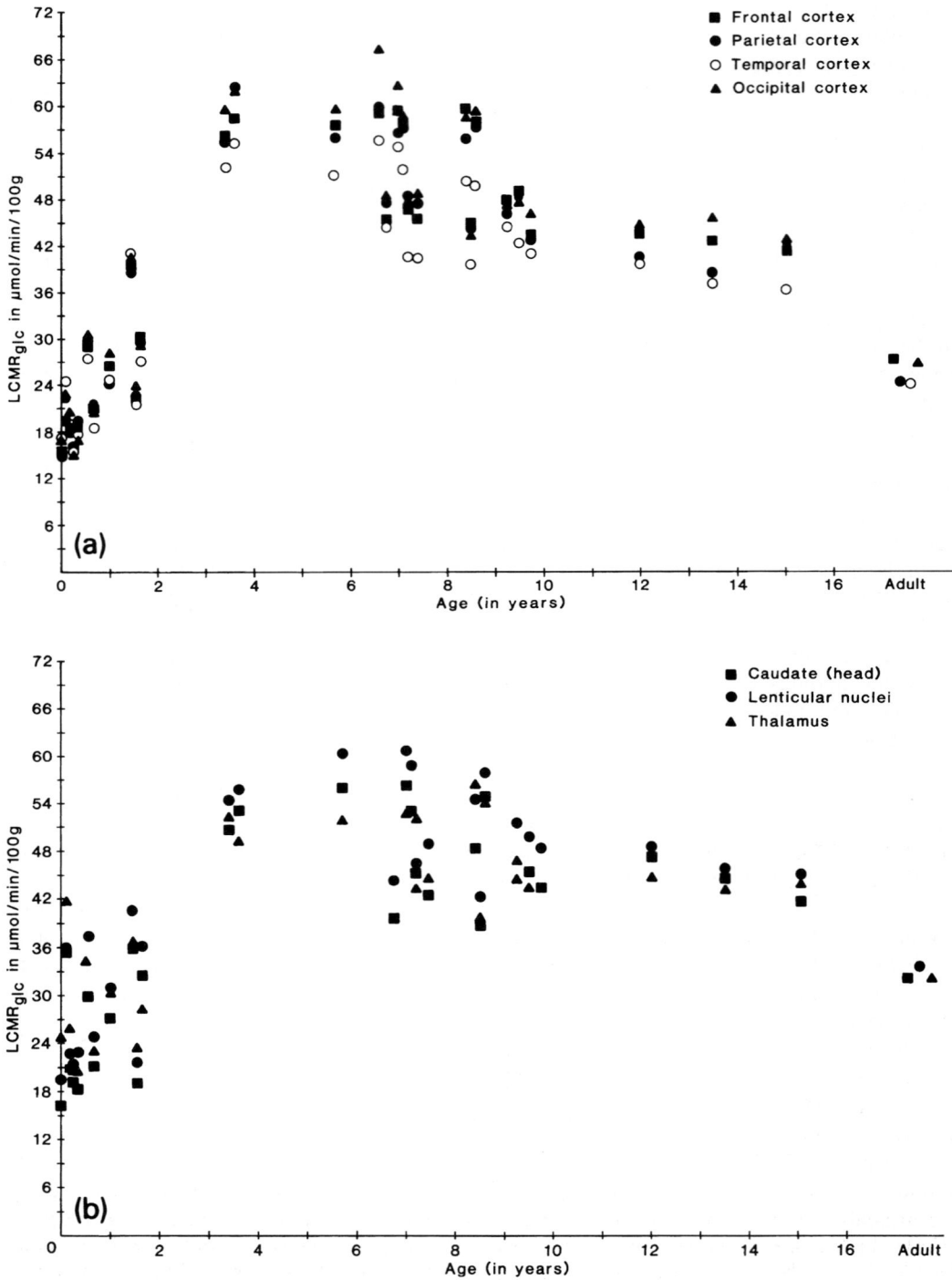

Fig. 5. Absolute rates of local cerebral glucose utilization plotted as a function of age. In the infants and children, points represent individual values of glucose utilization; in adults, points are mean values from 7 subjects.

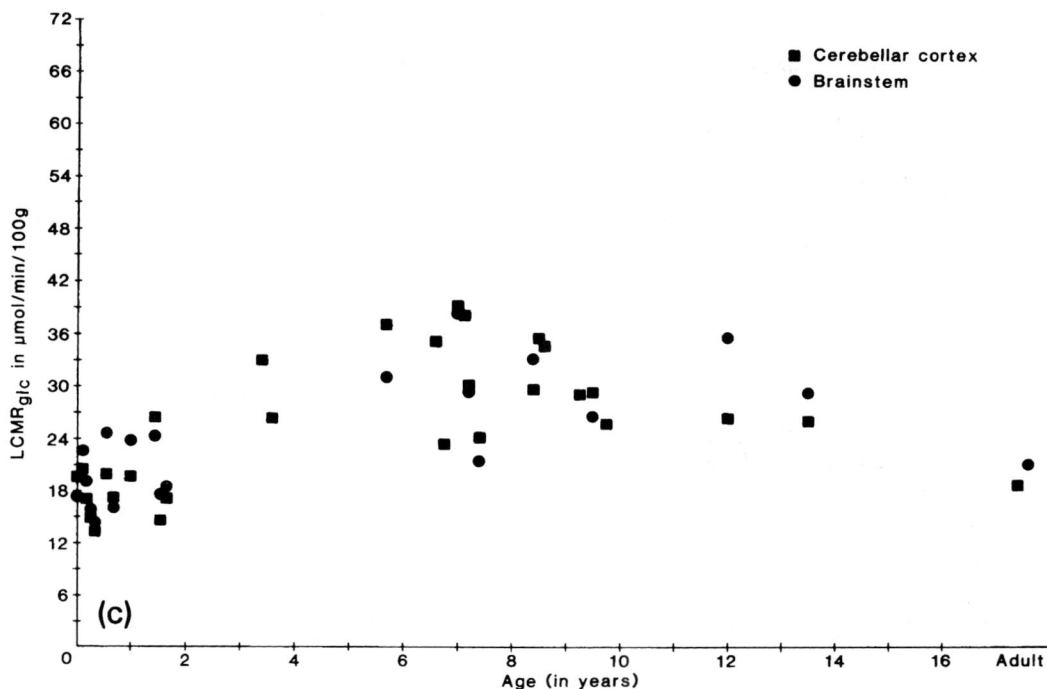

Fig. 5 (continued).

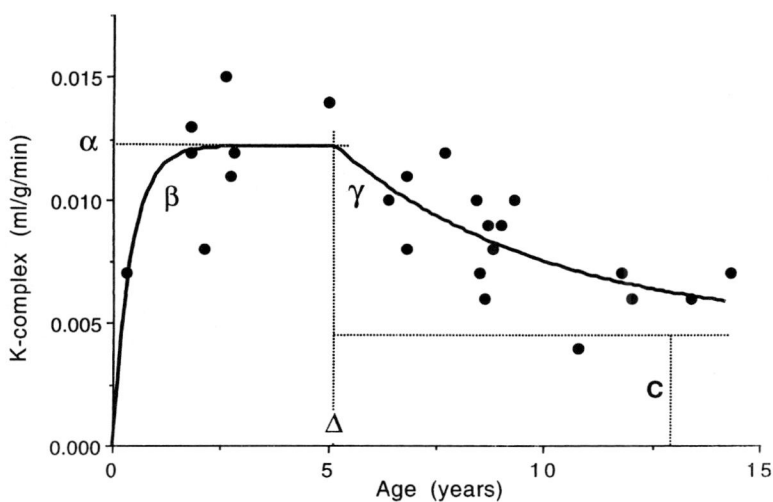

Fig. 6. Serotonin synthesis capacity plotted as a function of age. Serotonin synthesis capacity in non-autistic children ($n = 24$). Global brain values for the unidirectional uptake rate constant for α[$^{11}$C]methyl-L-tryptophan (K-complex; ml/g per min) for the siblings of autistic children and children with epilepsy were fitted according to a 5-parameter developmental model. Parameter $\alpha$ ($0.0122 \pm 0.0008$ SD) represents the magnitude of the plateau phase, and parameter $C$ ($0.0047 \pm 0.0064$ SD) describes adult values. The shape parameters $\beta$ and $\gamma$ represent the rate of increase ($\beta = 2.33 \pm 1.06$ SD) and decline ($\gamma = 0.2066 \pm 0.3177$ SD) of the developmental process with age. The parameter $\Delta$ ($5.16 \pm 2.03$ SD) indicates the age at which the plateau phase ends, and the decline to adult values begins.

peak at 2 months of age, followed by a slow decline until about 3 years of age, when puberty occurs
(Goldman-Rakic and Brown, 1982). The same group
of investigators has reported a similar time course
for expression of serotonin receptors (Lidow et al.,
1991). We (Chugani et al., 1999) measured whole-
brain serotonin synthesis capacity at different ages
using [$^{11}$C]AMT and PET in autistic children and
a comparison group comprised of 8 healthy non-
autistic children with an autistic sibling (6 males,
2 females, 2–14 years) and 16 epileptic children
without autism or pervasive features (9 males, 7 females, 3 months–13 years) (Fig. 6). For non-autistic
children, serotonin synthesis capacity was >200%
of adult values until the age of 5 years and then
declined toward adult values. Serotonin synthesis capacity values declined at an earlier age in girls than
in boys. These data suggest that humans undergo
a period of high brain serotonin synthesis capacity during childhood followed by a decline toward
adult values. However, caution must be used in the
generalization of these data because the majority of
children within the comparison group had medically
intractable seizures requiring at least one anticonvulsant medication. Patients with multiple anatomical
brain lesions were not included, e.g., those with
tuberous sclerosis. Younger or less cooperative children in both the autistic and non-autistic groups were
sedated with nembutal or midazolam during the scan.

### GABA$_A$ receptor expression

An understanding of human GABA$_A$ receptor ontogeny is highly relevant in elucidating the pathophysiology of neurodevelopmental disorders in
which GABAergic mechanisms play a role, as well
as understanding age-related differences in the pharmacology of drugs acting on this system. We have
measured age-related changes in the brain distribution of the GABA$_A$ receptor complex in vivo using
PET in epileptic children under evaluation for surgical treatment (Chugani, Muzik, Juhasz et al., 2001;
Fig. 7). PET imaging was performed using the tracer
[$^{11}$C]flumazenil (FMZ), a ligand which binds to α
subunits of the GABA$_A$ receptor. FMZ binding was
quantified using a two-compartment model yielding
values for the volume of distribution (VD) of the
tracer in tissue. All brain regions studied showed

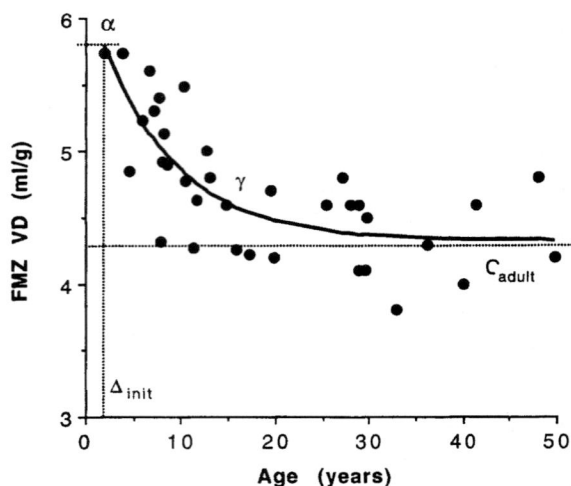

Fig. 7. GABA$_A$ receptor binding plotted as a function of age.
[$^{11}$C]flumazenil volume of distribution values vs. age in the
hemisphere contralateral to the seizure focus fitted to the 3-
parameter exponential model. Parameter $\alpha$ (5.79 ± 0.25 ml/g)
represents volume of distribution values at 2 years of age and
$C_{adult}$ (4.32 ± 0.11 ml/g) represents adult volume of distribution
values. Finally, the rate of decline is characterized by $\gamma$ (0.126 ±
0.041).

the highest value for FMZ VD at the youngest age
measured (2 years), and the values then decreased
exponentially with age. Medial temporal lobe structures, primary visual cortex and thalamus showed
larger differences between age 2 years and adult
values (approximately 50% decrease) as compared
to basal ganglia, cerebellum and other cortical regions (25–40% decreases). Furthermore, subcortical regions reached adult values earlier (14–17.5
years) compared to cortical regions (18–22 years).
The ontogeny data of FMZ VD from children may
contribute to understanding regional differences in
synaptic plasticity, and may improve rational therapeutic use of drugs acting at the GABA$_A$ receptor in
the pediatric population.

## Functional neuroimaging in developmental disorders

### Autism

#### Glucose metabolism
In the first study of cerebral glucose metabolism
in autism, Rumsey, Duara, Grady et al. (1985) re-

ported diffuse hypermetabolism by approximately 20% in a group of 10 autistic men compared to 15 healthy gender and age-matched control subjects. The finding of globally increased cerebral glucose metabolism in autism has not been replicated in subsequent FDG PET studies (De Volder, Bol, Michel et al., 1987; Herold, Frackowiak, Le Couteur et al., 1988; Siegel, Asarnow, Tanguay et al., 1992). However, there are methodological differences in subsequent studies and, therefore, differences in global cerebral glucose metabolism between normal and autistic adults cannot be discounted. For example, Herold et al. (1988) compared 6 male autistic subjects to 6 healthy males and 2 females. Similarly, Siegel et al. (1992) compared autistic adults (12 males, 4 females; 17–38 years) and normal controls (19 males, 7 female, mean age 27 years) mixed for gender, and found no difference in global cerebral glucose metabolism. Since there are known gender differences in cerebral glucose metabolism on the same order of magnitude (see Baxter, Mazziotta, Phelps et al., 1987) as those Rumsey et al. (1985) reported between autistic and normal men, the inclusion of females in control groups could mask a true global increase in cerebral glucose metabolism in autistic subjects. De Volder et al. (1987) reported no differences in global cerebral glucose metabolism using PET in 18 autistic children (11 male, 7 female, aged 2–18 years) compared to a control group which was comprised of children (3 normal children aged 7, 14 and 15 years; 3 children with unilateral pathology aged 9, 12 and 12.5 years) with various brain pathologies, as well as 15 adults (mean age 22 years). Few conclusions can be drawn from the De Volder study since glucose metabolism shows marked changes with age (Chugani et al., 1987, see above).

Horwitz, Rumsey, Grady et al. (1988) added four male autistic subjects to the series reported by Rumsey et al. (1985) and showed that the global brain glucose metabolic rate measured with PET was 12% higher in the autistic group, a difference which was statistically significant. In addition, Horwitz et al. (1988) performed a correlation analysis which showed significantly fewer positive correlations between frontal and parietal cortices, with the most notable discrepancy found between the left and right inferior frontal regions. Furthermore, the thalamus

and basal ganglia also showed less correlation with frontal and parietal cortices in the autistic group compared to the controls.

Focal abnormalities of glucose metabolism have been reported in a number of other PET studies in which global brain glucose metabolism was not addressed. Heh, Smith, Wu et al. (1989) measured glucose metabolism in the cerebellum based upon neuropathological data showing fewer Purkinje and granule cells in the cerebellum (Bauman and Kemper, 1985; Ritvo, Freeman, Scheibel et al., 1986) and vermal cerebellar hypoplasia measured on MRI (Courchesne, Courchesne, Press et al., 1988). However, Heh et al. showed no significant differences in mean glucose metabolic rates for cerebellar hemispheres or vermal lobes VI and VII in autistic subjects (5 males and 2 females; 19–36 years) compared to control subjects (7 males, 1 female; 20–35 years). Schifter, Hoffman, Hatten et al. (1994) studied a heterogeneous group of children (9 males, 4 females; 4–11 years) with autistic behavior coexisting with seizures, mental retardation and neurological abnormalities. Visual analysis of the FDG PET scans revealed that 5 of the 13 subjects had focal abnormalities located in different brain regions for each patient. Regions showing hypometabolism included: right cerebellum and left temporal–parietal–occipital cortices; right parietal cortex, bilateral thalamus and left occipital cortex; right parietal and left temporal–parietal cortices; right parietal–occipital and left occipital cortices; and bilateral temporal lobes.

Buchsbaum, Siegel, Wu et al. (1992) applied a visual continuous performance task, which was associated with greater right than left hemisphere metabolism in autistic subjects (5 males, 2 females; 19–36 years) than in their normal control subjects (13 males, mean age 24 years). Siegel et al. (1992) studied 16 high-functioning autistic adults (12 male, 4 female; 17–38 years) and 26 normal controls (19 males, 7 female, mean age 27 years) and reported that autistic subjects had a left > right anterior rectal gyrus (located in inferior frontal lobe) asymmetry, as opposed to the normal right > left asymmetry in that region. The autistic group also showed low glucose metabolism in the left posterior putamen and high glucose metabolism in the right posterior calcarine cortex. The same group (Siegel, Nuechterlein, Abel et al., 1995) studied glucose metabolism in 14 adults with a history of infantile autism (12 men, 3 women, aged 17–38 years, mean 24 years; 15 of 16 subjects previously reported by Siegel et al., 1992) and reported that autistic subjects showed abnormal thalamic glucose metabolism, and correlations of task performance with pallidal metabolism suggested subcortical dysfunction during the attentional task in autism. Recently, Haznedar, Buchsbaum, Metzger et al. (1997) performed MRI and glucose PET scans on 7 high-functioning autistic patients (5 males, 2 females, mean age 24.3 years) and 7 sex and age-matched normal adults. Right anterior cingulate was significantly smaller in relative volume and was metabolically less active in the autistic patients compared to the normal subjects. However, these data were not corrected for partial volume effects (Hoffman, Huang and Phelps, 1979) and, therefore, the possibility cannot be excluded that the right anterior cingulate cortex hypometabolism may be secondary to the volume decrease documented on MRI.

An association of autism in children with a history of infantile spasms has been long recognized (Riikonen and Amnell, 1981). Chugani, da Silva and Chugani (1996) reported that 18 children (7 males, 11 females; 10 months to 5 years of age) from a total of 110 children with a history of infantile spasms and normal MRI scans showed bilateral temporal lobe glucose hypometabolism on PET. Long-term outcome data were obtained for 14 of the 18 children; 10 of the 14 children met DSM-IV criteria for autism. All 14 children had continued seizures and mental retardation. Two temporal lobe regions, superior temporal gyrus and hippocampus, showed significant hypometabolism compared to age-matched controls. These observations are relevant not only because histological studies of postmortem brain tissue from autistic subjects show abnormalities in hippocampus (Bauman and Kemper, 1994), but also because recent studies using volumetric MRI in patients with fragile X syndrome have found abnormalities in hippocampus (increased volume) and superior temporal gyrus (decreased volume) (Reiss, Lee and Freund, 1994).

*Cerebral blood flow*
A number of studies of autistic subjects measuring cerebral blood flow with SPECT can be found in the literature reporting a variety of global and focal abnormalities. George, Costa, Kouris et al.

(1992) reported global cerebral hypoperfusion in the resting state in adult autistic men with seizures (4 males, 22–34 years) compared to control subjects (2 males, 2 females; 25–32 years). George et al. (1992) further observed pronounced hypoperfusion in the frontotemporal cortices, whereas McKelvey, Lambert, Mottron et al. (1995) localized most consistent hypoperfusion to the vermis and the right cerebellar hemisphere in 3 adolescent autistic subjects (2 males, 1 female; 14–17 years). Mountz, Tolbert, Lill et al. (1995) also reported hypoperfusion in autistic subjects (5 males, 1 female; 9–21 years) compared to the control group (5 males, 2 females; 6–20 years), but localized it primarily to the left temporoparietal and the right anterior temporal region.

Zilbovicius, Garreau, Tzourio et al. (1992) measured regional cerebral blood flow with SPECT and $^{133}$Xenon in 21 children (12 boys, 9 girls, aged 5–11 years, mean 7.4) with autism defined by DSM-III-R criteria. Five cortical brain areas including frontal, temporal, and sensory association cortices were examined. The children with autism showed no cortical regional abnormalities compared to an age-matched group of 14 non-autistic children with slight to moderate language disorders. While the autistic subjects in this study were sedated, the control group (those with language disorders) were not. In a longitudinal study, Zilbovicius, Garreau, Samson et al. (1995) also studied cerebral blood flow in pre-school autistic children. Five autistic children (3 males, 2 females) were studied at the age of 3–4 years and again 3 years later, in comparison to 2 age-matched groups of non-autistic children (5 children ages 3–4 years, and 7 children aged 6–12 years) with normal development. These investigators reported frontal hypoperfusion in the autistic children at ages 3–4 years, but not at the ages of 6–7 years, suggesting a delayed frontal maturation in childhood autism. Chiron, Leboyer, Leon et al. (1995) compared cerebral blood flow in 18 autistic children (14 males, 4 females; 4–14 years) to 10 control subjects (5 males, 5 females; 4–16 years), reporting that blood flow was greater in the left hemisphere in control subjects, but greater in the right in autistic patients. All but one of the autistic subjects were sedated with intrarectal pentobarbitone and, in some cases, intramuscular droperidol, while only 2 of the 10 control subjects were sedated. While barbiturates have been reported to decrease cerebral metabolism in adults (Theodore, di Chiro, Margolin et al., 1986), Chiron et al. (1992) showed that cerebral blood flow (measured using $^{133}$Xenon SPECT) was not significantly different from controls in children sedated with pentobarbitone.

*Task-activated brain mapping*

In a functional mapping study using [$^{15}$O]water PET, Happé, Ehlers, Fletcher et al. (1996) applied a 'theory of mind' task that required attributing mental states to the characters of a narrative. The statistical parametric mapping analysis showed that the Asperger's group (5 males, 20–27 years) showed a slightly different location of activation in inferior prefrontal cortex (Brodmann area 9 instead of 8) compared to the normal control group (6 males, 24–65 years).

Müller, Behen, Rothermel et al. (1999) studied auditory perception and receptive and expressive language in 5 high-functioning autistic adults (4 men, 1 woman; 18–31 years) compared to 5 normal men (23–30 years) using an [$^{15}$O]water activation paradigm. PET scans were performed at rest, and while subjects listened to tones, listened to short sentences, repeated short sentences and generated sentences. Analyses of peak activations revealed reduced or reversed dominance for language perception in temporal cortex, and reduced activation of auditory cortex and the cerebellum during acoustic stimulation in the autistic group. Data from the 4 autistic men and 5 normal men were reanalyzed (Müller, Chugani, Behen et al., 1998) to examine three predetermined regions of interest — dentate nucleus of the cerebellum, thalamus and Brodmann area 46 — based upon serotonin synthesis studies showing abnormalities in these three regions in autistic boys (Chugani et al., 1997). The results of this reanalysis showed that the dorsolateral prefrontal cortex (area 46) and thalamus in the left hemisphere and the right dentate nucleus all manifested less activation in the autistic men than in the control group during sentence generation. In contrast, with sentence repetition, increases in blood flow were significantly larger in left frontal cortex and right dentate nucleus in the autistic subjects than the control group. These data suggest that left frontal cortex, left thalamus and right dentate nucleus showed atyp-

ical functional changes with language tasks in high-functioning autistic men, consistent with the earlier findings of abnormal AMT uptake in these regions (Chugani et al., 1997).

Due to the small numbers of autistic subjects, all of the functional mapping studies thus far performed should be considered pilot studies. However, this is a promising approach for high-functioning subjects who are able to cooperate with the performance demands of this type of study.

*Neurotransmitter studies*

Studies investigating alterations in neurotransmitters, hormones and their metabolites in the blood, cerebrospinal fluid (CSF) and urine of autistic patients have been numerous and have provided some evidence for the potential involvement of several neurotransmitters in autism (for review see Anderson, 1994). Furthermore, given that there is evidence for dysfunction in widely distributed brain regions in autism (Minshew, Goldstein and Siegel, 1997), the monoamine neurotransmitters are interesting candidates to be examined due to their widespread modulatory role in the brain. To this purpose, functional imaging has been used to examine the role of two monoamine transmitters, dopamine (Ernst, Zametkin, Matochik et al., 1997) and serotonin (Chugani et al., 1997, 1999), in autism.

Ernst et al. (1997a) studied 14 medication-free autistic children (8 boys, 6 girls, mean age 13 years) and 10 healthy children (7 boys, 3 girls, mean age 14 years) with [$^{18}$F]-labeled fluorodopa (F-DOPA) using PET. F-DOPA is a precursor of dopamine which is taken up, metabolized and stored by dopaminergic terminals. Ernst and colleagues calculated the ratios of F-DOPA activity (as the activity within a region of interest divided by activity in occipital cortex) measured between 90 and 120 min following tracer administration. Regions sampled were the caudate, putamen, midbrain, lateral and medial anterior prefrontal regions, regions which are all rich in dopaminergic terminals, and occipital cortex, a region poor in dopaminergic terminals. They reported a 39% reduction of the F-DOPA ratio in the anterior medial prefrontal cortex/occipital cortex in the autistic group, but no significant differences in any of the other regions measured. These authors suggested that decreased dopaminergic function in prefrontal cortex may contribute to the cognitive impairment seen in autism.

Although there is evidence for the potential involvement of several other neurotransmitters in autism, the most consistent findings involve serotonin. Schain and Freedman (1961) first reported increased blood serotonin in approximately one-third of autistic patients, but studies of the serotonin metabolite 5-HIAA in CSF have failed to demonstrate consistent abnormalities of central serotonergic tone (for review see Anderson, 1994). Pharmacological treatments which decrease serotonergic neurotransmission, such as tryptophan depletion, have been reported to result in an exacerbation of symptoms in autistic subjects (McDougle, Naylor, Cohen et al., 1996a). Conversely, administration of serotonin re-uptake inhibitors appear to result in improvement of compulsive symptoms, repetitive movements and social difficulties in autistic adults (Cook, Rowlett, Jaselskis et al., 1992; Gordon, State, Nelson et al., 1993; McDougle, Naylor, Cohen et al., 1996b). Chugani et al. (1997, 1999) have applied [$^{11}$C]α-methyl-tryptophan ([$^{11}$C]AMT) as a PET tracer in autistic subjects. [$^{11}$C]AMT, which has been developed as a tracer for serotonin synthesis with PET (Diksic, Nagahiro, Sourkes et al., 1990), is an analogue of tryptophan, the precursor for serotonin synthesis. Following the administration of labeled or unlabeled α-methyl-L-tryptophan (AMT) in rats, the synthesis of α-methyl-serotonin in brain has been demonstrated by high-pressure liquid chromatography (Diksic et al., 1990; Missala and Sourkes, 1988). [$^{3}$H]α-methyl-serotonin synthesized in brain has been localized to serotonergic neurons and nerve terminals by combined autoradiography and tryptophan hydroxylase immunocytochemistry at the electron microscopic level (Cohen, Tsuiki, Takada et al., 1995). Furthermore, [$^{3}$H]α-methyl-serotonin present in nerve terminals could be released by $K^+$ induced depolarization, suggesting that this tracer is stored within the releasable pool of serotonin (Cohen et al., 1995). Since α-methyl-serotonin (AM-5HT), unlike serotonin, is not a substrate for the degradative enzyme monoamine oxidase (Missala and Sourkes, 1988), accumulation of AM-5HT occurs in serotonergic terminals. In addition, AMT, unlike tryptophan, is not incorporated into protein in significant amounts (Diksic et al., 1990; Madras and Sourkes,

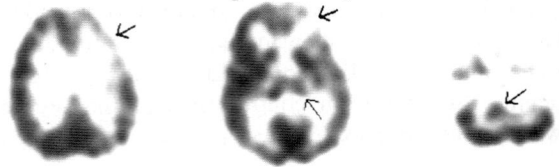

**A.   Autistic Boy (6.8 years old)**

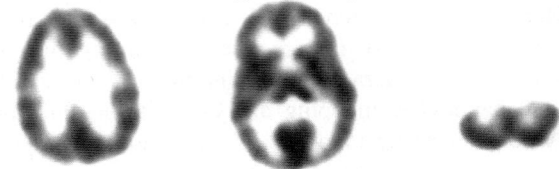

**B.   Male Sibling (9.4 years old)**

Fig. 8. α[$^{11}$C]methyl-L-tryptophan PET images of (A) a 6.8-year-old autistic boy and (B) a 9.4 year old male sibling (left side of image is the right side of the brain). Arrows denote decreased serotonin synthesis in left frontal cortex and left thalamus and increased serotonin synthesis in right dentate nucleus in the autistic child.

1965). These properties of AMT make it a suitable tracer substance for the measurement of serotonin synthesis in vivo in humans with PET (Chugani, Muzik, Chakraborty et al., 1998; Muzik, Chugani, Chakraborty et al., 1997; Nishizawa, Benkelfat, Young et al., 1997).

Chugani et al. (1997) used [$^{11}$C]AMT and PET to study healthy, seizure-free children with autism (7 males, 1 female, 4–11 years) and their healthy non-autistic siblings (4 males, 1 female, 8–14 years). All of the autistic subjects and 3 of the 5 siblings were sedated with nembutal or midazolam. Gross asymmetries of [$^{11}$C]AMT standard uptake value (SUV) in frontal cortex, thalamus and cerebellum were visualized in seven autistic boys, but not in the one autistic girl studied nor in four of the five siblings (Fig. 8). Decreased [$^{11}$C]AMT accumulation was seen in the left frontal cortex and thalamus in 5 of 7 autistic boys. This was accompanied by an elevated [$^{11}$C]AMT accumulation in the right cerebellum. The region of increased tracer accumulation in the cerebellum appeared to be in the dentate nucleus based upon coregistration with the MRI. In the remaining 2 autistic boys, [$^{11}$C]AMT accumulation was decreased in the *right* frontal cortex and thalamus and elevated in the left dentate nucleus. No asymmetries were seen in the frontal cortex or thalamus of the sibling group (Fig. 8); however, one sibling showed an increased [11C]AMT accumulation in the right dentate nucleus. Interestingly, this boy had a history of calendar calculation and ritualistically lined up his toys, behaviors commonly seen in autistic children. The overall difference in asymmetry scores between the autistic boys and their siblings was found to be statistically significant, and regional asymmetry scores in the frontal cortex and thalamus were also found to differ significantly. The specificity of these abnormalities to serotonin synthesis was apparent when comparing the [11C]AMT scans to the FDG PET and MRI scans, both of which were normal by visual examination in the children studied.

Chugani et al. (1999) also measured whole-brain serotonin synthesis capacity in autistic and non-autistic children at different ages using [11C]AMT and PET. Global brain values for serotonin synthesis capacity were obtained for 30 healthy, seizure-free autistic children (24 males, 6 females, 2–15 years), 8 of their healthy non-autistic siblings (6 males, 2 females, 2–14 years), and 16 epileptic children without autism (9 males, 7 females, 3 months–13 years). Children in the epilepsy group had medically intractable seizures, but patients with multiple anatomical brain lesions (e.g., tuberous sclerosis patients) were not included. Epileptic patients were taking at least one anticonvulsant medication. All of the autistic and epileptic subjects and 4 of the 8 siblings were sedated with nembutal or midazolam during the PET scan. For non-autistic children, serotonin synthesis capacity was >200% of adult values until the age of about 5 years and then declined toward adult values. Serotonin synthesis capacity values declined at an earlier age in girls than in boys. In autistic children, serotonin synthesis capacity increased gradually between the ages of 2 years and 15 years to values 1–1/2 times adult normal values and showed no gender difference. These data suggest that humans undergo a period of high brain serotonin synthesis capacity during childhood, and that this developmental process is disrupted in autistic children. Serotonin synthesis capacity was estimated also in four high-functioning autistic adults (3 males, 1 female; mean age 26.5, mean full scale IQ = 70) (Chugani, Muzik, Chakraborty et al., 1996). Values of serotonin synthesis capacity for different brain regions in one autistic woman studied fell within the range of values measured in normal adult females (*n* = 5). Comparisons made between autistic men and control men (*n* = 5) showed that mean serotonin synthesis capacity values were significantly higher for all brain regions in the autistic group. Interestingly, clomipramine, a tricyclic nonselective serotonin uptake inhibitor, has been shown to benefit autistic adults (Gordon, Rapoport, Hamburger et al., 1992 and Gordon et al., 1993; McDougle, Price, Volkmar et al., 1992), whereas treatment of 8 autistic children with clomipramine resulted in a worsening of behavior in 6 of the children, including increased tantrums, irritability, aggression, self-injury and crying spells (Sanchez, Campbell, Small et al., 1996). Differences in response of autistic symptoms to serotonergic drugs between autistic adults and children would be expected in light of the findings with [11C]AMT-PET that young autistic children have lower serotonin synthesis than normal children, whereas autistic men have higher serotonin synthesis than normal men.

### Attention deficit and hyperkinetic disorder (ADHD)

#### Glucose metabolism

The first PET study of ADHD was a study of glucose metabolism in adults with a history of hyperactivity in childhood and who continued to have symptoms of the disorder. Zametkin, Nordahl, Gross et al. (1990) measured global and regional glucose metabolism in 25 adults with ADHD (18 men and 7 women; mean age 37.4 ± 6.9 years) and compared the values to a group of 50 healthy adults (28 men and 22 women; mean age 36.3 ± 11.7 years). Global cerebral glucose metabolism was 8.1% lower in the ADHD group, and 30 of 60 regions measured showed significantly lower glucose metabolism in the ADHD group. The regions with the largest reductions in glucose metabolism were the premotor cortex and the superior prefrontal cortex, which are areas involved in control of attention and motor activity. The same investigators also examined the effects of chronic stimulant treatment on cerebral glucose metabolism in adults with ADHD. Matochik, Liebenauer, King et al. (1994) performed 2 PET studies in adults (mean age 35.5 years) with ADHD. They performed a baseline scan followed by a second scan 6 weeks following treatment with either methylphenidate ($n = 19$) or D-amphetamine ($n = 18$). No significant differences in whole-brain or regional glucose metabolic rate were observed with either drug treatment, despite significant behavioral improvement in both drug groups. Although these investigators were able to detect reduced global and regional cerebral glucose metabolism with PET in adults with ADHD, they did not find any significant differences in brain glucose metabolism in adolescents with ADHD as compared to an age-matched normal control group (Ernst, Cohen, Liebenauer et al., 1997; Zametkin, Liebenauer, Fitzgerald et al., 1993). Ernst et al. (1997b) suggested that gender and developmental interactions may have limited the sensitivity of the studies on the younger subjects.

*Neurotransmitter studies*
Ernst, Zametkin, Matochik et al. (1998) studied dopaminergic function with PET using the tracer [18F]fluorodopa in adults with ADHD. They measured the uptake of [18F]fluorodopa in prefrontal cortex, striatum and midbrain in 17 adults with ADHD (8 males and 9 females, $39.3 \pm 6.2$ years old) compared to 23 adult controls (13 males and 10 females, $33.7 \pm 10.5$ years old). [18F]fluorodopa uptake was decreased by approximately 50% in the medial and left prefrontal areas in the adults with ADHD as compared to the control group. In addition, there was a significant difference due to gender in prefrontal [18F]fluorodopa uptake. In the ADHD group, men showed significantly lower uptake than in women in prefrontal cortex, whereas the men showed higher prefrontal uptake than women in the control group. These investigators suggested that prefrontal dopaminergic function may mediate the symptoms of ADHD in adults.

*Dyslexia*

*Cerebral blood flow*
The first cerebral blood flow investigation of developmental dyslexia using a stimulation paradigm was performed by Rumsey, Andreason, Zametkin et al. (1992), who studied men with severe developmental dyslexia ($n = 14$, mean age 27 years) during an auditory phonological task compared to 14 matched controls. Paulesu, Frith, Snowling et al. (1996) con-

firmed and extended these findings by comparing brain regions activated by a rhyming and a short-term memory task with visually presented letters in 5 compensated adult dyslexic men (mean age 25.2 years) with 5 normal age and gender-matched controls ($n = 6$, mean age 27.2 years). During the rhyming task, control subjects showed activation of a constellation of left perisylvian structures including the inferior frontal gyrus, the posterior superior temporal gyrus, and portions of the insula. The main difference between the control and dyslexic subjects on this task was the failure of the dyslexic group to activate the insula. In the short-term memory task, controls activated similar regions to the rhyming task but also left supramarginal gyrus and left lingual gyrus. In comparison, the dyslexic group again failed to activate the insula and showed less activation than the control group in many regions, but most prominently in Broca's area. Paulesu et al. (1996) proposed that the phonological problems in dyslexia may be due to a dysfunctional left insula which may act normally as a bridge between Broca's area, superior temporal and inferior parietal cortices. More recently, functional disconnection of the left angular gyrus from the 'normal brain reading network' has been proposed by Horwitz, Rumsey and Donohue (1998). In order to assess difficulties in motor skills often present in dyslexic individuals, Nicolson, Fawcett, Berry et al. (1999) compared brain activation in 6 dyslexic adults with 6 matched controls using [15O]water PET during prelearned or novel sequences of finger movements. Activation of the right cerebellar cortex was significantly lower in the dyslexic group under both stimulation conditions.

*Tourette syndrome*

*Neurotransmitter studies*
Dopaminergic dysfunction has been implicated in Tourette syndrome, a chronic neurologic disorder characterized by involuntary motor and phonic tics, and often accompanied by symptoms of ADHD and obsessive compulsive disorder. Wong, Singer, Brandt et al. (1997) measured D2-like dopamine receptor density in the caudate nucleus of adults with Tourette syndrome using PET with the tracer [11C]3-N-methyl-spiperone. D2-like density was measured using 2 different techniques in 2 groups of adults

with Tourette syndrome (group I: $n = 9$ ages 19–35 years, mean 27.0 years; group II: $n = 20$ ages 19–52 years, mean $36.2 \pm 8.9$), as compared to normal adult controls (group I: $n = 44$, 22 men and 22 women ages 19–73 years; group II: $n = 24$, aged 18–83 years). Using the caudate/cerebellum ratio of $[^{11}C]3$-$N$-methyl-spiperone uptake method, neither Tourette group showed significant differences from the controls. However, a two-PET scan technique, used to calculate the maximum number of binding sites ($B_{max}$), showed that 4 of the 20 Tourette patients in group II had significantly elevated D2-like receptor number. Wong et al. (1997) concluded that a subgroup of patients with Tourette syndrome have elevated D2-like receptors in the caudate nucleus, but that the majority of adults with Tourette syndrome show normal D2 receptor binding. Ernst, Zametkin, Jons et al. (1999) studied dopaminergic function in adolescents with Tourette syndrome ($n = 11$) compared to healthy controls ($n = 10$ age, gender, handedness, sexual maturation and IQ-matched) with PET using the tracer $[^{18}F]$fluorodopa. They measured accumulation of $[^{18}F]$fluorodopa in caudate nucleus, putamen, frontal cortex and midbrain, and reported significantly increased uptake in left caudate nucleus (by 25%) and in right midbrain (by 53%) as compared to controls.

*Other cognitive disorders of childhood*

*Turner syndrome*
Though MRI studies have been unrevealing, a wide variety of cognitive and learning impairments have been identified in patients with Turner syndrome. Using PET with FDG, Clark, Klonoff and Hayden (1990), found a consistent pattern of bilateral occipital and parietal hypometabolism in adults with this syndrome. Elliott, Watkins, Messa et al. (1996) demonstrated similar hypometabolic patterns in children with Turner syndrome with additional temporal lobe hypometabolism in some patients. In the same study, Elliott et al. (1996) also found a general correlation between the neuropsychological profile and locations of the PET abnormalities.

*Spastic diplegic cerebral palsy*
Children who were born prematurely may have the type of cerebral palsy known as spastic diplegia where the legs are predominantly affected. These children have a high incidence of learning difficulties even though the MRI scans seldom show cortical abnormalities on visual assessment. Rather, CT and MRI scans show evidence of white matter damage close to the cerebral ventricles. FDG PET studies in children with spastic diplegia have revealed focal hypometabolism in the parietal–occipital cortex (Kerrigan, Chugani and Phelps, 1991) adjacent to the sites of white matter damage shown on CT and MRI. These investigators postulated that the presence of focal cortical hypometabolism in spastic diplegic children may be due to a disruption of white matter tracts and may be a marker of learning disabilities so commonly seen in these children. This interpretation is supported by recent MRI studies showing decreased volumes mainly in the parietal–occipital cortex (Inder, Huppi, Warfield et al., 1999).

**Summary and future prospects**

The application of functional neuroimaging with PET and SPECT have shed new light on changes in brain function and biochemistry in the developing brain during maturation, as well as on various developmental disorders of cognition. Increasing sensitivity of the new generations of scanners allows a reduction in the radioactive dose administered, thus increasing the predilection to apply these imaging modalities in children. Further development of novel radiolabeled tracers, guided by knowledge of the biochemical characteristics underlying childhood developmental disorders derived from basic and genetic studies, is the logical next step in the application of PET and SPECT in these disorders.

**References**

Anderson, GM: Studies on the neurochemistry of autism. In Bauman ML, Kemper TL (Eds), The Neurobiology of Autism. Baltimore, MD: Johns Hopkins University Press, pp. 227–242, 1994.

Andre-Thomas CY, Saint-Anne Dargassies S: The neurological examination of the infant. London: Medical Advisory Committee of the National Spastics Society, 1960.

Bailey A, Le Couteur A, Gottesman I et al.: Autism as a strongly genetic disorder: Evidence from a British twin study. Psychology Medicine: 25; 63–77, 1995.

Bauman M, Kemper TL: Histoanatomic observations of the brain in early infantile autism. Neurology: 35; 866–75, 1985.

Bauman ML, Kemper TL: Neuroanatomic observations of the brain in autism. In Bauman ML, Kemer TL (Eds), The Neurobiology of Autism. Baltimore, MD: Johns Hopkins Press, pp. 119–141, 1994.

Baxter LR, Mazziotta JC, Phelps ME et al.: Cerebral glucose metabolic rates in normal human females versus normal males. Psychiatry Research: 21; 237–245, 1987.

Boddaert N, Zilbovicius M: Functional neuroimaging and childhood autism. Pediatric Radiology: 32; 1–7, 2002.

Bookheimer SY: Methodological issues in pediatric neuroimaging. Mental Retardation and Developmental Disabilities Research Reviews: 6; 161–165, 2000.

Bronson G: The postnatal growth of visual capacity. Child Development: 45; 873–890, 1974.

Buchsbaum MS, Siegel BV, Wu JC et al.: Brief report: Attention performance in autism and regional brain metabolic rate assessed by positron emission tomography. Journal of Autism and Developmental Disorders: 22; 115–125, 1992.

Chiron C, Jambaque I, Nabbout R et al.: The right brain hemisphere is dominant in human infants. Brain: 120; 1057–1065, 1997.

Chiron C, Leboyer M, Leon F et al.: SPECT of the brain in childhood autism: Evidence for a lack of normal hemispheric asymmetry. Developmental Medicine and Child Neurology: 37; 849–860, 1995.

Chiron C, Raynaud C, Maziere B et al.: Changes in regional cerebral blood flow during brain maturation in children and adolescents. Journal of Nuclear Medicine: 33; 696–703, 1992.

Chugani DC, Muzik O, Behen ME et al.: Developmental changes in brain serotonin synthesis capacity in autistic and nonautistic children. Annals of Neurology: 45; 287–295, 1999.

Chugani DC, Muzik O, Chakraborty PK et al.: Brain serotonin synthesis measured with α[C-11]-methyl-tryptophan positron emission tomography in normal and autistic adults. Society for Neuroscience Abstracts: 22; 22, 1996.

Chugani DC, Muzik O, Chakraborty PK et al.: Human brain serotonin synthesis capacity measured in vivo with alpha-[C-11]methyl-L-tryptophan. Synapse: 28; 33–43, 1998.

Chugani DC, Muzik O, Juhasz C et al.: Postnatal maturation of human GABAA receptors measured with positron emission tomography. Annals of Neurology 49; 618–626, 2001.

Chugani DC, Muzik O, Rothermel R et al.: Altered serotonin synthesis in the dentatothalamo-cortical pathway in autistic boys. Annals of Neurology: 14; 666–669, 1997.

Chugani HT: Development of regional brain glucose metabolism in relation to behavior and plasticity. In Dawson G, Fischer KW (Eds), Human Behavior and the Developing Brain. New York: Guilford Publications, pp. 153–175, 1994.

Chugani HT. Neuroimaging of developmental nonlinearity and developmental pathologies. In Thatcher RW, Lyon GR, Rumsey J, Krasnegor N (Eds), Developmental Neuroimaging: Mapping the Development of Brain and Behavior. San Diego, CA: Academic Press, pp. 187–195, 1996.

Chugani HT. The ontogeny of cerebral metabolism. In Garreau B (Ed), Neuroimaging in Child Neuropsychiatric Disorders. Berlin: Springer, pp. 89–96, 1998.

Chugani HT, da Silva EA, Chugani DC: Infantile spasms:

III. Prognostic implications of bilateral hypometabolism on positron emission tomography. Annals of Neurology: 39; 643–649, 1996.

Chugani HT, Phelps ME: Maturational changes in cerebral function in infants determined by [18]FDG positron emission tomography. Science: 231; 840–843, 1986.

Chugani HT, Phelps ME, Mazziotta JC. Positron emission tomography study of human brain functional development. Annals of Neurology: 22; 487–497, 1987.

Clark C, Klonoff H, Hayden M: Regional cerebral glucose metabolism in Turner's syndrome. Canadian Journal of Neurological Sciences: 17; 140–144, 1990.

Cohen Z, Tsuiki K, Takada et al.: In vivo-synthesis of radioactively labelled α-methyl serotonin as a selective tracer for visualization of brain serotonin neurons. Synapse: 21; 21–28, 1995.

Cook EH, Rowlett R, Jaselskis C et al.: Fluoxetine treatment of children and adults with autistic disorder and mental retardation. Journal of the American Academy of Child and Adolescent Psychiatry: 31; 739–745, 1992.

Courchesne E, Courchesne RY, Press GA et al.: Hypoplasia of cerebellar vermal lobules VI and VII in autism. New England Journal of Medicine: 813; 1349–1354, 1988.

De Volder A, Bol A, Michel C et al.: Brain glucose metabolism in children with the autistic syndrome: Positron Tomography Analysis. Brain and Development: 9; 581–587, 1987.

Diemer K: Capillarisation and oxygen supply of the brain. In Lubbers DW, Luft UC, Thews G, Witzleb E (Eds), Oxygen Transport in Blood and Tissue. Stuttgart: Thieme, pp. 118–123, 1968.

Diksic M, Nagahiro S, Sourkes TL et al.: A new method to measure brain serotonin synthesis in vivo. I. Theory and basic data for a biological model. Journal of Cerebral Blood Flow and Metabolism: 9; 1–12, 1990.

Egelhoff JC, Ball WS Jr., Koch BL et al.: Safety and efficacy of sedation in children using a structured sedation program. American Journal of Roentgenology: 168; 1259–1262, 1997.

Elliott TK, Watkins JM, Messa C et al.: Positron emission tomography and neuropsychological correlations in Turner's syndrome children. Dev Neuropsychol: 12; 365–386, 1996.

Ernst M, Cohen RM, Liebenauer LL et al.: Cerebral glucose metabolism in adolescent girls with attention-deficit/hyperactivity disorder. Journal of the American Academy of Child and Adolescent Psychiatry: 36; 1399–1406, 1997b.

Ernst M, Freed ME, Zametkin AJ: Health hazards of radiation exposure in the context of brain imaging research: special consideration for children. Journal of Nuclear Medicine: 39; 689–698, 1998.

Ernst M, Zametkin AJ, Jons PH et al.: High presynaptic dopaminergic activity in children with Tourette's disorder. Journal of the American Academy of Child and Adolescent Psychiatry: 38; 86–94, 1999.

Ernst M, Zametkin A, Matochik J et al.: Low medial prefrontal dopaminergic activity in autistic children. The Lancet: 350; 638, 1997a.

Ernst E, Zametkin AJ, Matochik JA et al.: DOPA decarboxylase activity in attention deficit hyperactivity disorder adults. A

[Fluorine-18]fluorodopa positron emission tomographic study. Journal of Neuroscience: 18; 5901–5907, 1998.

Folstein SE, Rutter ML: Infantile autism: A genetic study of 21 twin pairs. Journal of Child Psychology and Psychiatry: 18; 297–321, 1977.

Fox PT, Mintun MA, Reiman EM et al.: Enhanced detection of focal brain responses using intersubject averaging and change-distribution analysis of subtracted PET images. Journal of Cerebral Blood Flow and Metabolism: 8; 642–653, 1988.

Friston KJ, Holmes AP, Worsley KJ et al.: Statistical parametric maps in functional imaging: A general approach. Human Brain Mapping: 2; 189–210, 1995.

Fuster JM: The Prefrontal Cortex: Anatomy, Physiology, and Neuropsychology of the Frontal Lobe. 3rd ed., Philadelphia, PA: Lippincott-Raven, pp. 177–178, 1997.

George M, Costa D, Kouris K et al.: Cerebral blood flow abnormalities in adults with infantile autism. Journal of Nervous and Mental Disease: 180; 413–417, 1992.

Goldman-Rakic PS: The frontal lobes: uncharted provinces of the brain. Trends in Neuroscience: 7; 25–429, 1984.

Goldman-Rakic PS, Brown RM: Postnatal development of monoamine content and synthesis in the cerebral cortex of rhesus monkeys. Developmental Brain Research: 4; 339–349, 1982.

Gordon CT, Rapoport JL, Hamburger SD et al.: Differential response of seven subjects with autistic disorder to clomipramine and desipramine. American Journal of Psychiatry: 149; 363–366, 1992.

Gordon CT, State RC, Nelson JE et al.: A double-blind comparison of clomipramine, desipramine and placebo in the treatment of autistic disorder. Archives of General Psychiatry: 50; 441–447, 1993.

Happé F, Ehlers S, Fletcher P et al.: 'Theory of mind' in the brain. Evidence from a PET scan study of Asperger syndrome. NeuroReport: 8; 197–201, 1996.

Haznedar M, Buchsbaum M, Metzger M et al.: Anterior cingulate gyrus volume and glucose metabolism in autistic disorder. American Journal of Psychiatry: 154; 1047–1050, 1997.

Heh CWC, Smith R, Wu J et al.: Positron emission tomography of the cerebellum in autism. American Journal of Psychiatry: 146; 242–245, 1989.

Herold S, Frackowiak R, Le Couteur A et al.: Cerebral blood flow and metabolism of oxygen and glucose in young autistic adults. Psychological Medicine: 18; 823–831, 1988.

Hoffman EJ, Huang SC, Phelps ME: Quantitation in positron emission computed tomography: 1. Effect of object size. Journal of Computer Assisted Tomography: 3; 299–308, 1979.

Hoffman EJ, Phelps ME: Positron emission tomography: principles and quantitation. In Phelps ME, Mazziotta JC, Schelbert HR (Eds), Positron Emission Tomography and Autoradiography: Principles and Applications for the Brain and Heart. New York: Raven Press, pp. 237–86, 1986.

Horwitz B, Rumsey JM, Donohue BC: Functional connectivity of the angular gyrus in normal reading and dyslexia. Proceedings of the National Academy of Sciences: 95; 8939–8944, 1998.

Horwitz B, Rumsey J, Grady C et al.: The cerebral metabolic landscape in autism. Intercorrelations of regional glucose utilization. Archives of Neurology: 45; 749–755, 1988.

Huang SC, Phelps ME, Hoffman EJ et al.: Noninvasive determination of local cerebral metabolic rate of glucose in man. American Journal of Physiology: 238; E69–E82, 1980.

Inder TE, Huppi PS, Warfield S et al.: Periventricular white matter injury in the premature infant is followed by reduced cerebral cortical gray matter volume at term. Annals of Neurology: 46; 755–60, 1999.

IRCP Publication 53. Radiation Dose to Patients from Radiopharmaceuticals. Annals of the International Commission on Radiological Protection. New York: Pergamon Press, p. 15, 1988.

Kagan J: Do infants think? Scientific American: 226; 74–82, 1972.

Kellaway P: An orderly approach to visual analysis: parameters of the normal EEG in adults and children. In Klass DW, Daly DD (Eds), Current Practice of Clinical Electroencephalography. New York: Raven, pp. 69–147, 1979.

Kennedy C, Sakurada O, Shinohara M et al.: Local cerebral glucose utilization in the newborn macaque monkey. Annals of Neurology: 12; 333–340, 1982.

Kennedy C, Sokoloff L: An adaptation of the nitrous oxide method to the study of the cerebral circulation in children; normal values for cerebral blood flow and cerebral metabolic rate in childhood. Journal of Clinical Investigation: 36; 1130–1137, 1957.

Kerrigan J, Chugani HT, Phelps ME: Regional cerebral glucose metabolism in clinical subtypes of cerebral palsy. Pediatric Neurology 7; 415–425, 1991.

Kinnala A, Suhonen-Polvi H, Äärimaa T et al.: Cerebral metabolic rate for glucose during the first six months of life: an FDG positron emission tomography study. Archives of Disease in Childhood: 74; F153–F157, 1996.

Kuhl PK, Williams KA, Lacerda F et al.: Linguistic experience alters phonetic perception in infants by 6 months of age. Science: 255; 606–608, 1992.

Langstrom B, Dannals RF: Carbon-11 compounds. In Wagner HN (Ed), Principles of Nuclear Medicine. 2nd ed., Philadelphia, PA: W.B. Saunders, pp. 166–178, 1995.

Lidow MS, Goldman-Rakic PS, Pakic P: Synchronized overproduction of neurotransmitter receptors in diverse regions of the primate cerebral cortex. Proceeding of the National Academy of Sciences USA: 88; 10218–10221, 1991.

Lipsitt LP: Learning in infancy: cognitive development in babies. Journal of Pediatrics: 109; 172–182, 1986.

Lou H, Henriksen L, Greisen G et al.: Redistribution of cerebral activity during childhood. Brain Development: 12; 301–305, 1990.

Madras BK, Sourkes TL: Metabolism of α-methyl-tryptophan. Biochemical Pharmacology: 14; 1499–1506, 1965.

Matochik JA, Liebenauer LL, King AC et al.: Cerebral glucose metabolism in adults with attention deficit hyperactivity disorder after chronic stimulant treatment. American Journal of Psychiatry: 151; 658–64, 1994.

McDougle CJ, Naylor ST, Cohen DJ et al.: Effects of tryptophan depletion in drug-free adults with autistic disorder. Archive of General Psychiatry: 53; 993–1000, 1996a.

McDougle CJ, Naylor ST, Cohen DJ et al.: A double-blind, placebo-controlled study of fluvoxamine in adults with autistic disorder. Archives of General Psychiatry: 53; 1001–1008, 1996b.

McDougle CJ, Price LH, Volkmar FR et al.: Clomipramine in autism: preliminary evidence of efficacy. Journal of the American Academy of Child and Adolescent Psychiatry: 31; 746–750, 1992.

McKelvey J, Lambert R, Mottron L et al.: Right-hemisphere dysfunction in asperger's syndrome. Journal of Child Neurology: 10; 310–314, 1995.

Merola C, Albarracin C, Lebowitz P et al.: An audit of adverse events in children sedated with chloral hydrate or propofol during imaging studies. Paediatric Anaesthesia: 5; 375–378, 1995.

Minshew NJ, Goldstein G, Siegel DJ: Neuropsychologic functioning in autism: profile of a complex information processing disorder. Journal of the International Neuropsychological Society: 3; 303–316, 1997.

Missala K, Sourkes TL: Functional cerebral activity of an analogue of serotonin formed in situ. Neurochemistry International: 12; 209–214, 1988.

Mountz J, Tolbert L, Lill D et al.: Functional deficits in autistic disorder: Characterization by technetium-99m-HMPAO and SPECT. Journal of Nuclear Medicine: 36; 1156–1162, 1995.

Müller RA, Behen ME, Rothermel RD et al.: Brain mapping of language and auditory perception in high-functioning autistic adults: a PET study. Journal of Autism and Developmental Disorders: 29; 19–31, 1999.

Müller RA, Chugani DC, Behen ME et al.: Impairment of dentato-thalamo-cortical pathway in autistic men: language activation data from positron emission tomography. Neuroscience Letters: 245; 1–4, 1998.

Muzik O, Ager J, Janisse J et al.: A mathematical model for the analysis of cross-sectional brain glucose metabolism data in children. Progress in Neuro-Psychopharmacology and Biological Psychiatry: 23; 589–600, 1999.

Muzik O, Chugani DC, Chakraborty PK et al.: Analysis of [C-11]alpha-methyl-tryptophan kinetics for the estimation of serotonin synthesis rate in vivo. Journal of Cerebral Blood Flow and Metabolism: 17; 659–669, 1997.

Muzik O, Chugani DC, Juhasz C et al.: Statistical parametric mapping: Assessment of application in children. Neuroimage: 12; 538–49, 2000.

Nicolson RI, Fawcett AJ, Berry EL et al.: Association of abnormal cerebellar activation with motor learning difficulties in dyslexic adults. Lancet: 353; 1662–1667, 1999.

Nishizawa S, Benkelfat C, Young SN et al.: Differences between males and females in rates of serotonin synthesis in human brain. Proceedings of the National Academy of Sciences USA: 94; 5308–5313, 1997.

Parmelee AH, Sigman MD: Perinatal brain development and behavior. In Haith M, Campos J (Eds), Biology and Infancy, Vol II. New York: Wiley, pp. 95–155, 1983.

Paulesu E, Frith U, Snowling M et al.: Is developmental dyslexia a disconnection syndrome? Evidence from PET scanning. Brain: 119; 143–157, 1996.

Phelps ME, Huang SC, Hoffman EJ et al.: Tomographic measurement of local cerebral metabolic rate in humans with (F-18)2-fluoro-2-deoxyglucose: validation of method. Annals of Neurology: 6; 371–388, 1979.

Poldrack RA, Pare-Blagoev EJ, Grant PE: Pediatric functional magnetic resonance imaging: progress and challenges. Topics in Magnetic Resonance Imaging: 13; 61–70, 2002.

Raichle M: Behind the scenes of functional brain imaging: a historical and physiological perspective. Proceedings of the National Academy of Sciences USA: 95; 765–772, 1998.

Ramsey NF, Kirkby BS, Van Gelderen et al.: Functional mapping of human sensorimotor cortex with 3D BOLD fMRI correlates highly with $H_2^{15}O$ PET rCBF. Journal of Cerebral Blood Flow and Metabolism: 16; 755–764, 1996.

Reiss AL, Lee J, Freund L: Neuroanatomy of fragile X syndrome: The temporal lobe. Neurology: 44; 1317–1324, 1994.

Riikonen R, Amnell G: Psychiatric disorders in children with earlier infantile spasms. Developmental Medicine and Child Neurology: 23; 747–760, 1981.

Ritvo ER, Freeman BJ, Scheibel AB et al.: Lower Purkinje cell counts in the cerebella of four autistic subjects: initial findings of the UCLA–NSAC autopsy research report. American Journal of Psychiatry: 143; 862–866, 1986.

Rosen BR, Buckner RL, Dale AM: Event-related functional MRI: past, present, and future. Proceedings of the National Academy of Sciences USA: 95; 773–780, 1998.

Rosenberg DR, Sweeney JA, Gillen JS et al.: Magnetic resonance imaging of children without sedation: preparation with simulation. Journal of the American Academy of Child and Adolescent Psychiatry: 36; 853–859, 1997.

Rumsey J, Duara R, Grady C et al.: Brain Metabolism in Autism. Resting cerebral glucose utilization rates as measured with positron emission tomography. Archives of General Psychiatry: 42; 448–455, 1985.

Rumsey JM, Andreason P, Zametkin AJ et al.: Failure to activate the left temporoparietal cortex in dyslexia. An oxygen 15 positron emission tomographic study. Archives of Neurology: 49; 527–534, 1992.

Sanchez LE, Campbell M, Small AM et al.: A pilot study of clomipramine in young autistic children. Journal of the American Academy of Child and Adolescent Psychiatry: 35; 537–544, 1996.

Schade JP, van Groenigen WB: Structural organization of the human cerebral cortex. Acta Anatomica: 47; 74–111, 1961.

Schain RJ, Freedman DX: Studies on 5-hydoxyindole metabolism in autism and other mentally retarded children. Journal of Pediatrics: 59; 315–320, 1961.

Schifter T, Hoffman J, Hatten H et al.: Neuroimaging in infantile autism. Journal of Child Neurology, 9; 155–161, 1994.

Siegel BV Jr., Asarnow R, Tanguay P et al.: Regional cerebral glucose metabolism and attention in adults with a history of childhood autism. The Journal of Neuropsychiatry and Clinical Neurosciences: 4; 406–414, 1992.

Siegel B, Nuechterlein K, Abel L et al.: Glucose metabolic correlates of continuous performance test performance in adults with a history of infantile autism, schizophrenics, and controls. Schizophrenia Research: 17; 85–94, 1995.

Slifer K, Bucholts J, Cataldo MD: Behavioral training of motion control in young children undergoing radiation treatment without sedation. Journal of Pediatric Oncology Nursing: 11; 55–63, 1994.

Slifer K, Cataldo MF, Cataldo M et al.: Behavior analysis of motion control for pediatric neuroimaging. Journal of Applied Behavior Analysis: 26; 469–470, 1993.

Sokoloff L, Reivich M, Kennedy C et al.: The [$^{14}$C] deoxyglucose method for the measurement of local cerebral glucose utilization: theory, procedure, and normal values in the conscious and anesthetized albino rat. Journal of Neurochemistry: 28; 897–916, 1977.

Steffenburg S, Gillberg C, Hellgren L et al.: A twin study of autism in Denmark, Finland, Iceland, Norway and Sweden. Journal of Child Psychology and Psychiatry and Allied Disciplines: 30; 405–416, 1989.

Stocklin G: Fluorine-18 compounds. In Wagner HN (Ed), Principles of Nuclear Medicine. 2nd ed., Philadelphia, PA: W.B. Saunders, pp. 178–194, 1995.

Ter-Pogossian MM: Positron emission tomography. In Wagner HN, Szabo Z, Buchanan JW (Eds), Principles of Nuclear Medicine. London: W.B. Saunders, pp. 342–346, 1995.

Thatcher RW, Walker RA, Giudice S: Human cerebral hemispheres develop at different rates and ages. Science: 236; 1110–1113, 1987.

Theodore WH, di Chiro G, Margolin R et al.: Barbiturates reduce human cerebral glucose metabolism. Neurology: 36; 60–64, 1986.

Tyler DB, van Harreveld A: The respiration of the developing brain. American Journal of Physiology: 136; 600–603, 1942.

Wong DF, Singer HS, Brandt J et al.: D2-like dopamine receptor density in Tourette syndrome measured by PET. Journal of Nuclear Medicine: 38; 1243–1247, 1997.

Zametkin AJ, Liebenauer LL, Fitzgerald GA et al.: Brain metabolism in teenagers with attention-deficit hyperactivity disorder. Archives of General Psychiatry: 50; 333–340, 1993.

Zametkin AJ, Nordahl TE, Gross M et al.: Cerebral glucose metabolism in adults with hyperactivity of childhood onset. New England Journal of Medicine: 323; 1361–1366, 1990.

Zilbovicius M, Garreau B, Samson Y et al.: Delayed maturation of the frontal cortex in childhood autism. American Journal of Psychiatry: 152; 248–252, 1995.

Zilbovicius M, Garreau B, Tzourio N et al.: Regional cerebral blood flow in childhood autism: a SPECT study. American Journal of Psychiatry: 149; 924–930, 1992.

CHAPTER 9

# Conceptual and psychometric issues in the neuropsychologic assessment of children: measurement of ability discrepancy and change

Robin D. Morris [a],[*], Jack M. Fletcher [b] and David J. Francis [c]

[a] *Department of Psychology, Georgia State University, University Plaza, Atlanta, GA 30303, USA*
[b] *Department of Pediatrics, University of Texas Health Science Center-Houston, Houston, TX, USA*
[c] *Department of Psychology, University of Houston, Houston, TX, USA*

## Introduction

Neuropsychological assessments of children are designed to measure human abilities objectively and reliably. Since abilities are developing in children, it is necessary to measure not only the concurrent relationships of different abilities, but also to capture changes in the level, rate, and interrelationship of abilities over time. In order to accomplish these tasks, neuropsychologists must select measures that meet appropriate psychometric standards and which derive from a conceptual understanding of the development of children's abilities and the disruption of these abilities due to neurologic and environmental factors. From this basis, neuropsychologists can complete evaluations that lead to treatment plans which can be monitored over time (Rourke, Fisk and Strang, 1986).

Neuropsychologic assessment of children is based on a set of explicit and implicit assumptions. The explicit assumptions are well known and involve understanding and documenting the 'psychometric properties' of the performance tests, rating scales, and other assessment procedures. In developmental neuropsychology, it is commonly acknowledged, many

times only by consensus, that certain procedures have proven reliability; and that the procedures measure a particular ability in a manner consistent across children and occasions. Criterion validity studies have shown that prescribed procedures discriminate relevant groups. Descriptive validity studies using variance partitioning techniques (e.g., factor analysis) have been used to assess the interrelationship of various procedures and constructs. Other explicit assumptions involve the nature, purpose, process, and outcome of such assessments.

There are also important concepts and assumptions in this area that are implicit and are rarely discussed explicitly. Of particular interest are the concepts of *ability discrepancy* (i.e., differences between measures of an individual's abilities) and *ability change*. These concepts, which are fundamental to neuropsychological assessment, assume that: (a) the assessment procedures are sufficiently reliable to detect ability discrepancies and/or ability changes; (b) these ability discrepancies/changes are related to biological and/or environmental variability; and (c) these ability discrepancies/changes can be used to design an intervention program. An additional assumption, implicit when assessing children, is that the ability discrepancy may change over time, particularly in children recovering from a brain insult.

---

* Corresponding author. E-mail: psyrdm@langate.gsu.edu

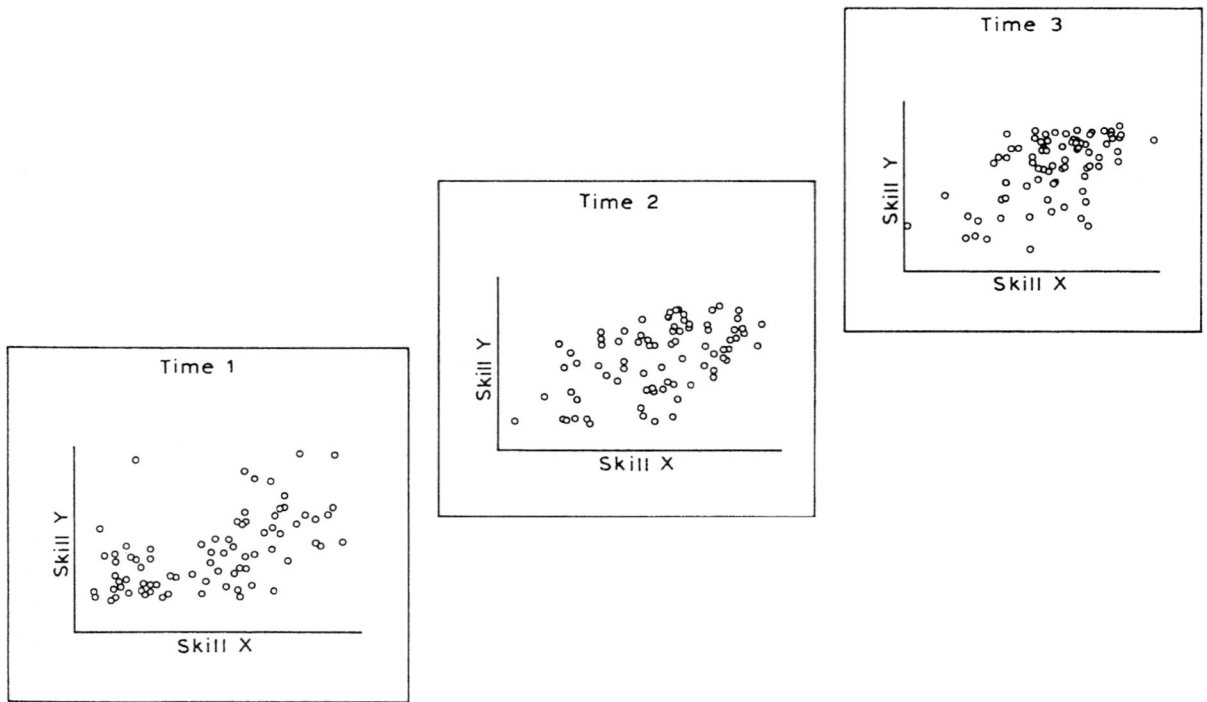

Fig. 1. Relation between two abilities ($X-Y$) over time.

The concepts of ability discrepancy and ability change are intimately linked in developmental neuropsychology and represent separate two-dimensional frameworks for understanding and assessing children; one framework is the relation between abilities, the other is the relation between time points (see Fig. 1). In children, the study of recovery of function and the evaluation of the effectiveness of various treatment paradigms are directly linked to understanding the changes in ability discrepancies over time. This represents a third framework which integrates the other two more traditional frameworks. In other words, the assessment of the similarities or differences among children's abilities (ability discrepancy) has at its core many of the same conceptual and psychometric issues as the assessment of change between two time points (ability change). In children, neuropsychologists recognize the need for a temporal perspective because of the developing nature of abilities and the potential for *change* in all abilities, whether or not two abilities are discrepant at some arbitrary point in time or not. Unfortunately, exactly what is meant by the concepts of discrepancy

and change in an individual child is often not well understood, and is only rarely researched. In particular, these concepts lead to significant measurement problems that are seldom subjected to empirical scrutiny. Consequently, such assumptions about discrepancies remain implicit, and investigations of ability change remain hampered by poor design and analysis, representing the failure to place these issues into a psychometric framework.

This chapter will discuss relationships between ability discrepancy and ability change in the context of a few critical measurement issues, and practical clinical and research problems underlying the neuropsychological assessment of children. We will show that the measurement of ability discrepancies and ability change are influenced by problems involving the reliability of measures, scaling, and construct validity. Methods for identifying ability discrepancies and change over time will also be briefly discussed. We will address the problematic role of ability discrepancy determination as the basis for definitions and classification of developmental learning and attention disorders. However, such discrepancies are also highly relevant for understanding relationships of neuropsychological performance with central nervous system (CNS) pathophysiology and environmental variation. These points will be further highlighted by a discussion of ability change as the basis for assessment of recovery of function and evaluation of treatment effectiveness in a child recovering from a brain insult.

## What is an ability discrepancy?

The presence or absence of a discrepancy in a child's abilities is often the key finding from a neuropsychological assessment. For example, the literature on children often emphasizes differences in WISC-R Verbal (VIQ) and Performance IQ (PIQ) scores, reading versus arithmetic scores, or lateralized motor and sensory deficit findings (Rourke et al., 1986). A related emphasis in the literature on children with various disabilities (i.e., learning disabilities or developmental language disorders) has been on the discrepancy in a child's current measured ability ('attainment') versus their potential ability in specific areas of interest (Fletcher and Morris, 1986). Such discrepancies have often represented the primary basis for both clinical and research definitions of disorders of learning and attention. For example, most policy-based definitions of reading disability require a measurable discrepancy of 1–2 standard deviations between a reading test score and an IQ test score (i.e., potential). In the absence of such a discrepancy, the child is considered to be 'normal' or a 'slow learner'. In other words, in the absence of an ability–potential discrepancy, children are considered to have achieved their expected potentials, even though their level of potential or attainment may be deficient (i.e., children with mental retardation) when compared with population norms (Fletcher and Morris, 1986).

Different definitions of 'ability–ability' (two different abilities compared at one point in time) and 'ability–potential' discrepancies may reflect variations in implicit assumptions concerning the reference points used for interpreting assessment results. As example, two concepts which have been used to describe ability profile characteristics are shape and/or elevation (Morris, 1988). When examining differences between a child's abilities, such as when

the VIQ is significantly higher than the PIQ, the focus is clearly on profile shape. The description and/or diagnosis is based on ability–ability discrepancy criteria. Clearly, one appropriate reference for such comparisons is the individual (an ipsative ability discrepancy), although normative-based scores play a role in such comparisons. The reference point is to population norms when the focus is on elevation of the child's test profile, as when comparing a child's VIQ, which is 69, to the average VIQ (which is 100). The description or diagnosis is based on the deviation of the individual child from the typical performance in the population of same-aged children (a normative ability discrepancy). If such discrepancy relationships are not clearly defined, then the basic underlying assumptions regarding the purposes and outcome of the assessments are confused.

What is often not recognized is the implicit assumption that individual ability profiles should be flat for a given child and constant across children. Attributing ability–ability discrepancies to biological factors (e.g., genetic), environmental factors (e.g., socioeconomic status), and measurement factors is tantamount to saying that, in the absence of intrinsic and extrinsic sources of variability and given perfect measurement reliability, all children would obtain the same profiles across tests, represented as a straight line. Another interpretation of this concept is that the underlying null hypothesis in developmental neuropsychological assessment is that there are 'no differences' between abilities. A key debate in the area has focused on what should be considered a significant ability difference for a child (either clinically or statistically) and how this difference should be defined.

## What is ability change?

Common approaches to the assessment of change also reflect the process of evaluating ability differences, but in a different conceptual plane. When one evaluates ability change between two time points, an 'ability–ability' discrepancy is being assessed, but it is one that occurs over time between two measures of the same ability. The perception of change as a difference in performance that occurs between two time points has led to a great deal of confusion regarding the measurement and analysis of change. We have earlier discussed alternative conceptualizations that treat change as "a continuous process which underlies performance. . . " (Francis, Fletcher, Stuebing et al., 1991). Much of the clinical use and research with children has employed 'incremental approaches' to the measurement of change by using difference scores between two time points.

There are many statistical and psychometric problems associated with the use of difference scores. In the literature on change, these problems concern (a) the inverse relationship between the reliability of the difference score and the correlation between the pre-test and post-test scores themselves, and (b) the correlation between the observed difference score and the pre-test score and the role this correlation plays in studying correlates of change (i.e., in answering questions like 'Do younger children show more change than older children in recovering from brain injury?'). There have been many alternative change scores recommended (residualized change scores, regression-based change scores, base-free measures of change; Zimmerman and Williams, 1982a). However, none of these approaches has been found to be free of all these problems.

It is perhaps ironic that these problems with difference scores have been focused on the study of change and not on the study of ability–achievement and ability–ability discrepancies. The focus on these problems in the study of change has often in the past influenced social scientists to eschew the very study of change for fear of being led astray by statistical and psychometric artifacts. Despite these problems, many clinicians carry on undaunted in the use of ability–achievement and ability–ability discrepancies in defining and diagnosing clinical disorders, even though similar criticisms apply to these 'difference' scores. Even more ironic is the fact that, in the case of studying behavior *change*, there is a simple solution to the problems associated with difference scores, which is to collect more than two time points of data (Francis et al., 1991). Unfortunately, there is no such simple solution to the conceptual, statistical, and psychometric problems associated with the use of 'difference' (i.e., discrepancy) scores in defining and diagnosing childhood disorders.

Defining ability change as the difference between scores at two time points suggests that change is an incremental process rather than a process of continuous development over time (Willett, 1988). If change is continuous, then the change that occurs between any two assessments is the result of the child's developmental trajectory at the time of these assessments. Unfortunately, with only two time points, one cannot tell whether the change is multiplicative or additive in nature.

Conceptually, the study of behavior change is made more feasible (not less) by the collection of more than two assessments, provided that one models change as a *continuous* rather than an incremental process. In fact, the precision with which change can be measured improves dramatically with the number of time points used (Willett, 1988). Moreover, with more than two assessments, the reliability of estimated change can also be estimated directly from the data. When only two time points have been collected, assessment of the reliability of the difference score must draw on information about measurement error that is typically external to the study at hand, or is not available at all.

This important information about the reliability of estimated change makes it possible to study correlates of change meaningfully by allowing the researcher to control for bias that results from errors of measurement. Just as in the case of ability–ability and ability–achievement discrepancies, the reliability of using estimated change difference scores is related to (1) the reliability of the individual measurements that make up the difference, and (2) the variance in true differences (i.e., variance in true change) (Rogosa, Brandt and Zimowski, 1982). Although it may be possible for the reliability of the difference score to exceed the reliability of the individual measures involved (Zimmerman and Williams, 1982b), the fact remains that the use of only two assessments limits the precision with which change is estimated and makes the investigation of change correlates difficult at best. Moreover, most developmental progressions are not consistently linear, except for very short periods of time, which further limits the usefulness of using just two time points to describe ability change in any child. At least three time points are typically required to describe linear change with one degree of freedom to estimate error; four or more time points are necessary to estimate non-linear change over time.

The collection of more than two time points also allows the researcher to adopt more sophisticated approaches to modelling individual growth than does the use of simple difference scores (Francis et al., 1991). Such methods facilitate the estimation of parameters that describe each individual's growth trajectory. These parameters can then be correlated to other variates of interest in order to study correlates of changes. A particular strength of these approaches is that they permit correlation between initial status and change, which makes it possible to evaluate change from any point on the initial assessment distribution.

## Measuring ability discrepancy over time

The notion of ability–ability discrepancies measured at a single time can be generalized to multiple time points. Such a generalization leads directly to questions about change in discrepancies, e.g., is the magnitude of the discrepancy between a particular child's achievement and IQ stable, or is it getting larger or smaller over time? Such questions are typically fashioned in terms of a direct comparison between discrepancies measured at two points in time (i.e., incremental change). Such questions concerning the relative magnitude of two discrepancies can be answered by direct comparison (i.e., repeated measures MANOVA) because the within-time discrepancies are unbiased estimates of the true discrepancies, and the difference between these estimates will likewise provide an unbiased estimate of the difference between discrepancies over time. However, individuals are usually interested in determining the relation between subject characteristics and the change in discrepancies. Do young children show larger changes in discrepancies over time than older children, i.e., is the change in the size of the discrepancy correlated with age? Such a finding could be used as evidence that younger children's skills become more comparable with time, or that younger children show a greater propensity than older children for their deficit skills to 'catch up'. Answers to such questions suffer from the same problems (brought on by measurement error) that limit the usefulness of the simple difference score for studying correlates of change, only in this case the problems are compounded by the presence of three

difference scores ($D_1 = X_1 - Y_1$, $D_2 = X_2 - Y_2$, and $D = D_2 - D_1$).

Interestingly, the notion that change in a single skill can be conceptualized as a continuous process can be generalized to change in multiple skills, where each skill is described by its own separate time-dependent function whose parameters vary across subjects. By conceptualizing change in this manner, the advantages brought to the study of single skill change can be extended to the study of changes in skill discrepancies. That is, the study of changes in skill discrepancies can also be approached from a model of continuous change. Imagine a simple situation where two skills are both changing at constant rates, but the rates of change are not equal. More concretely, suppose that for a particular subject skill $X$ is increasing at 1 standardized unit per month and skill $Y$ is increasing at 2 standardized units per month. Obviously, we are describing two lines with unequal slopes, i.e., the lines are not parallel. These lines must cross, as must be the case for two growth trajectories where the difference between skill levels is not constant over time. Hence, depending on the times at which measurement is made, the difference between skills could be getting smaller with time, but it will eventually get larger with time after the lines cross. This change in the difference between skills must occur in this case because the growth rates for the two skills are different.

In this example, the difference between $X$ and $Y$ at any point in time is a function of the two rates of change and the initial levels of the two skills. That is, the discrepancy at any point in time is directly determined from the four parameters that describe the two growth models: the slope and intercept describing the relation between skill $X$ and time, and the slope and intercept describing the relation between skill $Y$ and time. More importantly, considering each skill as a function of time tends to shift our focus away from the magnitude of the discrepancy at any point in time, and compels us to ask 'why is skill $X$ growing at a rate that is so much slower than skill $Y$?'. The important issue is not the size of the skill discrepancy at any particular point in time, but rather sizeable differences in the rates of skill development for this child. Of course, for such questions to be meaningfully addressed, the skills must be measured on an interval level over time, and the metric for the two skills must be comparable. These points are equally valid, although much less obvious, when discussing changes in the magnitude of discrepancies over time. We think that this shift in emphasis away from the magnitude of skill discrepancies at fixed time points to a focus on differences in developmental rates is at least as important as the shift away from incremental views of change in favor of a conceptualization of change as a continuous process (Francis et al., 1991).

Clearly, the focus on ability discrepancies in developmental neuropsychology implies that such discrepancies cause difficulties in adaptation for a child. Most interventions are focused on alleviating any ability discrepancies. In some situations, ability discrepancies may have positive adaptive influences on a child. Although the assessment issues in such children are the same, decisions regarding their impact are different. In addition, there may be treatment decisions in some children that are designed to maximize such discrepancies.

## Implicit requirements in developmental neuropsychological assessment

In addition to implicit assumptions concerning the measurement of discrepancy and change, the developmental neuropsychologist must make a series of additional decisions and interpretations regarding the results of any assessment he or she obtains from a child. These decisions and interpretations are rarely made explicit. The first implicit assumption includes deciding whether to reject the null hypothesis regarding the absence of ability discrepancies or changes in the child's abilities, depending on the type and purpose of the assessment being performed. If the null hypothesis is rejected and there are ability discrepancies, or changes in a child's abilities over time, the clinician must then decide whether such findings are related to (1) psychometric limitations in the assessment measures utilized, (2) variation due to environmental influences, or (3) variation due to biological influences. When making these decisions, clinicians are actually being asked to partition the discrepancy-related variance into the various influences on a child's test results (psychometric, environmental, biological, and error variances). The developmental neuropsychologist can have considerable data on the

impact of the known psychometric variance in accounting for the observed discrepancy, but may have only limited ability to understand the environmental factors (variance) involved, and almost no ability to understand the biological variance involved. This is one reason why the psychometric properties of the tests are of such interest.

Developmental neuropsychologists must also decide whether such discrepancies allow for the valid description, classification, or diagnosis of a particular child for the purposes intended. Once they have decided that such discrepancies are a valid index of the child's true state, they must then, based on this description, develop a predictive model and/or intervention strategy to assist the child's future development. Finally, once the predictive model is developed and intervention has been initiated or completed, they must evaluate whether the model and the intervention are effective. This latter step is completely dependent on assessing whether an ability discrepancy changes over time, again utilizing the underlying null hypothesis assumption of 'no difference (change) over time'. The best way to understand the measurement issues behind these implicit assumptions is to use a case example, presented with reduced details and information, for illustrative purposes.

### Case example

This case involves a 9-year-old boy who was in good health and performing well in school until he was involved in an automobile accident and sustained blunt trauma to the head. For purposes of an unrelated research project, he had limited testing performed approximately 2 weeks before his accident. On this evaluation, he obtained a WISC-R VIQ of 110, a PIQ of 102, and an FSIQ of 105. He also had been given the WRAT-R and had reading, spelling, and arithmetic scores which all fell at a standard score of 108.

Severity indices of this child's accident-related injury yielded a Glasgow Coma Scale score of 4 on the scene and 6 at 24 hours. The child was in coma for 7 days and had post-traumatic amnesia for 18 days. Neuroimaging studies were consistent with diffuse brainstem injury with evidence of shearing in the brainstem. There was also contusional injury to the fronto-temporal and temporal–parietal area of the left hemisphere but no subdural hematoma. No neurosurgical procedure was necessary.

During hospitalization, the child was referred for neuropsychological evaluation, which revealed expressive and receptive aphasia, right hemiparesis, and sufficient amnesia and disorientation to preclude test-based evaluation. The child was later discharged, received homebound instruction from school as well as occupational, physical, and speech therapies on an outpatient basis. By 4 months post-injury, the boy was fully oriented and ambulatory with no obvious signs of aphasia and considerable resolution of the right-sided hemiparesis. He was referred 6 months following his accident for neuropsychological evaluation to assess the extent of his recovery and to prepare for school placement. Since he was alert, ambulatory, and not obviously aphasic, the school was recommending that he return to regular classes with occupational therapy and speech therapy monitoring. The parents were concerned because his language seemed different and he also seemed forgetful and inattentive. When they discussed these issues with the school, they were told that the school was not obliged to provide services because of the head injury and would only serve the child if he met eligibility criteria as learning disabled (LD), speech and language handicapped (SLH), mentally retarded (MR), or emotionally disturbed (ED) on school-based discrepancy criteria. For either LD or SLH, the child would have to demonstrate scores on measures of academic achievement or language that were at least one standard deviation below the composite score (FSIQ) on an intelligence test.

The child received a complete neuropsychological evaluation that revealed the expected problems with short-term memory, attention, and motor coordination on the right side. However, the tests used to measure these abilities are not on the list accepted by the state education agency. To comply with their requirements, the child was administered the WISC-R, Wide Range Achievement Test-Revised (WRAT-R), and Test of Language Development-Primary (TOLD-P). The following scores were obtained: WISC-R VIQ = 72; PIQ = 84; FSIQ = 80; WRAT-R reading = 94; spelling = 94; arithmetic = 84; TOLD-P = 68. Because none of these test scores corresponded to the school-based criteria (>15 point discrepancy with FSIQ) for LD, SLH, MR, and because the neuropsychologist was not willing to label the child ED, the eligibility committee recommended placement in regular classes.

This case demonstrates several real-life, conceptual, and psychometric issues involved in determining ability discrepancies and change discrepancies in assessment results and scores. The first question is whether there has been a related change in this child's abilities 6 months after his head injury (time-based 'ability–ability' discrepancy). The second issue is whether this child can qualify, based on state discrepancy criteria, to receive special education services (within-time 'ability–achievement' discrepancy). The third issue is what kind of specific deficit, if any, has the child sustained regardless of whether or not the measured discrepancy meets state discrepancy criteria (within-time 'ability–ability' discrepancy).

Test results relevant to these issues include: (a) time 1 (pre-injury) vs time 2 (6 months post-injury) scores; (b) FSIQ vs WRAT-R scores; (c) VIQ vs PIQ; (d) FSIQ vs TOLD-P scores; and (e) differences among achievement scores. For issue (a) there were changes over time points between 18 and 38 standard score points, (b) FSIQ was 4–14 points below WRAT-R scores, (c) PIQ exceeded VIQ by 12 points, (d) TOLD-P was 12 points below FSIQ, and (e) arithmetic was 10 points below reading and spelling on the WRAT-R.

For each score comparison, the question is whether the discrepancy is large enough to be either clinically significant or to qualify the child for placement. Another way to consider this issue is to ask whether the discrepancy is real and statistically takes into account the errors of measurement of both test scores and their relations; if it is statistically real, then is the discrepancy clinically rare and meaningful? The comparison under (c) is sometimes made to compare left-hemisphere and right-hemisphere functions; the comparison under (a) can be used to estimate differences relative to premorbid levels of functioning; and the comparisons under (b) and (d) are typically used for special education eligibility purposes. For each comparison, the conclusions would change if the computation of discrepancy were made with regression techniques that corrected for the intercorrelation of the measures and took into account the reliability of the individual measures involved. As an example, we would conclude that VIQ was significantly lower than PIQ, suggesting the presence of significant left-hemisphere involvement in the case. We would also conclude that the child's present level of intellectual functioning was significantly lower than his premorbid functioning. Although we would not conclude that the child qualified as LD< we would conclude that he qualified as SLH based on the 12-point difference in FSIQ and TOLD-P scores. Note that these issues would not emerge if we simply compared these scores with age-based norms, as this child is generally functioning in the average range in all intellectual and academic areas and would not meet most 'deficient' cut-off scores based on the normal distribution. The one exception is that the TOLD-P language score would meet most cut-off score criteria as being deficient. These discrepancies emerge only because of the attempt to compare correlated tests. Such regression-based adjustments can be used to assess both within-time ability–ability and ability–achievement discrepancies and time-based ability–ability discrepancies.

Continuing our case, the parents, one year later, question whether their child's independent speech/language therapy has been effective. They are most concerned with his frustration surrounding the therapy and wonder if he really needs it. They ask for a reevaluation to assess whether the treatments being provided for their child are impacting his recovery. Although we will not discuss evaluation results, the assumptions underlying this assessment are quite important for the assessment of discrepancy and change.

**Assessing recovery of function and rehabilitation effectiveness**

Assessing recovery of function and rehabilitation effectiveness in such a child has both theoretical and practical significance for developmental neuropsychology. Studies focused on the natural recovery of children following brain injury are related to the theoretical concepts of plasticity, lateralization of function, and underlying development. Studies of the rehabilitation-influenced recovery of such children focus on the practical aspects of treating such

children's ability discrepancies. The primary purpose of the former is *predicting* cognitive or behavioral *outcome*, while the purpose of the latter is *influencing* cognitive or behavioral *outcome*, hopefully in a positive manner. The ability to assess rehabilitative treatments' influence on outcome can only be adequately assessed if one is able to accurately predict a child's natural outcome without such special treatment. This is because the concept of rehabilitation, or treatment outcome, has within it an explicit assumption that such intervention should change (i.e., improve) outcome above and beyond that which would occur by 'natural' recovery without it. Clearly these issues are directly linked to the discussion of ability discrepancy and ability change.

Taking this orientation to the study of recovery of function and rehabilitation effectiveness in children, one must additionally identify those subcomponents of ability change that are related to (1) normal developmental influences, (2) natural recovery process, and (3) recovery due to the influence of rehabilitation/treatment efforts. This model suggests that developmental neuropsychologists must be able to partition recovery (ability change) into variance components related to (1) age-related, normal developmental changes, (2) 'natural' recovery processes following acquired deficits, (3) rehabilitation/treatment-influenced changes, and (4) the amount of change due to interactions between the other three factors. This last component, the interaction effect, is easy to conceptualize, but is probably the most difficult component to assess and describe. The interrelationships between the three subcomponents of change over time must be addressed, all of which are typically in the same direction in children (i.e., improvement, growth).

Traditionally, the literature on recovery of function has focused on the biological/neurological components of a child's improved functioning in his environment, while the rehabilitation literature has focused on the environmental components for such improved functioning. It is likely that basic biological recovery will affect behavior, which in turn can influence the environment; but at the same time environmental influences can affect neurologic functioning. In other words, there is an interaction between the neurologic changes and the environmental changes.

The concept of 'recovery of function' in the developing (changing) child appears to be a more complex theoretical construct than seems the case for the adult. The most simple definition of recovery for a child following brain injury would be a return (ability change) to their pre-insult level of functioning. Such a definition, however, is not as clear in its meaning as it might appear since 'pre-insult level' is a moving target. This level could be interpreted as a child's performance on a specific test that is the same at a later point in time as it was before the child was injured. Thus, a child may obtain a raw score of 15 on a specific memory test after obtaining a score of 15 before his injury, some 6 months ago. Is this recovery? What is the child's baseline if age is increased by 6 months? It is entirely possible that the child achieved such a score on follow-up through a completely different strategy or process than had been used before. For example, he may have used verbal labelling strategies to remember the geometric shapes presented in the test, where he had not in the past. Some researchers might argue that such results do not represent recovery, but represent a form of compensation, whereby the child has learned a specific strategy to assist him with performing certain functions. Other researchers would argue that such results do represent recovery, because they are evidence of a child's ability to make use of his various capacities in an adaptive way. Or could a child naturally be changing cognitive strategies when performing such a task, such that he is beginning to use linguistic labels to assist with non-verbal memory processes as part of the normal developmental progression?

*Shifting baselines*

Another issue that should be apparent is that children achieving a similar raw score on a test 6 months later would typically be behind their age mates, as increased scores would be expected. Because of this, some proponents have suggested that recovery has only occurred when a child's age-scaled score at follow-up matches that at pre-injury (age-standard level recovery). Such results are easily described by the use of standard scores: the child, pre-injury, might have had a standard score of 100, but 6 months later the same raw score would represent a standard

score of 90. An even more important question is raised by following this child at 6-month intervals for the next 10 years and showing that at every evaluation, the child's standard score is 90. This would suggest that the child's actual rate of development (see Satz, Fletcher, Clark et al., 1981 for discussion of deficit, delay, lag, and rate constructs) is paralleling the normal developmental progression of children without brain injuries. In this model, recovery could actually be defined as that period when a child starts to *parallel* the normal developmental progression again (parallel recovery), regardless of level of functioning. The level of standard score in such a child would be a function of the length of time between injury and parallel recovery; thus, the longer the time to achieve such recovery, the lower the standard score for a child. The concepts behind techniques that allow for estimation of individual growth curve analyses would support this view of recovery within our framework of ability change (Francis et al., 1991).

Another difficulty with the parallel recovery definition for children is the situation that occurs when children are so severely injured that their level of functioning has regressed, or is so minimal that it is significantly below their pre-injury level. Such children may, after a period of time, begin to show parallel recovery, represented by a consistent rate of new functioning maintained over time. However, their level of functioning still remains well behind even their pre-injury level of functioning for many years. In the present case, such children would maintain their 80 FSIQ over the years. To do this, they clearly are developing new knowledge and abilities, and are doing so at an 'average' developmental rate, except that their pre-injury level of abilities was much higher. Conceptually, such children appear to be re-developing, retracing the developmental progression that was previously achieved in the past. Few researchers, or parents, would consider such children recovered.

*Components of recovery*

To address this conceptual dilemma, a child's abilities may be partitioned into two important components. The first component is previous and historical development, what he has *already achieved*, which we will call the pre-injury developmental progression and level. The second component represents his development in the *future*, which we will call the post-injury developmental progression and level. The concept of 'recovery' must encompass both components. One question may be whether a child's injury has resulted in his performing at a lower level than his pre-injury development (change discrepancy) or whether a child's injury has resulted in post-injury development being altered from what would have been predicted (change discrepancy). In other words, is the ability change, and therefore recovery, related to his past development, or future potential? Or, is it caused by a regression of functioning, restriction of potential functioning, or both? These are two very different, although interrelated concepts, which have become more and more important as research has begun to show that early developmental lesions may not have a measurable effect until a later age.

The issue is certainly relevant for children with head injuries (Fletcher and Levin, 1988). In the more severe head injuries, there is clearly a regression in some functions to lower ability levels, while in more mild head injuries there is no such regression, but there may be disruption of some memory functions. In the latter cases, there are often notable changes on achievement and IQ testing years later (usually lower standard scores) due to the *lack* of new learning over that time period in relationship to their peers. This raises the question of the definition of 'recovery'. Should a child be considered as 'recovered' only when the post-injury development measurements are the same as if the child had never been injured? Or should the environmental event (i.e., the injury) and all its consequences just be considered another effect on development (just as effects might be expected from other events such as changing schools or parents getting a divorce)? If the latter is assumed, then the expectation that a child would reach his or her pre-injury potential might not be valid.

*Abilities versus function*

In addition to these complexities, the construct 'function' also is very complex in the developing child. Typically, function is considered an ongoing process, and represents a label in a classification of related activities. Thus we can talk about memory functions,

or physiologic functions. Such a simple definition becomes more problematic when we consider that typically, in developmental neuropsychology, such functions represent an integrated system of various components (i.e., naming abilities are a function of the language system). Unfortunately, in children the actual components (abilities) of each system may change as the child develops, so the function one identifies at one age may be somewhat different from the function one identifies at another age, even though we may use the same label for it. In more analytic terms, the suggestion is that the underlying covariance matrix between functional system components can change with development, or there can actually be additions or deletions of various subcomponents. Again, as an abstract example, let us say that function A is made up of a system of components (abilities) we will call B1, B2, and B3. The child is injured, and we see a deficit in function A. On follow-up testing a year later, we see no deficit on A, and conclude that A has 'recovered'. This conclusion may be unwarranted because of normal developmental changes in the system of subcomponents during that year. As an example, it may be that only subcomponents B1 and B2 remain a part of function A. Therefore, whether the initially impaired subcomponent (B3) is still affected cannot be determined using a measure of function A. Whether the function that has recovered is the same function that was originally assessed is frequently open to debate. It is also evident that there is the possibility of misinterpretation of test results when, in fact, the subskill that was primarily impaired has actually not improved. Global measures of function, such as IQ scores, which are typically multifactorial, may be more prone to misinterpretation than more specific indices of components of the functional systems.

Given that we know a child's pre-injury level of functioning, we need clear prediction equations for (1) what the child would have been like without the injury, (2) what the child will be like given the injury and 'natural' recovery, and (3) what the child will be like given additional effective rehabilitation. For each of these predictions we need both ability *level* and *progression* (ability change) information for each specific function of interest, in addition to any interrelationships and interactions between functions or predictive components. It is because of the lack of accurate developmental information, the typical lack of pre-injury indices of a child's functioning, and the significant methodologic and design problems, that research on recovery of function and rehabilitation effectiveness will probably continue to provide limited information.

## Summary and conclusions

The ability to assess ability discrepancies and change accurately is central to advancing developmental neuropsychological theory, research, practice, and treatment. Making the current implicit assumptions regarding these constructs explicit will require a notable shift in current thinking. By considering ability change as a continuous process, with a focus on changes in skill discrepancies over time, there may evolve more sophisticated and superior models of developing brain–behavior relationships. These models will be facilitated by careful measures of the biologic and environmental correlates of the change parameters inherent in these models.

## References

Fletcher JM, Levin HS: Neurobehavioral effects of brain injury in children. In Routh D (Ed), Handbook of Pediatric Psychology. New York: Guilford Press, pp. 258–296, 1988.

Fletcher JM, Morris RD: Classification of disabled learning: Beyond exclusionary definitions. In Ceci S (Ed), Handbook of Cognitive, Social, and Neuropsychological Aspects of Learning Disabilities, Vol. 1. New York: Lawrence Erlbaum, pp. 55–80, 1986.

Francis DJ, Fletcher JM, Stuebing KK, Davidson KC, Thompson NM: Analysis of Change: Modeling Individual Growth. Journal of Consulting and Clinical Psychology: 59(1); 1991.

Morris RD: Classification of learning disabilities: Old problems and new approaches. Journal of Consulting and Clinical Psychology: 56; 789–794, 1988.

Rogosa DR, Brandt D, Zimowski M: A growth curve approach to the measurement of change. Psychological Bulletin: 90; 726–748, 1982.

Rourke BP, Fisk JL, Strang JD: Neuropsychological Assessment of Children: A Treatment Oriented Approach. New York: Guilford, 1986.

Satz P, Fletcher JM, Clark W, Morris R: Lag, deficit, rate and delay constructs in specific learning disabilities: a reexamination. In Answara A, Geschwind N, Galaburda A, Albert M, Gartrell N (Eds), Sex Differences in Dyslexia. Townson, MD: The Orton Dyslexia Society, pp. 129–150, 1981.

Willett JB: Questions and answers in the measurement of change. In Rothkopf EZ (Ed), Review of Research in Education: 15; 345–422, 1988.

Zimmerman DH, Williams RH: The relative error magnitude in three measures of change. Psychometrika: 47; 141–147, 1982a.

Zimmerman DH, Williams RH: Gain scores in research can be highly reliable. Journal of Educational Measurement: 19; 149–154, 1982b.

*Handbook of Neuropsychology*, 2nd Edition, Vol. 8, Part I
S.J. Segalowitz and I. Rapin (Eds)

CHAPTER 10

# Neuropsychological assessment in infancy

## Victoria Molfese * and Bernadette Price

*Center for Research in Early Childhood Education, College of Education and Human Development, University of Louisville,
Louisville, KY 40292, USA*

## Introduction

The brain and its functioning from the prenatal period across the life span are of great interest to clinicians and researchers from many disciplines. This interest in what has come to be called 'neuropsychology' or 'developmental neuropsychology' has grown as techniques for assessing behaviors began to be linked to neurological, physiological, and neuroanatomical techniques (e.g., electroencephalography, event-related potentials, functional magnetic resonance imaging, magnetoencephalography, positron emission tomography, etc.). Researchers interested in brain functioning and in behavioral processes have worked on parallel paths toward establishing bases on which different techniques are used to assess the functioning of individuals and to identify individuals exhibiting or at risk for displaying deviations from normal functioning.

Interest in neuropsychological assessment of infants and preschool children arose in part as a function of the increased numbers of infants surviving very low birth weight and preterm birth with many infants, including those born as early as 24 weeks gestational age, surviving, some without severe central nervous system (CNS) damage. More information on the cognitive and neurological status of these survivors was needed, particularly information that would permit greater precision in the early identi-

fication of infants with or at risk for neurological dysfunctions. There was also the need to improve the ability to identify infants with mild or moderate impairments since these more subtle impairments are frequently harder to detect in early life than more severe impairments. It was hoped that improved identification would lead to better methods of linking these infants to different types of interventions to reduce the risk or remediate the impairments.

Interest also arose because of the hope generated by the development of neonatal assessment scales that accurate assessments could be made in the neonatal period, and that these assessments could be useful for predicting development in later infancy and childhood. It was hoped that these assessment scales could be used to provide a baseline against which developmental changes as well as the effects of different intervention techniques could be evaluated. The development of Brazelton's Neonatal Behavioral Assessment Scale (NBAS, 1973), which combined neurological and behavioral assessments, contributed substantially to increasing the interests of clinicians and researchers in specialties outside of neurology and pediatrics in neonatal assessment and neuropsychology. A further contribution of the NBAS was the recognition that infant state or level of alertness and responsivity to events external to the infant were important considerations when evaluating infant performance on neuropsychological assessments. Many neuropsychological assessment scales now include consideration of infant state as a necessary part of the assessment protocol.

---
* Corresponding author. Tel.: +1 (502) 852-0582; Fax: +1 (502) 852-1497; E-mail: tori@louisville.edu

There have been two orientations taken to the development of neuropsychological assessments for infants and preschool children. The first orientation has focused on the behavior side of the brain–behavior relation. While the focus is on the assessment and prediction of behaviors, inferences about brain functioning are also made. Clinicians and researchers working in this area are seeking to link measures of behavioral functioning with brain functioning. The hope is that behavioral measures can be used to evaluate current behavior and to predict subsequent behaviors. The second orientation is on the brain side of the brain–behavior relation. Here the focus is on the identification of specific brain functions, their etiology and developmental course during the infancy and early childhood periods. Clinicians and researchers working in this area are often well trained in neurology and neuroanatomy and are seeking further information on brain functioning. These investigators are using neuropsychological information to develop valid and reliable links to brain functioning and the characteristic behaviors that are both manifestations and consequences of brain functioning. The hope is that these neuropsychological measures can also be used to evaluate the extent to which changes occurring in brain functioning due to development, time since injury or event and other causes are consequently reflected in related behaviors. These two orientations are not exclusive, although clinicians and researchers working in each area have typically not been interested in sharing assessment procedures because the types of assessment procedures appropriate to each orientation often do not satisfy the requirements of the other orientation.

For both orientations of brain–behavior relations a variety of pediatric neuropsychological assessment procedures have been developed that are consistent with the goals of each orientation. Interestingly, the assessment procedures of both orientations fit into the scheme described by Lewis and Fox (1983). This scheme contains three levels of assessment. The first level, 'primary assessment', serves as an initial screening for dysfunctions or risks for dysfunctions in which infants are initially classified as normal and abnormal, or, in some cases, as suspect, non-suspect and certain, based on behavioral assessments. Primary screening instruments are developed for use with populations of infants to identify those

at risk for abnormalities and as a means for referring those infants for further assessment. The second level of assessment, 'secondary assessment', is applied primarily to infants in the suspect and certain categories and involves more in depth screening to separate areas of function and dysfunction. Secondary assessments are more comprehensive than primary assessments in that they frequently cover a variety of developmental abilities, permit evaluations of individual skills and provide a scheme by which areas of function and dysfunction can be identified. Assessments that serve these purposes are more complex than primary assessments in the scope of the behaviors that are evaluated, and are more time consuming and expensive to administer. These secondary assessments typically lead to initial decisions about appropriate multidisciplinary interventions for the disability or impairment identified through the application of the secondary assessment.

Although primary and secondary assessments have different application purposes, they do share many similarities in underlying test theory and construction. Because they both are designed to be screening techniques applicable to populations or large groups of infants (often including both prematurely born and full-term infants), primary and secondary assessments are designed to be administered within a short time period (usually 10–30 min), and, therefore, are composed of a small number of items (usually ranging from less than 30 to around 50 items). The short administration time facilitates the use of these assessments with sick and preterm infants for whom lengthy testing periods would be stressful. Typically these assessments can be administered without the use of specialized equipment and without extensively trained examiners, although as noted below this may not be true of all secondary assessments. Evaluations of infants using these assessments are based on either a total scale score, which is composed of summed item scores, or on the infant's performance on specific items or clusters of items. Procedures which usually accompany the scales often permit a means by which scores can be categorized according to prognosis. For the most part, these assessments are designed to permit an evaluation of short-term status of the infant and a means by which changes can be determined over a short time period (frequently day-to-day changes or changes within a week or month). Long-term prediction is rarely the goal of primary and secondary assessments.

Many assessments designed for use in the early infancy periods would be classified as either primary or secondary assessments (see Table 1). Examples of primary assessments frequently used in neonatal and infant research and clinical practice are the Apgar Scale, Bayley Infant Neurodevelopmental Screener, Dubowitz Assessment of Gestational Age and various perinatal risk scales (e.g., High Risk Pregnancy Screening System, and Obstetric Complications Scale) that evaluate antepartum, intrapartum and postpartum events. Examples of secondary assessments include: Amiel-Tison Neurological and Adaptive Capacity Score, Dubowitz Neurological Assessment of the Preterm and Full-Term Newborn Infant, Neurobehavioral Assessment for Preterm Infants, Neonatal Neurological Examination. These scales have aspects of their test theory and construction that are appealing to both pediatric neuropsychology orientations described above.

The third level in the assessment scheme is applied to infants whose condition makes them likely to fall into the certain category, although these tertiary assessments are also applied to some suspect infants on whom detailed information is needed to further evaluate their status. Tertiary assessments are used to gain more information about the extent and type of dysfunction thought to be present and to provide a basis by which changes and progress in specific nervous system functioning, whether developmental or intervention-based, can be gauged. Tertiary assessments are more complex than primary or secondary assessments. These assessments typically require administration by specialists with extensive training, and they frequently involve the use of a variety of methodologies to distinguish between areas of function and dysfunction. The results of tertiary assessments ideally provide a basis for making a long-term prediction concerning the prognosis for the infant and for making recommendations concerning intervention.

Several neuropsychological assessments that would be considered to fall within the category of tertiary assessments have been frequently used in the newborn and preschool periods (see Table 1). Examples of these tertiary assessments are: Assessment of Preterm Infants' Behavior, Neonatal Be-

havior Assessment Scale, Neurological Examination of the Full-Term Newborn Infant. These scales are well known and some are considered to be standards against which pediatric neuropsychology assessments are evaluated.

All three levels of assessment are included in the focus of this chapter because all three levels contribute importantly to neuropsychological assessments in the infancy period. Indeed, it is not unusual to find published reports of studies in which primary assessments are combined with secondary and/or tertiary assessments to address a variety of research questions. Described below are examples of the frequently used primary, secondary and tertiary neuropsychological assessments scales designed for use with infants from birth to 2 years of age. Information is provided on the purpose for which each scale was developed, the types of items on the scales, administration methodology, administration time, scoring procedures and information on validity. Reliability information is not typically available on these scales and is presented to the extent that it is available. Examples of how some of these scales have been used in research studies in the infancy period are described in the subsequent section. Because of the prevalence in which pediatric neuropsychological assessments are being used in studies of drug-exposed infants and because often multiple types of neuropsychological assessment have been administered in these studies, they are used as examples of pediatric neuropsychological assessments in research.

## Primary assessment instruments

*Apgar method of evaluation of the newborn infant (Apgar, 1953)*

The Apgar Scale was designed to evaluate the postnatal status of the newborn infant. The scale consists of five items: appearance (color), pulse (heart rate), grimace (reflex irritability), activity (muscle tone), and respirations. The items are typically scored at 1 and 5 min after birth, although scores obtained at 10 min and beyond are not uncommon, particularly when initial scores are low. Each item can receive a maximum of two points, with a total score of ten reflecting optimal status. Scores of three or below at any time but especially at 5 min are indications of

TABLE 1

Neuropsychological assessment in infancy

| | Test description | Age | Items and scoring |
|---|---|---|---|
| *Primary* | | | |
| Apgar Scale (Apgar, 1953) | Assesses postnatal status of newborn infants. Judgments based on Appearance (color), Pulse (heart rate), Grimace (reflex), Activity (muscle tone), and Respirations | Newborn infants: 1 and 5 minutes after birth and at subsequent time points if initial scores are low | 5 items, 2 points per item. Optimal score is 10. Score of $\leq 3$ at 5 minutes indicates depressed physiological status |
| Bayley Infant Neurodevelopmental Screener (BINS, Aylward, 1995) | Assesses basic neurological functioning to detect developmental delay and neurological impairment in 4 areas: neurological, receptive, expressive, and cognitive functions. Contains a subset of Bayley Scale items. Assessment time: 10 minutes | Infants from 3 months to 24 months | Variable number of items by age to evaluate posture, tone, movement, elicited and observable behaviors. Scores of 0 or 1 for each item and summed across areas to indicate high, moderate, or low developmental delay |
| Dubowitz Assessment of Gestational Age (Dubowitz, Dubowitz and Goldberg, 1970) | Assesses infant gestational age at birth using neurological and physical items | Neonatal period | Items include 10 neurological signs and 11 physical characteristics. Item scores range 0–4 and are summed |
| High Risk Pregnancy Screening System (Hobel, Hyvarinen, Okada and Oh, 1973) | Assesses women and their infants for biomedical risks | Scored from medical record information | 126 items in 3 subscales (maternal antepartum, maternal intrapartum, and neonatal) Each item scored: 1, 5, or 10. Scores from subscales are used to determine risk. Scores within subscales: <10 is low risk and >10 is high risk |
| Obstetrics Complications Scale (Littman and Parmelee, 1978) | Assesses biomedical optimality of women and their infants | Scored from medical record information | 20 antepartum, 15 intrapartum, 6 infant items scored as 1 or 0; summed for total score |
| *Secondary* | | | |
| Amiel-Tison Neurological and Adaptive Capacity Scale (Amiel-Tison, Barrier, Shnider et al., 1982) | Assesses effects of obstetric medication on infants | Administered to full-term, newborn infants at birth | 20 items assess: tone, alertness, adaptive capacity, motor activity, cry, primary reflexes. Items are scored 0 (abnormal) to 2 (normal) and summed |
| Dubowitz Neurological Assessment of the Preterm and Full-Term Newborn Infant (Dubowitz and Dubowitz, 1981) | Assesses neurological functioning, emphasizing movement and tone | Full-term infants assessed within 3 days and preterm infants from birth to term | 33 items divided into habituation, movement and tone, reflexes, and neurobehavioral responses. 5-point rating scales. Item scores are evaluated individually. State and asymmetries are noted |
| Neurobehavioral Assessment for Preterm Infants (Korner and Thom, 1990) | Assesses maturity of functioning in preterm infants. Assessment time: 30 minutes | Preterm infants 32 to 37 weeks (conceptional age) | 7 items clusters: motor development and vigor, scarf sigh, popliteal angle, alertness and orientation, irritability, vigor of crying, and percent asleep ratings. Average cluster scores from 3 to 9 point ratings. Behavioral state is noted |

| Measure | Assesses | Population/Age | Item details |
|---|---|---|---|
| Neonatal Neurological Examination (Sheridan-Pereira, Ellison and Helgeson, 1991) | NEONEURO assesses neurological and neurobehavioral performance | NEONEURAL: first 48 hours after birth, after 72 hours, and up to 1 week | 32 items distributed: hypertonus, reflexes, tone, tremor, alertness and fussy. 2-, 3-, 5-point rating scales. Can be summed. Cut scores differentiate normal from abnormal groupings |
| Infant Neurological International Battery (Ellison, 1994) | INFANIB assesses infants, particularly premature and other risk infants. Untimed | INFANIB is administered from birth to 18 months | For INFANIB, 20 items in supine, prone, sitting, standing, or suspended positions. Item, subscale and total scores can be calculated |

*Tertiary*

| Measure | Assesses | Population/Age | Item details |
|---|---|---|---|
| Assessment of Preterm Infants' Behavior (Als, Lester, Tronick and Brazelton, 1982) | Assesses behavior in prematurely born infants in five areas: physiology, motor organization, state, attention/interaction, self-regulatory processes and reflexes | Infants once they are in an open crib up to one month post-term | 280 items scored on 9-point descriptive scales. Various scoring protocols can be used |
| Brazelton Neonatal Behavioral Assessment Scale (Brazelton, 1973; Brazelton and Nugent, 1995) | Assesses responses to and reactions to the environment in areas of physiological, motor, state, and attentional/interactional processes | Term infants, healthy preterm infants < 37 weeks gestational age, and preterm infants through 48 weeks post-conceptual age | 28 behavioral items and 18 reflex items plus 7 items for risk infants. Behavioral items scored on 9-point scale, reflex items on a 4-point scale. Optimal states are specified. Items grouped into packages: Habituation, Motor-Oral, Truncal, Vestibular, and Social-Interactive |
| The Neurological Examination of the Full Term Newborn Infant (Prechtl and Beintima, 1964; Prechtl, 1977) | Assesses nervous system abnormalities. Comprehensive exam that starts with an observational period and then items are administered | Newborn period | 5 items assess: state, posture, motor activity, appearance, reflexes, movements, motility, response threshold, crying, pathological movements, hemisyndrome, reaction type. Item states are specified. Items scored on a 2–4 point scales and summed |

*Outcome measures*

| Measure | Assesses | Population/Age | Item details |
|---|---|---|---|
| Bayley Scales of Infant Development (Bayley, 1969, 1993) | Assesses development of infants and children, including high risk and developmentally delayed. Three parts: Mental Development Index (MDI), Psychomotor Development Index (PDI), and Behavior Rating Scale. Assessment time: 25–60 minutes | Infants and children from 1 to 42 months of age | Age based items sets with varying numbers of items. Index scores and developmental age scores are calculated based on item scores: passed, not passed. 30 Behavior items rated on a 5-point scale and scores are categorized |
| Denver Developmental Screening Scale (Frankenburg and Dodds, 1967; 1992; Frankenburg, Dodds and Fandal, 1970) | Assesses children for developmental delay. Assessment time: 10–25 minutes | Infants and children birth to age 6 | 125 items assessing 4 function areas: Personal Social, Fine Motor Adaptive, Language and Gross Motor. Items are scored as advanced, normal, caution, and delay. Scores are used to assign children to normal, suspect or untestable groups |
| Stanford-Binet Intelligence Scale, Fourth Edition (Thorndike, Hage and Sattler, 1986) | Assesses general cognitive abilities in four areas: Verbal Reasoning, Abstract/Visual Reasoning, Quantitative Reasoning, and Short-Term Memory. A brief screening battery can also be given | Appropriate for children age 2 to adulthood | Items in each test are scored pass/fail and summed to derive subtest and subscale scores as well as a test composite score |

depressed physiological status and are often used as signs of morbidity or mortality. Significant correlations have been reported between low Apgar scores and incidence of neonatal mortality and neurological abnormality in a large sample of full-term infants from the Collaborative Project (Drage and Berendes, 1966) and from a meta-analysis of Apgar scores and adverse outcomes (van de Riet, Vandenbussche, Le Cessie and Keirse, 1999). A neonatal mortality rate of 15% has been found in infants with 1-min Apgar scores lower than three, although successful resuscitation of infants with Apgar scores of 0 at 1 and 5 min has been reported. However, with these infants successful outcomes were influenced by gestational age, birth weight and 10-min Apgar scores (Haddad, Mercer, Livingston et al., 2000). Neurological outcomes of infants with Apgar scores less than three are generally poor. Data from the National Collaborative Perinatal Project have been used to evaluate outcomes of children at age 7 years. Nelson and Ellenberg (1981) confirmed the relation between low Apgar scores and increased incidence of neonatal death and cerebral palsy. However, it was noted that for some children who were survivors of Apgar scores of 0 to 3 at 10 min, 80% had no major handicaps. Thus, use of Apgar scores as an absolute predictor of infant outcomes is not always possible (Golden, 1998).

When applied to preterm infants, the validity of the scores is uncertain since many of the behaviors evaluated on the Apgar Scale are negatively influenced by low gestational age (e.g., respiration, tone, cry). However, low Apgar scores at 1 and 5 min have been found predictive of mortality in low birth weight (<2000 g), preterm infants (Hegyi, Carbone, Artwar et al., 1998). Apgar scores have not been predictive of common complications associated with preterm birth, such as cerebral palsy (Topp, Langhoff-Roos and Uldall, 1997). It has also been reported that compared to physicians, nursing staff have difficulty assigning correct Apgar scores (Letko, 1996).

*Bayley Infant Neurodevelopmental Screener (BINS Aylward, 1995)*

Several neuropsychological screening scales have been developed for use with young infants. Most include assessments of posture, tone, movement and of specifically elicited or observed behaviors. The BINS was developed to enable infants 3–4 months, 5–6 months, 7–10 months, 11–15 months, 16–20 months and 21–24 months to be screened for developmental delay or neurological impairment. A subset of items from the Bayley Scales of Infant Development (Bayley, 1993) that have been linked to developmental delay are included as part of the assessment scale. Scoring is based on 0 (non-optimal) and 1 (optimal) for items representing four areas: neurological functions/intactness, receptive functions, expressive functions and cognitive processes. Scores are summed across areas and risk for developmental delay or neurological impairment is evaluated as high, moderate or low. These assessments were constructed to enable parents, nursing staffs and others assessing young infants to have a screening tool. Videotapes are available for training purposes and can be used with parents. The BINS provides a means by which parents might quantify their concerns and observations about their children's development.

Aylward, Verhulst and Bell (1994) report on the predictive utility of a previous version of the BINS, the Early Neuropsychological Optimality Rating Scales (ENORS), applied at 6, 12 and 24 months. ENORS scores, especially when combined with measures of the family socio-economic environment, were highly predictive of cognitive outcomes at 3 years of age. Aylward et al. (1994) provide an interesting and useful demonstration of the value to categorizing scores as optimal or non-optimal. An odds ratio approach was used which tested how children's 36 month score on the McCarthy Scales of Children's Abilities (MSCA) are influenced if children had optimal or non-optimal scores on the ENORS at 6, 12 or 24 months. Participants were 573 high-risk infants participating in a longitudinal study. The likelihood of a normal MSCA was increased by 2.4 to 10.7 times if ENORS-6 was optimal, 9.85 to 90.1 for optimal ENORS-12 and 10.5 to 54.5 for optimal ENORS-24. An optimal socio-economic environment contributed modestly to these ratios. Similar finding using the BINS with infants 6, 12 and 24 months and assessing outcomes at 36 months on the MSCA are reported by Aylward and Verhulst (2000).

*Dubowitz Assessment of Gestational Age (DAGA, Dubowitz, Dubowitz and Goldberg, 1970)*

The DAGA scale, which should not be confused with the Dubowitz Neurological Assessment of Preterm and Full-Term Newborn Infant (1981), was designed to enable the gestational age of infants to be determined with greater accuracy than is possible with other available techniques (e.g., maternal report of menstrual history, infant weight, appearance, neurological maturity). Many consider the determination of gestational age to be an important base against which the significance of neurological characteristics can be evaluated (Parmelee and Michaelis, 1971). The Dubowitz Scale is administered in the neonatal period and consists of a neurological component and a physical component, with items taken from scales by St-Anne Dargassies (1954), Amiel-Tison (1968) and Farr, Mitchell, Nilgian and Parkin (1966). The assessment includes 10 neurological signs (e.g., posture, ankle dorsiflexion, arm recoil, popliteal angle, and ventral suspension) and 11 physical characteristics (e.g., edema, skin texture, skin color, skin opacity). Scores of individual items vary from 0 to a maximum of 4. Item scores within each component are summed to achieve a total score. King, Perlman, Laptook et al. (1995) adapted the DAGA by reducing the number of items and summing scores into a total score to determine how cocaine exposure affected term and near-term infants. DAGA scores reflected no group differences between exposed and non-exposed infants.

A shorter version of the Dubowitz assessment has been developed (Ballard, Novak and Driver, 1979) for use with preterm infants. In many hospitals the Ballard scoring system is used routinely to determine gestational age in all newborn infants. Research reports show that the Dubowitz overestimates gestational age when applied to preterm infants (Spinnato, Sibain, Shaver and Anderson, 1984); however, moderate agreement has been shown between newborn Dubowitz scores and prenatal ultrasonic biparietal diameter measures in classifying infants as small-for-gestational age and preterm (Vik, Vatten, Markestad et al., 1997). It is common, however, for the Ballard to be used with preterm infants. The Ballard scale includes 12 of the 21 Dubowitz items and correlates highly ($r = 0.97$) with the longer Dubowitz. Though

not recommended as a replacement for the Dubowitz since it does not cover as many behaviors, the shorter Ballard test would be expected to cause less stress to the already stressed preterm infants. Assessments of gestational age of preterm infants using the Ballard has been found to be accurate with and without prior knowledge of other gestational age information (Smith, Dayal and Monga, 1999).

*High-Risk Pregnancy Screening System (HRPSS) (Hobel, Hyvarinen, Okada and Oh, 1973)*

Although the HRPSS contains more items than the typical number on primary screening instruments, the HRPSS was designed to screen large populations of women and their infants for biomedical risks and is frequently used in obstetrics settings. The 126 items contained on the scale were obtained from other biomedical risk scales or derived from the authors' clinical judgments. The items are divided into three subscales: maternal antepartum (51 items pertaining to cardiovascular, renal and metabolic problems, previous pregnancies, anatomical abnormalities, various diseases, drug use and maternal physical characteristics), maternal intrapartum (40 items pertaining to maternal conditions, placental problems, and specific fetal conditions), and neonatal (35 items pertaining to maturity, respiration, metabolic disorders, cardiac, hematologic, and CNS problems). Each item receives a score of 1, 5 or 10, based on the potential of the condition represented by the items for resulting in morbidity or mortality. Total scores and subscale scores are used to evaluate risk. Total scores less than 10 are assumed to indicate low risk while scores greater than 10 indicate high risk.

HRPSS has been used in numerous studies, including studies of cocaine-exposed infants. Group differences between cocaine-exposed and non-exposed infants have been reported on the neonatal subscale of the HRPSS (e.g., Alessandri, Bendersky and Lewis, 1998; McGrath, Sullivan, Lester and Oh, 2000) but not by all investigators (e.g., Tronick, Frank, Cabral et al., 1996). Increased neonatal medical risk as measured by the HRPSS has been reported from a combination of effects due to prenatal cocaine exposure, birth weight, antepartum and intrapartum risks (Bendersky and Lewis, 2000).

The original HRPSS was reconfigured into the Problem-Oriented Perinatal Risk Assessment System (PROPAS). The PROPAS contains most of the same items as the HRPSS but does have some different items and includes a listing of maternal postpartum items. Because the postpartum items are unweighted it is not possible to derive a risk score from them. The PROPOAS is frequently used in hospital obstetric units as a standard medical record form.

### Obstetric Complications Scale (OCS) (Littman and Parmelee, 1978)

This scale is based on Prechtl's optimality concept and contains all but one of the items on the Prechtl Scale of Optimal Obstetric Complications (Prechtl, 1967). In contrast to most scales including the HRPPS which are developed to identify and quantify conditions that place infants at-risk for mortality and morbidity, optimality based scales examine medical conditions within a narrowly defined range of values that are likely to result in minimal risk for infants.

The OCS contains 41 items divided into 20 antepartum, 15 intrapartum, and 6 infant items. Items are scored as optimal (1) or non-optimal (0) and item scores are summed to obtain a total score. The total scores are divided by the number of items scored to compensate for missing data. Validity has been assessed in correlations with the Postnatal Complications Scale (PNCS) and the Pediatric Complications Scale (PCS) also developed by Littman and Parmelee. However, the between-scale score correlations have been low. Scafidi, Field, Wheeden et al. (1996) have reported sensitivity (the number of true positives) of the OCS to group differences in cocaine-exposed and non-exposed infants, but group differences were not found on the PNCS. The OCS, PNCS, PCS have been used extensively in research, especially in conjunction with the Brazelton Neonatal Behavioral Assessment Scale.

### Secondary assessment instruments

The scales described in this section share significant overlaps in the items they contain and in much of their test theory and construction. The item overlap is the result of the limited behavioral repertoire of young infants and because the items were primarily taken from a larger set of neurological assessment items devised by leaders in neurological assessments of neonates and infants: Peiper (1963), Prechtl (1977) and St. Anne Dargassies (1977). Both the range and overlap of items on the four scales described in this section are illustrated in Table 1. These scales have also frequently combined the classic neurological items with some behavioral assessment items taken from developmental assessment scales (e.g., the Bayley Scales, the Brazelton Scales, etc.). The similarities across scales in this section also extend to some similarities in test construction. The similarities exist despite differences across scales in the specific assessment purposes for which each scale was constructed.

### Amiel-Tison Neurological and Adaptive Capacity Score (NACS, Amiel-Tison, Barrier, Shnider et al., 1982)

This is a screening exam specifically designed to evaluate the effects of obstetrical medications, and separate these effects on the newborn from effects due to perinatal asphyxia, neurological disease or birth trauma on the behaviors of full-term, newborn infants. The NCAS was designed to be administered in the delivery room shortly after birth and contains items thought to be sensitive to obstetric medications, perinatal asphyxia and birth trauma (e.g., tone items). The scale contains items and features derived from the Brazelton BNAS (1973), the Scanlon Einstein Neonatal Neurobehavioral Assessment Scale (Scanlon, Brown, Weiss and Alper, 1974) and the Amiel-Tison Neurological Examination (Amiel-Tison, 1976). The 20 items reflect passive and active tone, primary reflexes, adaptive capacity and a general assessment component which evaluates alertness, quality of cry and motor activity. Scale items are scores 0 (abnormal) to 2 (normal) based on the infant's responses. The items are summed to produce a total score. The exam can be administered in 5 min. Readministration is recommended after 2 hours and again after 24 hours in case of low scores (i.e., total scores less than 34) or in the presence of abnormalities. Amiel-Tison et al. (1982) report that the NACS produces results which are similar to results produced by the ENNS.

From its publication, the Amiel-Tison has been criticized (Michenfelder, 1982; Tronick, 1982) on a number of grounds: sensitivity, validity, and lack of research support. Despite these criticisms the NACS is widely used especially in research on effects of obstetric anesthesia (Camann and Brazelton, 2000). Reasons for the popularity of the NACS have included its simplicity, non-invasiveness, and speed of administration. However, calls continue for studies of determine the validity of the NACS for differentiating neonates with impaired functioning from those with normal functioning. Brockhurst, Littleford, Halpern and Fisher (2000) published the results of an extensive literature review on reliability, validity and sensitivity of the NACS. While the findings are not clearly positive with regard to the validity of the NACS, it does appear from some studies that scores of infants exposed to intrapartum anesthesia receive lower NACS scores and that these scores are related to subsequent behaviors in the newborn period. However, additional research is needed with this popularly used but not well researched assessment instrument and with the increasing popularity of epidural anesthesiology during labor and delivery, the time might be right for such research.

### Dubowitz Neurological Assessment of the Preterm and Full-Term Newborn Infant (NAPFI, Dubowitz and Dubowitz, 1981)

Considered a comprehensive neurological examination, this scale draws items and scoring procedures from NBAS (Brazelton, 1973), Howard, Parmelee, Kopp and Littman (1976), NEFNI (Prechtl, 1977), and St. Anne Dargassies (1977) scales into an examination designed to be part of the routine examination of newborn infants. The scale items emphasize assessment of movement and tone. There are 33 items divided into habituation, movement and tone, reflexes, and neurobehavioral responses. Infant state and the presence of asymmetries are noted when scoring, along with an evaluation of the infant's responses to items. Each item has a five-point rating scale consisting either of descriptions of responses or stick figure drawings of possible responses. The examination is designed to permit an administration time of 10–15 min and can be used with full-term infants within the first three days and with preterm

infants from birth to term. The scale developers encourage repeated assessments as important for obtaining valid scores and for observing changes in neurological signs that occur over time, particularly in preterm infants as they mature. The item scores are used individually, rather than summed into a total score, so that the focus is on the pattern of responses.

Various efforts have been made to develop a quantified version of the NAPFI for use in research. Dubowitz, Mercuri and Dubowitz (1998) have revised the NAPFI by eliminating some and adding other items and including an optimality score to be useful for research studies. Cut scores (less than 10%) based on item performance in a sample of term infants were used as the basis for establishing the overall optimality score. 'Suboptimal' scores are used to identify children needing reassessment. Eyler, Delgado-Hachey, Woods and Carter (1991) also sought to quantify the NAPFI for use in research and explored the quantification of NAPFI by applying scores to each items and grouping of items into clusters: habituation, orientation, range of state, regulation of state, autonomic regulation, motor performance and abnormal reflexes. Regression models involving NAPFI factor scores and Bayley scores at 6, 12, 18 and 24 months resulted in little predictive utility.

Recently, Haataja, Mercuri, Regev et al. (1999) have developed a variation of the NAPFI for use with older infants (2 to 24 months of age). This assessment consists of 33 items divided into neurologic signs, development of motor function, and state of behavior. Items are scored as 0 to 3, with high score as optimal. Scores on items are thought to represent percent observed in normal populations, with scores of 3 obtained by 75% of the normal population to scores of 0 observed in 10% or less of the normal population. Descriptions of responses or stick figure drawings of possible responses are used for item scoring. A global score is obtained by summing the items scores. Results of frequency distributions at 12 and 18 months are reported with a cohort of children with normal birth histories.

### Neurobehavioral Assessment for Preterm Infants (NAPI, Korner and Thom, 1990)

The NAPI was developed as a research instrument useful for addressing developmental issues affecting preterm infants. The instrument can be used with preterm infants through 37 weeks conceptional age. Seven clusters of items are included in the assessment: motor development and vigor, scarf sigh, popliteal angle, alertness and orientation, irritability, vigor of crying and percent asleep ratings. Items are administered in an invariant order and behavioral state is assessed throughout. Average cluster scores are obtained from 3- to 9-point scales for individual clusters. Test–retest reliability is reported to be 0.60. Training in administration and scoring procedures are recommended. Korner, Stevenson, Forrest et al. (1994) has shown that motor development and vigor, irritability and vigor of crying scores on the NAPI are affected by medical conditions, while scores on alertness and orientation and neurobehavioral functions were not affected.

Recent applications of the NAPI have involved assessments of drug-exposed infants. Espy, Riese and Francis (1997) reported that preterm neonates prenatally exposed to cocaine and alcohol differed in NAPI performance compared to matched non-exposed control infants. Cocaine-exposed infants showed attention deficits which persisted across assessment days while alcohol-exposed infants showed deficits in motor development but these deficits were reduced over time. Other effects of cocaine, alcohol and effects of tobacco use on other NAPI cluster scores were not found. Brown, Bakeman, Coles et al. (1998) studied the effects of cocaine–polydrug use, alcohol use and non-drug use on the NAPI performance of preterm and full-term infants. Prenatal exposure to cocaine, alcohol or both was found to affect performance on NAPI alertness/orientation and irritability scores. Amount of cocaine used was related to motor development scores but amount of alcohol and tobacco used was not related to NAPI scores.

*Neonatal Neurological Examination (Neoneuro,
Sheridan-Pereira, Ellison and Helgeson, 1991)*

The Neoneuro assesses neurological and neurobehavioral performance of full-term newborn infants. Thirty-two items, most from the Prechtl NEFNI and Dubowitz NAPF, are distributed across seven factors: hypertonus, primitive reflexes, limb tone, neck support, reflexes and tremor, alertness and fussy.

Items are administered when infants are in a quiet alert state. Items are scored on 2-, 3- or 5-point scales and factor scores as well as total scores can be obtained. Cut scores are provided to differentiate normal, mildly abnormal, moderately abnormal, severely abnormal from assessments administered in the first 48 hours after birth and after 72 hours to 1 week. Sheridan-Pereira et al. (1991) report that infants from birth to one week of age have been assessed with high reliability (0.73).

The infant Neurological International Battery (INFANIB, Ellison, 1994) is a neurological assessment instrument for use with infants, especially premature and other at-risk infants, and resembles the Neoneuro. The battery contains 20 items administered in supine, prone, sitting, standing or suspended positions and can be administered to infants from birth to 18 months. Infants can be grouped as normal, transiently abnormal and abnormal neurological development based on scores. Item, subscale and total scores can be created (Ellison, Horn and Browning, 1985). Petersen, Sommerfelt and Markestad (2000) report the use of the INFANIB to classify infants at 4, 7, 13 and 18 months as normal, dystonic, hypotonic or suspected cerebral palsy (CP). Performance scores on the Bayley (1969) Mental Development and Motor Development Index at 13 months and Fagan Test (Fagan and Shepherd, 1987) at 7 months were compared across groups. Although no differences between groups were found on Fagan scores, group differences were found on Bayley Motor Index scores and were found for infants weighing less than 1500 g at birth as well as for infants weighing less than 2000 g at birth who had been diagnosed as hypotonic and suspected CP. These authors note that only 36% of the infants with CP were identified at or before 7 months of age and suggest that general movement assessment such as that suggested by Cioni, Ferrari, Einspieler et al. (1997) might enable earlier detection.

**Tertiary assessment instruments**

These instruments have been developed through extensive research and clinical activities. The process of scale development, efforts to refine the scales, establish their reliability and study their validity have been reported extensively in the literature. Because of such extensive literature, these aspects of the instruments will not be generally reported here.

### Assessment of Preterm Infants' Behavior (APIB, Als, Lester, Tronick and Brazelton, 1982)

The APIB was designed to serve the same assessment functions as the NBAS but with consideration of the competency and adaptive limitations of prematurely born infants and ill full-term infants. The APIB is designed to be applied to infants once they are in an open crib and includes evaluations of five systems: physiology, motor organization, state, attention/interaction and self-regulatory processes plus a reflex summary score. Items in each system, which includes items from Brazelton's NBAS (1973), are scored using a 9-point descriptive rating scale. There are 280 items, including behavioral and reflex items. Various scoring protocols are reported, including some allowing individual items to be grouped into 31 summary variables and other scoring 18 summary variables.

Various studies have reported the validity of the system scores. Als and her colleagues (Als, Duffy and McAnulty, 1988; Duffy, Als and McAnulty, 1990) report that preterm infants are less well organized on system scores than full-term newborn infants. Sell, Figueredo and Wilcox (1995) used confirmatory factor analysis with the system scores to verify the existence of several behavioral domains: overall modulation of behavior, motor competencies, availability, sociability, habituation during sleep, autonomic competency and reactivity. Results confirmed six of the seven domains (all but autonomic competency) and provided a means for a more simplified scoring system than has been used by Als. The APIB has been used extensively to evaluate the effectiveness of intervention approaches with preterm infants, especially the Neonatal Individualized Developmental Care Program (NIDCAP, Als, Lawhon, Duffy et al., 1994). NIDCAP has been reported to improve the outcomes of preterm infants, particularly time on ventilator, onset of nipple feed, duration of hospital stay, reduced incidence of lung disease, retinopathy, and severe intraventricular hemorrhages, and neurodevelopmental outcomes, including APIB and qualitative EEG measures (Buehler, Als, Duffy et al., 1995). A review of five stud-

ies using the NIDCAP reported outcome differences between Developmental Care infants and control infants, including improvements on APIB, NBAS and Bayley Scale scores (Lotas and Walden, 1996). However, Ariagno, Thoman, Boeddiker et al. (1997) report that although APIB scores of experimental and control infants were different, with experimental group infants attaining higher scores, the development of sleep patterns, 36-week NAPI scores and Bayley scores at 4, 12 and 24 months were not different between the two groups.

### Brazelton Neonatal Behavioral Assessment Scale (NBAS, Brazelton, 1973; Brazelton and Nugent, 1995)

The NBAS was developed to evaluate the behaviors of full-term neonates and it has been widely used for research and clinical purposes. First published in 1973, the most recent version of the NBAS retains its orientation toward research and clinical applications. The goal of the NBAS is to identify and describe individual differences in infants' responses to and effects on their environment. Physiological, motor, state, and attentional/interactional processes are assessed. Emphasis is placed on the interactive nature of the infant's behaviors. Infants are assessed on 28 behavioral items and 18 reflex items, which screen for gross neurological abnormalities. In addition, seven supplement items designed to assess the behaviors of at risk infants are included. Behavioral items are evaluated on a 9-point scale and reflexes are scored on a 4-point scale. Items are grouped into 'packages' (habituation, motor–oral, truncal, vestibular, social-interactive) and are designed to be administered in a specified (but 'not invariant') order since infant state is important. Optimal states for all item are specified. The range of infants for whom the NBAS is designed are term infants, healthy preterm infants less than 37 weeks gestational age, and for preterm infants through 48 weeks post-conceptional age.

Changes since the 1973 version of the NBAS include some additions to the reflex items, the addition of the supplemental items, changes is optimal state specified for some items, changes in the description and scoring of some items, and more extensive information on the clinical uses of the NBAS, particularly with families. Standardization information is not provided.

*The Neurological Examination of the Full-Term Newborn Infant (NEFNI, Prechtl, 1977; Prechtl and Beintema, 1964)*

This screening scale, originally published by Prechtl and Beintema and later republished by Prechtl alone, was developed to make a diagnosis for nervous system abnormalities at birth or soon after. The scale is clearly the most comprehensive of all newborn neurological exams. The examination begins with an observation period followed by the administration of over 50 items which permit assessment of state, resting posture, spontaneous motor activity, appearance, reflex elicitation, passive and active movements, motility, response threshold, crying, pathological movements, hemisyndrome, and reaction type. Each item has a specified state which the infant must attain to permit administration. Items are score on 2- to 4-point scales based on both observation and elicitation of responses. Item scores can be summed to provide information on neurological functioning and combinations of individual items can be used to diagnose clinical syndromes.

Work by Prechtl and associates (Cioni, Ferrari, Einspieler et al., 1997) as shown the advantage of including assessments of general movement as part of the NEFNI. Results show that general movement is strongly correlated with neurological scores in preterm and full-term infants, but general movement scores had higher sensitivity (the number of true positives) and specificity (the number of true negatives) than neurological scores for preterm infants. In a related publication, Prechtl, Einspieler, Cioni et al. (1997) reported that 'fidgety movements' (e.g., 'an ongoing stream of small, circular, and elegant movements of neck, trunk and limbs') had a higher specificity and sensitivity (96% and 95%, respectively) for neurological outcomes at 2 years of age than neurological outcomes determined by ultrasound-scan (83% and 80%, respectively). Prechtl (1984) has recommended that the general movement scores be used alone if neurological examination is difficult to conduct. However, a more recent study of developmental outcomes of preterm infants found that neonatal NEFNI scores but not general movement

scores were predictive of neurological and developmental outcomes at 2 years of age (Maas, Mirmiran, Hart et al., 2000).

The NEFNI has been used extensively in research. For example, Lou, Hansen, Nordentoft et al. (1994) found that severely stressful life-events in pregnancy in combination with a poor social network resulted in low NEFNI scores in 4- to 14-day-old infants compared to infants of mothers who were not stressed and had supportive social networks. Maternal education had a positive effect on NEFNI scores.

**Infant outcome measures**

Several standardized scales have been developed to assess the developmental status of infants. With the exception of the Denver Developmental Screening Scale (Frankenberg and Dodds, 1992) which is devised to be an aid in the initial screening of large populations of infants, these scales are designed to provide in-depth evaluations of the developmental status of infants in a number of different behavioral domains. These scales have been used frequently to aid in quantifying the current development status of children and in the prediction of development in later childhood. This section contains descriptions of some of the scales frequently used in research and which have been used by researchers to evaluate the validity of assessments of pediatric neurological functioning on the attainment of specific skills later in development. Thus, most of the scales described below relate specifically to assessments in the infancy period, although the Stanford–Binet is most appropriate for assessment in early childhood (ages 2 years and beyond). The Stanford–Binet, however, has been frequently used in longitudinal studies spanning the neonatal and early childhood periods. The information contained in this section on developmental assessment scales and their administration procedures should be helpful in considering the results of the predictive studies reported in this chapter.

*Bayley Scales of Infant Development (BSID, Bayley, 1969, 1993)*

Of all the current infant assessment scales, the Bayley has been used most frequently with both full-term and prematurely born infants. First published in

1963, the Bayley Scales were restandardized and revised in 1993. The BSID are designed for the evaluation of children's developmental status from 1 to 42 months of age, including high-risk and developmentally delayed infants. It is composed of three parts: Mental Development Index, Psychomotor Development Index, and the Behavior Rating Scale. The Mental Development Index (MDI) contains items assessing development of perception, problem solving, number concepts, language and personal/social abilities. The Psychomotor Development Index (PDI) contains items assessing development of movement quality, sensory integration and perceptual–motor integration abilities. The Bayley Scales also include a Behavior Rating Scale in which the examiner uses information from the caregiver and from observations during the assessment period to rate the child on attention/arousal, orientation engagement, emotional regulation and motor quality. These items, rated on a 5-point scale, provide a qualitative assessment of the child's test taking behaviors. The Behavior Rating Scale scores are categorized as non-optimal, questionable and within normal limits.

The BSID is organized into item sets with items within each set organized according to increasing difficulty. Basal and ceiling points are established within item sets with fewer than five passed items indicating that a lower item set should be administered and all but two or fewer passed items indicating that a higher item set should be administered. Items are similar to those contained on the 1963 version, although some items have been renamed, some dropped and some new items added. Instructions for computing developmental index scores and developmental age, along with interpretative guidelines are provided.

### Denver Developmental Screening Scale (DDSS, Frankenberg and Dodds, 1967, 1992; Frankenberg, Dodds and Fandal, 1970)

This scale was designed to be an easily administered screening tool for the early identification of children from birth to age six years with developmental problems. The scale contains 125 items covering four function areas: Personal Social, Fine Motor Adaptive, Language and Gross Motor. A separate section (Test Behavior) asks the assessor to evaluate the child's behavior during assessment in areas of compliance, interest in surroundings, fearfulness and attention span. A subset of the 125 items which fall within a range around the child's chronological age are administered or scored based on parental report. The test is useful for children suspect for and at risk for developmental problems but is primarily used as a screener applied to asymptomatic children often during routine pediatric examinations. Norms are provided for comparison with the child's performance on each item. Items are scored as advanced (item passed earlier than the normed age range where 100% are expected to pass), normal (item passed within the normed age range), caution (item failed or refused that 75% or more of children than age can pass) and delay (item is failed or refused that falls below the normed age range). Performance on the entire test is considered when assigning children to normal, suspect or untestable categories based on presences/absences of item scores reflecting cautions and delays. Rescreening is recommended for suspect and untestable categories.

The accuracy of the Denver II in identifying and classifying infants has been the subject of several studies. Glascoe, Byrne, Ashford et al. (1992) report an 83% accuracy rate in identifying 3- to 72-month-old infants with language disabilities, mild mental retardation and functional delay, but a low specificity rate (43%) resulting in a high overreferral rate. Items in the language function area were identified as more accurate in discriminating children with and without disabilities. Glascoe (2001) has questioned whether the overreferral rates produced by screening tests is a problem. Children aged 7 months to 8 years were administered at least two developmental screening tests, including the Denver II, and diagnostic assessments intelligence, language and academic achievement in children over the age of 2 1/2 years. Interestingly of the four screening tests (Parents Evaluations of Developmental Status, Brigance Screens, Battell Developmental Inventory Screening Test, and Denver-II), the Denver II had the highest false-positive rate (45%, compared to 22%, 27% and 22%, respectively). However, it was also reported that children identified as false positive perform much like true negative children on measures of intelligence, language and academic achievement and would not be considered at risk.

There has been much interest in all versions of the DDSS because of the focus on developmental milestones. These milestones have been used by physicians and parents as indicators of developmental status of infants, although there is little evidence that differential attainment rates of these milestones is related to intelligence beyond what is indicated by attainment (or non-attainment) per se (Capute and Accardo, 1991). Attention is turning to factors which influence the attainment of developmental milestones. Specifically, sleep position has been linked with attainment of developmental milestones, such as rolling prone to supine, tripod sitting, creeping, crawling and pulling to stand. While supine sleepers were found to lag behind prone sleepers in attaining these developmental milestones, they still attained the milestones within the normal developmental range (Davis, Moon, Sachs and Ottolini, 1998).

### Stanford–Binet Intelligence Scale, Fourth Edition (SB IV, Thorndike, Hagen and Sattler, 1986)

This scale assesses the general intellectual abilities of children from 2 years through adulthood. The scale scores can be used to obtain a composite score as well as factor or subscale scores for Verbal Reasoning, Abstract/Visual Reasoning, Quantitative Reasoning, and Short-Term Memory. In all there are 15 subtests but the number of subtests administered varies according to the age and ability of the child. The items in each test are arranged in levels with increasing difficulty across levels and are administered in a fixed order. The Vocabulary test is given first and uses chronological age to determine the level at which testing should begin. Performance on the vocabulary test and chronological age are used to determine the entry level for the other tests. Basal and ceiling levels are established for each test given. Although there are 15 subtests, the number of subtests administered varies by chronological age and vocabulary test performance. The Stanford–Binet also permits a quick screening battery to be administered. A total score can be obtained using scores from four tests (vocabulary, bead memory, quantitative, and pattern analysis). These four tests are representative of the four areas of cognitive abilities. This screening battery takes about 30–40 min to administer. If information on the pattern of cognitive abilities in needed, it is recommended that two additional tests (memory for sentences and comprehension) be added to the four tests indicated above. For both screening batteries, the vocabulary test is used as the routing test, and both basal and ceiling levels are established for each test.

Preschool children typically receive eight tests (vocabulary, comprehension, absurdities, pattern analysis, copying, quantitative, bead memory and memory for sentences) from the four subscales. However, it is not clear that the four-factor structure of the SBIV is appropriate for representing the intelligence of preschool children. Molfese, Yaple, Helwig et al. (1992) found that a three-factor model or a two-factor model was the best fit to the data obtained from three-year-old children. The results using exploratory factor analysis and confirmatory factor analysis differed in the number of factors identified; however, two of the three factors identified by exploratory factor analysis are easily identified as 'verbal' based on the subtests loading on the two factors. The other factor is clearly 'nonverbal'. The two-factor model identified through confirmatory factor analysis is composed of verbal and nonverbal abilities. These results are consistent with the findings of Reynolds, Kamphaus and Rosenthal (1988), Ownby and Carmin (1988), Kline (1989) and Thorndike (1990) as findings from all four studies identified factor structures in the SB4 for three-year-old children that contained two factors (one verbal and one nonverbal).

## Applications neuropsychological assessments in infancy

While the assessments described above have been used individually in studies on newborn infants and young children, multiple assessments involving different instruments and methodologies are often used within a study to characterize participants and to obtain measures of dependent variables for predictive modeling. The studies described below were selected from among a vast body of published literature dealing with the effects of prenatal drug expose on infant outcomes. This literature is particularly pertinent to this chapter because of the numerous published studies of the effects of prenatal drug exposure on central nervous system (CNS) development. For example, drug exposure has been found to affect habituation scores on the NBAS, infant state, reflexes and motor maturity, and sleep states of infants, all of which are thought to reflect CNS functioning (DiPetro, Suess, Wheeler et al., 1995; Mayes, Granger, Frank et al., 1993; Richardson, Hamel, Goldschmidt and Day, 1996). Provided here are some examples of studies using multiple neuropsychological assessment of infants using both behavioral and physiological assessments.

Brown et al. (1998) studied the effects of drug exposure to determine whether premature infants are more impacted by exposure to maternal drug use than full-term infants. In this study, multiple neuropsychological assessments and two measures of physiological responses were administered: maternal medical risks were assessed using the Littman and Parmelee Obstetric Complications Scale (OCS), medical risks of infants were evaluated using the Neonatal Medical Index (NMI, Korner et al., 1994) and using Apgar scores, gestational age was determined using the Ballard scoring system, the Neurobehavioral Assessment for Preterm Infants (NAPI) was used for the neuropsychological examination of the infants, and reactivity to handling was evaluated using physiological measures of changes in heart and respiratory rates. Maternal self-report, medical records and maternal and infant urine samples were used to determine the drug exposure of the 87 premature and 148 full-term infant participating in the study. Infants participating in the study were classified as having been exposed to cocaine and some combination of alcohol, tobacco and marijuana, or to alcohol only or to none of these. Compared to the non-drug-using group, drug (including alcohol) using mothers had lower (less optimal) OCS scores, but their infants did not differ on NMI, Apgar, nor Ballard scores. The drug-exposed infants, however, did differ in NAPI scores on orientation and irritability, and on respiratory rate and change in respiratory rate. Premature, drug-exposed infants were more irritable than drug-exposed full-term infants.

Van Baar, Soepatmin, Gunning and Akkerhuis (1994) studied the longitudinal development of a group of 35 drug-exposed and 35 non-exposed infants from birth through age 5.5 years. Drug-exposed infants were poly-drug-exposed to methadone, heroin, cocaine and other drugs during pregnancy. At different ages infants were assessed on a variety of instruments, including EEG, the Dubowitz NAPFI, the Brazelton NBAS, and the Bayley Scales of Infant Development. Group differences were seen at birth on EEG measures and Dubowitz scores, at 4 weeks (but not at birth) on some NBAS items, and on 24- and 30-month scores on the Bayley MDI. Interestingly, no group differences were found on EEG at 6 and 12 months, nor on a neurological exam administered at 6 and 12 months. While there were early group differences in neuropsychological scores, these differences did not persist beyond the newborn period. However, group differences in cognitive abilities did persist throughout the period of the study. Scher, Richardson and Day (2000) investigated the effects of prenatal cocaine exposure on infant neuropsychological development. Full-term infants were classified based on their mother's trimester of drug use or nonuse. Perinatal complications were assessed at birth using a combination of Hobel's HRPSS, the Littman and Parmelee OCS, and a scale developed by Zax, Sameroff and Babigian (1977), infant status was assessed using Apgar and Dubowitz's DAGA, and sleep EEG. At one year, the Bayley Scales of Infant Development were administered. Results showed some maternal demographic and maternal medical risk differences between drug groups, but there were no differences for the infant neuropsychological assessment scores. Cocaine/crack and poly-drug use did affect spectral power in sleep EEG measures at birth and one year of age, which remained a significant finding even after covariates of prenatal drug use were statistically controlled. Interhemispheric correlations between homologous brain regions were also reduced. These findings were interpreted as reflecting effects on interhemispheric synaptic connections which may reflect fewer interhemispheric neuronal connections in utero or a delay in interconnections in the drug-exposed infant.

Together these three studies illustrate the importance to multiple assessments of neuropsychological functioning in infants. While effects of prenatal drug exposure were found, findings were not significant between groups for all of the measures taken nor at all the ages at which assessments were administered. The best approach to neuropsychological assessments in infancy is clearly one that combines behavioral and physiological techniques. Yet a caution is needed as well. There are many neuropsychological assessments available in the literature, of which those reviewed here are a subset of those most frequently used in published work. We must be cautious in considering research approaches to neuropsychological assessments in infancy to guard against the use of lengthy batteries of behavioral assessments and the use of numerous neurological, physiological, and neuroanatomical techniques in our efforts to assess infants. Sound theoretical and methodological rationales underlying what information is needed and how each measure contributes to the gathering of that information are needed.

### Assessment and intervention

Up to this point, the focus of the chapter has been on assessment of neuropsychological functioning in infancy, yet assessment should not exist without a consideration of the purpose for which the assessment is undertaken. Intervention, which is the intended link with assessment, typically receives far less consideration in the infant neuropsychological literature compared to the attention given to assessment. Indeed, rarely in the development and implementation of new assessment techniques is there a consideration of what specific intervention techniques are indicated in light of the assessment results.

Kaye (1986) has argued that in a clinical setting assessment and intervention must be considered together since both involve issues of importance which intersect. First, both assessment and intervention involve questions of costs and benefits. For assessment the question is 'assessment for what?' In attempting to answer this question, assessments must be designed that can identify conditions which truly lead to a poor prognosis if not treated (cost), and identify the conditions for which a treatment exists that actually improves the prognosis (benefit). It makes little sense to assess individuals for risk conditions if the question of treatability is unknown or if options for treatment are undeveloped. Kaye argues that many assessment scales have been developed for which treatability is either unknown or not considered. For intervention, the cost/benefit question focuses on 'intervention with whom?' Since a variety of possible interventions exist, the choice of an intervention strategy involves issues of what the cost of the intervention will be (both in terms of applying the intervention and not applying it) and how much benefit will be gained for applying the intervention. Clearly, 'what' is assessed must be a condition for which intervention makes cost/benefit sense to treat.

Second, for both assessment and intervention techniques the cost of the technique is often far too expensive to permit its use with large populations. Thus, decisions must be made as to who will be assessed and who will receive the intervention. These decisions are not made easily and are rarely addressed in these terms. Most frequently, assessment techniques are evaluated in terms of sensitivity and specificity, where sensitivity is the proportion of true positives identified and specificity is the proportion of true negatives. Ideally, the most efficient use of assessment techniques is to maximize their sensitivity and specificity so that maximal benefit will be obtained for those individuals to whom the assessment technique is applied. Attaining this goal is difficult and usually involves the manipulation of the scale scores used to effectively identify positive and negative cases. For intervention, effectiveness is evaluated based on the attainment of specified outcome criteria by individuals identified as most likely to benefit from the intervention. Frequently, however, beneficial effects are found for subgroups of individuals but not for the group as a whole. Identifying which subgroups are most likely to benefit has been problematic, but is important to improving the efficiency of the intervention technique.

Third, decisions on administering assessment techniques or providing intervention techniques frequently involve decisions as to what types of cases should have highest priority. Kaye argues that it makes little sense to develop and administer assessment and intervention techniques without knowing what their payoffs will be, and frequently the payoff is not known with any certainty. These payoffs can only be properly evaluated with consideration of a variety of different issues. For example, in developmental neuropsychology behaviors indicative of abnormal functioning must be separated from normal developmental processes. Such a separation is difficult since baselines are difficult to establish that are comprehensive enough to cover the range of behaviors needed. Further, the ability to clearly specify what the outcomes of a particular case would be without intervention is difficult since naturally occurring control cases, appropriate to the situations, are rarely available. Thus, prioritizing cases by focusing on maximizing payoffs is fraught with difficulties.

What is needed is a closer link between assessment and intervention techniques such that evaluation based on assessments can be used in a prescriptive sense for specific intervention programs. Kaye describes this notion as using assessment techniques as 'placement tests' for intervention programs. Close study then needs to be made of the relation between the initial assessment performance and the influence of the intervention on subsequent assessment performances. Ideally, longitudinal samples of infants would be followed by repeated assessment and intervention phases as long as they were needed to obtain the desired outcomes. It is only through repeated assessments of infants that it is possible to isolate changes in the status due to the effects of intervention from those due to normal, developmental processes. Further, as many of the research reports have indicated, not all neuropsychological problems are detectable at birth, and not all neuropsychological problems detectable at birth persist into later infancy. One-time assessments simply will not satisfy the need to accurate evaluations of infant neurological status.

Additional effort is needed to promote the needs for and benefits from early assessment and early intervention. The American Academy of Pediatrics (1994) has called for greater efforts from pediatricians in the early identification of infants with developmental disabilities which might benefit from early intervention. Such early identification could take place during the 12 well-child visits that occur during the first five years of life. Glascoe, Foster and Wolraich (1997) have responded to this call by looking at the costs of different approaches to the early identification of developmental disabilities. The first level of identification they used was based on parental responses to a 2-item questionnaire followed by direct screening of different subgroups of infants using either the Denver II or the Battelle Developmental Inventory Screening Test (Newborg, Stock, Wnek et al., 1984). Diagnostic evaluations were administered to children suspected of develop-

mental delay based on screening. Costs of administering the screening tools and interpreting results, of diagnostic evaluations were calculated. The use of parental concerns as one level of screening was identified as effective and was cited as one way in which the cost of direct screening can be reduced. Glascoe et al. suggest that self-administered parent questionnaires that can be completed while waiting for physician appointments might be feasible. Consistent with this suggestion is Aylward's BINS which has been developed as tool which parents can use to report the developmental abilities of their children and the inclusion of the Denver Prescreening Developmental Questionnaire which can be used by parents as part of the Denver II. Beyond this initial screening, the costs greatly increase. The costs are variable for the professional staff time for direct screening, depending on the screening tool used, but costs are high for screening interpretation and diagnostic evaluations by physicians or other highly trained professionals. Health plan or other payment coverage for these latter costs is problematic. Thus, while the long-term cost savings and personal and societal benefits gained from the early identification of developmental disabilities coupled with effective intervention are high, there are potential conflicts driving the ability of pediatricians to put the early identification call into practice.

## Conclusions

Great progress has been made toward the assessment of neuropsychological functioning in infancy. These assessments, many of which have been devised within the past decade, have generally received a considerable amount of psychometric attention but most have been underutilized in large-scale longitudinal studies effectively designed to permit the study of changes in neurological and developmental functioning. In addition, there is still the need for assessments that meet criteria pertaining to administration issues and address issues of validity. Vohr (1999) summarized the criteria needs as "easy to administer, has a reasonable administration time, is a norm-referenced measurement, is reliable, has interrater reliability and has accepted concurrent and predictive validity." (page 140). While many of the assessments listed above meet these criteria, several do not, although recent revisions to well-established neuropsychological assessment instrument have incorporated some of the criteria identified by Vohr. What is also needed is for clinicians and researchers to select from the neuropsychological assessment instruments already established those that best match their intended usage and to apply them carefully in combination with appropriate interventions. Only through further study can the required progress be made in linking assessment with appropriate interventions that reduce risks for neurological dysfunction and remediate impairments.

# References

Alessandri S, Bendersky M, Lewis M: Cognitive functioning in 8- to 18-month-old drug-exposed infants. Developmental Psychology: 34; 565–73, 1998.

Als H, Duffy F, McAnulty B: Behavioral differences between preterm and full-term newborns as measured with the APIB system scores. Infant Behavior and Development: 11; 305–318, 1988.

Als H, Lawhon G, Duffy F, McAnulty B, Gibes-Grossman R, Blickman J: Individualized developmental care for the very low-birth-weight preterm infant: Medical and neurofunctional effects. Journal of the American Medical Association: 272; 853–858, 1994.

Als H, Lester B, Tronick E, Brazelton T: Manual for the assessment of preterm infants' behavior (APIB). In Fitzgerald H, Lester B, Yogman M (Eds), Theory and Research in Behavioral Pediatrics. New York: Plenum Press, pp. 65–132, 1982.

American Academy of Pediatrics: Committee on Children with Disabilities. Screening infants and young children for developmental disabilities. Pediatrics: 93; 863–865, 1994.

Amiel-Tison C: Neurological evaluation of the maturity of newborn infants. Archives of Diseases of Childhood: 43; 89–90, 1968.

Amiel-Tison C: A method for neurological evaluation within the first year of life. Current Problems in Pediatrics, Vol. 111. Chicago, IL: Year Book Medical Publishers, 1976.

Amiel-Tison C, Barrier G, Shnider S, Levinson G, Hughes S, Stefani S: A new neurologic and adaptive capacity scoring system for evaluating obstetric medications in full-term newborns. Anesthesiology: 56; 340–350, 1982.

Apgar V: A proposal for a new method of evaluation of the newborn infant. Current Research in Anesthesia and Analgesia: 32; 260–267, 1953.

Ariagno R, Thoman E, Boeddiker M, Kugener B, Constantinou J, Mirmiran M, Baldwin R: Developmental care does not alter sleep and development of premature infants. Pediatrics: 100; 1026–1027, 1997.

Aylward GP: The Bayley Infant Neurodevelopmental Screening Manual. San Antonio, TX: The Psychological Corporation, 1995.

Aylward G, Verhulst S: Predictive utility of the Bayley Infant Neurodevelopmental Screener (BINS) risk status classifications: Clinical interpretation and application. Developmental Medicine and Child Neurology: 42; 25–31, 2000.

Aylward GP, Verhulst SJ, Bell S: Enhanced prediction of later normal outcome using infant neuropsychological assessment. Developmental Neuropsychology: 10; 377–393, 1994.

Ballard J, Novak K, Driver M: A simplified score for assessment of fetal maturity of newly born infants. Journal of Pediatrics: 95; 769, 1979.

Bayley N: The Bayley scales of infant development: Birth to two years. New York: Psychological Corporation, 1969.

Bayley N: Bayley Scales of Infant Development, 2nd ed. San Antonio, TX: Psychological Corporation, 1993.

Bendersky M, Lewis M: Prenatal cocaine exposure and neonatal condition. Infant Behavior and Development: 22; 353–366, 2000.

Brazelton T: Neonatal Behavioral Assessment Scale. Philadelphia, PA: Lippincott, 1973.

Brazelton T, Nugent J: Neonatal Behavioral Assessment Scale, 3rd ed. Clinics in Developmental Medicine No. 137. London: Mac Keith Press, 1995.

Brockhurst N, Littleford J, Halpern S, Fisher D: The neurologic and adaptive capacity score: systematic review of its use in obstetric anesthesia research. Anesthesiology: 92; 237–246, 2000.

Brown J, Bakeman R, Coles C, Sexson W, Demi A: Maternal drug use during pregnancy: Are preterm and full-term infants affected differently? Developmental Psychology: 34; 540–554, 1998.

Buehler D, Als H, Duffy F, McAnulty G, Liederman J: Effectiveness of individualized developmental care for low-risk preterm infants: Behavioral and electrophysiologic evidence. Pediatrics: 96; 923–932, 1995.

Camann W, Brazelton T: Use and abuse of neonatal neurobehavioral testing. Anesthesiology: 92; 3–5, 2000.

Capute A, Accardo P: Developmental Disabilities in Infancy and Childhood. Baltimore: Paul H. Brookes Publishing, 1991.

Cioni G, Ferrari F, Einspieler C, Paolicelli P, Barbani T, Prechtl H: Comparison between observation of spontaneous movements and neurologic examination in preterm infants. Journal of Pediatrics: 130; 704–711, 1997.

Davis B, Moon R, Sachs H, Ottolini M: Effects of sleep position on infant motor development. Pediatrics: 102; 1135–1140, 1998.

DiPetro J, Suess P, Wheeler J, Smouse P, Newlin B: Reactivity and regulation in cocaine-exposed neonates. Infant Behavior and Development: 18; 407–414, 1995.

Drage J, Berendes H: Apgar scores and outcome of the newborn. Pediatric Clinics of North America: 107; 635–643, 1966.

Dubowitz L, Dubowitz V: The Neurological Assessment of the Preterm and Full-Term Newborn Infant. Philadelphia, PA: Lippincott, 1981.

Dubowitz L, Dubowitz V, Goldberg C: Clinical assessment of

gestational age in the newborn infants. Journal of Pediatrics: 77; 1–10, 1970.

Dubowitz L, Mercuri E, Dubowitz V: An optimality score for the neurologic examination of the term newborn. Journal of Pediatrics: 133; 406–416, 1998.

Duffy F, Als H, McAnulty G: Behavioral and electrophysiological evidence for gestational age effects in healthy preterm and full-term infants suited two weeks after expected due date. Child Development: 61; 1271–1286, 1990.

Ellison P: The Infantib. San Antonio, TX: Psychological Corporation, 1994.

Ellison P, Horn J, Browning C: Construction of an infant neurological international battery (Infantib) for assessment of neurological integrity in infancy. Physical Therapy: 65; 1326–1331, 1985.

Espy K, Riese M, Francis D: Neurobehavior in preterm neonates exposed to cocaine, alcohol and tobacco. Infant Behavior and Development: 20; 297–309, 1997.

Eyler F, Delgado-Hachey M, Woods N, Carter R: Quantification of the Dubowitz Neurological Assessment of Preterm Neonates: Developmental outcome. Infant Behavior and Development: 14; 451–469, 1991.

Fagan J, Shepherd P: The Fagan test of infant intelligence. Cleveland, OH: Infanttest, Corp., 1987.

Farr V, Mitchell R, Nilgian G, Parkin J: The definition of some external characteristics used in the assessment of gestational age in the newborn infant. Developmental Medicine and Child Neurology: 8; 507, 1966.

Frankenberg W, Dodds J: The Denver Developmental Screening Test. Journal of Pediatrics: 71; 181–191, 1967.

Frankenberg W, Dodds J: Denver II. Denver: Denver Developmental Materials, 1992.

Frankenberg W, Dodds J, Fandal: The revised Denver Developmental Screening Test manual. Denver: University of Colorado Press, 1970.

Glascoe F: Are overreferrals on developmental screening tests really a problem? Archives of Pediatrics and Adolescent Medicine: 155; 54–59, 2001.

Glascoe F, Byrne K, Ashford L, Johnson K, Chang B, Strickland B: Accuracy of the Denver-II in developmental screening. Pediatrics: 89; 1221–1225, 1992.

Glascoe F, Foster E, Wolraich M: An economic analysis of developmental detection methods. Pediatrics: 99; 830–837, 1997.

Golden G: Comments on Apgar scores as predictors of chronic neurological disability by Nelson KB and Ellenberg JH. Pediatrics: 102; 262–264, 1998.

Haataja L, Mercuri E, Regev R, Cowan F, Rutherford M, Dubowitz V, Dubowitz L: Optimality score for the neurological examination of the infant at 12 and 18 months of age. Journal of Pediatrics: 135; 153–161, 1999.

Haddad B, Mercer B, Livingston J, Talati A, Sibai B: Outcome after successful resuscitation of babies born with Apgar scores of 0 at born 1 and 5 minutes. American Journal of Obstetrics and Gynecology: 183; 1210–1214, 2000.

Hegyi T, Carbone T, Artwar M, Ostfeld B, Hiatt M, Koons A,

Pinto-Martin J, Paneth N: The Apgar score and its components in the preterm infant. Pediatrics: 101; 79–81, 1998.

Hobel C, Hyvarinen M, Okada D, Oh W: Prenatal and intrapartum high risk screening. I. Prediction of the high risk neonate. American Journal of Obstetrics and Gynecology: 117; 1–9, 1973.

Howard J, Parmelee A, Kopp C, Littman B: A neurological comparison of preterm and full term infants at term conceptional age. Journal of Pediatrics: 88; 995–1002, 1976.

Kaye K: A four-dimensional model of risk assessment and intervention. In Farrani D, McKinney I (Eds), Risk in Intellectual and Psychosocial Development. New York: Academic Press, pp. 273–286, 1986.

King T, Perlman J, Laptook A, Rollins N, Jackson G, Little B: Neurologic manifestations of in utero cocaine exposure in near-term and term infants. Pediatrics: 259–264, 1995.

Kline R: Is the fourth edition Stanford–Binet a four-factor test? Confirmatory factor analyses of alternative models for ages 2 through 23. Journal of Psychoeducational Assessment: 7; 4–13, 1989.

Korner A, Stevenson D, Forrest T, Constantinou J, Dimiceli S, Brown B: Preterm medical complications differentially affect neurobehavioral functions: Results from a new Neonatal Medical Index. Infant Behavior and Development: 17; 37–43, 1994.

Korner A, Thom V: Neurobehavioral Assessment of the Preterm Infant. San Antonio, TX: Psychological Corporation, 1990.

Letko M: Understanding the Apgar score. Journal of Obstetric, Gynecologic and Neonatal Nursing: 25; 299–303, 1996.

Lewis M, Fox N: Issues in infant assessment. In Brown C (Ed), Childhood Learning Disabilities and Prenatal Risk. New York: Johnson and Johnson, 1983.

Littman B, Parmelee A: Medical correlates of infant development. Pediatrics: 61; 470–474, 1978.

Lotas M, Walden M: Individualized developmental care for very low-birth weight infants: A critical review. Journal of Obstetric, Gynecologic and Neonatal Nursing: 25; 681–687, 1996.

Lou H, Hansen D, Nordentoft M, Pryds O, Jensen F, Nim J, Hemmingsen R: Prenatal stressors of human life affect fetal brain development. Developmental Medicine and Child Neurology: 36; 826–832, 1994.

Maas Y, Mirmiran M, Hart A, Koppe J, Ariagno R, Sekreijse H: Predictive value of neonatal neurological tests for developmental outcome of preterm infants. Journal of Pediatrics: 137; 100–106, 2000.

Mayes L, Granger R, Frank M, Schottenfeld R, Bornstein M: Neurobehavioral profiles of neonates exposed to cocaine prenatally. Pediatrics: 91; 778–783, 1993.

McGrath M, Sullivan M, Lester B, Oh W: Longitudinal neurologic follow-up in neonatal intensive care unit survivors with various neonatal morbidities. Pediatrics: 106; 1397–1405, 2000.

Michenfelder J: Accept, revise, reject or punt: An example of the latter (editorial). Anesthesiology: 56; 337, 1982.

Molfese V, Yaple K, Helwig S, Harris L, Connell S: Stanford–Binet Intelligence Scale (4th ed.): Factor structure and verbal subscale scores for three year olds. Journal of Psychoeducational Assessment: 10; 47–58, 1992.

Nelson K, Ellenberg J: Apgar scores as predictors of chronic neurological disability. Pediatrics: 68; 36–44, 1981.

Newborg J, Stock J, Wnek L, Guidubaldi J, Svinicki J: Battelle Developmental Inventory Screening Test. Allen, TX: DLM Teaching Resources, 1984.

Ownby R, Carmin C: Confirmatory factor analyses of the Stanford–Binet Intelligence Scale, 4h ed. Journal of Psychoeducational Assessment: 6; 331–340, 1988.

Parmelee A, Michaelis R: Neurological examination of the newborn. In Hellmuth J (Ed), Exceptional Infant, Vol. 2. New York: Brunner/Mazel, pp. 3–23, 1971.

Petersen S, Sommerfelt K, Markestad T: Early motor development of premature infants with birthweight less than 2000 grams. Acta Paediatrics: 89; 1456–1461, 2000.

Peiper A: Cerebral Function in Infancy and Childhood. New York: Consultants Bureau, 1963.

Prechtl H: Neurological sequelae of prenatal and perinatal complications. British Medical Journal: 4; 763–767, 1967.

Prechtl H: The Neurological Examination of the Full Term Newborn Infant. Philadelphia, PA: Lippincott, 1977.

Prechtl H: Motor behavior of preterm infants. In Prechtl H (Ed), Continuity of Neural Functions from prenatal to Postnatal Life. Oxford: Blackwell, pp. 79–92, 1984.

Prechtl H, Beintema D: The neurological examination of the full term newborn infant. Philadelphia, PA: Lippincott, 1964.

Prechtl H, Einspieler C, Cioni G, Bos A, Ferrari F, Sontheimer D: An early marker for neurological deficits after perinatal brain lesions. The Lancet: 349; 1361–1363, 1997.

Reynolds C, Kamphaus R, Rosenthal B: Factor analysis of the Stanford–Binet Fourth Edition for ages 2 through 23. Measurement and Evaluation in Counseling and Development: 21; 52–63, 1988.

Richardson G, Hamel S, Goldschmidt L, Day N: The effects of prenatal cocaine use on neonatal neurobehavioral status. Neurotoxicology and Teratology: 18; 519–528, 1996.

Scafidi F, Field T, Wheeden A, Schanberg S, Kuhn C, Symanski R, Zimmerman E, Bandstra E: Cocaine-exposed preterm neonates show behavioral and hormonal differences. Pediatrics: 97; 851–855, 1996.

Scanlon J, Brown W, Weiss J, Alper M: Neurobehavioral responses of newborn infants after maternal epidural anesthesia. Anesthesiology: 40; 121–128, 1974.

Scher M, Richardson G, Day N: Effects of prenatal cocaine/crack and other drug exposure on electroencephalographic sleep studies at birth and one-year. Pediatrics: 105; 39–48, 2000.

Sell E, Figueredo A, Wilcox T: Assessment of preterm infants' behavior (APIB): Confirmatory factor analysis of behavioral constructs. Infant Behavior and Development: 18; 447–457, 1995.

Sheridan-Pereira M, Ellison P, Helgeson V: The construction of a scored neonatal neurological examination for assessment of neurological integrity in full-term neonates. Developmental and Behavioral Pediatrics: 12; 25–30, 1991.

Smith LN, Dayal V, Monga M: Prior knowledge of obstetric gestational age and possible bias of Ballard scores. Obstetrics and Gynecology: 93; 712–714, 1999.

Spinnato J, Sibain B, Shaver D, Anderson G: Inaccuracy of Dubowitz gestational age in low birth weight infants. Obstetrics and Gynecology: 63; 491–495, 1984.

St-Anne Dargassies S: Methode d'examen, neurologique du nouveau-né. Etudes Neonatal: 3; 101–123, 1954.

St. Anne Dargassies S: Neurological Development in the Full Term and Preterm Neonate. New York: Elsevier–North Holland, 1977.

Thorndike RL: Would the real factors of the Stanford–Binet Fourth Edition please come forward? Journal of Psychoeducational Assessment: 8; 412–435, 1990.

Thorndike R, Hagen E, Sattler J: Stanford–Binet Intelligence Scale: Fourth Edition. New York: Riverside Publishing Company, 1986.

Topp M, Langhoff-Roos J, Uldall P: Preterm birth and cerebral palsy. Predictive value of pregnancy complications, mode of delivery and Apgar scores. Acta Obstetricia et Gynecologica Scandinavica: 76; 843–848, 1997.

Tronick E: A critique of the neonatal neurologic and adaptive capacity score (NACS). Anesthesiology: 56; 338–339, 1982.

Tronick E, Frank D, Cabral H, Mirochnick M, Zuckerman B: Late dose–response effects of prenatal cocaine exposure on newborn neurobehavioral performance. Pediatrics: 98; 76–83, 1996.

Van Baar A, Soepatmin S, Gunning W, Akkerhuis G: Development after prenatal exposure to cocaine, heroin and methadone. Acta Pediatrics Supplement: 404; 40–46, 1994.

Van de Riet J, Vandenbussche F, Le Cessie S, Keirse M: Newborn assessment and long-term adverse outcome: A systematic review. American Journal of Obstetrics and Gynecology: 180; 1024–1029, 1999.

Vik T, Vatten L, Markestad T, Jacobsen G, Bakketeig L: Dubowitz assessment of gestational age and agreement with prenatal methods. American Journal of Perinatology: 14; 369–373, 1997.

Vohr B: The quest for the ideal neurologic assessment for infants and young children. Journal of Pediatrics: 135; 140–142, 1999.

Zax M, Sameroff A, Babigian H: Birth outcomes in the offspring of mentally disordered women. American Journal of Orthopsychiatry: 47; 218–230, 1977.

*Handbook of Neuropsychology*, 2nd Edition, Vol. 8, Part I
S.J. Segalowitz and I. Rapin (Eds)

CHAPTER 11

# Neuropsychological assessment of the preschool child

## Angela Garcia O'Shea, Brian Harel and Deborah Fein [*]

*Department of Psychology, University of Connecticut, 406 Babbidge Road, U-1020, Storrs, CT 06269-1020, USA*

## Introduction

In the past 20 to 30 years, increasing attention has been focused on brain–behavior relationships in the pediatric population. There is a greater awareness of the number of children who experience brain insults at a very young age and who require appropriate assessment and care. In addition, many psychiatric and behavioral disorders of childhood have been found to have neurological and developmental bases. The perspective and expertise of pediatric neuropsychologists, therefore, have become critical for understanding and treating children with a wide variety of these disorders.

Evaluation measures in child neuropsychological assessment have developed considerably over the last several decades. The neuropsychological assessment of children began as a single-test approach where the goal was to differentiate brain-damaged children from normally developing children. The field, however, was led to more of a battery/lesion-specification approach when single test scores were found to be variably reliable discriminators between normal and brain-damaged children. Examining a broad range of functions from a battery of tests was also shown to have limited validity for lesion localization in children (Baron, Fennell and Voeller, 1995; Teeter and Semrud-Clikeman, 1997; Tramontana and Hooper, 1988). This finding shifted the field of pediatric neuropsychology, once again, to the approach

it generally adopts today, the functional organizational approach (Fletcher and Taylor, 1984). Here, the emphasis is placed on specifying the behavioral effects of specific types of central nervous system (CNS) dysfunction and the goals are to describe: (1) the sequence and rate of normal development; (2) how neuropsychological disorders disrupt such development; and (3) the consequent patterns of spared and impaired abilities in individual children, and in particular disorders, over time (Fletcher and Taylor, 1984; Teeter and Semrud-Clikeman, 1997). In addition to the emphasis on the functional profile, there is a growing concern with providing ecologically valid neuropsychological assessments. Such assessments not only provide parents, teachers, and physicians with a profile of a particular child's neuropsychological strengths and weaknesses, but also indicate how this profile affects academic and behavioral functioning and translates into treatment recommendations. Also, more recently, an emphasis has been placed on the use of psychological tests in conjunction with more direct measures of brain function, such as structural and functional magnetic resonance imaging (MRI), electroencephalography (EEG) techniques, positron emission tomography (PET), and computerized tomography (CT) scans. The ability to investigate brain activity in children with developmental and neurological disorders has greatly enhanced the field of child neuropsychological assessment (Baron and Gioia, 1998; Teeter and Semrud-Clikeman, 1997).

The focus of this chapter will be on the neuropsychological assessment of the preschool child, specifically children aged 2 to 5 years. Several factors have

---
[*] Corresponding author. Tel.: +1 (860) 486-3518;
E-mail: fein@uconnvm.uconn.edu

converged to compel neuropsychologists to evaluate and assist children in their early years. Cognitive processes, specifically attention and memory, which are crucial for acquiring and retaining all of the skills and knowledge which the child needs to successfully navigate the tasks of later childhood, change dramatically in the preschool years. There are also profound changes in motor processes and in the schemata children use to understand their world, with enormous development in symbolic functions such as language, play, and drawing (Edwards, 1999).

Advances in medical knowledge and technology have brought about increased survival of children whose conditions, or their treatment, have a potentially adverse impact on the developing brain; these include, for example, extreme prematurity, brain malignancies, and traumatic brain injury. This has contributed to a growing population of young children who need neuropsychological assessment and remediation. With the increased knowledge of brain growth and development, the pediatric neuropsychologist can play an important role in a multidisciplinary team, bringing to the team an orientation that integrates psychological and medical factors as well as rehabilitative strategies and programs (Baron et al., 1995).

In the United States, the passage of Public Law 94-142, the Education of All Handicapped Children's Act, its amendments (P.L. 99-457), and its reauthorizations (P.L. 101-476 and P.L. 105-17), which mandate early intervention and preschool programs for children from birth to age 5, reflect the national focus on children with delays and disorders by the American federal government (Nuttall, Nuttall-Vasquez and Hampel, 1999). These children require early intervention programs; their initial disabilities may become more disabling, and secondary handicaps may appear if these children are left unaided. Using autism as an example, Mundy and Crowson (1997) argue that in the natural course of developmental disorders, the primary neural dysfunction can lead to environmental deprivation and to reduced opportunity for learning. These, in turn, can lead to secondary neural dysfunction, which may be even more devastating in its long-range consequences. The role of aggressive early intervention, they argue, can be to avert this secondary neurological dysfunction and its consequences.

Early intervention programs for the infant and early childhood populations are focusing more attention on the cognitive, behavioral, and social–emotional needs of young children in their natural environments, including family, preschool, and community settings. Consequently, comparisons of children's developmental acquisitions to those of their age peers have become more routine, and primary practitioners are more aware of risk factors in the preschool age group (Baron and Gioia, 1998). As a result, pediatric neuropsychologists have been asked to play important roles in the identification of neurodevelopmental disorders and in the creation of appropriate educational plans for preschool children (Tramontana and Hooper, 1988).

In this chapter, we will provide an introduction to some of the most pressing issues facing the pediatric neuropsychologist who sees the preschool child. We will review some of the more general issues, such as assessing delay vs. disorder and examining the validity of the predictions one can make from preschool neuropsychological evaluations. We will then present some of the approaches and models used in early neuropsychological assessment and provide a brief introduction to some specific assessment issues for the most common conditions referred for early neuropsychological evaluation. In the next sections, domains of neuropsychological assessment and assessment procedures are outlined. Some principles for presenting useful recommendations are then provided, followed by some ideas for future directions. As will be obvious to the reader, each of these sections could be (and has been) the subject of entire books; therefore, the discussions here should be regarded as brief overviews. It is hoped that some of the references provided will enable the reader to pursue these topics in more depth.

## General issues in neuropsychological assessment of the preschool child

### Delay vs. disorder

Although preschool children are quite varied in their development of cognition, language, social interaction skills, motor ability, and self-help skills, some of these young children are clearly developing outside the parameters of the normal range. For some, the difference or delay is clear enough to necessitate a diagnosis during infancy. For others, disability may not be clearly manifest until the preschool period, while for still others, only the behavioral and cognitive demands of school will make the disability apparent. In many cases, however, a known etiology such as prematurity will alert clinicians to the fact that the apparently normal child is at risk for later difficulties (Lifter, 1999).

Since developmental lag or deviance may indicate pathology, it is important to ascertain the age at which a specific behavior ceases to be developmentally appropriate or fall within normal limits; adjustments must be made, however, for individual circumstances related to environment, growth, and development (Baron et al., 1995). Satz, Fletcher, Clark and Morris (1981) describe the concept of *delay* as the onset of behavior in one group occurring later than in another. Risser and Edgell (1988) suggest that a developmental delay could result in defective organization of cognitive skills, thus causing low levels of performance. In their estimation, mental retardation in the absence of a specific known etiology might be considered the clearest example of delayed maturation. *Lag*, on the other hand, is defined as a difference in performance level on a particular behavior between two groups or individuals at one time in development that recedes at a later time in development (Satz et al., 1981). In other words, the lower group eventually catches up to the other group. In practice, it can be difficult to maintain the distinction between delay and lag. Therefore, in order to obtain a full picture of the development of a skill, it is necessary to specify age of onset, rate of acquisition at various points in time, and, ultimately, the final level of performance.

Some skills in some disorders cannot be described as delayed in onset or slowed in rate of acquisition because they do not follow a normal developmental sequence. *Deviance* in development can be considered the abnormal order of acquisition of abilities within a domain (Satz et al., 1981). Children with autism, for example, were found to show abnormal sequences of skill development in the communication and socialization arenas (VanMeter, Fein, Morris et al., 1997). VanMeter et al. point out, however, that whether a skill appears delayed or deviant depends on the width of the domain being evaluated. For ex-

ample, a child with expressive language delays might be found to have development that is slowed but follows a normal sequence if only expressive language skills were considered. If the broader communication domain was considered, however, including expressive and receptive skills, then developmental steps would appear to be out of sequence.

In sum, quantifying or categorizing the degree of delay, lag, or deviance is important because it may indicate the degree of need for intervention.

*Purposes of assessment*

Neuropsychological assessment can be an integral part of the diagnostic process. This type of evaluation is particularly important in the first few years of life since subtle difficulties can easily be overlooked in a general neurological examination, in global developmental indices, or in a routine pediatric screening, and may be precursors of subsequent learning or behavioral difficulties (Aylward, 1988).

The major purposes for obtaining a neuropsychological assessment include (1) defining the outcome of a known CNS insult or disorder (e.g., head injury, Down's syndrome, hydrocephalus), (2) investigating possible reasons for cognitive or behavioral difficulties, (3) obtaining a detailed profile of cognitive and behavioral strengths and weaknesses, (4) determining whether this profile is consistent with a suspected disorder or syndrome (e.g., Landau–Kleffner syndrome, Asperger's disorder), (5) characterizing aspects of the child's learning style, such as approach to problem-solving, preferred modality of information, response to reinforcers, flexibility, persistence, and sustained attention, (6) using assessment data to help formulate effective treatment strategies or management plans, (7) helping to assess the child's prognosis and risk for certain developmental outcomes (e.g., assessing the stability of IQ over time, where a consistently low IQ over several years would indicate a developmental trajectory ending in significant retardation), and (8) conducting ongoing assessments of change over the course of development and in response to particular interventions (e.g., worsening performance indicating neurological deterioration or ineffective education or treatment) (Kaplan, Fein, Kramer et al., 1999; Risser and Edgell, 1988; Tramontana and Hooper, 1988).

*Limitations in assessing the preschool child*

*Maturational factors*

CNS insults and disorders may have differing outcomes depending on age of onset. Early views held that brain insults occurring early in life are not as threatening as those occurring later in life (Kennard and McCulloch, 1944), and that early brain damage affects later performance of language-related skills, but not sensory and motor capacities (Hebb, 1949). Data accumulated since these early theories were put forth, however, present a much more complicated picture, one that results in no overarching principle, but rather one that depends on factors such as age, etiology, specific function (sensorimotor, language), and environmental stimulation or deprivation.

According to Kolb, Gibb and Gorny (2001), frontal lobe injury in children is often associated with more recovery than after a similar injury in adults. However, even in children, recovery appears to be closely related to developmental age, where the least ideal time for cortical injury to occur is before the first year of life and the most favorable time is around 1 to 2 years of age. Recovery from acquired aphasia in children also suggests a large difference between children and adults in capacity for brain reorganization and behavioral plasticity, with children having an enormous capacity for preserving function in the face of catastrophic brain injury. As with frontal lobe injury, there seem to be limitations on plasticity in children (see Aram, 1998; Aram and Eisele, 1992). Kolb and Whishaw (1990) indicated that injury between 1 and 5 years frequently results in reorganization of functions and recovery of language ability, whereas the periods both before and after this age range often result in more significant impairment. Similarly, aggressive behavior treatment applied before the age of 5, or possibly even 4, arguably produces the best outcome for children on the autism spectrum (Green, 1996).

Diamond and Goldman-Rakic (1986, 1989) have shown experimentally that primates can 'grow into' the cognitive and behavioral manifestations of early acquired lesions, and this appears to be true for some functions in children as well. Abnormal development may not be clinically manifested until the child must engage in a behavior that depends on the affected area. In fact, given the continued development of myeli-nation and brain connectivity and the progressively greater reliance on top-down processing during later childhood, behavioral expression of the brain insult may not be evident until years later (Baron and Gioia, 1998). Although this has been shown experimentally only for specific lesions of prefrontal cortex (Diamond and Goldman-Rakic), it may be speculated that developmental conditions such as ADHD, in which symptoms may appear after age 3, and autism, in which symptoms may appear at 15 to 18 months, represent the same developmental phenomenon.

*The neuropsychological evaluation*

Although neuropsychological examination of preschoolers has a similar format to that of older children, there are some significant differences. In preschoolers, maturational level affects the planning, execution, and interpretation of neuropsychological evaluation, including the range of behaviors that can be examined, the choice of test instruments, and the evaluation of performance on any one measure (Baron et al., 1995). At younger ages, children exhibit a relatively limited response repertoire and their performance is more variable and state-dependent. This, of course, becomes less of a problem in the later preschool years as the child approaches school age. Developmental progression, however, also complicates treatment evaluation, since one must disentangle the effects of successful intervention from maturational changes occurring during the treatment period (Baron et al.).

Pediatric neuropsychologists must be mindful of the poor psychometric status of early preschool assessment measures since many of the tests designed for preschool use are severely limited in floor, item gradient, and reliability, especially at the lower age levels (Bracken, 1987; Flanagan and Alfonso, 1995). There should be relatively less reliance on standardized test measures in assessing preschoolers as there are functional areas where standardized instruments are not available. Also, instruments designed for adults may be testing skills that have not yet developed in children. Reliance on observation and caregiver reports, therefore, will increase the validity and accuracy of evaluations (Nuttall et al., 1999).

Many pediatric neuropsychologists caution against making strong predictions from preschool data. Aylward, Gustafson, Verhulst and Colliver (1987) point out that while deficits involving motor function tend to be relatively stable over time, cognitive functioning may show considerable variability from infancy through early childhood. Wilson (1992) noted that, with the exception of severe CNS abnormality, it is difficult to make predictions regarding the ultimate level of cognitive development in the preschool child. Similarly, Baron et al. (1995) caution that evaluation of young children does not allow strong predictions for long-term success or failure, and "the risks for making erroneous statements about a child's future functioning are great" (p. 195). Ongoing neuropsychological assessment, therefore, can be used to monitor the child's developmental progress.

There are limitations in clinical practice that contribute to the tentative nature of predictions from the assessment of cognitive functioning of preschoolers and render the reliability of assessment in this age group less certain. One of these limitations concerns premorbid data for preschool children often being sparse. Another involves the significant chance of behavioral variability within the preschool age range that may affect the validity of an assessment; children of preschool age are usually more sensitive to surroundings than are older or younger children. The preschool child's performance on any one day may not be an accurate reflection of typical behavior, and performance in an unfamiliar setting, such as the neuropsychologist's office, may be unrepresentative of behavior in other settings. Other factors producing variability include fatigue, hunger, temperament, variable attentional capacity, psychological comfort, activity level, the child's mood and affect during testing, and the timing of an assessment (Baron and Gioia, 1998; Baron et al., 1995; Wilson, 1992). Therefore, the interpretation and diagnostic formulation are significantly improved with multiple test sessions, different time samples, multiple sources of information, and with the evaluation of behavior in multiple contexts (Baron and Gioia, 1998).

Finally, a resulting diagnostic formulation for young children based on neuropsychological evaluation, is eschewed by some clinicians, teachers, and child advocates. Such diagnoses, they feel, can unnecessarily stigmatize the child, present social barriers, create lowered expectations, reduce intervention efforts, and create unnecessary distress in the family. Although the usefulness of specific diagnostic labels continues to be debated, they have served both clinical and research purposes in (1) allowing specific description of various syndromes, (2) aiding in prognosis, (3) investigating the effectiveness of therapies for specific disorders, (4) guiding parents to appropriate support groups and literature, and (5) obtaining educational and treatment resources for the affected children.

## Models of assessment

Pediatric neuropsychology differs from adult neuropsychology primarily in its strong developmental orientation. It is therefore essential that measures and techniques be developed and utilized from the neonatal period upwards, rather than simply downscaling adult neuropsychological techniques to preschool children (Aylward, 1997). The following section will discuss the current approaches to and models of neuropsychological assessment in preschool children.

### Fixed battery vs. process-oriented approaches

The two most widely used general approaches to neuropsychological assessment are the fixed-battery approach and the selection of a flexible battery in conjunction with the process-oriented approach to interpretation. The fixed-battery approach attempts to provide a comprehensive assessment of neuropsychological function using a fixed set of validated test procedures. The tests used are not dependent upon the clinical hypothesis or the presenting problems of the client. The goal is to administer as many of the components of the battery as is possible given the client's condition. It is thought that individual variability will be represented sufficiently well if the battery taps into a broad range of cognitive capabilities. The benefit of using a fixed-battery approach is to allow comparisons among different clinical groups by providing a standard database (Tramontana and Hooper, 1988).

The process-oriented approach incorporates both quantitative and qualitative methods in neuropsychological assessment. The quantitative approach is concerned with selecting standardized tests to develop an initial screening battery that will cover a broad range of functions. The qualitative approach is concerned with the individual's method of solving a particular task and is also concerned with analysis of how the individual behaves as he or she passes or fails a particular task (Kaplan, 1988). As an amalgam of the two, the process-oriented approach often uses a core set of standardized tests in order to develop an initial picture of the patient's general pattern of function and dysfunction. The results are then used to develop hypotheses about the nature of the individual's deficits. These hypotheses are checked through the use of additional tests selected for the individual patient, which can include standardized tests and new components designed to separate the cognitive demands of standardized tests, and the careful observation of the patient's approach to each task (Tramontana and Hooper, 1988).

The strength of the process-oriented approach lies in its ability to tap into the different component processes that are used during test taking. This approach focuses on identifying the strategies employed by the child to solve a particular task as well as examining the nature of the errors made, the particular context in which they occurred, and the nature of the stimulus that evoked particular errors (Kaplan, 1988). Thus, the process-oriented approach could bring to light the need for different diagnostic decisions, treatment interventions, and teaching strategies in two children with identical test scores. The process approach as developed by Edith Kaplan, sometimes called the Boston Process Approach (White and Rose, 1997), is exemplified by the Wechsler Adult Intelligence Scale-Revised as a Neuropsychological Instrument (WAIS-R NI; Kaplan, Fein, Morris and Delis, 1991) for adults and the Wechsler Intelligence Scale for Children, Third Edition, Process Instrument (WISC-III PI; Kaplan et al., 1999) for school-age children. Such an instrument, providing a means for neuropsychologically analyzing and extending the standardized IQ test has not yet been developed for preschoolers, but the NEPSY: A developmental neuropsychological assessment (Korkman, Kirk and Kemp, 1997) has many such properties and provides a very useful set of neuropsychological measures for preschool-age children.

At preschool ages, the debate between the fixed-battery and the process-oriented camps is less vigorous than with older patients. For one thing, fixed batteries do not generally extend downward to pre-school ages. Further, many experienced clinicians reject the fixed battery as too limiting for young children (Baron et al., 1995). The collection of subtests included in the NEPSY were designed by the authors with a hypothesis-testing approach in mind and were therefore meant to be used as a set of tasks from which the tester can select rather than as a fixed battery (more detailed information on the NEPSY in the section 'Domains of assessment'). Finally, as mentioned above, since scores tend to be less reliable and the child less capable of testing at the preschool level, the evaluator is forced to rely more on observation and interview, which de facto constitutes a more qualitative and hypothesis-testing approach.

*The IQ construct*

Most neuropsychological assessments of preschool children include an IQ measure. This serves two main purposes: (1) it provides a rough index of general cognitive function, against which specific functions can be assessed; and (2) the subtests of IQ measures can themselves be interpreted as tools for neuropsychological assessment of a sampling of cognitive functions such as motor speed, accuracy, and word retrieval.

Although IQ as a construct is both definable and measurable, there are various difficulties with its use in preschool children. First, IQs obtained during early childhood have low predictive power, particularly in children who have sustained damage to the central nervous system (Wilson, 1992). Second, any attempt to determine functional deficits may be difficult since each subtest requires a variety of functions for successful performance (Wilson). In addition, the IQ subtests often have much lower reliability than the overall IQ score. Third, the IQ construct loses its validity as a function of heterogeneity among subtests. With a flat subject profile, an IQ score derived from these subtests is meaningful, but with increasingly uneven subtest scores, common in atypically developing children, the IQ scores will be correspondingly meaningless. Perhaps most important, intelligence tests have been used to label children as more limited than they may, in fact, be, especially children from culturally diverse backgrounds (Rey-Casserly, 1999). This misguided information can have consequent dramatic impact on the child's educational opportunities. Because of these factors, some authors (Neisworth and Bagnato, 1992) argue against the use of intelligence tests with young children. Regardless of whether or not an IQ score is included, it is imperative that pediatric neuropsychologists conduct comprehensive evaluations bolstered by qualitative observation. Rey-Casserly highlighted the importance of predicting with caution, increasing the validity of predictions by using multiple assessment points and considering social factors, and not overgeneralizing about the child's cognitive potential from test scores.

Another important issue to consider when testing preschool-aged children is the principle of increased differentiation. This principle suggests that as children age, their cognitive abilities become more specific and differentiable, and that this is based upon sufficient neurophysiological development and differentiation, as well as the prior experience necessary for the ability being assessed. The Differential Abilities Scales (DAS; Elliott, 1990) draws its theoretical basis from this principle. Children between the ages of 2 years, 6 months (2-6) and 3-5 receive only a General Conceptual Ability score, whereas children between the ages of 3-6 and 5-11 also receive the more differentiated Verbal Ability and Nonverbal Ability subtest scores.

*Aylward's early neuropsychological assessment model*

Aylward (1988, 1997) developed a classification schema for neuropsychological assessment that could be extended to the neonatal and early childhood periods. He pointed out that although there is much overlap between functions and between classes of functions, certain functions may not be fully developed until later ages and therefore are not able to be tested. For this reason, he believes that neuropsychological assessment models must be age-specific and that functions should not be measured equally at each age. Aylward's schema involves basic neurological functions, receptive functions (visual, auditory, tactile), expressive functions (fine motor, oral motor, gross motor), processing (memory/learning, reasoning), and mental activity. In the preschool period, the focus is on receptive, expressive, and processing functions (see Aylward, 1997 for a more comprehensive review of this schema).

*Wilson's branching model*

Wilson's (1992) model was developed based on the premise that a fixed-battery approach to pediatric neuropsychological assessment would be ineffective. Therefore, a process-oriented approach was adopted, focusing primarily on the cognitive functions or behavior to be assessed as opposed to the tests to be used to make the assessment. The clinical approach is directed by a hypothesis testing framework based on the child's presentation, which helps in both selecting tests and in interpreting results. Wilson's model assumes that "various aspects of neuropsychological function are able to be described in terms of constructs. . . , and that these constructs may be defined operationally" (Wilson, 1992, p. 379). The neuropsychological constructs addressed in Wilson's model include such processes as auditory discrimination, formulation of language, auditory-sequential memory, short-term auditory memory, word retrieval, auditory cognition, auditory–visual cognition, visual discrimination, visual–spatial function, visual–sequential memory, visual cognition, fine motor skills, graphomotor skills, and praxis (Wilson, 1992). Like Aylward, Wilson noted that neuropsychological functions are not independent, but rather have considerable overlap with each other. Therefore, when an initial assessment uncovers a deficit in a complex neuropsychological function, the results can be interpreted to help refine the measures used in order to get a more specific pattern of dysfunction (Wilson, 1992). For example, a child with language formulation difficulties might be found to have good auditory discrimination but poor auditory cognition, or might be found to have good auditory discrimination but poor sequential memory in both auditory and visual domains, with implications for differential remediation. Wilson's model, including assessment instruments for each construct, is described in Wilson (1992).

*Systemic developmental approach of Children's Hospital, Boston*

Another process-oriented model of neuropsychological assessment, more broadly theoretical and less specific in its content than that of Wilson, has been developed at Children's Hospital in Boston (Bernstein, 2000; Bernstein, Prather and Rey-Casserly, 1995; Holmes-Bernstein and Waber, 1990; Rey-Casserly, 1999). This approach advocates assessment which is dynamic and systemic, concerned not with test performance per se but with the overall adaptation of the child. The child is the central focus of analysis and "reflects the theoretical framework within which the data will be collected and interpreted" (Bernstein, p. 411). A comprehensive history and observations from various sources together form the basis for hypotheses, which are then tested through further observation and quantitative and qualitative analysis of test performance. A 'systems' approach such as that used in behavioral neurology is adapted to review the systems resulting from the nature and timing of the child's neurological insult, the resulting compensations and unique developmental path, and the environmental challenges and supports provided by the family and other cultural contexts. The resulting picture of the *whole child* in adaptation to the environment then lends itself to recommendations for treatment interventions and provides strategies for management and risk assessment. Rey-Casserly describes an extension of this model for preschool children, which she calls the *tripartite model*, referring to the integration of information obtained from history, observation, and testing. These three areas are accorded equal weight and together promote the overall adjustment of the child rather than emphasize deficits. From each of these sources, information is obtained about general cognition, language processes, nonverbal processes, executive functions, memory, social–emotional adjustment, preacademic skills, and motor functions.

## Major categories of disorders and special populations

The clinician should be familiar with disorders of children that he/she will evaluate. The presence of a specific disorder may alert the clinician to areas of expected deficit, to important diagnostic questions, and to behavioral challenges that the child may present. This section will briefly review some aspects of the disorders and special populations that the neuropsychologist working with preschool children may encounter most often: traumatic brain in-

jury, pervasive developmental disorders, attention-deficit/hyperactivity disorder, language disorders, mental retardation, cultural differences, and visual and hearing impairments. For those conditions covered in more detail in this volume, we will restrict our discussion to some specific assessment issues. For more information on these conditions as well as those not covered here such as epilepsy, hydrocephalus, and medical and genetic disorders, the reader is referred to Yeates, Ris and Taylor (2000).

### Traumatic brain injury

Approximately one million children in the United States sustain closed head injuries each year (Teeter and Semrud-Clikeman, 1997). Moreover, it appears that individuals up to 24 years old are more likely to sustain head injuries than older individuals and that males receive injuries twice as often as females (Kraus, 1995). Unlike many disorders, traumatic brain injury (TBI) can produce very different neurobehavioral sequelae depending on the injury type (e.g., falls versus high velocity motor vehicle accidents), age at which injury occurred, severity of the injury, possible neurological complications, and treatment protocol (Fletcher, Levin and Landry, 1984).

Despite the variability that characterizes TBI there are certain generalizations that can be made about its common sequelae in *adults and later childhood*. The neurobehavioral sequelae of head injury often include declines in nonverbal intelligence, visual–motor impairment, attentional and memory deficits, decreases in oral fluency, comprehension, and verbal association, achievement declines in reading, and an increase in psychiatric disorders (Ewing-Cobbs, Fletcher and Levin, 1986). Mild head trauma, in particular, often results in mild and rapidly improving deficits in the areas of attention and memory. Conversely, moderate to severe head trauma often results in the manifestation of significant neuropsychological deficits across a wide range of functions (Smith, Barth, Diamond and Giuliano, 1998).

The neurobehavioral sequelae of TBI in *preschoolers* are less well understood than in later childhood and adulthood. Ewing-Cobbs, Fletcher, Levin et al. (1997) examined neuropsychological outcome in children aged 4 months to 7 years by comparing performance on (1) composite IQ and motor skills, (2) receptive and expressive language abilities, and (3) Verbal and Performance IQ scores. The results of this study indicated that severe traumatic brain injury in preschoolers resulted in deficient scores across all domains, with motor scores lower than IQ scores. Conversely, after mild to moderate traumatic brain injury it was found that Verbal IQ scores were significantly lower than Performance IQ scores. In addition, expressive language scores were lower than receptive language scores. With regard to reading, Barnes, Dennis and Wilkinson (1999) found that children who sustained head injuries in the preschool years, before basic word decoding skills are acquired, or in the early elementary grades when decoding skills are being taught, were most at risk for difficulties in acquiring basic word decoding and reading comprehension skills.

When evaluating preschool children, it is important to consider both the development of brain function (Kolb and Fantie, 1989) and the external changes in demands and expectations of the environment (Ylvisaker, Hartwick and Stevens, 1991). As indicated earlier, damage to certain areas of the brain, especially the frontal regions, may not become apparent until some months or years later since some functions of these areas do not manifest until later in life when the functions are mature and when the environment demands their execution. Thus young children may 'grow into a deficit', making it difficult to assess the impact of early injuries, and making it important to follow even the children who appear to be doing well. Injury to prefrontal cortex very early in life, in particular, may be increasingly apparent as the demands for socialization and rule-governed behavior increase in preschool and kindergarten settings.

Three stages of recovery from TBI have been identified in adults: acute (0–3 months), middle (3–12 months), and late (12 months and on) (Stuss and Buckle, 1992; Williams, 1992). The acute phase consists of a period of unconsciousness followed by a confusional state during which the individual is disoriented and shows generalized attentional and memory deficits. The middle phase is characterized by recovery from the generalized confusional state and the manifestation of specific cognitive deficits. During this phase of recovery Smith et al. (1998) rec-

ommend administering a comprehensive neuropsychological battery, emphasizing that head-injured patients may manifest practically any neuropsychological deficit during their recovery, depending on the nature and severity of the neurological impairment. During the late phase, they recommend retesting with a comprehensive neuropsychological battery in order to follow the progress of recovery and to determine the approximate point at which recovery is no longer occurring.

It has been found that children progress through the same stages as adults, although the initial stages are completed more rapidly (Smith et al., 1998). The assessment of head injury in preschool children, however, is complicated by a decrease in the appropriateness of traditional neuropsychological procedures for this age group. In general, it is important to measure overall cognitive functioning, motor functions, and receptive and expressive language abilities in children recovering from TBI. It is also crucial to assess attention and executive impairment in this population of children, although these are more difficult to assess in preschool children. Nevertheless, one can observe the behavior of the child under changing stimulus conditions and can utilize parent/teacher reports and behavioral observations of sustained and selective attention, distractibility, concentration, frustration tolerance, and behavioral disinhibition.

### Pervasive developmental disorders

Pervasive developmental disorders are characterized by severe and pervasive impairment in several areas of development including reciprocal social interaction skills and communication skills, and by the presence of stereotyped behavior, interests, and activities (American Psychiatric Association, 1994). Some of the pervasive developmental disorders include autistic disorder and Asperger's disorder. For a more detailed account of autism refer to Minshew and Dunn (2003, this volume).

Recent data (Stevens, Fein, Dunn et al., 2000) suggest that cognitive functioning in preschool children with autistic disorder is a much more potent prediction of school-age outcome than are preschool behavioral abnormalities. This underscores the importance of cognitive assessment in this population at preschool ages as a predictor and as an index of treatment effectiveness. Assessment and diagnosis of children with autistic disorder are complicated by a pattern of development in which certain milestones are achieved at age-appropriate times whereas others are not. In some children, the first year or two of life are developmentally normal followed by regression in language and functioning, while in others, cognitive and language (but not usually motor) development is already delayed in the first year. Assessment is also complicated by extreme behavioral and cognitive heterogeneity. Children with autism can either be low-functioning or high-functioning, and recent evidence suggests that these two groups (separated by a nonverbal IQ of about 70) show quite different patterns of functioning (Fein, Stevens, Dunn et al., 1999; Rapin, 1996; Stevens et al.). Siegel (1998) notes that children with low-functioning autism can show symptoms often associated with mental retardation (e.g., restricted play, poor social skills, stereotypic movements, echolalic speech).

The purposes of assessment with young children with autistic disorder, as with many other children, include diagnostic and prognostic decision-making, ascertaining current functioning levels, identifying asset and deficit patterns, obtaining information for planning educational and therapeutic interventions, and evaluating progress (Siegel, 1998). Information about both the level and pattern of performance is important as this will indicate if functioning is within normal variation or atypical, as well as reveal relative strengths and weaknesses across various domains of functioning.

Cognitive profiles in preschool children with low-functioning autism tend to be rather flat, although language may still show relative impairment (Fein, Dunn, Allen et al., 1996). Preschool children with high-functioning autism have individual profiles, but as a group tend to show strengths in rote learning and rote and single word language, visuospatial skills and motor skills, and deficits in comprehension and formulation of complete language, verbal memory for meaningful language, and complex reasoning.

Significant and chronic impairments of social interactions and/or repetitive patterns of behavior also characterize Asperger's disorder (American Psychiatric Association, 1994). Unlike autistic disorder, children with Asperger's are not impaired in the domain of language, and cognitive development may be age-appropriate. Regarding assessment of children with suspected Asperger's disorder, Ehlers and Gillberg (1993) suggest including neuropsychological, intelligence, language, and neuropsychiatric (e.g., parent/teacher interviews and rating scales) measures. A two-tiered approach is recommended by Gillberg and Gillberg (1989), with the first stage consisting of screening for social impairments, narrowness of interests, the presence of repetitive routines, speech and language problems, nonverbal communication difficulties, and motor difficulties, i.e., a detailed assessment of the core and strongly associated features. The second stage entails using a more comprehensive assessment, which relies on reports from the child's teachers and parents as well as testing of the child.

Testing a child with a pervasive developmental disorder can be very challenging. These children are often not motivated to perform to the best of their ability in a testing situation. Furthermore, many of these children do not gain a sense of accomplishment from doing a task well. For these reasons it is important to use incentives. Garretson, Fein and Waterhouse (1990) found that incentives can sometimes normalize performance to a striking degree. In order to determine which incentives will be most reinforcing and the most effective way to explain the reinforcement contingency to the child (e.g., "first work, then M and M's"), it is important to question caregivers or teachers about how the child has been taught.

In addition to using appropriate reinforcers, children with pervasive developmental disorders should be given ample time to acclimate to the testing environment prior to testing. It may also help to have a caregiver or teacher present during testing so that the child feels more comfortable and so that behavior will be under better control. Since children with pervasive developmental disorders also often have marked difficulty with receptive and expressive language, it may be necessary to simplify the test instructions in order to ensure that the child understands the directions. Keeping work sessions short and interspersing easier tasks among more difficult ones may also help to sustain attention, which is deficient among many children with these disorders.

*Attention-deficit/hyperactivity disorder*

According to the DSM-IV, "a persistent pattern of inattention and/or hyperactivity–impulsivity that is more frequent and severe than is typically observed in individuals at a comparable level of development" is considered to be the essential feature of attention-deficit/hyperactivity disorder (ADHD) (American Psychiatric Association, 1994). Conceptually this is seen as a disturbance in attention span, self-regulation, activity, and impulse control (Teeter and Semrud-Clikeman, 1997). (For a more detailed account of ADHD, see Tannock, 2003, this volume.)

In conducting a neuropsychological evaluation of a preschool child with known or suspected ADHD, emphasis should be placed on specific domains of functioning (in addition to any domains indicated to be problematic for the individual child); these include the ability to sustain attention, other executive skills such as planning, organizing, deducing rules, and set shifting, which are best examined by behavioral observations in this age group, fine and gross motor skills, motor sequencing and speed, visual–motor integration, and visual and verbal memory (see Table 1 for specific tests).

A diagnosis of ADHD does not depend on neuropsychological findings; these findings, however, can be useful for confirmation of diagnosis, assessment of severity, and evaluation of treatment effectiveness. In addition, a neuropsychological assessment of ADHD should be able to assist in the differential diagnosis of this disorder as well as in delineating specific subtypes (Slomka, 1998). Although there is a paucity of research on the neuropsychological manifestation of ADHD in the preschool population, Mariani and Barkley (1997) found that clinic-referred, preschool-age boys with ADHD performed significantly worse than did children in a community comparison group on tests of academic achievement, motor control, and working memory. They found the early deficits in motor control and working memory to be an inherent part of the syndrome, supporting the conceptualization of ADHD as involving deficits in executive functions beyond the problems in behavioral inhibition and sustained attention.

Young children with disordered attention or hyperactivity are difficult to test. These children will often have difficulty staying on task when presented with tests requiring considerable mental effort and may be inclined to give up easily. Just as with children with pervasive developmental disorders, it may help to intersperse easier tests among the more difficult ones. Also, using appropriate reinforcers, such as stickers or edibles, may help keep the child motivated and engaged. Since these children are easily distracted and have short attention spans it is also important to minimize distractions and give breaks when necessary. Allowing the child to choose the order in which the tasks are done or which reinforcer they wish to earn may help prevent oppositional behavior. In addition, if the child has trouble sitting still (a common characteristic in children with disordered attention or hyperactivity), the tester should allow the child to move elsewhere or stand and stretch between tasks so long as it does not encourage out-of-control behavior. Many children with disordered attention or hyperactivity need extra time switching their attention from one task to another. For these children it is important to give instructions slowly and clearly, and allow extra time, if necessary, between tasks. Children with attention difficulties also show inconsistency in test performance because their performance may vary from day to day, depending on internal factors. If the examiner has reason to suspect that the child's performance may not reflect his or her best efforts, he/she may choose to readminister specific items or subtests, if possible, on a different day.

The above modifications will promote the most cooperative behavior and the highest test performance among preschool children. It should be remembered, however, that the children's home or preschool environments may not be inclined or able to make these modifications to normal behavioral demands. Because the typical testing environment is highly structured, novel, and provides intensive one-on-one adult attention, the child with ADHD may demonstrate levels of attention and information processing that are above usual, thus providing false negative results. It is important to inform parents or teachers that the evaluation results may represent the child's highest, rather than typical, performance. If the child was frankly uncooperative, on the other hand, parents should be informed that test performance probably represents an underestimate of their capacity. Observation of behavior under conditions of difficulty or frustration, although not representing the child's cognitive potential, may give the examiner valuable insight into his/her behavior and personality, which may limit the child with ADHD more than cognitive difficulties.

*Language impairment*

There is a great deal of controversy regarding the etiology, diagnosis, and methods of intervention for children with specific language impairments (SLI). For a more detailed account of language impairment, see Rapin, Dunn and Allen (2003, this volume).

In order to assess a child with SLI it is necessary to first determine what aspects of language will be assessed, and the diagnostic and exclusionary criteria to be used. Although both expressive and receptive language must be assessed, there is no consensus as to the optimal tests that can be used to assess these functions (Bishop, 1997; Cole, Dale and Thal, 1996). In order to be psychometrically sound, a test must be valid, reliable, and adequately standardized on the appropriate population. In this regard recent research has brought into question the utility of some of the measures currently used to assess language impairment in preschoolers (Williams, Voelker and Ricciardi, 1995). For a description of some of the more widely used assessment measures, refer to Bishop (1997) and Cole et al. (1996), and see Table 1.

In addition to a thorough evaluation of language processes, certain other functions should be routinely assessed in the child referred for possible or known language disorder. Assessment of nonverbal cognitive processes is crucial, since it will reveal the extent to which normal or above-average intelligence can be used to help compensate for the linguistic disability. Play and social skills should also be considered since they are often mildly to moderately deficient in children with language impairments. Verbal memory can be expected to be impaired, and should be assessed against nonverbal aspects of memory. Lastly, features of pervasive developmental disorders should be ruled out, as should the possibility of comorbid ADHD.

*Mental retardation*

According to the DSM-IV (American Psychiatric Association, 1994), mental retardation consists of three essential features: (1) significantly subaverage general intellectual functioning (approximately two standard deviations below the mean on one or more standardized tests of intelligence); (2) deficits in at least two areas of adaptive functioning such as communication, social skills, self-care skills, etc.; and (3) onset in the developmental period (before 18 years). The DSM-IV further categorizes mental retardation by degrees of severity based on IQ: mild (50–55 to about 70); moderate (35–40 to 50–55); severe (20–25 to 35–40); and profound (below 20 or 25). These categorizations are important in so far as they affect the method of intervention that is used and suggest ultimate levels of functioning that can be attained (Sparrow and Carter, 1992). The American Association on Mental Retardation's (AAMR, 1992) classification system includes children with IQ's from 70 to 75 in order to allow for measurement error. They also describe subcategories of mental retardation. Their classification system, however, is based on level of support needed by individuals in order to function (intermittent, limited, extensive, pervasive).

The classification of mental retardation requires an evaluation that includes standardized measures of both intelligence and adaptive functioning. An overall approximate level of retardation can be estimated from standard batteries or IQ tests as long as basal levels are reached. There are several issues that need to be considered carefully, however, when assessing preschool children with mental retardation. The first is the reliability and validity of the tests being used. It is often difficult to determine an accurate mental age because of failure to establish a basal level of performance. In addition many of the currently used psychometric tests may not offer the opportunity for the preschooler to demonstrate age-appropriate behaviors (Huang, Hunter, Reinert and Wishon, 1992). In fact, it has been proposed that there may be no measure of intelligence capable of diagnosing mental retardation in children who are less than 3 to 4 years of age (Sparrow and Carter, 1992). The younger or lower-functioning a child, the harder it is to accurately differentiate among cognitive abilities. Another issue concerns the appropriateness of standard assessment techniques. Preschoolers who are severely mentally retarded often require that modifications be made to the tests, such as allowing the child to respond by eye blinking, pointing, or nodding. It is also important to determine individual characteristics of the child that may adversely affect test performance. In particular, it is important to be aware of problems in attention, concentration, motivation, anxiety, and compliance. These problems are prevalent in children with mental retardation and may make it difficult to obtain an accurate estimate of cognitive functioning. In fact, at very young ages, especially the first year or two of life, adaptive functioning scales, which measure a child's ability to cope with social demands in a given social environment (Huang et al., 1992), may be more predictive of later functioning than cognitive measures. For this reason, it may be more useful to rely on adaptive functioning scores (Sparrow and Carter, 1992). Of course, observing behavior in different settings and at multiple time points increases reliability of adaptive behavior results. Furthermore, careful assessment of adaptive behavior within the child's cultural context will help to avoid mislabeling children (Bucy, Smith and Landau, 1999).

In addition to intelligence and adaptive functioning instruments, Bucy et al. (1999) highlight the importance of including academic readiness measures in the assessment of a preschooler who is mentally retarded. These measures are typically curriculum-based or criterion-referenced tests. According to Huang et al. (1992), curriculum- and criterion-based instruments are often sensitive to deficits that may not be detected by a standardized psychological test. The Peabody Developmental Motor Scales (PDMS; Folio and Fewell, 1983), for example, can be used as a criterion-referenced measure of motor patterns and skills with young children with severe mental retardation who do not respond to standardized procedures.

Preschoolers with mental retardation will demonstrate delays in all areas of development including the acquisition of cognitive, language and social skills and, to a less consistent degree, motor skills. However, it is important to realize that the level of severity may be related to the specific function that is affected. For example, mild mental retardation in preschool children often manifests as difficulties in language development. These difficulties mostly involve language form, content, and use, as opposed to speech production. Early warning signs of difficulty in the development of language in preschool children include prolonged persistence of babbling, primarily one-word utterances past the age of 2.5 to 3 years, excessive crying as a means of gaining attention, and difficulty understanding spoken words and following verbal directions (Huang et al., 1992).

An assessment of a preschool child with suspected mental retardation, therefore, should include a comprehensive history of development, assessment of overall cognitive ability, receptive and expressive language abilities, and adaptive skills, including motor ability. In addition to being aware of attention, memory, and compliance effects on testing, the examiner should also attend to history factors that may affect behavior such as head injury, seizures, illness, fatigue, allergies, and medications.

*Cultural diversity*

The population of culturally and linguistically diverse preschool children in the United States is rapidly growing (Li, Walton and Nuttall, 1999). In order to be effective, clinicians must approach the assessment process differently when working with young children who may be racially or culturally different from themselves and who may not have the same native language as the neuropsychologist. First, they should attempt to learn about the preschooler's culture and ethnic group so that the child's responses can be put into the appropriate context. It is also necessary for the clinician to be aware of any preconceived notions he or she may have about a particular ethnic group in order to help prevent any possible stereotypes from influencing the assessment procedures (Sattler, 2001). Moreover, psychologists need to be aware of possible differences in styles and patterns of behavior (Nuttall et al., 1999), and also be aware of the child's experiences in his or her particular environment. For example, there may be a weakness in motor processes in a particular child, specifically graphomotor skills, that is due mainly to that child's lack of experience with using a pencil (Gopaul-McNicol and Thomas-Presswood, 1998). Making accommodations to the testing situation by taking extra time to build rapport with both parents and children will increase the child's motivation and comfort and, ultimately, will improve validity of test performance.

TABLE 1

Tests for preschoolers

---

**General neuropsychological measure**

*NEPSY: A developmental neuropsychological assessment* (Korkman et al., 1997), designed to assess neuropsychological development in children ages 3 to 12 in five functional domains: (1) attention/executive functions, (2) language, (3) sensorimotor functions, (4) visuospatial processing, and (5) memory and learning. There are separate forms for children ages 3 to 4 and for those ages 5 to 12.

**General cognitive ability**

*Bayley Scales of Infant Development, Second Edition* (BSID-II; Bayley, 1993), designed to assess the cognitive development of infants and toddlers ages 1 to 42 months. Items on this test comprise the Mental, Motor, and Behavior Rating scales.

*Differential Ability Scales* (DAS; Elliott, 1990), used for individuals ages 2-6 to 17-11 years, but is especially useful in the late toddler and early childhood range. The DAS is divided into two age levels for preschool children (lower preschool level 2-6 to 3-5; upper preschool level 3-6 to 5-11) with different subtests comprising the General Conceptual Ability composite.

*Kaufman Assessment Battery for Children* (K-ABC; Kaufman and Kaufman, 1983), designed to measure intelligence and achievement in children ages 2-6 to 12-6. The subtests comprise two factors: sequential processing and simultaneous processing.

*Leiter International Performance Scale, Revised* (Leiter-R; Roid and Miller, 1997), designed as a test of nonverbal intellectual ability of individuals aged 2-0 to 20-11 years. Consists of 20 subtests in the primary domains of visualization, reasoning, attention, memory, and memory span, and relies on the use of perceptual tasks.

*McCarthy Scales of Children's Abilities* (McCarthy, 1972), applicable to children between the ages of 2-6 to 8-6 years. Provides five area scores: verbal, perceptual-performance, quantitative, motor, and memory.

*The Miller Assessment for Preschoolers* (MAP; Miller, 1988), designed to identify preschoolers ages 2.9 to 6 years who are at risk for developmental delay. Items are grouped into five performance areas: neural foundations, coordination, verbal, nonverbal, and complex tasks which fall into three main categories: sensory and motor, cognitive, and combined abilities.

*Mullen Scales of Early Learning* (MSEL; Mullen, 1995), measures the cognitive functioning of young children from birth to 68 months. Normative data can be derived from five specific scales: Gross Motor, Visual Reception, Fine Motor, Receptive Language, Expressive Language.

*Stanford–Binet Intelligence Scale, Fourth Edition* (SB : FE; Thorndike, Hagen and Sattler, 1986), used to assess the cognitive functioning of individuals from ages 2 through adulthood. Yields four scores in the areas of Verbal Reasoning, Abstract/Visual Reasoning, Quantitative Reasoning, and Short-Term Memory.

*Wechsler Preschool and Primary Scale of Intelligence, Revised* (WPPSI-R; Wechsler, 1989), used for the cognitive assessment of children ages 3-0 to 7-3. Contains 10 core battery subtests that combine to form the Verbal and Performance scales.

*Woodcock–Johnson III Tests of Cognitive Abilities* (WJ-III COG; Woodcock, McGrew and Mather, 2001b), designed to assess cognitive ability in individuals ages 2 through adulthood. This test includes specific early development subtests that are applicable to preschool children and provides guidelines for accommodations to be used while administering this test to preschoolers.

NOTE: Specific subtests of the general cognitive ability tests just presented will not be individually listed under the domains; only relevant subtests of the NEPSY will be presented.

An asterisk indicates tests that are only applicable to the upper limit of the preschool period in this chapter (i.e. children 5 years of age)

**Language/speech**

*Clinical Evaluation of Language Fundamentals, Preschool* (CELF-Preschool; Wiig, Secord and Semel, 1992), a downward extension of the CELF-R; this test assesses communication skills in preschool and early elementary children aged 3-0 to 6-11 years. This test specifically focuses on receptive and expressive language abilities in the areas of word meanings, word and sentence structure, and recall of spoken language.

*Comprehensive Assessment of Spoken Language* (CASL; Carrow-Woolfolk, 1999a), designed for assessing oral language knowledge, processes, and skills in individuals aged 3 to 21 years. The test focuses on language knowledge (structure) and language performance (processing) (see text).

*Early Language Milestone Scale, Second Edition* (ELM Scale-2; Coplan, 1993), assesses speech and language development during infancy and early childhood; specifically measures language development from birth to 36 months of age and intelligibility of speech from 18 to 48 months of age. It was designed to screen for language or speech delays as early as possible in a child's development.

*Expressive One-Word Picture Vocabulary Test, Revised* (EOWPVT-R; Gardner, 1990), designed to obtain an estimate of verbal intelligence for children ages 2-0 to 11-11. The test appears to best serve the purpose of measuring the child's ability to utilize language, that is, expressive vocabulary.

*Expressive Vocabulary Test* (EVT; Williams, 1997), designed to assess expressive vocabulary and word retrieval in individuals ages 2-6 through adulthood (see text).

*Peabody Picture Vocabulary Test, Third Edition* (PPVT-III; Dunn and Dunn, 1997) designed to measure receptive vocabulary in individuals aged 2-0 to adulthood.

TABLE 1 (continued)

*Preschool Language Scale-3* (PLS-3; Zimmerman, Steiner and Pond, 1992), measures the receptive and expressive language ability of children from birth to 6 years, 11 months (6-11). Yields scores in auditory comprehension and expressive communication focusing on four language aspects: language precursors, semantics, structure, and integrative thinking skills.
*Receptive One-Word Picture Vocabulary Test* (ROWPVT; Gardner, 1985), designed to evaluate the receptive vocabulary of children ages 2-0 to 11-11.
*Sequenced Inventory of Communication Development, Revised Edition* (SICD-R; Hedrick, Prather and Tobin, 1984) designed to assess communication abilities of children ages 4 to 48 months. Includes a Receptive Scale (sound and speech discrimination, awareness, and understanding) and Expressive Scale (imitating, initiating, and responding behavior; verbal output and articulation).
*Test for Auditory Comprehension of Language, Third Edition* (TACL-3; Carrow-Woolfolk, 1999b), designed to measure auditory comprehension of language in children ages 3-0 to 9-11 and is organized into three sections: (1) word classes and relations, (2) grammatical morphemes, and (3) elaborated phrases and sentences. This test also helps to identify individuals having receptive language disorders.
*Test of Early Language Development, Second Edition* (TELD-2; Hresko, Reid and Hammill, 1991), designed to assess the early development of oral language in the areas of receptive and expressive language, syntax, and semantics in children ages 2-0 to 7-11.
*Test of Language Development–Primary, Third Edition* (TOLD-P:3; Newcomer and Hammill, 1997), used to determine specific strengths and weaknesses in language development of children aged 4-0 to 8-11 by screening children's expressive and receptive competencies in major linguistic areas. The purpose is to identify English-speaking children who show significant delays in language proficiency.
*NEPSY Language Domain subtests* — Body Part Naming, Phonological Processing, Comprehension of Instructions, Verbal Fluency, Oromotor Sequences, * Speeded Naming (5+ years), * Repetition of Nonsense Words (5+ years)

**Visual–spatial abilities**
*Developmental Test of Visual Perception, Second Edition* (DTVP-2; Hammill, Pearson and Voress, 1993), measures visual–perceptual and visual–motor integration abilities in children ages 4-0 to 10-11.
*Test of Visual Perceptual Skills (non-motor), Revised* (TVPS-R; Gardner, 1996), assesses how a child visually perceives non-language forms by measuring visual discrimination, spatial relationships, form constancy, figure–ground, and closure in children aged 4-1 to 13-0 years.
*NEPSY Visuospatial Domain subtests* — Design Copying, Block Construction, * Arrows (5+ years), * Route Finding (5+ years)

**Motor functioning**
*Beery–Buktenica Developmental Test of Visual–Motor Integration, Fourth Edition* (VMI; Beery, 1997), used to screen for visual–motor problems in individuals aged 3-0 to 17-11 years by assessing the extent to which children can integrate visual and motor skills as evidenced by copying a set of increasingly difficult geometric designs.
*Peabody Developmental Motor Scales* (Folio and Fewell, 1983), assesses gross and fine motor functions in children from birth to 7 years.
*Purdue Pegboard* (Tiffin, 1948), assesses fine motor ability related to eye–hand coordination and finger dexterity with norms (Wilson, Iacoviello, Wilson and Risucci, 1982) beginning at age 2 years, 6 months and continuing into adulthood.
*Test of Visual–Motor Skills, Revised* (TVMS-R; Gardner, 1995), designed to assess visual motor integration skills in children ages 3 to 13 years. The test requires the child to visually perceive and replicate 25 increasingly difficult geometric designs in order to assess eye–hand motor accuracy, motor control, motor coordination, and/or the child's gestalt interpretation.
*NEPSY Sensorimotor Domain subtests* — Imitating Hand Positions, Visuomotor Precision, Manual Motor Sequences, * Fingertip Tapping (5+ years), * Finger Discrimination (5+ years).

**Learning and memory**
* *Children's Memory Scale* (CMS; Cohen, 1997), designed to evaluate learning and memory functioning in children ages 5 to 16 years. The test yields several indices including general memory, visual and verbal immediate and delayed, delayed recognition, learning, and attention/concentration.
* *California Verbal Learning Test — Children's Version* (CVLT-C; Delis, Kramer, Kaplan and Ober, 1994), designed to assess strategies and processes involved in learning and recalling verbal material in children ages 5 to 16.
*NEPSY Memory and Learning Domain subtests* — Narrative Memory, Sentence Repetition, * Memory for Faces (5+ years), * Memory for Names (5+ years)
*TVPS-R subtests* — Visual Memory, Visual Sequential Memory

**Attention**
*Child Behavior Checklist — Attention Problems Scale* (Achenbach, 1991), examines behaviors such as attention, behavioral control, and task performance in children aged 4 to 18 years (see Social/Emotional Functioning).
*Conners' Behavior Rating Scales* (Conners, 1997), provides cognitive problems/inattention, hyperactivity, and ADHD indices in children ages 3 to 17 (see Social/Emotional Functioning).

TABLE 1 (continued)

---

*Conners' Kiddie Continuous Performance Test* (K-CPT; Conners, 2001), computer-administered test designed to identify attention problems and to measure treatment effectiveness in children aged 4 to 5 years. This test takes approximately 7.5 min to administer and provides indices of reaction time, variability of reaction time, and error rates including omission and commission error types (see text).
*Early Childhood Attention Deficit Disorders Evaluation Scale* (ECADDES; McCarney, 1995), designed to assess ADHD in children aged 24 to 72 months through observation of behavior in both the home and the school.
*Gordon Diagnostic System* (Gordon, 1996), a visual continuous performance test that consists of a Preschool Delay Task, Preschool Vigilance '0' Task, and Preschool Vigilance '1' Task for children ages 3 to 5.
*Test of Variables of Attention* (TOVA; Greenberg, Corman and Kindschi, 1996), designed to assess attention and impulse control in individuals aged 4 years through adulthood. The test uses computerized visual and auditory stimuli to assess attention.
\* *CMS* — Attention/Concentration Index (5+ years)

**Executive functions**
\* *Behavior Rating Inventory of Executive Function* (BRIEF; Gioia, Isquith, Guy and Kenworthy, 2000), a questionnaire for parents and teachers to assess executive function behaviors in both the home and school in children ages 5 to 18 years. Yields the following eight scales: Inhibit, Shift, Emotional Control, Initiate, Working Memory, Plan/Organize, Organization of Materials, and Monitor.
*NEPSY Attention/Executive Domain subtests* — Visual Attention, Statue, \* Tower (5+ years), \* Auditory Attention and Response Set (5+ years), \* Design Fluency (5+ years), \* Knock and Tap (5+ years)

**Pre-academic skills**
*Boehm Test of Basic Concepts, Preschool Version* (Boehm, 1986), designed to measure knowledge of basic relational concepts in children ages 3 to 5. These concepts include size, direction, position in space, quantity, and time, and are considered necessary for achievement in the beginning years of school.
\* *Key Math Diagnostic Inventory of Mathematics, Revised* (Connolly, 1988), measures understanding and application of math skills and concepts for children from kindergarten through grade nine. Sequences of skills are organized according to the domains of Basic Concepts, Operations, and Application.
*Metropolitan Readiness Test* (MRT; Nurss and McGauvran, 1986), series of tests that measure fundamental competencies for reading, mathematics, and language-based activities in young children. Level I is designed for preschool children prior to entering kindergarten and for children in the beginning and middle of kindergarten and includes subtests such as auditory memory, beginning consonants, and visual matching.
*Test of Early Reading Ability-2* (TERA-2; Reid, Hresko and Hammill, 1989), designed to assess early reading behaviors (e.g., relational vocabulary, knowledge of the alphabet and its functions, letter naming) in children ages 3-0 to 9-11.
*Test of Early Written Language, Second Edition* (TEWL-2; Hresko, Herron and Peak, 1996), measures early writing ability consisting of a basic writing portion and a contextual writing portion in children ages 3-0 to 10-11; can be used to determine the strengths and/or weaknesses of a student's writing ability.
*Woodcock–Johnson III Tests of Achievement* (WJ-III ACH; Woodcock, McGrew and Mather, 2001a), designed for individuals ages 2 through adulthood. For young children, an Early Developmental Scale is available which includes 12 subtests measuring the following areas: Reading, Mathematics, and Knowledge. Subtests also measure short- and long-term retrieval and oral comprehension. The WJ-III ACH provides guidelines for accommodations to be used while administering this test to preschoolers.

**Social/emotional functioning**
*Behavior Assessment System for Children, Revised; Teacher Rating Scale, -Preschool — Parent Rating Scale, Preschool* (BASC-R; Reynolds and Kamphaus, 1998), the preschool specific measures are designed to assess the behavioral and emotional functioning of children aged 2.5 to 5 years. The Externalizing, Internalizing, and Attention Problems scales, Behavioral Symptoms Index, and Adaptive and Social Skills scales allow for measurement of both adaptive and clinical dimensions of a child's behavior.
*Child Behavior Checklist* (CBCL; ages 2 to 3; Achenbach, 1992) (CBCL; ages 4 to 18; Achenbach, 1991), used to assess the competencies (e.g., activities, social) and problems (e.g., withdrawal, anxiety/depression, aggressive behavior) of children and adolescents through the use of ratings and reports by different informants.
*Conners' Behavior Rating Scales, Revised: Conners' Parent Rating Scales and Conners' Teacher Rating Scales* (CPRS; CTRS; Conners, 1997), used to assess problem behaviors in children ages 3 to 17. These include oppositional behavior, cognitive problems/inattention, hyperactivity, anxiety, social problems, etc. The scale also yields an ADHD index and DSM-IV Inattention, Hyperactivity/Impulsivity, and Total factors.
*Preschool Evaluation Scale* (PES; McCarney, 1992), designed to assess behavior (e.g., muscle skills, expressive language, self-help skills) related to developmental delays in children between birth and 72 months.
*Preschool and Kindergarten Behavior Scales* (PKBS; Merrell, 1994), a behavioral rating instrument used to evaluate social skills and problem behaviors in preschool and kindergarten children ages 3 to 6; used as a screening tool for the early detection of social–emotional problems.

TABLE 1 (continued)

*Social Skills Rating System: The Social Skills Rating System, Teacher; and the Social Skills Rating System, Parent* (SSRS-T; SSRS-P; Gresham and Elliott, 1990), used to screen and evaluate the social skills of children in preschool through high school in different settings and to assist in the development of interventions when social skill deficits are identified; items are made up of prosocial behaviors (e.g., makes friends, controls temper) and problem behaviors (e.g., temper tantrums).

*Vineland Social–Emotional Early Childhood Scales* (Sparrow, Balla and Cicchetti, 1998), used to assess the social–emotional functioning of children from birth through 5 years, 11 months. Three scales are yielded: Interpersonal Relations, Play and Leisure Time, and Coping Skills, along with a Social–Emotional Composite.

**Adaptive behavior**

*Home Observation for the Measurement of the Environment* (HOME; Caldwell and Bradley, 1984), designed to screen for sources of potential environmental risk. Includes an Infant/Toddler Home Inventory for children from birth to 3 years and an Early Childhood Inventory for children ages 3 to 6 years.

*Scales of Independent Behavior, Revised* (SIB-R; Bruininks, Woodcock, Weatherman and Hill, 1996), used to assess the independent functioning of individuals from early infancy to late adulthood in home, school, and community settings. There is an Early Development Form used for young children and individuals with developmental functioning levels below 8 years.

*Vineland Adaptive Behavior Scales* (VABS; Sparrow, Balla and Cicchetti, 1984), used to assess adaptive behavior in individuals from birth to age 19 in four specific domains: (1) Communication, (2) Daily Living Skills, (3) Socialization, and (4) Motor Skills. These scales also include an Adaptive Behavior Composite and a Maladaptive Behavior scale.

**Play**

*Play Observation Scale* (Rubin, 1989), used to assess free play preferences (social and cognitive play and non-play categories) in an unstructured environment in preschool children aged 2 to 6 years.

*Symbolic Play Checklist* (Westby, 1980), integrates language, cognitive, and social aspects of play in children ages 9 to 60 months old.

*Symbolic Play Test, Second Edition* (Lowe and Costello, 1988), developed to assess early concept formation and symbolization in children ages 1 to 3 years based on a child's spontaneous, nonverbal play activities with specified sets of miniature objects.

Many culturally diverse children who live in the United States are also bilingual and English may not be their first language. Lack of mastery of English may adversely affect standardized test scores for these children and these scores may be inappropriately interpreted by the clinician as a true measure of the child's accumulated knowledge or ability (Sattler, 2001). According to Rhodes, Kayser and Hess (2000), language development issues are essential to the differential diagnosis of language impairments and normal language differences in Spanish-speaking preschool children. Since the neuropsychological assessment of young children who speak Spanish places emphasis on the language through which the assessment is conducted, issues regarding the translation and adaptation of instruments and the use of interpreters are underscored. Li et al. (1999) recommend first attempting to find a neuropsychologist who speaks the child's native language. If one is not available, then, and only then, should an interpreter who has been trained appropriately be enlisted. Furthermore, tests that have language adaptations in the preschool child's particular language should be utilized whenever possible (see Li et al. for appropriate tests to be used with culturally diverse preschoolers).

When dealing with culturally different children, both language and non-language performance scales should be administered, when possible. This will help to ensure that the child's full repertoire of abilities is measured since language ability will rarely be equal in both languages, even for fully bilingual children. Clinicians should also be aware, however, that even nonverbal assessment involving motor or perceptual tasks is not culture-free (Armour-Thomas, 1992). Therefore, test results and behavioral observations must always be interpreted within the linguistic and cultural context of the preschool child. For a more complete review of this literature the reader is referred to Gopaul-McNicol and Thomas-Presswood (1998) and Suzuki, Ponterotto and Meller (2001).

*Hearing and vision impairments*

*Hearing impaired preschoolers*

Hearing loss in preschool children has far-reaching implications for their development of language and communication skills. Depending on the level of intervention and degree of hearing loss, young children will adopt different modes of communication. For a more detailed account of hearing impairment and its implications, see Mayberry (2003, this volume).

The crucial components of a comprehensive assessment for preschoolers with hearing loss include assessments of audiological functioning, language and communication skills, cognitive functioning, adaptive behavior, and social–emotional functioning. In order to guarantee that each component is thoroughly assessed using the appropriate measures, it is necessary to utilize the resources and expertise of a multidisciplinary diagnostic team (Mullen, 1999). When using standardized assessment measures, it will be important for the examiner to reduce background noise, keep visual distractions to a minimum and be sensitive to visual cues from the preschool child, speak clearly and avoid obstructing his/her mouth (i.e., untrimmed beard, hands, etc.), and avoid complicated language or idioms. The psychologist should also check to make sure the child understands what is being said by asking questions or by having the child repeat back directions when possible, and observe the child's behaviors in order to understand how the child copes (Mullen, 1999). Furthermore, given the difficulties with standardized assessment measures, an ecological approach to assessment has been recommended for use with deaf, or hard of hearing, preschoolers. In this way, a greater amount of information can be gathered from a greater number of sources thus increasing the chance that the child will receive appropriate intervention.

*Visually impaired preschoolers*
The assessment of visually impaired children is fraught with numerous difficulties. Like many of the other special populations discussed, standardized measures are not generally normed on visually impaired children. Thus the validity and reliability of any conclusions drawn from the results must be questioned, and interpretations must be made with caution. In addition, few clinicians have been properly trained to work with, and be sensitive to, these children's special needs. For a more detailed account of the implications of visual impairment, see Warren and Hatton (2003, this volume).

Given that the sense of sight is the primary means by which individuals interact with their environment, visually impaired children are at a significant disadvantage in the quality and quantity of their experiences compared to sighted children. Because visual impairments can be manifest across a broad spectrum of behaviors, it is important to thoroughly assess these children, especially including the areas of cognitive development, psychosocial development, language development, and motor development.

A comprehensive assessment requires that the assessor gathers information from numerous sources including observational and objective data from parents, medical specialists, teachers, and any other professionals who interact with the child and family. There are also important considerations which need to be addressed when working with children with visual impairments such as ensuring that the child is wearing glasses if he/she needs them prior to assessment, allowing the child to have extra time to explore the testing environment, and using both tactile and verbal reinforcements (Moore, 1999).

As mentioned earlier, most assessment measures were not normed on children with visual impairments. Consequently, any conclusions drawn from such data may result in erroneous assumptions regarding the child's cognition. It is therefore also the responsibility of the evaluator, through appropriate recommendations, to ensure that results are not used to inappropriately lower expectations for the child. For a review of commonly used assessment instruments for the visually impaired preschooler, refer to Moore (1999).

**Domains of assessment**

The goal of the neuropsychological evaluation is to ensure that all important areas of functioning are assessed. Evaluations for preschool children with suspected or known neurodevelopmental or acquired disorders should include tests from the following broad functional areas: general cognitive ability, language/speech functions, visual–spatial abilities, motor functions, learning and memory, attention, executive functions, pre-academic skills, social–emotional functioning, adaptive behavior, and play. Some areas, such as language functioning, visuospatial abilities, and motor abilities are easier to evaluate because they are associated with specific tasks. Other abilities, such as problem-solving, attention, and executive processing are more general functions which affect performance in many areas and must be monitored through several tests and behavioral observations (Wainwright, Fein and Waterhouse, 1991).

The assessment of *general cognitive ability* in preschool children is usually accomplished by using measures that attempt to sample all relevant domains, including abstract reasoning and conceptual skills. For example, the WPPSI-R (Wechsler, 1989) and the Differential Ability Scales (DAS; Elliott, 1990) (see Table 1) are intelligence tests that yield summary scores. As mentioned earlier, however, these overall scores are frequently misleading and can be meaningless when there is significant discrepancy between subtests. Therefore, it is frequently the interpretive conceptual framework or task analysis of subtests that makes the assessment of general cognitive ability *neuropsychological*. This can be accomplished by focusing on how or why a child performed in a particular manner (e.g., attention, motor skills, conceptualization problems), rather than on the actual score obtained (Aylward, 1997). It is important to make use of the neuropsychological application of intelligence and developmental tests because excessive length and noncomparable abilities prevent a downward scaling of neuropsychological batteries from adults or older children to preschoolers (Aylward, 1997).

A test that deserves particular mention here, however, is the NEPSY (Korkman et al., 1997). The NEPSY consists of a series of subtests that measure neuropsychological development in children ages 3 to 12 in five functional domains: (1) attention/executive functions, (2) language, (3) sensorimotor functions, (4) visuospatial processing, and (5) memory and learning. This is the first attempt at creating a comprehensive neuropsychological measure specifically for children and there is no doubt that these tests are extremely clinically useful. Although the NEPSY is relatively new, researchers have begun to use it and many find it to be a strong developmental neuropsychological instrument based on sound theory and research (Benedict, 1999; Kolk and Talvik, 2000).

*Language* and *speech* are two important components of the communication process. Language refers to the code that represents the information to be communicated, while speech serves as a major modal-ity for expressing language (Wyatt and Seymour, 1999). There are specific linguistic rules that make up language systems; these rules involve syntactic, semantic, and pragmatic aspects. Preschoolers' difficulties with communication are typically manifested as an inability to efficiently produce speech and/or problems with acquisition of the linguistic rules that make up their particular language system (Wyatt and Seymour, 1999).

There are several formal measures of language available for use with preschoolers, such as the Peabody Picture Vocabulary Test, Third Edition (PPVT-III; Dunn and Dunn, 1997) and the Expressive One-Word Picture Vocabulary Test (EOWPVT; Gardner, 1990), which examine receptive and expressive vocabulary, respectively, at the single-word level. The PPVT-III is co-normed with the Expressive Vocabulary Test (EVT; Williams, 1997). Although this pair of tests is very useful, some of the items on the EVT require the child to produce synonyms rather than simple labels for pictures, which may become too conceptually difficult for children with developmental disabilities thus resulting in an inaccurate picture of their expressive vocabulary skills. A receptive companion for the EOWPVT is the Receptive One-Word Picture Vocabulary Test (ROWPVT; Gardner, 1985). This pair of tests could also be used for measuring receptive and expressive vocabulary in children.

There are also measures examining different aspects of the comprehension of language (e.g., oral language, syntax vs. semantics). The Test for Auditory Comprehension of Language, Third Edition (TACL-3; Carrow-Woolfolk, 1999b), for example, measures the child's understanding of vocabulary, grammatical morphemes, and syntax through the selection of correct pictures. The Preschool Language Scale-3 (PLS-3; Zimmerman, Steiner and Pond, 1992) tests auditory comprehension and expressive ability, sampling four skills in each of these domains at 6-month age intervals. One of the newest measures of language that can be used in young children is the Comprehensive Assessment of Spoken Language (CASL; Carrow-Woolfolk, 1999a), which is designed to assess oral language knowledge, processes, and skills in children as young as age three. The development of this test was guided by the concept that language reflects two dimensions: (1) language knowledge, which encompasses structural categories such as semantics and pragmatics; and (2) language performance, which encompasses the three major processing systems of auditory comprehension, oral expression, and retrieval (Carrow-Woolfolk, 1999a,b). All CASL tests are orally administered and require only oral or pointing responses. Although no studies to date have been conducted on the CASL, the clinical utility of this test appears to be extremely positive and the subtest on pragmatics fills a real need in this area. In addition to using formal instruments of language, examiners can also screen specific language skills with observations from spontaneous conversation (e.g., stuttering, misperceived verbal instructions) (Baron et al., 1995).

*Visual–spatial function* refers to the ability of a child to analyze, synthesize, and appreciate structural similarities and differences in visually presented stimuli (Wilson, 1992) (see Table 1 for specific tests). The perceptual system enables children to interpret information that will be used in cognitive and motor tasks (Dunn, 1999). For preschoolers, these tasks generally require constructional abilities and can involve representational or nonrepresentational stimuli (e.g., NEPSY Design Copying and Block Construction).

*Motor function* in the preschool years involves both gross and fine motor development, including visual–motor integration skills. In addition to formally assessing a child's motor skills, the neuropsychologist should observe gross motor activity, including the child's sense of balance and equilibrium, coordination, and gait. The same should be done with fine motor skills, including observation of the child's pencil grip (is it mature or immature? is the palm of the hand or a fist being used to hold the pencil?) and placement of paper on written tests. It is also important to note whether definite hand preference has been established. In addition, any unusual motor movements, such as tics or twitches, must be documented. All of these observations should be evaluated in light of the child's history (Baron et al., 1995).

The *memory* domain is extremely important in young children at risk for neuropsychological dysfunction. The most important aspects of memory to measure include immediate vs. delayed, recall vs. recognition, and learning ability. It is also important to compare different modalities of presentation (i.e. visual vs. verbal). There are very few learning/memory tasks available for the preschool population (particularly for the younger children). Only measures of immediate memory span (e.g., sentence repetition, motor/hand movements) appear to be sufficiently developed for the preschool child (Baron and Gioia, 1998).

The construct of *attention* comprises several elements, including the abilities to *focus* and *sustain* attention (Mirsky, Anthony, Duncan et al., 1991; Willmott, Anderson and Anderson, 2000), which are important in assessing the preschool child. Problems with focusing attention are apparent when the child cannot engage with the material and only gives it brief attention. The ability to sustain attention can be observed in the context of natural activities or through the completion of formal tasks, such as continuous performance tests. The Conners' Kiddie Continuous Performance Test (K-CPT; Conners, 2001) is a very new measure that appears to meet the need for the early identification of attention disorders. Although it follows the same basic format as most continuous performance tests, two aspects make this test extremely suitable for preschool children. These include the brief administration time and the presentation of pictures of objects rather than letters, thereby preventing the interference of any possible letter recognition difficulties that young children may exhibit. During any type of continuous performance task, the examiner should note duration of attention span, distractibility, vigilance, and any disparity between different time periods of testing (Baron et al., 1995). The degree to which the examiner is required to provide frequent prompts to stay on task can also serve as an indication of sustained attention (Baron and Gioia, 1998). For children with many disorders, including ADHD and PDD, there is a marked discrepancy between excellent sustained attention for preferred activities vs. poor attention to adult imposed tasks. The nature of tasks that provoke inattention can also serve as clinical cues to other dysfunctions; for example, children with language disorders may become restive and uncooperative when language tasks are introduced.

The key *executive control* functions for young children include initiation, inhibition, and flexibility.

The child's inhibitory capacity is a critical function that becomes more important through the preschool years (Baron and Gioia, 1998). The young child's abilities to shift from one activity to the next are behaviors that comprise the flexibility subdomain. Observation is key in assessing executive functioning in this population of children. The examiner should observe the child during periods of transition, which can reveal potential problems in flexibly shifting set (Baron and Gioia, 1998). The examiner should also observe the child's ability to reason and plan by taking note of how the child approaches tasks (is he/she impulsive? can he/she develop alternative strategies?) (Baron et al., 1995).

*Pre-academic skills* are important to assess in preschool children in order to ascertain whether they are developing the necessary skills and knowledge in preparation for functioning in a school environment. According to Boehm (1986), when children begin school, their knowledge of basic concepts is critical for understanding the teacher's directions and communicating with others. Therefore, a child's mastery of basic concepts can serve as an indication of school readiness and help spot possible developmental delays (Boehm).

The assessment of *social–emotional functioning* is critical during the preschool years because skills in this area impact children's later functioning in various settings. Assessment attempts to identify children's behavior in several areas, such as anxiety, impulse control, depression, attentional problems, aggressive behavior, and also prosocial behavior. Any attempts to measure a preschooler's social–emotional behaviors or reactions will begin with parent and/or teacher concern and descriptions of the child's behavior. Direct observations should then be made of the child, followed by formal measures of social–emotional functioning (typically consisting of parent and teacher report) in order to obtain a clearer picture of the child's reported behaviors.

*Adaptive behavior* involves a child's use of developmentally appropriate communication skills, self-care skills, and social interaction skills in order to function sufficiently in the environment. One of the most widely used parent interview scales of adaptive behavior is the Vineland Adaptive Behavior Scales (VABS; Sparrow, Balla and Cicchetti, 1984). This measure provides developmental scores in the areas of communication, socialization, daily living skills, and motor functioning, as well as a global index of adaptive behavior and a maladaptive behavior scale. The Home Observation for the Measurement of the Environment (HOME; Caldwell and Bradley, 1984) is a combination of observation and interview, designed to evaluate the home environment. In addition to formal instruments, it will be important for the examiner to observe the preschoolers' comprehension of nonverbal social cues and gestures, and display of socially inappropriate actions such as age-inappropriate aggression, withdrawal, or anxiety (Baron et al., 1995). It also will be useful for the examiner to note emotional maturity by observing the ease or difficulty of separation from parent, reaction to failure, cooperativeness, and response to praise.

The assessment of *play* can provide a wealth of information about a child's developmental level as well as his or her curiosity and willingness to engage with others. According to Trawick-Smith (1994), play is an essential aspect of learning, resulting in increases in cognitive, language, and social development, problem-solving, and creativity. For this reason, the assessment of play is an important component of the neuropsychological evaluation and mostly involves observations of the child in a natural or contrived play setting.

The development of age-appropriate play can fall under different categories (e.g., pretend, functional) and involves different factors such as the incorporation of schemas into play (see Westby, 2000, for more detail). Play develops along several dimensions simultaneously. It becomes more complex, progressing from simple schemata (holding a toy telephone to the ear) to sets of related schemata (feeding each of several dolls in turn, or feeding, diapering and putting a doll to bed), culminating in extended fantasy role play in the preschool years. It becomes less self-centered, progressing from pretending with the self to pretending with or animating toy figures. Play objects also become more divorced from reality, with early toys being representative of what they signify (toy telephone), to less representative (a stick for a gun), to totally imaginary objects. Deficits in appropriate play have been widely documented among children with developmental disabilities. However, there has been little research on the development of play or the relation between play and adaptive behavior in such children. Sigafoos, Roberts-Pennell and Graves (1999) found that observed play in children with developmental disabilities was primarily functional and exploratory, with less constructive and pretend play. These results suggest little overall relation between appropriate play and other major domains of adaptive behavior.

Table 1 provides a sampling of measures that are available for the assessment of the domains described above in the preschool child. These tests are by no means intended to comprise an exhaustive list, and only brief descriptions of the measures are included, since reviews on the reliability and validity of these measures is beyond the scope of this chapter.

## Assessment procedures

### Record review and interview

In preparation for conducting an assessment, the examiner should review the child's available records, which may include medical documents. These records encompass information pertaining to any complications or special circumstances related to the mother's pregnancy and baby's delivery (e.g., the newborn's need for placement in a neonatal intensive care unit (NICU) or extended hospital stay at birth); also included might be injuries, illnesses, surgeries, and visits to specialists (Kalesnik, 1999). Consideration of neuropsychological findings in light of the child's early history is necessary in pediatric neuropsychological assessment because of the frequent congruence between events occurring in the child's medical history and neuropsychological results. In fact, early medical/biological risk has been associated with subsequent learning disabilities, ADHD, and behavior problems (Aylward, 1997).

Other relevant documents that should be reviewed, if possible, include preschool records and reports from any previous evaluations or treatment conducted by psychologists, pediatricians, or early intervention providers. Parents, past and present-day care or preschool teachers, pediatricians, and any other pertinent professionals should be involved in the assessment process (Romero, 1999). It is extremely important that the parents of the preschooler be interviewed. The most useful types of questions to be asked in the interview setting are highly specific

yet open-ended (e.g., how would your child let you know if he/she wanted a snack or toy that was out of reach?), and general answers should be checked by asking for specific examples. The information obtained in the interview with the parents should include an early history of the child (e.g., pregnancy, delivery, infancy, sleeping, eating, temperament, developmental milestones, illness, injuries), family history (e.g., genetic risk factors), family background (e.g., family structure, socioeconomic status, particular stressors, coping style, support system, type of discipline used), family history of neurological and psychiatric disorders, and school history, if applicable (e.g., special education services; academic, social, and behavioral problems). The interview should also cover information regarding any initial concerns, prior diagnoses or recommendations, problem behaviors, and current medications.

When past records have been reviewed, parents have been interviewed and asked to complete child history forms, and clarifications regarding any discrepancies between parent report and previous records have been made, the background information should provide a reasonably comprehensive picture of birth, medical history, developmental milestones (Kalesnik, 1999), and the child's social and cultural context (Rey-Casserly, 1999).

### Behavioral observations

In addition to interviews and reviews of school and medical records, valuable information regarding the child's strengths as well as weaknesses that cannot be obtained through standardized test scores can be derived from direct observation of the preschooler's behavior during the formal administration of tests. Some of these observations have already been noted, but it is useful to mention them once again. During the behavioral observation, the examiner should observe the child's greeting behavior, eye contact, ability to separate from his or her caretaker, response to the examiner, reciprocal interaction, play behavior, activity level, pragmatic use of language, and general emotional tone. Testing behaviors that should be noted include the child's ability to shift from one task to another, attention span, prompts needed, ability to comprehend directions, consistency, cooperativeness, motivation, response to praise, self-correction of errors, task approach, differential response to tasks, and reaction to failure. The pediatric neuropsychologist should be particularly alert to signs of anxiety or fear of failure on the child's part. Observation of the preschool child's spontaneous and symbolic play either through observation or contrived play sessions is equally important, as it may have prognostic value in children with developmental disabilities (Wainwright et al.). Observations made in the classroom, on the playground, or at home, when feasible, help to complete the impression of the child (Wainwright et al., 1991).

### Testing situation

Preschoolers come to the testing situation with different levels of maturation and with different experiences and cultural backgrounds. Examiners must be flexible and creative in order to elicit cooperation and to determine accurately what the young child knows. In addition, the examiner must provide the preschool child with clear, positive directions and enough structure to help him or her complete tasks successfully (Romero, 1999). The physical testing situation is also very important when testing the preschooler (Wilson, 1992); the testing room should be brightly lit and free of distractions, and tables and chairs should be of appropriate size for preschool children (Romero, 1999).

Examiners who have experience with preschoolers and knowledge of standardized testing procedures will be able to discern more clearly a child's intent and motives and know whether a child is being uncooperative, is truly frightened, or is sincerely trying but still failing. Parents may also be helpful in clarifying the child's demonstrated capacities if they are present in the room, which is more likely to happen with 2- to 3-year-olds. Parents can provide information regarding how typical the child's behavior is and how it compares to capacities seen in other settings. Again, accuracy of parent report will be increased by asking for specific events and examples rather than accepting general assertions of competence (Romero, 1999).

The examiner must be aware of the child's behavior throughout the testing session, as the length of a session is dependent upon the ability of the preschooler to sustain attention and motivation. Prior to beginning testing, toys and materials such as picture books and large crayons can be used for establishing rapport (Romero, 1999). There also may be times during testing when standard procedures will need to be modified in order to elicit the highest level of performance of an uncooperative, frustrated, or anxious child. For example, one may choose to present subtests from a battery in an alternative order so that a task that is enjoyable for the child will follow a particularly difficult portion of the testing. A variety of reinforcement contingencies can also be used during testing in order to enhance performance and help identify the strengths of a child. These include providing the child with food or sticker reinforcers, frequent breaks, and/or verbal praise (Wainwright et al., 1991), where praise is contingent on effort and not success (Romero).

### Interpretation and communication of results

Historical, observational, and test data must be brought together to complete the full picture of the child's strengths and weaknesses. In general, the younger the child, the less predictive standardized test scores will be of later school-age test scores and academic performance. Systematic observation of how the child responds and copes with the assessment, therefore, will aid in making important inferences about how that child functions. Furthermore, since the preschool child's mental abilities do not readily arrange themselves in clear functional groupings, the examiner can probe particular areas where the child appears to be having difficulties by using the approach of *testing the limits*. This approach calls for readministration of test items with which the child had difficulty in order to ascertain how the items need to be changed for the child to succeed. This results in better understanding of why a child is having difficulty and can lead to recommendations that address how best to teach the child (Schnell and Workman-Daniels, 1992).

The effective communication of results is crucial in identifying and obtaining appropriate services for a child in need of special services. Findings should be summarized and translated into workable recommendations with the specification of behaviors that are essential for a particular child to develop in order to be successful in kindergarten or first grade in his or her school system. Effective communication of results may be facilitated by fostering a comfortable, supportive atmosphere, by using descriptive behavioral levels, by using diagnostic labels sensitively, and by clearly recognizing and exploring the parents' concerns, fears, and desires for their child (Laroche and Kruger, 1999; Wainwright et al., 1991).

## Recommendations

The strong interest in pediatric rehabilitation is evidenced by the recently formed Section of Pediatric Rehabilitation Psychology in the American Psychological Association's Division 22. This section is of interest to pediatric neuropsychologists, in particular, because discussion and activity focus on the functional correlates of neuropsychological profiles, implications for rehabilitation and educational planning, and the impact of disability on child development. In addition, this section provides a forum for pediatric rehabilitation-related issues and many child neuropsychologists play significant roles in rehabilitation teams.

Historically, the purpose of neuropsychological assessment was primarily to identify the presence and nature of brain dysfunction, as mentioned in the introduction, but the emphasis in clinical neuropsychology, and especially pediatric neuropsychology, has shifted to the functional and ecological assessment of the individual in order to recommend appropriate interventions. Major difficulties in achieving this important clinical goal, however, continue to involve diagnostic systems that were developed for descriptive rather than prescriptive purposes, inadequacies in the content, predictive, and ecological validities of standard neuropsychological tasks, and very limited research on treatment efficacies for different types of children (Lyon, Moats and Flynn, 1988).

Rourke, Fisk and Strang (1986) provided some guidelines for intervention that call specific attention to both immediate and long-term demands of the environment placed on the child and to the availability of resources in a particular educational setting. Focusing on these factors will allow for the development of more realistic recommendations and their implementation. In developing recommendations for an individualized plan, it is important to clearly specify the child's learning style and sug-

gest compensatory actions that draw on the child's strengths. It is best to offer teachers, parents, and others involved specific strategies and/or programs for accomplishing the plan's objectives (Laroche and Kruger, 1999). These may include contingency management techniques, specific learning strategies involving memory and attention, peer tutoring procedures, specific programs such as daily living skills or social skill programs, and specific placement recommendations (e.g., mainstreaming in preschool for a specific number of hours per week in a particular classroom size) (Teeter and Semrud-Clikeman, 1997).

Recommendations will be based on a child's current performance capabilities. The ideal approach to providing recommendations is to concentrate on both the strengths and weaknesses of a child's abilities. Depending on the orientation of the clinician, however, a program may be designed to improve only the child's weaknesses, or may emphasize and build only on the child's strengths, or as just mentioned, concentrate on both. The utilization of any one of these approaches will obviously affect both the techniques employed and the course of the intervention (Teeter, 1997).

Attempts to remediate the child's weaknesses seem to be most beneficial when deficits are pervasive in nature (Teeter, 1997). Remediation techniques have historically included perceptual–motor training and direct teaching of language skills. Although these techniques may produce little improvement in the child's academic performance, modest success has been documented with a few specific disorders (Teeter and Semrud-Clikeman, 1997). For example, one commonly used remedial technique for children with developmental disabilities, specifically autism, that has demonstrated success is Applied Behavior Analysis (ABA). This approach breaks down skills to be learned into very small components, including foundation skills such as attention and compliance, and teaches them systematically, using sophisticated principles of learning theory. Research suggests that such intensive behavioral intervention, beginning in the preschool years, can have a significant and lasting positive impact (Green, 1996). ABA is therefore the treatment of choice for many young children with autism as its potential for dramatic improvement is greatest with the youngest of children.

Another technique designed to target weakness that is becoming more widespread is a tool called FastForWord®Language (Scientific Learning Corporation, 1997), based upon Tallal's research (e.g., Tallal, Miller and Fitch, 1993; Tallal, Stark and Mellits, 1985) on temporal auditory processing of information in children. FastForWord®Language is an intervention program that uses computer games to treat children with language learning impairments in the ability to process auditory temporal information. This occurs by training specific auditory or phonological skills related to speech and language acquisition that are considered to be prerequisites for reading. FastforWord®Language is designed for use with 5- to 12-year-olds. However, there is a recent version designed for preschoolers that is an attempt to build early learning skills, such as attention and focus, phonological awareness, and organization skills. Although the results are described as encouraging with reported increases in overall language abilities, auditory processing speed, phonological awareness, and listening and comprehension skills (Veale, 1999), the underlying assumptions of this remediation tool that temporal processing deficits cause language-learning impairments and that this technique trains the brain by engaging brain plasticity mechanisms have been questioned (Gillam, 1999). Therefore, claims about treatment effectiveness need to be empirically validated through independent examination.

Some arguments against the use of remediation techniques in isolation arise from the experience that there may be some improvement in the process itself, but there is typically not a positive generalization of learning to other areas since the focus is on training specific processing deficits (Teeter, 1997). An example involves children with social skill difficulties who have been trained in social skill strategies; they often display appropriate social interaction in controlled, therapeutic settings, but fail to generalize these skills to natural settings (Teeter and Semrud-Clikeman, 1997). Similarly, many experienced neuropsychologists feel that trying to remediate global deficits such as attention is of little use because children seem to generalize least in those areas that are hardest for them (Wainwright et al., 1991).

Concentrating whenever possible on the child's strengths, in addition to remediation, identifies the child's most intact abilities, and an intervention program that focuses on those strengths can be planned (Teeter, 1997). The purpose of this approach is to build self-esteem and feelings of confidence and success, which are essential in order for the child to be motivated (Wainwright et al., 1991). When only focusing on deficits, a child may begin to feel frustrated and lose self-confidence. Teaching to the child's strengths, on the other hand, reduces the possibility of the child falling farther and farther behind peers (Teeter, 1997). Rourke and Del Dotto (1992) recommend combined intervention approaches that are primarily compensatory in nature. Developmental stages, severity of the dysfunction, and the emotional and adaptive capacity of the child will ultimately influence which orientation is initiated.

Educational planning is necessary for preschool children, including making placement decisions, particularly for 4- to 5-year-olds, and even some 3-year-olds. The neuropsychologist should help parents consider the range of possibilities for these placements, such as fully mainstreamed classrooms, partially mainstreamed classrooms, substantially separate classrooms with opportunities for mainstreaming, separate day schools, and residential placements. This requires taking care to explain intervention options thoroughly, teaching parents about child development, training parents to participate actively in school planning meetings and to become effective advocates for their child (Laroche and Kruger, 1999). A key element to keep in mind during program planning is the cultural, social, and educational differences among families. In other words, programs that work well with one family or setting may be impractical or ineffective with another, therefore there is a need to recognize individual differences when prescribing and coordinating services (Laroche and Kruger, 1999).

Some assessments suggest the need for other professionals to be involved, especially when the neuropsychologist feels that certain areas are beyond his/her training or competence. For example, if there is possible seizure activity, mental deterioration, motor symptoms or delays, or unusual facial structure, a referral to a pediatric neurologist is in order. In fact, any child with significant neurodevelopmental delay or disorder should be seen by a neurologist at least once. Significant language problems may indicate a comprehensive evaluation by a speech and language pathologist preceded by an audiological exam. Similarly, an occupational therapist may be consulted if motor deficits exist (Wainwright et al., 1991). The neuropsychologist must also remain clinically sensitive to the state of family functioning and, after achieving good rapport with parents, should not hesitate to refer them to a family therapist for issues related or unrelated to the child's disability. Children with significant behavior issues may benefit from ongoing consultation or therapy from a behavioral psychologist, while mood disorder or severe attention difficulty might dictate referral for ongoing supportive or cognitive therapy, or for a psychiatric consultation in order to address the possible use of psychotropic drugs.

Psychopharmacological treatment may be needed by some preschoolers. There has been some debate, however, concerning how early in life stimulants may be used without compromising the safety and well-being of the child. There is little research on the effects of stimulants on preschoolers (Santosh and Taylor, 2000). In general, the clinical efficacy of stimulants has been more variable and limited in preschoolers than in older age groups. Musten (1998) reported that cognitive and parent report measures of inattention were found to improve more than measures of impulsivity or noncompliance in preschoolers on stimulant medication. Byrne, Bawden, DeWolfe and Beattie (1998), however, reported improvement in behavior as well as in attentional functioning. A significant concern is the incidence of side effects such as dysphoria, anorexia, insomnia, increased solitary play, and poor peer relationships that have been particularly high in preschool children and somewhat different from the side effects reported for school-age children (Firestone, Musten, Pisterman et al., 1998). For this reason, psychopharmacological intervention is rarely advised in isolation. Most childhood disorders are complex and medications may not uniformly improve all areas of the child's functioning. Pharmacological interventions should therefore be combined with psychosocial interventions, such as behavioral treatments, individual or group therapy for the child, parent training, and/or family therapy (Teeter and Semrud-Clikeman, 1997).

Establishing and maintaining open channels of communication among the parents, school, and other providers (e.g., neuropsychologist, physician, occupational therapist) is necessary in order to monitor the success of placement programs or interventions. This is extremely important when several different professionals are involved and all are targeting the same symptoms. In these cases, efforts must be coordinated so that all of the necessary services will be delivered efficiently (Laroche and Kruger, 1999).

Neuropsychological assessment of the preschool child must continually be thought of as an ongoing process. Follow-up assessments can be useful in identifying the developmental progress of a child and in clarifying the effectiveness of a particular intervention program with the intent of modifying intervention plans, if necessary (Baron et al., 1995; Rourke and Del Dotto, 1992; Wainwright et al., 1991). During follow-up evaluations, pediatric neuropsychologists must be mindful of the child's maturational level, as certain skills and/or deficits may become more visible over time and any new areas of weakness (whether due to ineffective treatment or true limitations) may need additional interventions (Aylward, 1997). In fact, Teeter and Semrud-Clikeman (1997) recommend regular follow-up at 6-month intervals because treatment recommendations may not always be carried out adequately. In general, children in early intervention programs or special preschool classrooms should be reassessed periodically (every 6–12 months) in order to monitor their rate of growth.

## Future directions

Pediatric neuropsychology is in its own early childhood. It has emerged only recently as an independent field of study and practice, standing at the intersection of adult neuropsychology, child neurology, psychiatry, pediatrics, developmental psychology, and cognitive neuroscience, and was forged out of knowledge from all of these disciplines.

One could try to imagine what a highly developed pediatric neuropsychology would look like. It would have a comprehensive description of nervous system development, in what ways each stage or process could go awry, what biological and social factors could influence each of these processes, and the range of outcomes produced by each combination of events. This is obviously impossible, even given unlimited time and resources, since the combinations of such events and processes are virtually unlimited. On the other hand, we do not see an unlimited number of outcomes, but a somewhat discrete set of developmental pathway abnormalities; therefore, these syndromes must represent the final common pathway of multiple possible etiologies and moderating variables. In this light, the enormous task of unraveling the pathways of normal and abnormal development, while daunting, seems a little less impossible. To further this goal, we need advances in the fundamentals of developmental cognitive neuroscience (see Johnson, 1997, for an overview of the current state of this knowledge regarding specific functions). It seems clear that advances in functional neuroimaging will play a major role in the growth of this knowledge, especially when technical developments allow its routine use with young children.

The second branch of this ideal pediatric neuropsychology would entail the development of our clinical assessment and treatment skills. Our understanding of the development of cognition and emotion is far from complete but even the extensive information that has been gathered in the last 50 years is not generally put to use in our assessment instruments or in our treatment and educational recommendations. Information from the basic sciences about the development of the nervous system and about the development of the mind informs clinical assessment and treatment to a very limited degree. Most assessment techniques for preschool children still represent downward extensions of assessment procedures for older children or adults; for example, standardized tests tend to catalogue specific skills rather than examine the quality of the child's play or thinking with a Piagetian orientation. The literature on efficacy of specific interventions with specific developmental syndromes is limited indeed. With few exceptions, our recommendations are guided by our clinical experience and beliefs, rather than by controlled outcome studies. We sorely need such studies, so that our recommendations and intervention programs can rest on solid empirical grounds.

All of these desired developments require extensive cross-disciplinary collaboration. The limits of disciplinary isolation and the fruitfulness of collaboration can be seen in the interesting discovery, by Diamond and Goldman-Rakic (Diamond and Doar, 1989; Diamond and Goldman-Rakic, 1986, 1989; see Johnson, 1997, chapter 7, for a review of some of this work) that their respective disciplines of developmental psychology and primate neurobiology had for years been using an identical, simple, working memory paradigm, under different names, to study cognition in infants and monkeys. The resulting application of what had been learned about the development and prefrontal localization of this skill in monkeys to human infant development gave great impetus to studies of human frontal lobe development. Therefore, the possibility for similar discoveries in the field of pediatric neuropsychology is not only exciting, but quite possible indeed.

## References

Achenbach TM: Manual for the Child Behavior Checklist/4–18 and 1991 Profile. Burlington, VT: University of Vermont, Department of Psychiatry, 1991.

Achenbach TM: Manual for the Child Behavior Checklist/2–3 and 1992 Profile. Burlington, VT: University of Vermont Department of Psychiatry, 1992.

American Association on Mental Retardation: Definitions, Classifications, and Systems of Supports (9th ed.). Washington, DC: Author, 1992.

American Psychiatric Association: Diagnostic and Statistical Manual of Mental Disorders (4th ed.). Washington, DC: Author, 1994.

Aram DM: Acquired aphasia in children. In Sarno MT (Ed), Acquired Aphasia (3rd ed.). San Diego, CA: Academic Press, pp. 451–480, 1998.

Aram DM, Eisele JA: Plasticity and recovery of higher cognitive functions following early brain injury. In Rapin I, Segalowitz SJ (Eds), Handbook of Neuropsychology, Vol. 6: Child Neuropsychology. New York, NY: Elsevier, pp. 73–92, 1992.

Armour-Thomas E: Intellectual assessment of children from culturally diverse backgrounds. School Psychology Review: 21; 552–565, 1992.

Aylward GP: Infant and early childhood assessment. In Tramontana MG, Hooper SR (Eds), Assessment Issues in Child Neuropsychology. New York, NY: Plenum Press, pp. 225–248, 1988.

Aylward GP: Infant and Early Childhood Neuropsychology. New York, NY: Plenum Press, 1997.

Aylward GP, Gustafson N, Verhulst SJ, Colliver JA: Consistency in the diagnosis of cognitive, motor, and neurologic function over the first three years. Journal of Pediatric Psychology: 12; 77–98, 1987.

Barnes MA, Dennis M, Wilkinson M: Reading after closed head injury in childhood: Effects on accuracy, fluency, and comprehension. Developmental Neuropsychology: 15; 1–24, 1999.

Baron IS, Gioia GA: Neuropsychology of infants and young

children. In Goldstein G, Nussbaum PD, Beers SR (Eds), Neuropsychology. Human Brain Function: Assessment and Rehabilitation. New York, NY: Plenum Press, pp. 9–34, 1998.

Baron IS, Fennell E, Voeller K: Pediatric Neuropsychology in the Medical Setting. New York, NY: Oxford University Press, 1995.

Bayley N: Bayley Scales of Infant Development (2nd ed.). San Antonio, TX: The Psychological Corporation, 1993.

Beery KE: Beery-Buktenica Developmental Test of Visual Motor Integration (4th ed.). Parsippany, NJ: Modern Curriculum Press, 1997.

Benedict NJ: Reactive attachment disorder: A neuropsychological study. Dissertation Abstracts International: 59; 3680, 1999.

Bernstein JH: Developmental neuropsychological assessment. In Yeates KO, Ris, MD, Taylor HG (Eds), Pediatric Neuropsychology. New York, NY: The Guilford Press, pp. 405–438, 2000.

Bernstein JH, Prather PA, Rey-Casserly C: Neuropsychological assessment in preoperative and postoperative evaluation. Neurosurgery Clinics of North America: 6; 443–454, 1995.

Bishop DVM: Uncommon Understanding: Development and Disorders of Language Comprehension in Children. Hove: Psychology Press, 1997.

Boehm AE: Boehm Test of Basic Concepts, Preschool Version. San Antonio, TX: The Psychological Corporation, 1986.

Bracken BA: Limitations of preschool instruments and standards for minimal levels of technical adequacy. Journal of Psychoeducational Assessment: 4; 313–326, 1987.

Bruininks RH, Woodcock RW, Weatherman RF, Hill BK: Scales of Independent Behavior, Revised. Itasca, IL: Riverside Publishing, 1996.

Bucy JE, Smith T, Landau S: Assessment of preschool children with developmental disabilities and at-risk conditions. In Nuttall EV, Romero I, Kalesnik J (Eds), Assessing and Screening Preschoolers: Psychological and Educational Dimensions (2nd ed.). Boston, MA: Allyn and Bacon, pp. 318–339, 1999.

Byrne J, Bawden H, DeWolfe N, Beattie T: Clinical assessment of psychopharmacological treatment of preschoolers with ADHD. Journal of Clinical and Experimental Neuropsychology: 20; 613–627, 1998.

Caldwell BM, Bradley RH: Home Observation for Measurement of the Environment. Little Rock, AR: Center for Research on Teaching and Learning, University of Arkansas, 1984.

Carrow-Woolfolk E: Comprehensive Assessment of Spoken Language. Circle Pines, MN: American Guidance Service, 1999a.

Carrow-Woolfolk E: Test for Auditory Comprehension of Language (3rd ed.). Austin, TX: Pro-Ed, 1999b.

Cohen MJ: Children's Memory Scale. San Antonio, TX: The Psychological Corporation, 1997.

Cole K, Dale P, Thal D (Eds): Communication and Language Intervention Series, Vol. 6: Assessment of Communication and Language. Baltimore, MD: Paul H. Brookes Publishing, 1996.

Conners CK: Conners' Rating Scales –Revised Technical Manual. Toronto, ON: Multi-Health Systems, 1997.

Conners CK: Conners' Kiddie Continuous Performance Test. Toronto, ON: Multi-Health Systems, 2001.

Connolly A: Key Math Diagnostic Inventory of Essential Math-

ematics, Revised. Circle Pines, MN: American Guidance Service, 1988.

Coplan J: Early Language Milestone Scale, (2nd ed.). Austin, TX: Pro-Ed, 1993.

Delis DC, Kramer JH, Kaplan E, Ober BA: California Verbal Learning Test, Children's Version. San Antonio, TX: The Psychological Corporation, 1994.

Diamond A, Doar B: The performance of human infants on a measure of frontal cortex function: the delayed response task. Developmental Psychobiology: 22; 271–94, 1989.

Diamond A, Goldman-Rakic PS: Comparative development in human infants and infant rhesus monkeys of cognitive functions that depend on frontal cortex. Society for Neuroscience Abstracts: 12; 742, 1986.

Diamond A, Goldman-Rakic PS: Comparison of human infants and infant rhesus monkeys on Piaget's AB task: Evidence for dependence on dorsolateral prefrontal cortex. Experimental Brain Research: 74; 24–40, 1989.

Dunn LM, Dunn LM: Peabody Picture Vocabulary Test (3rd ed.). Circle Pines, MN: American Guidance Service, 1997.

Dunn W: Assessment of sensorimotor and perceptual development. In Nuttall EV, Romero I, Kalesnik J (Eds), Assessing and Screening Preschoolers: Psychological and Educational Dimensions (2nd ed.). Boston, MA: Allyn and Bacon, pp. 240–261, 1999.

Edwards CP: Development in the preschool years: The typical path. In Nuttall EV, Romero I, Kalesnik J (Eds), Assessing and Screening Preschoolers: Psychological and Educational Dimensions (2nd ed.). Boston, MA: Allyn and Bacon, pp. 9–24, 1999.

Ehlers S, Gillberg C: The epidemiology of Asperger syndrome: A total population study. Journal of Child Psychology and Psychiatry and Allied Disciplines: 34; 1327–1350, 1993.

Elliott CD: Differential Ability Scales. San Antonio, TX: The Psychological Corporation, 1990.

Ewing-Cobbs L, Fletcher JM, Levin HS: Neurobehavioral sequelae following head injury in children: Educational implications. Journal of Head Trauma Rehabilitation: 1; 57–65. 1986.

Ewing-Cobbs L, Fletcher JM, Levin HS, Francis DJ, Davidson K, Miner E: Longitudinal neuropsychological outcome in infants and preschoolers with traumatic brain injury. Journal of the International Neuropsychological Society: 3; 581–591, 1997.

Fein D, Dunn M, Allen DA, Aram DM, Hall N, Morris R, Wilson BC: Neuropsychological and language data. In Rapin I (Ed), Clinics in Developmental Medicine, No. 139: Preschool Children with Inadequate Communication: Developmental Language Disorder, Autism, Low IQ. London: Mac Keith Press, pp. 123–154, 1996.

Fein D, Stevens M, Dunn M, Waterhouse L, Allen D, Rapin I, Feinstein C: Subtypes of pervasive developmental disorder: Clinical characteristics. Child Neuropsychology: 5; 1–23, 1999.

Firestone P, Musten L, Pisterman S, Mercer J, Bennett S: Short-term side effects of stimulant medication are increased in preschool children with attention-deficit/hyperactivity disorder: A double-blind placebo-controlled study. Journal of Child and Adolescent Psychopharmacology: 8; 13–25, 1998.

Flanagan DP, Alfonso VC: A critical review of the technical characteristics of new and recently revised intelligence tests for preschool children. Journal of Psychoeducational Assessment: 13; 66–90, 1995.

Fletcher JM, Levin HS, Landry HS: Behavioral consequences of cerebral insult in infancy. In Almli CR and Finger S (Eds), Early Brain Damage, Vol. 1: Research Orientations and Clinical Observations. Orlando, FL: Academic Press, pp. 189–213, 1984.

Fletcher JM, Taylor HG: Neuropsychological approaches to children: Towards a developmental neuropsychology. Journal of Clinical Neuropsychology: 6; 39–56, 1984.

Folio MR, Fewell RR: Peabody Developmental Motor Scales. Allen, TX: DLM Teaching Resources, 1983.

Gardner MF: Receptive One-Word Picture Vocabulary Test. Novato, CA: Academic Therapy Publications, 1985.

Gardner MF: Expressive One-Word Picture Vocabulary Test–Revised. Novato, CA: Academic Therapy Publications, 1990.

Gardner MF: Test of Visual–Motor Skills, Revised. Burlingame, CA: Psychological and Educational Publications, 1995.

Gardner MF: Test of Visual Perceptual Skills (non-motor), Revised. Burlingame, CA: Psychological and Educational Publications, 1996.

Garretson HB, Fein D, Waterhouse L: Sustained attention in children with autism. Journal of Autism and Developmental Disorders: 20; 101–114, 1990.

Gillam RB: Treatment for temporal processing deficits: Computer-assisted language intervention using FastForWord®: Theoretical and empirical considerations for clinical decision making. Language, Speech, and Hearing Services in Schools: 30; 363–370, 1999.

Gillberg IC, Gillberg C: Asperger syndrome: Some epidemiological considerations: A research note. Journal of Child Psychology and Psychiatry and Allied Disciplines: 30; 631–638, 1989.

Gioia GA, Isquith PK, Guy SC, Kenworthy L: Behavior Rating Inventory of Executive Function: Professional Manual. Odessa, FL: Psychological Assessment Resources, 2000.

Gopaul-McNicol S, Thomas-Presswood T: Working with Linguistically and Culturally Different Children: Innovative Clinical and Educational Approaches. Boston, MA: Allyn and Bacon, 1998.

Gordon M: Gordon Diagnostic System. DeWitt, NY: Gordon Systems, 1996.

Green G: Early behavioral intervention for autism: What does research tell us? In Maurice C, Green G, Luce SC (Eds), Behavioral Intervention for Young Children with Autism: A Manual for Parents and Professionals. Austin, TX: Pro-Ed, pp. 29–44, 1996.

Greenberg LM, Corman CL, Kindschi CL: Test of Variables of Attention. Los Alamitos, CA: Universal Attentions Disorders, 1996.

Gresham FM, Elliott SN: Social Skills Rating System Manual. Circle Pines, MN: American Guidance Service, 1990.

Hammill DD, Pearson NA, Voress JK: Developmental Test of Visual Perception (2nd ed.). Austin, TX: Pro-Ed, 1993.

Hebb DO: Organization of Behavior. New York, NY: Wiley, 1949.

Hedrick D, Prather E, Tobin A: The Sequenced Inventory of Communication Development, Revised Edition. Los Angeles, CA: Western Psychological Services, 1984.

Holmes-Bernstein J, Waber DP: Developmental neuropsychological assessment: The systemic approach. In Boulton AA, Baker GB, Hiscock M (Eds), Neuromethods, Vol. 17: Neuropsychology. Clifton, NJ: Humana Press, pp. 311–371, 1990.

Hresko WP, Herron SR, Peak PR: Test of Early Written Language (2nd ed.). Austin, TX: Pro-Ed, 1996.

Hresko WP, Reid DK, Hammill DD: Test of Early Language Development (2nd ed.). Austin, TX: Pro-Ed, 1991.

Huang AM, Hunter LR, Reinert HR, Wishon PM: Assessment of children with mental retardation and other handicapping conditions. In Nuttall EV, Romero I, Kalesnik J (Eds), Assessing and Screening Preschoolers: Psychological and Educational Dimensions. Boston, MA: Allyn and Bacon, pp. 311–326, 1992.

Johnson MH: Developmental Cognitive Neuroscience: An Introduction. Malden, MA: Blackwell, 1997.

Kalesnik J: Developmental history. In Nuttall EV, Romero I, Kalesnik J (Eds), Assessing and Screening Preschoolers: Psychological and Educational Dimensions. Boston, MA: Allyn and Bacon, pp. 94–111, 1999.

Kaplan E: A process approach to neuropsychological assessment. In Boll T, Bryant BK (Eds), The Master Lecture Series, Vol. 7: Clinical Neuropsychology and Brain Function: Research, Measurement, and Practice. Washington, DC: American Psychological Association, pp. 127–167, 1988.

Kaplan E, Fein D, Kramer JH, Delis DC, Morris R: WISC-III as a Process Instrument. San Antonio, TX: The Psychological Corporation, 1999.

Kaplan E, Fein D, Morris R, Delis DC: WAIS-R as a Neuropsychological Instrument. San Antonio, TX: The Psychological Corporation, 1991.

Kaufman AS, Kaufman NL: Kaufman Assessment Battery for Children (K-ABC). Circle Pines, MN: American Guidance Service, 1983.

Kennard MA, McCulloch WS: Functional organization of frontal pole in monkey and chimpanzee. Journal of Neurophysiology: 7; 37–40, 1944.

Kolb B, Fantie B: Development of the child's brain and behavior. In Reynolds CR, Fletcher-Janzen E (Eds), Handbook of Clinical Child Neuropsychology. New York, NY: Plenum Press, pp. 17–39, 1989.

Kolb B, Gibb R, Gorny G: Cortical plasticity and the development of behavior after early frontal cortical injury. Developmental Neuropsychology: 18; 423–444, 2001.

Kolb B, Whishaw IQ: Fundamentals of Human Neuropsychology (3rd ed.). San Francisco, CA: WH Freeman, 1990.

Kolk A, Talvik T: Cognitive outcome of children with early-onset hemiparesis. Journal of Child Neurology: 15; 581–587, 2000.

Korkman M, Kirk U, Kemp S: NEPSY: A developmental neuropsychological assessment. San Antonio, TX: The Psychological Corporation, 1997.

Kraus JF: Epidemiological features of brain injury in children: Occurrence, children at risk, causes and manner of injury, severity, and outcomes. In Broman SH, Michel ME (Eds), Traumatic Head Injury in Children. New York, NY: Oxford University Press, pp. 22–39, 1995.

Laroche M, Kruger LJ: Implementing the results of preschool assessments: Transforming data and recommendations into action. In Nuttall EV, Romero I, Kalesnik J (Eds), Assessing and Screening Preschoolers: Psychological and Educational Dimensions (2nd ed.). Boston, MA: Allyn and Bacon, pp. 407–420, 1999.

Li C, Walton JR, Nuttall EV: Preschool evaluation of culturally and linguistically diverse children. In Nuttall EV, Romero I, Kalesnik J (Eds), Assessing and Screening Preschoolers: Psychological and Educational Dimensions (2nd ed.). Boston, MA: Allyn and Bacon, pp. 296–317, 1999.

Lifter K: Descriptions of preschool children with disabilities or at-risk for developmental delay: How should a child be called? In Nuttall EV, Romero I, Kalesnik J (Eds), Assessing and Screening Preschoolers: Psychological and Educational Dimensions (2nd ed.). Boston, MA: Allyn and Bacon, pp. 25–49, 1999.

Lowe M, Costello AJ: The Symbolic Play Test (2nd ed.). Windsor: NFER-Nelson Publishing Company, 1988.

Lyon GR, Moats L, Flynn JM: From assessment to treatment: Linkage to interventions with children. In Tramontana MG, Hooper SR (Eds), Assessment Issues in Child Neuropsychology. New York, NY: Plenum Press, pp. 113–142, 1988.

Mariani MA, Barkley RA: Neuropsychological and academic functioning in preschool boys with attention deficit hyperactivity disorder. Developmental Neuropsychology: 13; 111–129, 1997.

Mayberry RI: Cognitive development in deaf children: the interface of language and perception in neuropsychology. In Segalowitz SJ, Rapin I (Eds), Child Neuropsychology, Handbook of Neuropsychology, 2nd Edition, vol. 8, part II. Amsterdam: Elsevier, chapter 20, 2003.

McCarney SB: Preschool Evaluation Scale. Columbia, MO: Hawthorne Educational Services, 1992.

McCarney SB: Early Childhood Attention Deficit Disorders Evaluation Scale. Columbia, MO: Hawthorne Educational Services, 1995.

McCarthy D: McCarthy Scales of Children's Abilities. San Antonio, TX: The Psychological Corporation, 1972.

Merrell KW: Preschool and Kindergarten Behavior Scales. Austin, TX: Pro-Ed, 1994.

Miller LJ: Miller Assessment for Preschoolers. San Antonio, TX: The Psychological Corporation, 1988.

Minshew NJ, Dunn M: Autism specturm disorders. In Segalowitz SJ, Rapin I (Eds), Child Neuropsychology, Handbook of Neuropsychology, 2nd Edition, vol. 8, part II. Amsterdam: Elsevier, chapter 33, 2003.

Mirsky AF, Anthony BJ, Duncan CC, Ahearn MB, Kellam SG: Analysis of the elements of attention: A neuropsychological approach. Neuropsychology Review: 2; 109–145, 1991.

Moore MC: Assessing the preschool child with visual impairment. In Nutall EV, Romero I, Kalesnik J (Eds), Assessing and Screening Preschoolers: Psychological and Educational Dimensions (2nd ed.). Boston, MA: Allyn and Bacon, pp. 360–380, 1999.

Mullen EM: Mullen Scales of Early Learning. Circle Pines, MN: American Guidance Service, 1995.

Mullen Y: Assessment of the preschool child with a hearing loss. In Nutall EV, Romero I, Kalesnik J (Eds), Assessing and Screening Preschoolers: Psychological and Educational Dimensions (2nd ed.). Boston, MA: Allyn and Bacon, pp. 340–359, 1999.

Mundy P, Crowson M: Joint attention and early social communication: Implications for research on intervention with autism. Journal of Autism and Developmental Disorders: 27; 653–676, 1997.

Musten L: Efficacy of stimulant medication treatment of attention deficit hyperactivity disorder in preschool-aged children. Dissertation Abstracts International: 59; 1374, 1998.

Neisworth JT, Bagnato SJ: The case against intelligence testing in early intervention. Topics in Early Childhood Special Education: 12; 1–20, 1992.

Newcomer PL, Hammill DD: Test of Language Development–Primary (3rd ed.). Austin, TX: Pro-Ed, 1997.

Nurss J, McGauvran M: Metropolitan Readiness Assessment Program. San Antonio, TX: The Psychological Corporation, 1986.

Nuttall EV, Nuttall-Vasquez K, Hampel A: Introduction. In Nutall EV, Romero I, Kalesnik J (Eds.), Assessing and Screening Preschoolers: Psychological and Educational Dimensions (2nd ed.). Boston, MA: Allyn and Bacon, pp. 1–8, 1999.

Rapin I: Practitioner review: Developmental language disorders: A clinical update. Journal of Child Psychology and Psychiatry and Allied Disciplines: 37; 643–655. 1996.

Rapin I, Dunn M, Allen DA: Developmental language disorders. In Segalowitz SJ, Rapin I (Eds), Child Neuropsychology, Handbook of Neuropsychology, 2nd Edition, vol. 8, part II. Amsterdam: Elsevier, chapter 22, 2003.

Reid DK, Hresko WP, Hammill DD: Test of Early Reading Ability (2nd ed.). Austin, TX: Pro-Ed, 1989.

Rey-Casserly C: Neuropsychological assessment of preschool children. In Nuttall EV, Romero I, Kalesnik J (Eds), Assessing and Screening Preschoolers: Psychological and Educational Dimensions (2nd ed.). Boston, MA: Allyn and Bacon, pp. 281–295, 1999.

Reynolds CR, Kamphaus RW: Behavior Assessment System for Children, Revised. Circle Pines, MN: American Guidance Service, 1998.

Rhodes RL, Kayser H, Hess RS: Neuropsychological differential diagnosis of Spanish-speaking preschool children. In Fletcher-Janzen E, Strickland TL, Reynolds CR (Eds), Handbook of Cross-Cultural Neuropsychology: Critical Issues in Neuropsychology. New York, NY: Kluwer Academic/Plenum Publishers, pp. 317–333, 2000.

Risser AH, Edgell D: Neuropsychology of the developing brain: Implications for neuropsychological assessment. In Tramontana MG, Hooper SR (Eds), Assessment Issues in Child Neuropsychology. New York, NY: Plenum Press, pp. 41–65, 1988.

Roid G, Miller L: Leiter International Performance Scale–Revised. Wood Dale, IL: Stoelting Company, 1997.

Romero I: Individual assessment procedures with preschool children. In Nuttall EV, Romero I, Kalesnik J (Eds), Assessing and Screening Preschoolers: Psychological and Educational Dimensions. Boston, MA: Allyn and Bacon, pp. 59–71, 1999.

Rourke BP, Del Dotto JE: Learning disabilities: A neuropsychological perspective. In Walker CE, Roberts MC (Eds), Handbook of Clinical Child Psychology (2nd ed.). Oxford: Wiley, pp. 511–536, 1992.

Rourke BP, Fisk JL, Strang JD: Neuropsychological Assessment of Children: A Treatment-Oriented Approach. New York, NY: The Guilford Press, 1986.

Rubin KH: Play Observation Scale. Waterloo, ON: University of Waterloo, 1989.

Santosh P, Taylor E: Stimulant drugs. European Child and Adolescent Psychiatry: 9(Suppl. 1); I27–43, 2000.

Sattler J: Assessment of children: Cognitive applications (4th ed.). La Mesa, CA: Jerome M. Sattler, 2001.

Satz P, Fletcher J, Clark W, Morris R: Lag, deficit, rate, and delay constructs in specific learning disabilities: A re-examination. In Ansara A, Geschwind N, Galaburda A, Albert M, Gatrell N (Eds), Sex Differences in Dyslexia. Towson, MD: The Orton Dyslexia Society, pp. 129–150, 1981.

Schnell RR, Workman-Daniels K: Intellectual assessment of preschoolers. In Nuttall EV, Romero I, Kalesnik J (Eds), Assessing and Screening Preschoolers: Psychological and Educational Dimensions. Boston, MA: Allyn and Bacon, pp. 145–192, 1992.

Scientific Learning Corporation: FastForWord® Language. Oakland, CA: Author, 1997.

Siegel DJ: Evaluation of high-functioning autism. In Goldstein G, Nussbaum PD, Beers SR (Eds), Neuropsychology. Human Brain Function: Assessment and Rehabilitation. New York, NY: Plenum Press, pp. 109–134, 1998.

Sigafoos J, Roberts-Pennell D, Graves D: Longitudinal assessment of play and adaptive behavior in young children with developmental disabilities. Research in Developmental Disabilities: 20; 147–161, 1999.

Slomka G: Attention deficit hyperactivity disorder. In Snyder PJ, Nussbaum PD (Eds), Clinical Neuropsychology: A Pocket Handbook for Assessment. Washington, DC: American Psychological Association, pp. 124–140, 1998.

Smith RJ, Barth JT, Diamond R, Giuliano AJ: Evaluation of head trauma. In Goldstein G, Nussbaum PD, Beers SR (Eds), Neuropsychology. Human Brain Function: Assessment and Rehabilitation. New York, NY: Plenum Press, pp. 135–170, 1998.

Sparrow SS, Balla DA, Cicchetti D: Vineland Adaptive Behavior Scales. Circle Pines, MN: American Guidance Service, 1984.

Sparrow SS, Balla DA, Cicchetti DV: Vineland Social–Emotional Early Childhood Scales. Circle Pines, MN: American Guidance Service, 1998.

Sparrow SS, Carter AS: Mental retardation: Current issues related to assessment. In Rapin I, Segalowitz SJ (Eds), Hand-

book of Neuropsychology, Vol. 6: Child Neuropsychology. New York, NY: Elsevier, pp. 439–452, 1992.

Stevens MC, Fein DA, Dunn M, Allen D, Waterhouse LH, Feinstein C, Rapin I: Subgroups of children with autism by cluster analysis: A longitudinal examination. Journal of the American Academy of Child and Adolescent Psychiatry: 39; 346–352, 2000.

Stuss DT, Buckle L: Traumatic brain injury: Neuropsychological deficits and evaluation at different stages of recovery and in different pathologic subtypes. Journal of Head Trauma Rehabilitation: 7; 40–49, 1992.

Suzuki LA, Ponterotto JG, Meller PJ (Eds): Handbook of Multicultural Assessment: Clinical, Psychological, and Educational Applications (2nd ed.). San Francisco, CA: Jossey-Bass, 2001.

Tallal P, Miller S, Fitch RH: Neurobiological basis of speech: A case for the preeminence of temporal processing. In Tallal P, Galaburda AM, Llinas RR, von Euler C (Eds), Annals of the New York Academy of Sciences, Vol. 682: Temporal Information Processing in the Nervous System: Special Reference to Dyslexia and Dysphasia. New York, NY: New York Academy of Sciences, pp. 27–47, 1993.

Tallal P, Stark RE, Mellits ED: Identification of language-impaired children on the basis of rapid perception and production skills. Brain and Language: 25; 314–322, 1985.

Tannock, R: Neuropsychology of attention disorders. In Segalowitz SJ, Rapin I (Eds), Child Neuropsychology, Handbook of Neuropsychology, 2nd Edition, vol. 8, part II. Amsterdam: Elsevier, chapter 28, 2003.

Teeter PA: Neurocognitive interventions for childhood and adolescent disorders. In Reynolds CR, Fletcher-Janzen E (Eds), Handbook of Clinical Child Neuropsychology (2nd ed.). New York, NY: Plenum Press, pp. 387–417, 1997.

Teeter PA, Semrud-Clikeman M: Child Neuropsychology: Assessment and Interventions for Neurodevelopmental Disorders. Boston, MA: Allyn and Bacon, 1997.

Thorndike RL, Hagen EP, Sattler JM: The Stanford–Binet Intelligence Scale: Fourth Edition. Chicago, IL: The Riverside Publishing Company, 1986.

Tiffin J: Manual for the Purdue Pegboard. Chicago, IL: Science Research Associates, 1948.

Tramontana MG, Hooper SR: Child neuropsychological assessment: Overview of current status. In Tramontana MG, Hooper SR (Eds), Assessment Issues in Child Neuropsychology. New York, NY: Plenum Press, pp. 3–38, 1988.

Trawick-Smith J: Interactions in the Classroom: Facilitating Play in the Early Years. New York, NY: Merrill, 1994.

VanMeter L, Fein D, Morris R, Waterhouse L, Allen D: Delay versus deviance in autistic social behavior. Journal of Autism and Developmental Disorders: 27; 557–569, 1997.

Veale T: Targeting temporal processing deficits through FastForWord®: Language therapy with a new twist. Language, Speech, and Hearing Services in Schools: 30; 353–362, 1999.

Wainwright L, Fein D, Waterhouse L: Neuropsychological assessment of children with developmental disabilities. In Amir N, Rapin I, Branski D (Eds), Pediatric and Adolescent Medicine, Vol. 1: Pediatric Neurology: Behavior and Cognition of the Child with Brain Dysfunction. New York, NY: Karger, pp. 146–163, 1991.

Warren DH, Hatton DD: Cognitive development in children with visual impairments. In Segalowitz SJ, Rapin I (Eds), Child Neuropsychology, Handbook of Neuropsychology, 2nd Edition, vol. 8, part II. Amsterdam: Elsevier, chapter 18, 2003.

Wechsler D: Wechsler Preschool and Primary Scale of Intelligence–Revised. San Antonio, TX: The Psychological Corporation, 1989.

Westby CE: Symbolic Play Checklist: Assessment of cognitive and language abilities through play. Language, Speech, and Hearing Services in the Schools: 11; 154–168, 1980.

Westby CE: A scale for assessing children's play. In Gitlin-Weiner K, Sandgrund A, Schaefer C (Eds), Play Diagnosis and Assessment (2nd ed.). New York, NY: Wiley, pp. 15–57, 2000.

White RF, Rose FE: The Boston process approach: A brief history and current practice. In Goldstein G, Incagnoli TM (Eds), Contemporary Approaches to Neuropsychological Assessment: Critical Issues in Neuropsychology. New York, NY: Plenum Press, pp. 171–211, 1997.

Wiig EH, Secord W, Semel E: Clinical Evaluation of Language Fundamentals–Preschool. San Antonio, TX: The Psychological Corporation, 1992.

Williams JM: Neuropsychological assessment of traumatic brain injury in the intensive care and acute care environment. In Long CJ, Ross LK (Eds), Handbook of Head Trauma: Acute Care to Recovery. New York, NY: Plenum Press, pp. 271–292, 1992.

Williams JM, Voelker S, Ricciardi PW: Predictive validity of the K-ABC for exceptional preschoolers. Psychology in the Schools: 32; 178–185, 1995.

Williams K: Expressive Vocabulary Test. Circle Pines, MN: American Guidance Service, 1997.

Willmott C, Anderson V, Anderson P: Attention following pediatric head injury: A developmental perspective. Developmental Neuropsychology: 17; 361–379, 2000.

Wilson BC: The neuropsychological assessment of the preschool child: A branching model. In Rapin I, Segalowitz SJ (Eds), Handbook of Neuropsychology, Vol. 6: Child Neuropsychology. New York, NY: Elsevier, pp. 377–394, 1992.

Wilson BC, Iacoviello JM, Wilson JJ, Risucci D: Purdue Pegboard performance in normal preschool children. Journal of Clinical Neuropsychology: 4; 19–26, 1982.

Woodcock RW, McGrew KS, Mather N: Woodcock-Johnson III Tests of Achievement. Itasca, IL: Riverside Publishing, 2001a.

Woodcock RW, McGrew KS, Mather N: Woodcock-Johnson III Tests of Cognitive Abilities. Itasca, IL: Riverside Publishing, 2001b.

Wyatt TA, Seymour HN: Assessing the speech and language skills of preschool children. In Nutall EV, Romero I, Kalesnik J (Eds), Assessing and Screening Preschoolers: Psychological and Educational Dimensions (2nd ed.). Boston, MA: Allyn and Bacon, pp. 218–239, 1999.

Yeates KO, Ris MD, Taylor HG (Eds): Pediatric Neuropsychology: Research, Theory, and Practice. New York, NY: The Guilford Press, 2000.

Ylvisaker M, Hartwick P, Stevens M: School reentry following head injury: Managing the transition from hospital to school. Journal of Head Trauma Rehabilitation: 6; 10–22, 1991.

Zimmerman IL, Steiner VG, Pond RE: Preschool Language Scale-3. San Antonio, TX: The Psychological Corporation, 1992.

CHAPTER 12

# Neuropsychological assessment of school-aged children

Steven Mattis * and Dana Zaret Luck

*Mattis and Luck Center for Neuropsychological Services, LLP, 34 South Broadway, Suite 100, White Plains, New York, 10601, USA*

## Chapter overview

In the past decade, the neuropsychological assessment of school-aged children has become a growth industry. Technological advances have enabled neuroscientists to untangle many complexities concerning brain–behavior relationships. There have been significant breakthroughs in the understanding of cognitive development in children. A broader application of the biopsychosocial model in psychiatry has blurred the traditional boundary between normal and abnormal behavior in childhood, requiring clinicians to assess each child's development across multidimensional systems incorporating biological, psychological, and social aspects of functioning. Psychopharmacological developments have enabled physicians to fine-tune individualized treatment regimens for children, often involving the administration of multiple psychotropic medications that require careful monitoring. A multitude of new syndromes and disorders in children have been identified, defined, and treated. The need for greater accuracy in performing a differential diagnosis, monitoring responses to medication, and helping to develop multidisciplinary treatment plans has become paramount. The neuropsychologist has become a critical partner to the neurologist and psychiatrist in identifying and treating neuropsychiatric disorders in children.

_____

* Corresponding author. E-mail: mattiss@aol.com

## Reasons for referral

A neuropsychological evaluation helps to determine the presence, nature, and severity of central nervous system impairment, to delineate the nature of the aberrant cognition and behavior attributable to this impairment, and to develop strategies for intervention, remediation, and management. The neuropsychological data provide critical quantitative and qualitative information about a child's level of cognitive, behavioral, and social–emotional functioning. Follow-up evaluations can measure the child's response to medication and intervention, as well as determining the degree of illness progression.

## Referral questions

There have been significant changes in the referral questions that bring a school-age child to neuropsychological attention in recent years. There has been an increase in referrals of children with behavioral and psychiatric problems known or highly suspected to be secondary to central nervous system dysfunction. Thus, children with attention-deficit/hyperactivity disorder (ADHD), oppositional defiant disorder (ODD), mood disorders, obsessive–compulsive disorder (OCD), Tourette Syndrome, and pervasive developmental disorder (PDD) comprise an increasing proportion of children referred for neuropsychological evaluation. This population presents difficult differential diagnostic dilemmas requiring inclusion of a careful developmental, social, and behavioral history, adaptive scales and structured interviews, and scales of emotional and personality development. The referrals can best be categorized according to the following four groups.

## Group I: children with specific learning disabilities

Ten years ago, the most common referral for a neuropsychological evaluation involved children presenting with learning and behavior difficulties in school. The diagnosis of a specific learning disorder independent of mood or attentional difficulty relies heavily on several factors: (1) the presence of a problem in academic achievement (i.e. academic achievement discrepant from that expected on the basis of IQ); (2) deficits in specific cognitive processes necessary for the acquisition or execution of the academic skill; and (3) a history indicating that the primary cognitive deficit was present in the preschool or early school grades. For example, in the case of a suspected reading disability, the history usually includes developmental delays in language milestones and/or a history of early difficulty acquiring decoding skills. The child usually presents with a variant of an underlying language disorder with a phonic awareness deficit or, very rarely, a visual perceptual disorder that causes confusion in the discrimination of specific lower case letters. While signs of a fine motor dyscoordination problem may also be present, this is usually a non-contributing factor to the reading disability, although it is likely to contribute to spelling and writing difficulties because such dyscoordination makes graphic production effortful in its own right.

Over the years, the schools have developed better procedures for identifying children with specific learning disorders. The classification system has been refined, and children with special education needs are provided with detailed individualized educational programs. While the special education system has assisted in the neuropsychological assessment of specific learning disabilities in children, many cases are more complicated and require more specialized neuropsychological evaluation.

## Group II: children with complicated learning disorders

Currently, the most common reason for referral for a formal neuropsychological evaluation occurs when the child presents with a complicated learning disability, or when there is confusion or conflict among school personnel, parents, and outside professionals with respect to the appropriate classification and treatment plan. In these cases, the neuropsychologist serves as a consultant to review background records and existing test data, to perform a full or partial neuropsychological evaluation, and to help to develop an integrated remedial program that most likely includes both school-based and private interventions.

The major difficulty in the differential diagnosis of children with complicated learning disorders is the fact that there is often significant co-morbidity between learning disorders and other clinical entities such as attention-deficit/hyperactivity disorder (ADHD), executive function disorder, and/or anxiety and mood disorders. The problem is confounded by the observation that not only are neuropsychological deficits demonstrated by children with each of these clinical entities, but that there is some overlap in their patterns of neuropsychological deficits.

The presence of independent or confounding attentional difficulties with and without hyperactivity is the most common co-morbid clinical condition seen in children with complicated learning disorders. The diagnosis of ADHD relies heavily on school and parent observations of impulsive, overly active, and inattentive behavior combined with a history of such behavior beginning in the preschool years. The overactivity is of such severity and constancy as to interfere with the child's ability to sustain sedentary activity. The inability to sustain attention results in difficulty attending to details, following instructions, and organizing one's school work. The presence of impulsivity with or without a high level of motor activity can make it difficult for the child to withhold comments, to screen inappropriate verbal observations, to accompany his or her parents to the supermarket, or to attend a movie without incident. Apparently, playing computer or handheld action games does not present a problem, but engaging in role playing games does. There is a spectrum of such activity ranging from the fidgety child who remains in his/her seat in school, to the child who must wander up and down the aisles in the classroom, touching or talking to other children, and having significant difficulty remaining in the class.

There is some controversy concerning the diagnosis of ADHD within the psychiatric and neurological communities. Some neurologists are more likely to view the disorder within its historic neurologic framework as a Hyper-Kinetic Syndrome (HKS), viewing HKS as a motor-executive disinhibition syndrome in which the attentional component is conceptualized as a praxic disorder, i.e. a disorder of intention rather than attention (Denckla, 1996). The findings by Mostofsky, Reiss, Lockhart and Denckla (1998) that ADHD children demonstrate decreased volume of posterior vermis in the cerebellum, with particular involvement of the inferior posterior lobules VII–X, suggest that cerebellar-to-prefrontal systems may be implicated in ADHD rather than the frontal–striatal systems generally considered when discussing executive deficits. Berquin, Giedd, Jacobsen et al. (1998) corroborated the Mostofsky et al. findings and support the contention that a cerebello-thalamo-prefrontal circuit dysfunction underlies the motor dyscontrol, disinhibition, and executive deficits observed in ADHD with hyperactivity. Barkley (1997) similarly suggests that a model of prefrontal lobe executive dysfunction best explains the cognitive and behavioral deficits associated with ADHD.

This view of the children's disorder as a hyperkinetic syndrome with or without attentional disorder has a lot of merit. It focuses primarily on the presence or absence of executive function difficulties, and it allows one to consider a wider range of diagnostic options when encountering the child with attentional difficulty who does not exhibit signs of hyperactivity or impulsivity. Thus, one can view the reported inattention to detail, failure to complete assignments, and difficulty in organizing tasks as behavior secondary to obsessive personal preoccupations, and/or mood disorder, and/or an ideational perseverative disorder. There is sufficient evidence of differences in the distribution of neuropsychological strengths and deficits in children with ADHD with hyperkinetic behavior and those with inattention alone that it might be better to consider these two as separate disorders than to continue to insist on a single hypothetical cause for the attentional disorder for both groups (see Clarke, Barry, McCarthy and Selikowitz, 2001 and Lockwood, Marcotte and Stern, 2001; and, in adults, see Gansler, Fucetola, Krengel et al., 1998 and Hesslinger, Thiel, Tebartz van Elst et al., 2001).

## Group III: children with recently acquired neurological damage

The third most common referral for neuropsychological evaluation involves the child who has incurred a probable encephalopathic event with neuropsychological sequelae. The rate of referral for this type of assessment has not changed significantly over the past decade. Although the school-related difficulties of these children are initially still apt to be detected and assessed within the school system, a more detailed neuropsychological evaluation is essential in order to explain the intricacies of specific brain–behavior relationships and their impact on a child's functioning, both inside and outside the classroom. Moreover, with increasing numbers of neurologically impaired students entering mainstream classrooms through the process of inclusion, the neuropsychologist serves as an important resource for general classroom teachers and individual aides who work with these children.

The most common causes of recently acquired neurological impairment include head trauma, stroke, encephalitis, and other acute brain insults. Unlike adults, children with acquired focal brain lesions generally experience significant recovery of function and a positive outcome due to the neuroplasticity of adjacent and contralateral regions in the young brain (Aram and Ekelman, 1986; Hecaen, 1983; Taylor, 1987). In contrast, the effects of early childhood head trauma produce more diffuse and subcortical brain involvement, often resulting in more persistent decrements in general intelligence and executive functions (Fletcher, Miner and Ewing-Cobbs, 1987; Levin, Ewing-Cobbs and Eisenberg, 1995). It also seems that the effects of some encephalopathic events that occur in early childhood may not emerge until later stages of brain development, at which time underlying problems involving neuronal myelinization and dendritic arborization interfere with the acquisition of higher cortical functions. Such damage might not emerge on a neuropsychological evaluation for some time following the insult, and, depending on the area of brain involved, some cognitive deficits secondary to such early trauma might not emerge fully until adolescence. The natural process of cognitive development in children involves rapid development and integration of specific skills. Therefore the target behavior one is measuring is likely to change over time as the brain matures. Finally, environmental factors play a significant role in facilitating cognitive development and in fostering recovery or rehabilitation. Thus, the basic principles concerning the effects of early brain damage in childhood on neuropsychological test performance still reflect (1) the locus and extent of brain tissue damage at the time of the encephalopathic event, (2) the extent to which uncommitted tissue remains available and accessible, (3) the nature of experienced environmental events fostering the development of specific cognitive–motor processes, and (4) the amount of time elapsed between insult and evaluation during which plasticity of function could develop. For children with recently acquired neurological damage, it is especially important to obtain a detailed developmental history across discrete cognitive domains prior to undertaking a neuropsychological evaluation. Moreover, serial neuropsychological evaluations of these children are generally undertaken at various time intervals, so that the results of an initial baseline neuropsychological assessment can be compared to the results of serial follow-up evaluations.

## Group IV: children with mood and/or social–emotional difficulties

The fourth group of children who are currently referred for neuropsychological evaluation includes those who present with significant behavioral, mood, and/or social–emotional difficulties that interfere with their functioning at home and at school. Referrals of this type have increased in recent years, primarily due to the tremendous growth in knowledge concerning the biochemical basis and the accompanying cognitive and affective sequelae of psychiatric disorders occurring in childhood. It is becoming increasingly clear, as research in the neuropsychological profile of psychiatric disorders of childhood is rigorously pursued, that many of the 'psychiatric disorders' have a wide range of associated cognitive and behavioral deficits. These children may exhibit prominent signs of attentional difficulties and executive function disorders that interfere with organizational skills, self-monitoring, regulation of mood and behavior, and interpersonal relationships.

The neuropsychological evaluation provides critical information concerning the differential diagnosis of psychiatric disorders in children, their major clinical repercussions, and the efficacy of treatment approaches. Thus, for example, the child who presents with a major depression is likely to exhibit disorders in the acquisition of academic skills that are not necessarily attributable to a constriction of motivation. Rourke (1988, 1989) has described a nonverbal learning disability in children for whom social ineptitude is a cardinal feature. A child with a nonverbal learning disability or Asperger's syndrome may present with social adjustment difficulties that mimic a depressive reaction. Current research and clinical data suggest that there will soon be a developmental neuropsychology model of affective and social skills deficits in children, although we presently possess very few instruments of neuropsychological significance to assess such processes.

## The nature of the neuropsychological evaluation

Despite the changes in the reasons for referral for neuropsychological evaluation, the basic nature of the neuropsychological evaluation has remained fairly consistent over the past ten years. It continues to be a labor-intensive practice that must be undertaken by, or under the close supervision of, a highly skilled clinical neuropsychologist who has a comprehensive understanding of both CNS development and damage. It requires extensive knowledge concerning (1) the normal ontogeny of the central nervous system, cognition, and affect, (2) the effects and functional recovery of damage to the CNS and distortions in the development of cognition and affect, (3) the nature of tests and instruments of clinical appraisal of all these processes, (4) the differential diagnosis of specific neurological and psychiatric disorders, and (5) methods of cognitive remediation and other treatment interventions.

In recent years, there has been a significant increase in the development, promotion, and use of standardized tests and rating scales to assess specific aspects of cognitive and behavioral functioning. This single chapter is not designed to acquaint the reader with a comprehensive listing of diagnostic neuropsychological tests, and the reader is referred to several excellent references that provide compendiums of these measures and their applications to clinical neuropsychology (Lezak, 1995; Spreen and Strauss, 1998). Many psychologists, educational specialists, and other professionals may be qualified to administer and summarize the findings of particular tests and measures. However, in order to be of value as an instrument of differential diagnosis, a battery of neuropsychological measures must be designed to test specific neuropsychological hypotheses, and the findings must be interpreted by a well-trained clinical neuropsychologist with knowledge of brain–behavior relationships and patterns of deficit associated with specific disease processes. The further differentiation of neuropsychological syndromes from behavioral syndromes and reactive emotional disorders requires additional training and experience in a clinical psychiatric or clinical psychological setting.

## Neuropsychological evaluation procedures

While the basic procedures employed to conduct a neuropsychological evaluation of the school-aged child have not changed significantly in the past ten years, it has become increasingly important to refine the specific referral question prior to undertaking the evaluation. Since more and more children are coming to clinical attention earlier, by the time they enter elementary school a number of children who come to neuropsychological attention have already undergone some form of prior evaluation by a developmental pediatrician, neurologist, speech and language therapist, occupational therapist, psychiatrist, school psychologist, and/or learning specialist. In the initial telephone contact with the parent, it is important to determine whether or not any previous evaluations have been undertaken, and, if so, it is important for the parent to have all formal records forwarded to the neuropsychologist. The evaluation begins with a clinical interview of the parents and child to determine the presenting problem. This is supplemented by a detailed interview concerning the child's developmental history, medical history, academic experience, family history, and social–emotional adjustment. Next comes an assessment period, during which the child undergoes a formal examination, which includes the administration of a battery of tests that is designed to address the particular referral question presented by that child. The

test data are then scored, analyzed and interpreted by the examiner. Feedback is provided to the parents during an informing interview, when specific recommendations for intervention are discussed. The findings are then shared with appropriate professionals through either a verbal or written report, which may be edited for specific academic or clinical purposes.

## Domains of assessment

A neuropsychological evaluation is designed to assess multiple domains of discrete cognitive abilities in order to discern discriminating patterns of performance that are associated with specific syndromes or disorders. Depending upon the referral question, the neuropsychological evaluation of children generally incorporates assessment of the following specific cognitive domains: attention, perception, memory and learning, language, conceptualization, spatial-construction skills, executive processes, motor skills, and social–emotional functioning. General domains of assessment include verbal and nonverbal intelligence and basic academic skills. Suggested tests and instruments designed to meet the diagnostic needs of each of the four referral groups will be provided later in the chapter, following a discussion of some general considerations regarding the nature of the clinician–child contract and presentation of the decision tree model of assessment.

## The nature of the clinician–child contract

While there is no morbidity or mortality rate associated with a neuropsychological evaluation, it necessitates the exploration of areas of deficit in children who are often quite sensitive and vulnerable to feelings of frustration and inadequacy. In order for the clinician to determine the precise nature and extent of CNS impairment exhibited by a child during a neuropsychological evaluation, the child must fail a specific task in a specific way that is pathognomonic of CNS impairment. To gain the child's cooperation, the clinician must establish a strong working relationship. From the outset, it is our practice to include the child in the process of discovery concerning his area(s) of difficulty. During the initial interview, the child is offered an opportunity to express his perspective on the presenting problem(s). Following a discussion of the presenting problem, a contract is established between the clinician and child in which the child agrees to persist at all tasks presented to him, and the clinician invites the child to serve as a co-investigator in teasing out the critical aspects of cognitive functioning that are underlying his difficulty. Rather than beginning the evaluation with relatively 'safe' tasks that circumvent the child's areas of deficit, we have found it most productive to 'zero-in' on suspected areas of weakness early on in the evaluation process, and to follow-up by mapping out areas of cognitive strength and weakness together with the child. Throughout the testing sessions, the child is invited to offer his perspective on the process. He is assured that the nature of his difficulties and suggestions for intervention will be provided to him at the conclusion of the evaluation.

## Strategies of assessment

For any given child, the reason for referral guides the examiner in developing an individualized battery of neuropsychological measures designed to assess both specific and general cognitive domains. This method is often referred to as a flexible battery approach, since it permits the examiner to select specific domains for evaluation, and to choose from an array of standardized measures and techniques to assess the child's performance in each domain. The flexible battery approach has largely replaced the fixed battery (such as that promoted by Reitan and Davison, 1974), in which every child is examined with the same fixed number of specific tasks that cover the most commonly evaluated cognitive domains. The flexible battery approach can be augmented by incorporating aspects of the process approach, which applies a more hypothetico-deductive model that encourages an in-depth assessment of specific problematic domains in order to gain a better quantitative and qualitative appreciation of the child's difficulties.

## The decision-tree approach

The model of evaluation most frequently utilized at our center continues to involve a 'decision-tree' approach (Fig. 1). In this model, the school-aged child undergoes a neuropsychological evaluation process that incorporates three phases. At the end of each stage, sufficient data are accumulated so that the examiner may decide (1) to stop accruing data because the initial referral questions have been answered, (2) to continue the assessment, or (3) to refer the child to another specialist who may be better able to answer the referring questions.

### Phase 1: the clinical interview and review of records

A careful review of background records and a clinical interview with the parents (and, in most cases, the child) precede any formal testing of the child. It is extremely helpful to the clinician if the parents have completed a structured questionnaire relating the nature of the chief complaint, gestational and delivery history, developmental milestones, family history as to learning and psychiatric disorders, and any medications the patient is taking. In the case of a chief complaint describing significant behavioral, social, and/or mood disorders, the interview can be quite lengthy. When the history suggests good social skills and relatedness and the complaint is limited to specific academic achievement difficulty, then the interview rarely takes more than a half hour. At the end of this interview, the clinician should have obtained (1) a good idea as to the nature and history of the chief complaint, (2) a developmental history, and (3) a brief review of prior testing (which often has already answered the referral question when re-interpreted within a neuropsychological framework). Sufficient data should be available to allow the clinician to make a reasonable decision as to whether or not neuropsychological testing is warranted. Most secondary or tertiary consultation work is conducted within this framework. Thus, in the case of the child who has undergone multiple prior evaluations — though somewhat flawed either in the analysis of data or the clarity of explication of findings — there might, nonetheless, be sufficient valid findings available to answer the referring questions without further testing. The clinical situation might be resolved with only a lengthy informing interview with the parents in which the results of the previous work-ups and their relationships to the child's behavior and the parental concerns are clarified in detail.

The Decision Tree

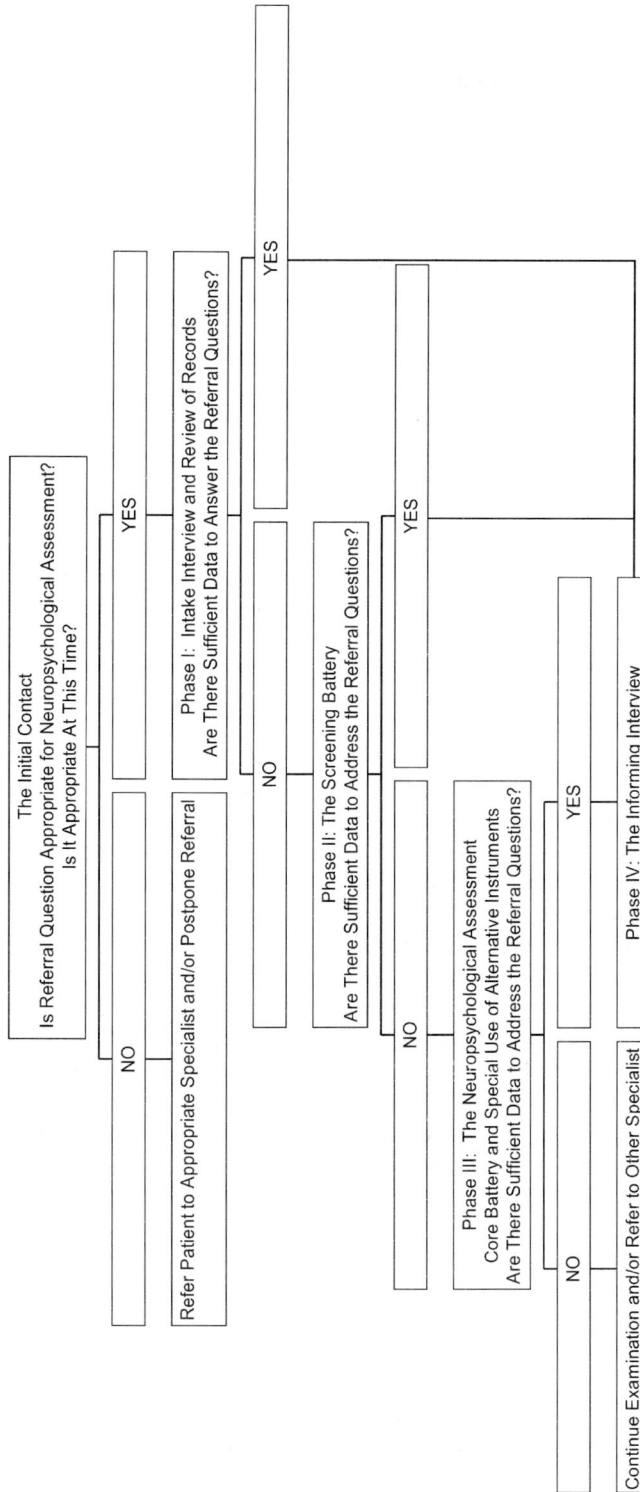

Fig. 1. The decision tree approach flow chart

*Phase 2: the screening battery*

If further testing is deemed necessary, the second stage is entered in which a screening battery is administered to the child, augmented by a critical test of the process implicated in the chief complaint (if this process is not specifically assessed by the screening battery). While the screening battery is similar to a 'core' battery in that it is given to every child as part of the neuropsychological evaluation, it does not necessarily serve the purpose of briefly assessing each of the specific cognitive abilities of general interest to most neuropsychologists. In general, the background data and prior evaluations usually contain enough elements to constitute a screening battery. In most cases, what is required is augmentation of the screening battery with more detailed exploration of the deficient neuropsychological processes and/or greater exploration of the social–emotional development factors reactive to or interacting with the existing deficits. The screening battery, as the name implies, should be composed of tasks which are sensitive to, and therefore screen for, the presence of cognitive dysfunction of the kind usually referable to CNS impairment. Screening tasks usually are contaminated by being relatively complex and requiring several neuropsychological processes for solution. The trick in developing such a screening battery is to reduce the frequency of false negatives without prohibitively increasing the rate of false positives. Once one has developed such a screening device based on the distribution of chief complaints and base-rate differential diagnoses in the population, then one should, on the basis of the findings of this examination, be able to make a decision as to whether or not to continue the neuropsychological evaluation, to shift to a more 'clinical' psychological strategy, or to refer the patient further to another specialty for further study.

*Phase 3: the neuropsychological assessment*

If one decides to continue the neuropsychological evaluation, then a brief core battery designed to augment the screening instrument is administered, and an extensive array of reasonably pure 'process-oriented' tasks is selected or developed and administered. The specific content of each of the three stages will vary as a function of the chief complaint and reason for referral. The application of the decision-tree approach to each of the four referral groups discussed above will be provided below.

## The neuropsychological assessment of the child with specific learning disabilities (Group I)

*Introduction*

If one has proceeded to this level of evaluation, it is often quite unclear as to whether one should pursue nature or nurture issues as the primary etiology of the child's disorder. Thus, the evaluation of behavior and learning difficulties for psychoeducational and psychological–psychiatric treatment entails the assessment of both neuropsychological and psycho-social parameters. The frequency with which both behavior and learning disturbances are the major chief complaints makes it incumbent upon the clinician to assess each factor for its specific and interactive contributions to the child's distress, and to generate specific recommendations for treatment or disposition on the basis of these contributions. Too often the clinician, after pursuing only one of these parameters, is willing to explain all of the chief complaints on the basis of the partial positive findings. Just as frequently, after pursuing one realm of parameters to a negative conclusion, the clinician is too willing to assume that the unexplored parameter is the primary contributing factor. It is really a rather weak argument to diagnose by exclusion. Thus, the school-aged child with school and social disturbances often presents the need for a very lengthy, seemingly exhaustive, evaluation. The child with a specific learning disability affecting school performance in the presence of at least average performance on measures of general intellectual abilities will present one of four syndromes, i.e. (1) a dyslexia with agraphia, (2) an agraphia with reading relatively intact, (3) a dyscalculia, often with an agraphia, and (4) a more diffuse language disorder manifesting as a dyslexia, dysgraphia, and dyscalculia.

*Phase 1: the clinical interview and review of records*

The initial contact is generally made over the phone, at which time the clinician might wish to obtain his first statement of the chief complaint and reason for referral, with special attention paid to the question of 'why at this time?' Most clinicians will establish the initial office visit with the parents sufficiently far in advance to allow the parents to fill out a questionnaire and/or forward school and prior evaluations. The purpose of this phase is to answer the question, 'Is it necessary for the child to undergo a (another) lengthy and costly neuropsychological evaluation?' On the basis of the nature of the chief complaints (as raised by the parents and often the school), the history of the complaints, the developmental and psychosocial history, school records, and any prior evaluations, it should be possible to answer the question of whether or not there is any substantial yield to be expected from a further evaluation. As school districts increasingly provide extensive psychoeducational diagnostic services, many clinicians find themselves in the position of providing a second opinion to the parents concerning their diagnoses and educational planning decisions. In a surprising number of cases, data equivalent to that obtained by the screening battery are readily available. If the clinician is in agreement with the prior conclusions or has minor revisions in diagnosis or treatment planning, then he/she serves best as an explicator of the prior assessments and an independent observer, in the future, of the efficacy of treatment.

## Phase 2: the screening battery

For the school-aged child with a possible specific learning disability, the neuropsychological screening battery should consist of an estimate of (1) general verbal and nonverbal intellectual abilities, (2) a test of naming, (3) motor coordination, and (4) academic achievement.

### WISC-III

In almost all cases, the WISC-III (Wechsler, 1991), if it has not been given in the last one or two years, is deemed the most widely used measure of verbal and nonverbal intellectual abilities. While all concede that the individual subtests, with rare exceptions, are multifactorial tasks and not specific to any given neuropsychological process, the WISC-III nonetheless serves as an excellent screening test of cognitive abilities, and inter-test and verbal–performance dis-

crepancies may raise concerns about the intactness of CNS functions.

### Naming

A naming test is included in the screening battery because of the prevalence of dysnomia in the learning disabled (LD) population. It has been estimated that, depending on the investigator and population studied, 50–90% of the LD population present some disorder in language development. A highly sensitive index of language disorder, which concurrently possesses a high degree of specificity, is a confrontation naming test. We continue to screen with the Mattis Naming Test, a 30-item naming test of objects, colors, and body parts (Mattis, French and Rapin, 1975) for which we have developed local norms. We also include the Boston Naming Test (Cohen, Town and Buff, 1988; Kaplan, Goodglass and Weintraub, 1978, 1983; Halperin, Healy, Zeitschick et al., 1989), even though it often produces false positives in children with lower I.Q. scores. As an alternative, we often use the Expressive One-Word Picture Vocabulary Test, 2000 (Brownell, 2000a; Gardner, 1981).

### Motor coordination

There are three classes of motor coordination that one might wish to examine, gross-, fine-, and graphomotor. The examination of gross motor coordination is difficult to learn only because of the large number of normally developing children of different ages one has had to observe to develop good internal norms for each age. Observation of rapid gait (undertaken normally, on toes, and on heels), tandem walking (undertaken as if walking on a straight line heel to toe), hopping in place on each foot, standing on each foot for longer than 5 seconds, and skipping is especially useful in determining the level of development of gross motor coordination and balance. Essentially one looks not only for the ability to perform these acts but also for extraneous movements and posturing of the arms and trunk.

Fine motor coordination is most frequently assessed by requiring the child to perform simple repetitive sequenced movements of the fingers, such as rapidly touching his index finger to his thumb and touching each of the fingers in turn to the thumb. One looks not only for the regularity, accuracy and fluency with which the task is performed but also for the presence of excessive extraneous and mirror movements on the non-performing hand. One might wish to review the PANESS (Physical and Neurological Examination for Soft Signs) which has norms for the timed performance of a number of fine and gross motor tasks (Denckla, 1973; Guy, 1976; Werry and Aman, 1976). Within the armamentarium of neuropsychological tests, the most commonly used fine motor tasks are the Grooved Pegboard (Klonoff and Low, 1974), Purdue Pegboard (Costa, Scarola and Rapin, 1964; Gardner and Broman, 1979), and finger tapping test (Klonoff and Low, 1974). As a screening task, in our setting, we have found the Purdue Pegboard (Purdue Research Foundation, 1948) to be most sensitive to the presence of neurologically significant fine motor dyscoordination, especially that administration requiring the pegs to be placed simultaneously with both hands.

Graphomotor coordination is a peculiar term and it is generally used only in those settings in which the child's difficulties frequently involve poor handwriting and/or spelling. One wishes to observe whether or not the child has adequate motor control of a pencil under circumstances requiring neither complex planning and construction skills nor language skills. We generally use a measure derived from the copying administration of the Benton Test of Visual Retention (Jantzen and Mattis, 1986; Mattis et al., 1975). In brief, the patient's reproduction of design cards III, V, VIII, and IX is scored for gaps or overshoots when two lines meet, the roundness of circles, and the presence of tremor. The sum of such line quality errors results in a graphomotor dyscoordination score. This score appears to be specific to motor deficiencies in that it correlates only in the low twenties with the Benton Copying correct and error scores, but discriminates children with high-risk birth histories and specific learning disabilities from those without such histories and diagnoses.

*Academic achievement*

There are a number of widely used tests of academic achievement which differ as to time of administration and the adequacy of the normative data. We continue to use the Wide Range Achievement Test, 3rd Edition (Wilkinson, 1993) as a screening measure. However, with rare exceptions — primarily the hyperlexic child — the WRAT-3 Reading standard

score tends not to overestimate decoding skill, the spelling score has always proven to be fairly accurate, and the paper and pencil arithmetic standard score has correlated well with national achievement tests of quantitative skills. If, by history, one suspects hyperlexia, then one might want to supplement the WRAT-3 Reading Test with the Gates–MacGinite Reading Comprehension Test (MacGinite, MacGinite, Maria and Dreyer, 2000) to get an accurate measure of silent reading comprehension in a multiple-choice format.

To reiterate, the screening battery for the school-aged child referred for assessment of learning and behavior disorders consists of the WISC-III, the Mattis or Boston Naming Test, the WRAT-3, and tests of gross-, fine-, and graphomotor skills.

*Criteria for further testing*

A good screening battery should highlight the fact that a problem requiring further evaluation exists and, to some degree, should direct your attention to the probable trouble areas. In the above battery, the following findings are definite indications that further neuropsychological evaluation is necessary: (1) if any subtest is performed at a level 2 or more standard deviations below the mean for age; or (2) if a discrepancy of greater than 2 standard deviations exists between obtained academic achievement and that expected by either Verbal or Performance IQ. Further evaluation, possibly neuropsychological, is indicated if the patient's behavior and/or affective expression during testing is bizarre for age and setting or stereotypical. The obligation for further evaluation is lessened by less definitive abnormal findings. For example, in the event that one or several subject scores are more than 1 standard deviation but less than 2 standard deviations from the mean for age, then the clinical significance of the pattern or profile in light of the child's test behavior, history and chief complaint should be evaluated before one arrives at a decision to continue the examination.

In our experience, it is rare for a school-aged child presenting with a possible learning disability to have negative findings on the above screening tests and then turn out to be a false negative on an extensive subsequent examination or at a later point in his/her academic progress. In general, a child in the third grade or above who does not already demonstrate a significant discrepancy between obtained and expected achievement scores will rarely be found to have a cluster of neuropsychological deficits likely to cause any clinically significant limitation of functions. This battery will result, however, in a number of false positives, but at an acceptable rate. For example, a child with a conduct disorder and school truancy will tend to have a significant discrepancy between obtained IQs and academic achievement that will require further evaluation. Generally, children with chronic psychiatric disorders present an achievement pattern in which reading levels are within normal limits, spelling scaled scores or percentiles are lower, and paper and pencil arithmetic achievement scores are even poorer (Greenblatt, Mattis and Trade, 1990). Nevertheless, their WISC-III Arithmetic subtest scaled score, while perhaps lower than Similarities, is most often well within normal limits.

There are a number of positive findings which, indeed, do indicate a deficiency in higher cortical functions but may not automatically obligate one to conduct an extensive examination because they do not necessarily limit the acquisition of academic skills. Among such common positive findings are (1) a constructional apraxia, which, no matter how severe, does not, by itself, limit achievement in any course except geometry, (2) an anomia, which, in the mild to moderate range and as an isolated deficit, will not be related to achievement discrepancies, and (3) an attention deficit–hyperactivity disorder, which will not necessarily be associated with achievement deficits. It should be noted, however, that the frequently observed concurrent motor dyscoordination and conduct disorders are associated with limitations in writing and arithmetic achievement. In some negative cases, one finds that the discrepancy between actual achievement and expectancy and/or the magnitude of an observed specific neuropsychological deficit is surprisingly mild given the nature of the chief complaint. Upon full examination, one often discovers that the child presents both a mild cognitive deficit (perhaps, by itself, unrelated to academic failure) and a mild psychogenic disorder, in conjunction with a clinically more significant interaction effect of both these components. For example, a child with mild graphomotor dyscoordination, who

unfortunately begins his/her academic career in a basal reader series that is heavily invested in writing letters before learning to otherwise use them, is likely to develop strong aversive reactions to the language arts portion of the school day. The extended battery should therefore always include a clinical interview and tests designed to elucidate the nature and significance of childhood anxieties and fears in addition to the usual cognitive tasks.

### Phase 3: the neuropsychological evaluation

At this point, one should have already assessed the reliability and validity of the chief complaints, 'ruled out' the more unlikely etiologic factors underlying the reason for referral, and developed a fairly good idea as to the nature of the hypotheses one is going to pursue. Among children with learning disabilities, a significant number have some variant of a developmental language disorder. It behooves the clinician, therefore, to include several tests of language development in his/her core battery, since the likelihood is high that these same tests will be required in the eventual investigation of the process disorders presented by the child. Described below are the tests and instruments of clinical appraisal suggested for the neuropsychological evaluation of learning disabled children.

### General intelligence

The construct of intelligence and its measurement present special problems for neuropsychology. The concept of general intelligence, given its various definitions, presumes that a given individual possesses a specific level of general problem-solving skill or adaptive behavior efficiency relative to an appropriate peer group across differing tasks. Accordingly, knowledge of an individual's problem-solving skill in one sphere of adaptive behavior should allow one to predict that individual's relative efficiency in another sphere of activity relative to same-age peers. Thus one should be able to predict an individual's score on a vocabulary test reliably if one knows that individual's ability to construct puzzles and designs, his/her general fund of information, or his/her reading ability. In general, assessment of children whose CNS is presumed intact supports the notion of a high correlation among at least the school-related cognitive skills measured by most IQ tests. However, in individuals whose CNS is not intact, the concept of general intelligence is not applicable. For example, how would one characterize the individual for whom one obtains a Verbal IQ of 125, a Performance IQ of 75 and a Full Scale IQ of 100? Would one conclude, on the basis of his Full Scale IQ, that this is a child of average intellectual abilities? That would be like having one hand in a pail of ice water and the other on a hot stove and saying 'Well, on average, I feel fine.' When the central nervous system is not intact, one cannot predict reliably from one subtest to the other and from one global measure of intelligence to academic performance. Under these circumstances, the Full Scale IQ not only is not the best measure of central tendency of intellectual abilities, but it is actually an irrelevant measure of intellectual abilities. Indeed, it is the observation that specific measures of intellectual abilities do not correlate in the usual manner that raises the first index of suspicion that the central nervous system may not be intact.

### Core battery tests and instruments

The measure of general intelligence used most widely in neuropsychological practice is the Wechsler Intelligence Scale for Children-3rd Edition (WISC-III, Wechsler, 1991).

### Special use of alternative instruments

The Raven Coloured Progressive Matrices and Standard Progressive Matrices (Raven, 1938, 1947, 1965) serve as untimed, non-constructional measures of visual reasoning, and they are widely accepted as relatively culture-free measures of general intellectual functioning. The Test of Nonverbal Intelligence (TONI-2) (Brown, Sherbenor and Dollar, 1990) is another measure of nonverbal intelligence that correlates with the WISC-III Performance IQ in children with developmental language disorders. The Stanford–Binet Intelligence Scale, 4th Edition (Thorndike, Hagen and Sattler, 1986) is still another measure of general intelligence that correlates highly with academic achievement in the normal population, but lacks the necessary research background in clinical populations to be useful at present as a neuropsychological instrument.

### Attention

Disorders of attention in childhood are often referable to anxiety and personal preoccupations and are usually secondary to intrapsychic and psychosocial factors. There are, however, classes of disorders of neurogenic etiology in which there is compromise of the neuroanatomic substrates for attentional processes. Attentional disorders are common with substance abuse, sleep deprivation, posttraumatic brain injury, and ADHD.

### Core battery tests and instruments

The WISC-III Freedom from Distractibility index (which is derived from the Arithmetic and Digit Span subtests) is usually considered to be a quick measure of immediate or working memory. Since the WISC-III results are readily available, this index score often alerts the examiner to explore attentional processes more fully.

The Continuous Performance Test (CPT) was first demonstrated to be a useful attentional measure in adults by Rosvold, Mirsky, Sarason et al. (1956), and later became widely applicable to children due to the availability of personal computers (Halperin, Wolf, Pascualvaca et al., 1988). The most recent version of this test, the CPT-II Computer Program for Windows (Conners and Staff, 2000) offers expanded norms, including ones for neurologically impaired individuals. The CPT procedure presents the child with a series of letters presented one at a time for a very brief interval. The child is required to press the space bar as soon as possible for every letter that appears except for the letter 'X'. When the letter 'X' appears, the child must inhibit the tendency to respond by pressing the space bar. The computer program measures a number of variables, including reaction time to hits and false alarms, and the number of hits and false alarms. The signal detection statistics d' and beta can therefore be computed for the total time period (approximately 15 minutes) and for discrete epochs. Due to its ease of administration and the availability of computerized scoring and report-generating capabilities, the CPT has become a widely used research tool.

### Special use of alternative instruments

An auditory continuous performance test (ACPT, Keith, 1994) is also available. Another widely used computerized continuous performance test that has visual and auditory versions is the Test of Variables of Attention (TOVA and TOVA-A, Greenberg, Leark, Dupuy et al., 1998a,b), which can also run on a personal computer. Somewhat more cumbersome, but quite sensitive, is the Gordon Diagnostic System (Gordon, 1986). Several subtests that assess aspects of short-term and working memory are included in the Broad Attention cluster of the new Woodcock–Johnson-III Tests of Cognitive Abilities (WJ-III, Woodcock, McGrew and Mather, 2001b).

*Perception*

In the presence of intact acuity, visual and auditory perceptual disorders are actually very infrequently observed, although very frequently implicated on the basis of deficiencies in perceptual–motor performance. Somatosensory impairments appear, in our experience, to be more prevalent in children who come to clinical attention because of learning or behavior problems.

*Core battery tests and instruments*
*Somatosensory.* The Halstead–Reitan sensory–perceptual tasks (Reitan and Davison, 1974) require the child to identify numbers, letters, and forms drawn on his fingertips. The Kinsbourne–Warrington Test of Finger Order and Differentiation (Kinsbourne and Warrington, 1962) was developed as a measure of finger agnosia. It has several sections, but only the two administrations not requiring special equipment are used in the core battery. In one administration, the examiner, using two of his fingers, touches one or two adjacent fingers of the child's hand. With his eyes closed, the child is required to detect whether 1 or 2 fingers are being touched. In another administration, two of the child's fingers on one hand are always touched. The child is asked to detect the number of fingers 'in between' the fingers touched. In this procedure 0–3 fingers may be 'in between'.

*Visual.* The Raven Coloured Progressive Matrices (Raven, 1947, 1965) for children up to age 11 years has been especially useful. This is an analogies task utilizing patterned visual stimuli and requiring no constructional or skilled motor output. The Coloured

Progressive Matrices is composed of three sets of twelve-item subtests. The first set contains perceptually complex tasks requiring perceptual extrapolation for solution. In contrast, the last set is perceptually simple, presenting simple gestalts but in conceptually complex analogistic relations. Individuals with visual perceptual disorders often perform at defective levels on the first set but, paradoxically, breeze through the 'harder' last set.

*Special use of alternative instruments*
*Visual.* There are a number of visual processing tasks which, in the adult literature, are deemed to be differentially impaired with posterior, especially non-dominant hemisphere, lesions. While one would not wish to invoke the localizing data, nonetheless the tasks themselves have clinical utility. The Benton Line Orientation Test (Benton, Hannay and Varney, 1975) and Facial Recognition Test (Benton and Van Allen, 1983) are both sensitive to disruption of visual perceptual processing, with the line orientation task having a seemingly higher attentional loading in children.

*Auditory.* The Auditory Skills Test (Goldman, Fristoe and Woodcock, 1976) is a relatively widely used standard instrument. This test requires a good auditory delivery system, has a signal in background (cafeteria) noise administration that has exceptional ecologic validity. A useful nonverbal auditory skills task is the timbre discrimination subtest of the Seashore Test of Musical Abilities (Seashore, Lewis and Saetveit, 1960).

*Memory and learning*

Marked amnesias in children are rare outside of patients with acute encephalitis and head trauma. The patient with a marked disability in acquiring new information because of an early encephalopathic event is more likely to present with retardation than with a specific learning disability or focal impairment. Nonetheless, extra-limbic system disability can result in relatively inefficient learning, without the difficulty being considered evidence of an amnesia. It should be noted that both verbal and nonverbal memory can be assessed in any modality. It is most convenient, especially with children, to test verbal mnestic processes using an auditory input and requiring a vocal output, and easier to assess non-verbal mnestic processes by presenting visual stimuli and requiring a motor output. Thus, verbal memory tasks usually present the child with a list of words or a paragraph and ask for oral recall of this material at some later point. In the older child or adult, it may be just as convenient to present the patient with a written word list or paragraph and ask for a written reproduction of the target material. Similarly, rather than present the patient with a relatively nonverbal geometric design to reproduce from memory (a visual input–motor output task), one might wish to present him with a melodic tune to hum at a later time (auditory input–vocal output). In brief, the limbic mnestic system appears to be organized in a lateralized manner along verbal and nonverbal continua rather than being sensory modality specific. As a rule of thumb, finding modality-specific differential memory deficits should raise one's index of suspicion concerning the integrity of the modality before seriously embarking on an exploration of a modality-specific mnestic deficit.

*Core battery tests and instruments*

There are very few good tests of recent memory for children. The more commonly used verbal memory tests generally are variants of the Buschke Selective Reminding (Buschke, 1974; Clodfelter, Dickson, Wilkes and Johnson, 1987; Said, Shores, Batchelor et al., 1990) procedure for children. We use a ten-item selective reminding test with 15 trials and a recognition probe at the very end. There are good norms for the Rey Auditory Verbal Learning Test for Children (Bishop, Knights and Stoddart, 1990; Schmidt, 1998). The California Verbal Learning Test, Children's Version (Delis, Kramer, Kaplan and Ober, 1994) offers the benefit of a computerized scoring program (Fridlund and Delis, 1998).

Among the nonverbal memory tasks, there are several useful instruments. The Benton Test of Visual Retention, Administration A (Benton, 1974) is frequently used. There are ten cards, the first presents one figure, the rest each present three geometric figures. Each card is presented for 10 seconds, removed, and the child is then asked to reproduce the designs from memory. We are presently using two recognition memory variants of this task. In one, the card is presented for 5 seconds, removed, and the child is then asked to select the target from among four alternatives. In the other variant, the target is presented for 10 seconds, removed, and, after a 15-second delay, the child is asked to detect the target from among the alternatives. In the adult literature, recognition memory is relatively robust and is relatively unimpaired in depression. The 5-second exposure procedure is more heavily loaded on attentional factors and the 15-second delay on mnestic processes. Administering both conditions often allows one to observe the differential effects of each neuropsychologic process on a similar task.

*Special use of alternative instruments*

Many clinicians use a procedure in which the child is asked to draw from memory a design or series of designs they have initially copied. The Bender Gestalt (Bender, 1938; Koppitz, 1963) and the Rey–Osterreith Complex Figure (Waber and Holmes, 1986) are both excellent examples of such methodologies. The major caveat to bear in mind in using such procedures is that the adult literature strongly suggests that procedural and 'motor' memory may relate more to the integrity of basal ganglia than limbic structures. To the extent that such structures are involved in the initial copying procedure, this method may not directly assess the mnestic processes under investigation. An updated version of the Rey Complex Figure Test and Recognition Trial (RCFT, Meyers and Meyers, 1995) provides a multiple-choice recognition trial that does not require motor output. The Wide Range Assessment of Memory and Learning (WRAML, Adams and Sheslow, 1990) is another measure that includes both verbal and visual memory subtests.

*Language*

The majority of children who come to the attention of educators because of failure to acquire reading skills tend to present one of several forms of developmental language disorders. Therefore, children seen for evaluation of learning and behavior problems should have a thorough language examination as part of the routine work-up. In general, examination for the presence of language disorder consists of assessment of word finding ability, language comprehension–semantics, syntax and grammar, imitative speech, central auditory processing of linguistic material, motor expressive speech, verbal fluency, pragmatics of spontaneous or discursive speech, assessment of oral speech mechanisms, and reading and writing skills.

*Core battery tests and instruments*
*Naming.* There are only a few reasonable naming tests for children. The three that we use most frequently include the Mattis Naming Test, the Boston Naming Test, and the Expressive One-Word Picture Vocabulary Test, all of which were described above.

*Sentence repetition.* The Spreen–Benton Sentence Repetition Test assesses this skill very well with quite usable norms (Spreen and Benton, 1969). An alternative might be the memory for sentences items of the Stanford–Binet-IV.

*Language comprehension.* The Token Test (DiSimoni, 1978) uses circles and squares (2 different sizes, 5 different colors). The child manipulates these objects in response to requests of increasing syntactic complexity. The Receptive One-Word Picture Vocabulary Test, 2000 Edition (Brownell, 2000b) is an alternative method of assessing a child's receptive vocabulary.

*Motor speech.* In addition to listening to the cadence, inflection, and rate of speech during the total testing period, one is obligated to examine directly for dyspraxias of speech. In examining an adult, each clinician has his/her own version of 'Methodist–Episcopal'. In children, there is an equivalent test called the Test of Verbal Dyspraxia (Blakeley, 1980), which uses target words such as 'linoleum', 'aluminum', and 'statistics', as well as consonant vowel configurations such as 'ta', 'pa', and 'ka' performed as diadokinetic tasks and rapidly sequenced syllables. Task difficulty asymptotes as one approaches adolescence, and the norms are only fair and need re-examination. In addition, one needs to be careful of dialect and regional differences. For example, 'linoleum' in much of Westchester County, NY, is a nonsense word.

*Verbal fluency.* The Controlled Oral Word Association Test (COWAT, Spreen and Benton, 1969, 1977) is a widely used measure of verbal fluency in which the individual is given three 1-minute trials to generate as many words as possible beginning with certain target letters of the alphabet (e.g. F, A, S). In addition to child COWAT norms (Gaddes and Crockett, 1975), there are also good child norms (Halperin et al., 1989) for categorized word fluency trials (using animals, foods, and words beginning with 'sh' as the target items).

In the adult, reading and writing skills are generally assessed as part of the aphasia examination, but, because these skills are often the focus of the reason for referral in children, they are addressed in a separate academic skills subsection presented below.

*Special use of alternative instruments*
Central auditory processing skills are often examined in children suspected of presenting a language disorder. This examination consists of a carefully controlled administration of verbal and, at times, nonverbal auditory events presented to each ear as competing stimuli. Dichotic stop consonants and staggered spondaic words, as well as a careful acoustosensory investigation, are part of this examination, often conducted by speech and language pathologists (see Hood and Berlin, 2003, this volume).

There are several well-respected multifactorial batteries for the evaluation of language processing in children. These include the Clinical Evaluation of Language Fundamentals, Third Edition (CELF-3, Wiig, Secord and Secord, 1995) and the Comprehensive Assessment of Spoken Language (CASL, Carrow-Woolfolk, 1999). The CELF-3 provides a comprehensive assessment of expressive and receptive language skills, while the CASL is particularly useful in evaluating pragmatic language and oral language skills. The Test of Pragmatic Language (TOPL, Phelps-Terasaki and Phelps-Gunn, 1992) assesses six aspects of pragmatic language, including physical setting, audience, topic, purpose, visual–gestural cues, and abstraction.

Several subtests from the Woodcock–Johnson III Tests of Cognitive Abilities (Woodcock et al., 2001b) are particularly useful in the assessment of phonological processing.

*Executive functions*

*Core battery tests and instruments*
In the assessment of executive functioning, a number of psychometric instruments derived from the study of adults have proven to have heuristic value in child evaluations. The most common include the Wisconsin Card Sorting Test, the Trail Making Test and the Stroop Color and Word Test. Included in our standard work-up are the Purdue Pegboard (with special attention paid to pegs placed simultaneously with both hands), and Luria's (1966) assessment of praxis, perhaps similar to the Hand Movement subtest on the Kaufman Assessment Battery for Children (K-ABC, Kaufman and Kaufman, 1983). Finally, an assessment of 'soft-signs', including choreiform movements of the upper extremities (Prechtl's movements) and possible indications of motor overflow as observed on the PANESS, is required.

*The Wisconsin Card Sorting Test (WCST, Heaton, 1981).* The WCST is one of the better measures of the processes involved in decision making that is normed for children (Chelune and Baer, 1986; Chelune and Thompson, 1987). On this task, the child is presented with four target cards depicting simple geometric designs, each of which differs from the others in at least one specific attribute. The child is then presented with a series of 128 comparable cards. When each card is presented, the child is asked to match the card to the target card with which it belongs. The principle for matching (sorting) the card is not told to the child, but must be induced from the feedback provided concerning the correctness of each match. Once the principle has been detected, as demonstrated by a specified number of successive correct matches, the 'rule' of sorting is then changed without warning and the child must both recognize the advent of a new rule and induce the new rule. Thus, this task assesses the ability to abstract an operating principle, to maintain that principle as long as it is effective, and to shift to another principle when appropriate. A computer-assisted administration format is available (Heaton and Staff, 1999), which is enjoyable for the child to take and easy for the examiner to score and analyze.

*The Trail Making Test (Reitan, 1979).* The Trail Making Test is a measure of mental flexibility and working memory with significant motor and visual search components. Trails A is a simple connect-the-dot task which presents circles distributed on a page, each containing a number. The child is asked to connect the circles in ascending numerical order. Trails B also presents circles distributed on a page, however, the circles contain either a number or a letter. The child is asked to start at number 1, then go to A, then to 2, then to B, alternating numbers in ascending order and letters in alphabetical order. The child is therefore required to shift set rapidly from numeric to alphabetic order. In general, Trails B is completed without error and the time to completion is the salient measure. Norms for the intermediate form of this test are appropriate for children (Spreen and Strauss, 1998).

*The Stroop Color and Word Test.* The Stroop Color and Word Test has some norms that apply to children (Golden, 1978). On the Stroop, the names of four colors are randomly repeated on a page, each name randomly printed in one of the four colors. Initially, the color names must be read aloud as quickly as possible to obtain a baseline measure of reading speed and to set the child for a reading response. On the critical interference task, the child is presented with a set of similar stimuli but must call out the color in which the word is printed, suppressing the more potent response of reading the word. The time to complete this task and the number of errors are the salient measures.

*Sequenced hand movements.* For both the Luria and Kaufman hand movements, the observation of a disassociation between the child's ability to say aloud the command for each of the hand positions in the correct sequence and the child's ability to perform the sequence adequately is often interpreted as 'hard' evidence of frontal dysfunction.

*Special use of alternative instruments*
*The Cambridge Neuropsychological Test Automated Battery* (CANTAB, Owen, Downes, Sahakian et al., 1990), is a computerized battery of executive functions tasks initially designed for use with adults. However, it appears to have a good deal of promise

for use with children. It consists of five subtests: Spatial Span; Spatial Working Memory; Tower of London (planning task); Attentional Set Shifting; and Simultaneous and Delayed Matching to Sample.

*The Delis–Kaplan Executive Function System* (Delis, Kaplan and Kramer, 2001) has nine tests designed to measure aspects of executive functions including: flexibility of thinking, inhibition, problem solving, planning, impulse control, concept formation, abstract thinking, and creativity in both verbal and spatial modalities.

*The Tower of Hanoi* (Pennington, Groissir and Welsh, 1993; Simon, 1975) is a sequential planning task that requires the child to adhere to specific rules for transfer of pieces.

*The Six Elements Test* (Burgess, Alderman, Evans et al., 1996) is a simplified version of the Behavioral Assessment of the Dysexecutive Syndromes that is appropriate for administration to children.

*The Hayling Sentence Completion Test* (Burgess and Shallice, 1997) is a sentence completion task that requires the individual to complete a sentence with an appropriate word on half the items and to complete the sentence with a word that does not apply on the other half. The sentences are constructed so that they generate a specific word with a very high degree of probability. The time to generate the novel words minus the time to generate the high probability words is the salient score. This task is similar in many ways to the Stroop.

*Go–No-Go Tasks* measure response inhibition (Christensen, 1979; Luria, 1966). Some of these techniques have been applied to the evaluation of attentional disorders in children (Trommer, Hoeppner, Lorber and Amstrong, 1988).

While *Controlled Oral Word Association Test (COWAT)* was described in the language section as a measure of verbal fluency, it is also considered to be an executive function skill.

### Conceptualization

This is a very difficult area to investigate in children. In adults, acquired brain damage might result in a deficit in the general ability to abstract or in a specific disturbance in comparative verbal or nonverbal relations, with localizing significance for the specific conceptual deficit. While a general inability to abstract can be observed in some children who have incurred brain damage several years prior to evaluation, in most cases the relationship between the nature and extent of tissue involvement and the nature of deficiencies in conceptualization is difficult to document. This lack of documentation seems likely to be due to two major factors: (1) the specific concepts to explore at different ages are not readily defined operationally; and (2) early damage might result in atypical or idiosyncratic acquisition of specific concepts rather than a distinct failure to acquire the concept.

Among those tasks requiring abstract ability and ideational flexibility, the Category Test (Klonoff and Low, 1974; Reitan and Davison, 1974) continues to enjoy widespread use. The Raven Coloured and Standard Progressive Matrices (Raven, 1938, 1947, 1965) overlap to some degree with the Category Test, but they do not focus on equivalent functions.

### Constructional skills

Traditionally, in the adult literature, constructional disorders are listed among the apraxias, i.e. disorders in purposeful movement. However, the prevalence of a chief complaint of handwriting, drawing, and/or three-dimensional constructional difficulties in childhood is so high that it warrants separate evaluation. The increasing complexity of imitative and spontaneous constructions, available to children as they mature, strongly suggests that constructional ability might be classifiable as a higher order conceptual ability in children, equivalent to verbal conceptual development. The most frequently observed constructional disorder is usually elicited on drawing tasks. In most circumstances, a deficiency involving the copying of geometric designs in the face of intact performance on a task such as the WISC-III Block Design subtest is not suggestive of a visual perceptual disorder. Rather, upon further evaluation, drawing difficulties are most often found to reflect underlying dyscoordination problems, or they occasionally represent a true visual–motor integration disorder, i.e. a constructional dyspraxia. In most cases, one would like to see both three-dimensional and two-dimensional construction to be impaired before one is willing to conclude that the patient has a constructional dyspraxia.

*Core battery tests and instruments*
The most commonly used tests to assess the ability to construct or reconstruct target items using manipulative materials are the Block Design and Object Assembly subtests of the WISC-III.

Of those drawing tests that require the child to copy geometric designs, the Beery–Buktenica Developmental Test of Visual–Motor Integration (Beery, 1997) contains the largest number of items appropriate for presentation to children under age 7, and it therefore provides the largest potential sample of clearly deficient constructions. It also includes some very complex gestalts at the upper age levels, and it has excellent norms. The only disadvantage is the degree to which the criteria for adequacy of construction are dependent on the integrity of graphomotor coordination.

*Special use of alternative instruments*
The Benton Test of Visual Retention (Benton, 1974) is normed for children over the age of 8 years; it contains items that are simple gestalts; and the adequacy of its construction is not highly skewed by graphomotor factors. The Benton does not seem to be as sensitive a measure of graphic skills as is the Beery or the Rey–Osterreith Complex Figure Test (Osterreith, 1944; Waber and Holmes, 1985). However, the Benton's specificity is such that, if the child is having difficulty on this test, the chances are exceedingly high that he/she is demonstrating a constructional apraxia and not a motivational or extrapyramidal disorder.

The Rey–Osterreith Complex Figure Test presents a complex design to recall and an even more complex scoring system (Waber and Holmes, 1986). It is not highly recommended for children below the teens.

The Bender Gestalt (Bender, 1938; Koppitz, 1963) is an excellent drawing test for the older school-aged child. However, one serious drawback to its use as a primary neuropsychological instrument is the patient's freedom to place the designs anywhere on the page. Proper placement demands the type of organizational and planning skills that are frequently compromised by those same psychogenic factors that are often part of the differential diagnosis. Without clear criteria — to discriminate the transient motivational factors affecting organizational relationships among the gestalts, the trait factors affecting the

same relationships, and the neurogenic factors affecting the adequacy of the gestalts themselves — the Bender is of limited specific use. Because of the probable regional aberration of the interpretation of drawing errors, the Bender does not occupy its otherwise rightful place as a part of our core battery. In a non-psychiatric setting, the Bender might serve as part of a second phase screening battery where the psychiatric false positive may be less significant.

A commonly used task in a psychiatric context is the Draw-a-Person Test (Goodenough and Harris, 1963; Naglieri, McNeish and Bardos, 1991). However, the specificity for neurogenic factors is so poor in a population of children with a modest base rate of primary psychosocial and psychiatric disorders as to offer little added information.

*Motor skills*

Perinatal anoxic events are among the most common risk factors encountered in our clinical population. In general, such anoxic events tend to compromise those systems that are metabolically most active (i.e. Betz cells, Purkinje cells, and basal ganglia, in particular caudate and putamen). It is not surprising, therefore, to observe some aspect of motor dyscoordination as a prevalent finding in this patient population.

*Core battery tests and instruments*
The evaluation of gross-, fine-, and graphomotor coordination was discussed earlier in this chapter.

*Academic achievement*

When children are referred for the assessment of possible learning disabilities, it is often necessary to obtain an estimate of academic achievement that is independent from the records provided by the school system. It is also important to obtain additional measures of specific subprocesses underlying the more complex achievement tasks. Regardless of the reason for referral, the child's school performance represents his/her relative success in an endeavor that occupies a quarter to a third of his/her waking life. Assessing a child's performance on standardized tests of academic achievement provides an objective estimate of his/her level of functioning.

## Core tests and instruments

The Wide Range Achievement Test, 3rd ed. (Wilkinson, 1993) offers word recognition, spelling, and arithmetic skills scores. To the extent that one is satisfied with age-based but not grade-based standard scores and percentiles, the WRAT-3 offers a fast reliable measure of achievement.

The Gates–MacGinite (MacGinite et al., 2000) reading comprehension subtest uses the customary booklet format in which the child reads a paragraph silently and responds to multiple-choice questions. This task requires the child to work independently for 35 minutes.

The Decoding Skills Test (Richardson and DiBenedetto, 1985) offers an excellent analysis of phonetic skills and should be used whenever a reading disorder is indicated by low achievement scores.

An improved understanding of phonological awareness problems (Torgesen and Mathes, 2000) and phonemic discrimination and sequencing issues (Lindamood, 1997; Lindamood, Bell and Lindamood, 1992) has resulted in the development of several evaluation and treatment programs to address these issues.

## Special use of alternative instruments

There are a number of comprehensive instruments designed to measure various aspects of academic functioning. Depending upon the presenting problem, one can administer the entire battery or specific subtests. Among the most widely used are the Woodcock–Johnson Tests of Achievement, 3rd ed. (WJ-III, Woodcock, McGrew and Mather, 2001a) and the Wechsler Individual Achievement Test, 2nd ed. (WIAT-II, The Psychological Corporation, 2001). The Gray Oral Reading Test, 4th ed. (GORT-4, Wiederholt and Bryant, 2001) offers several subtests that are read aloud by the child. The Test of Written Language, 3rd ed. (TOWL-3, Hammill and Larsen, 1996) assesses a child's writing competence by means of eight subtests.

Many school districts offer periodic assessments of the academic achievement of their students using tests with normative data derived from large numbers of same-aged and same-grade peers. These achievement test scores are readily available. For the amount of time they consume in the diagnostic session, general achievement tests do not add much

more than could be learned by obtaining the child's achievement scores on any of the state-wide exams common to all school systems. Only when one suspects an encapsulated psychiatric disorder specific to performing in a group, or attention deficits grossly affecting group testing, will the state-wide tests differ significantly from the office examination. In most instances the achievement tests are given so as to allow the clinician to observe directly the nature and level of performance.

## Social–emotional functioning

There is high co-morbidity of neuropsychological disorders and psychiatric disorders, although a surprisingly small number of studies exist documenting the nature and number of such disorders (Spreen, 1989). In general, the co-morbidity is thought to be due to one of several non-mutually exclusive factors: (1) reaction to successive failures results in deep feelings of inadequacy and subsequent depressive feelings; (2) the presence of cognitive deficits severely limits the defensive repertoire used to combat stress, resulting in greater frequency and severity of experienced raw affect; and (3) the same etiologic factors which caused the cognitive deficits are at work on those subcortical structures modulating relatedness, thought organization, and response to stress.

There are a number of procedures used to assess disorders of personality and affective state. They fall into one of three categories of instruments: questionnaire, structured interview, and projective tests. The validity of all such instruments for appraisal of psychiatric disorders does not meet criteria generally considered acceptable in the neuropsychology literature. Some of the more widely used instruments that focus on attentional and behavioral issues include the parent and teacher versions of the revised Conners' Rating Scales (Conners, 1997a). There is also a self-administered version that can be completed by children between ages 12 and 17 (Conners and Wells, 1997). Brown has also developed rating scales focusing on attentional and behavioral difficulties for children and adolescents (Brown, 2001). More general behavioral and affective symptomatology is addressed by the Behavioral Assessment Scale for Children (BASC, Reynolds and Kamphaus, 1992). The Yale–Brown Obsessive Compulsive Scale (YBOCS, Goodman, Price, Rasmussen et al., 1989a,b) is specific to behaviors that are associated with obsessive–compulsive difficulties.

The longstanding traditional projective measures for children continue to include the Thematic Apperception Test (Murray, 1938), the Rorschach inkblot technique (Rorschach, 1942), the Draw-a-Person Test (Goodenough and Harris, 1963; Naglieri et al., 1991), and a semi-structured sentence completion task.

## The neuropsychological assessment of the child with a complicated learning disorder (Group II)

### Introduction

The most common co-morbid diagnosis in children with complicated learning disorders is a disorder of attention. While psychiatry seems content to come to a diagnostic conclusion based on presenting symptoms and observations reported on third-party questionnaires, most neuropsychologists find it difficult to conclude pathology and to come to a diagnosis without positive findings derived from their examination. This presents a problem. To the extent that one seriously views ADHD cognition and behavior as reflecting dysfunction in basal ganglia and prefrontal systems, it would seem reasonable to assume that the presence of findings associated with dysfunction in these systems would corroborate the diagnosis, and the absence of findings peculiar to these systems would contradict the diagnosis, or, at the very least, minimize its likelihood.

The neuropsychological examination of ADHD in children tends to focus upon difficulties in sustained attention, executive skills deficiencies, frequently observed fine motor dyscoordination, and soft signs on such examinations as the PANESS. For many in the psychiatric community, the absence of corroborative findings on neuropsychological examination does not appear to lessen the certainty of the diagnosis. However, somewhere along the way, if a child is given a diagnosis of ADHD and one cannot find evidence on examination of an attentional disorder, executive disorder, and/or motor disinhibition, one might wish to reconsider the diagnosis and

pursue other etiologic factors underlying the child's situational inattentiveness and/or high activity level.

A complicating disorder often seen in children with ADHD and social–emotional difficulties is a disorder of executive processing. Executive processes refer to those processes recruited while making a decision and executing the decided plan of action. In general, one is interested in problem analysis, including working memory, abstraction, creative problem solving, execution of the solution, ongoing observation of the efficacy of the solution, and flexibility in developing alternative solutions should the initial one no longer be applicable or useful. In the adult literature, disorders in executive functions tend to be associated with lesions to frontal systems. In the adult literature, there is no single 'frontal lobe syndrome'. Likewise, in the pediatric neuropsychological literature, there is no single cluster of executive disorders. Executive disorders have been attributed to a wide spectrum of pediatric neurologic and psychiatric diagnoses, when disinhibition of behavior, affect, and/or attention, difficulty 'transitioning' between activities, inability to initiate activities and/or rapid cycling between behaviors and/or affective states have been central to the chief complaint. ADHD, Bipolar Disorder, Tourette Syndrome, and OCD have in common evidence of executive function deficits. Unfortunately for the purposes of differential diagnosis, there is no specific cluster of executive function deficits that seems to be incontrovertibly pathognomonic of any one diagnostic disorder. Nevertheless, the identification of a specific executive dysfunction or cluster of deficits in a given child allows the clinician to utilize the replicable specific deficit in executive function to explain the aberrant behavior associated with a number of complex psychiatric disorders.

### Phase 1: the clinical interview and review of records

Most hyperactive children come to clinical attention early in life, either at preschool and nursery school levels, when their activity level limits their ability to sit quietly during circle time. Difficulty making transitions is usually noted by kindergarten. In first grade, the necessity to be in class a full day within a structured setting strains their capacity, and those children with mild to moderate hyperactivity usually come to clinical attention within a few months. The clinical interview should be focused on the history of the chief complaint of overactive behavior. It is important to ascertain the most common early observations of the hyperkinetic child, i.e. 'colicky baby. . . difficult to soothe', 'ran before he walked', 'runs and runs and runs, but still has difficulty falling asleep', 'sitter can't keep up with him', 'can't take him to a supermarket', 'more interested in the commercials. . . when the show goes on he gets up and walks around and starts talking'. Most clinicians prefer to have the parents and teachers fill out a questionnaire concerning the school-aged child's behavior. Brown (2001) and Conners (1997b) have forms with excellent psychometric properties for both parents and teachers. It is also very important to get a good family history to ascertain the heritable ADHD behaviors and mood disorders within the family trees. HKS appears to have a greater genetic loading than does ADHD, primarily inattentive type, again supporting separate etiologic factors in the two disorders.

## *Phase 2. The screening battery*

In ADHD, combined type, predominantly hyperactive–impulsive type, or predominantly inattentive type, the nature of the chief complaint, the family history, and the rating scales comprise 'the screening battery'. If both the teachers and the parents endorse behaviors consistent with a possible diagnosis of ADHD, then the examination should continue. If the parents do not endorse the symptomatology but are seeking consultation because the school personnel have observed the target behaviors, then it is still possible to entertain the hypothesis of ADHD with the assumption that the home environment has sufficient flexibility or lack of structure that the target behaviors do not come to parental attention. If the teachers do not endorse the hyperkinetic behavior or inattention in the highly structured, achievement-oriented classroom setting, but the parents observe such aberrant behavior at home, it is difficult to maintain a diagnosis of ADHD and one should pursue alternative hypotheses for the site-specific inappropriate behavior. Parents of children with mood disorders, primarily Juvenile Onset Bipolar Disorder, often report attentional, hyperkinetic, oppositional/defiant,

and aggressive behavior at home, with peak conflict focused upon issues of homework and getting the child up and ready for school, in contrast with reports of reasonably socially appropriate behavior at school.

## *Phase 3: the neuropsychological assessment*

### *Core battery tests and instruments*
When the history and current observation allow one to seriously entertain the diagnosis of ADHD or HKS, the tasks critical to supporting the diagnosis are tests of attentional processes, both immediate and sustained, tests of executive functioning, and assessment of motor disinhibition and neurodevelopmental 'soft signs'. Thus, at minimum, one must conduct an assessment of attentional processes, which might include the WISC-III subtests comprising the Freedom from Distractibility index and the Processing Speed index, and a measure of sustained attention (such as the CPT).

### *Differential diagnosis of ADHD*

What one would like to see on neuropsychological evaluation to bolster one's confidence in the validity of the diagnosis of ADHD is:
(1) Evidence of an attentional disorder, especially fast reaction time with abnormally high errors of commission, significant variability in reaction time, and significant differences between performance levels at the beginning and end of the task.
(2) Evidence of deficiencies on tasks of executive function, including ideational errors, such as perseverative errors and failure to maintain set on Wisconsin and Towers, poor set flexibility on Trails B, an inability to inhibit 'reading the word' on the Stroop, and poor phonemic fluency on the COWAT.
(3) Evidence of motor disinhibition on tasks such as the Purdue Pegboard, rapid sequential movements of the upper extremities on the Luria and/or Kaufman hand movements, and physiologically aberrant motor disinhibition, such as motor clumsiness and overflow, elicited on direct examination, such as on the PANESS.

If the above findings are observed, then the confidence in the diagnosis should be high. Depending on the nature of the chief complaint or referring questions, one might be able to stop the evaluation at this point, having answered the diagnostic question. On the other hand, attentional difficulty, irritability, and high activity levels are also the manifest behaviors of a number of other pathologic processes associated with the social/emotional disorders seen in Referral Group IV (described below). Children with ADHD present a high co-morbidity for ODD, OCD, specific learning disabilities, tic disorders, and mood disorders. Often, the exclusion criteria are so extensive that a core battery cannot contain sufficient information to come to a diagnostic conclusion with a high degree of confidence. Moreover, ADHD symptomatology in a child with primary social skills deficits and a language disorder is usually the least of the child's problems, and an extensive understanding of these developmental disabilities is necessary to aid in treatment planning and parent counseling.

If (1) the evidence of attentional disorder on the CPT is limited to slow reaction time, diminished 'hits' but few errors of commission, a very conservative response bias, and a latency of response that is somewhat independent of inter-stimulus interval, (2) there is no evidence of executive skills deficits, and (3) there is little evidence of motor disinhibition, then one might wish to entertain a mood disorder, primarily depression, and/or anxiety-driven personal preoccupations as alternative diagnostic hypotheses to be pursued. Moreover, if (1) the evidence of attentional disorder on the CPT is limited to diminished 'hits' but few errors of commission, a somewhat liberal response bias, a latency of response that is somewhat independent of inter-stimulus interval, and the overall attentional index is within normal limits or only mildly atypical, (2) there is evidence of executive skills deficits, and (3) there is little evidence of motor disinhibition, then one might wish to entertain a mood disorder, primarily bipolar disorder, as an alternative diagnostic hypothesis to be pursued.

## Neuropsychological assessment of the child with recent CNS impairment (Group III)

When the child has a known or suspected recent central nervous system injury, the questions raised and the procedures followed are very similar to those employed when assessing an adult with a similar neurologic disorder. Most school age children presenting with suspected or demonstrated recently acquired CNS impairment have sustained a head injury or infectious disease. With any etiology it is necessary to conduct a careful assessment of the presence of multi-focal and diffuse impairment, with an emphasis on abnormalities in memory, language, and mood. A rather comprehensive broad-based assessment is required, therefore, to avoid missing a significant deficit. One will have the occasion, at some time, to see a child with focal damage, in which case one might wish to allot as much time as possible to the in-depth analysis of locus-specific disorders rather than utilizing an omnibus procedure.

*Phase 1: the clinical interview and review of records*

In the evaluation of the school-aged child who has incurred a recent encephalopathic event, it is important to obtain as much objective evidence as possible documenting the child's premorbid cognitive and behavioral status. In an office practice, one tends to see the child at some point beyond the acute encephalopathic event. It is important, therefore, to get some objective evidence of premorbid functioning, of acute change in cognitive and behavior status, and of the course of recovery since the event. In addition, one needs to get information about the nature and intensity of any past or ongoing treatment or rehabilitation. It is difficult for parents to be objective about such data. While an interview will generate information about premorbid functions, there may be one of two tendencies that most parents demonstrate and that might bias their report. The 'everything is O.K.' posture will result in observations that both minimize the extent of decrement in functioning and distort the level of premorbid functioning with comments such as 'he always had trouble with that'. On the other hand, the posture of 'mourning the lost child' tends to result in an exaggeration of the extent of deficit and an idealization of premorbid functioning. Parents usually do not present at one or the other extreme; but it is rare not to see some aspect of these two presentations as the predominant tone. Moreover, sometimes one parent is mourning while the other is minimizing, with neither one comforting the other or working towards a common goal for their child. It is often necessary, therefore, to obtain data from the school records, paying close attention to the child's performance on state or national achievement tests and to behavioral comments made by the teacher on the report cards. If rehabilitative treatment had been initiated, then intake conference notes, treatment progress notes, and any pre- and posttreatment evaluations should be reviewed.

Even when all the material is available to the examiner, one rarely feels comfortable concluding the clinical assessment procedure without conducting one's own examination. At the very least, no matter how extensive the previous work-ups, one prefers to administer, at a minimum, the equivalent of a screening battery. In a forensic practice, there are, at times, exceptional circumstances, when the patient is not physically available and an opinion is requested for something other than the diagnosis derived from personally conducted clinical examination. In general clinical practice, Phase 1 should not be accepted as a terminal assessment stage in the evaluation of children with recently acquired brain damage.

## Phase 2: the screening battery

When one is in a 'specialty clinic' setting, the patient population presents a limited number of somewhat circumscribed clinical disorders and there usually exists a relatively finite set of possible alternative diagnoses. Under these circumstances, it is possible to determine (1) sets of typical patterns of neuro-cognitive disorders associated with the specialty clinic's most common neurologic disorders, (2) the nature of the changes in these target neuropsychological profiles over the course of the disease, and (3) the nature of psychogenic and other neurogenic disorders that can mime the target profiles. Thus, if one could focus upon the neuropsychological presentation of a few specific neurologic entities, then one could begin to gather the necessary information to develop a useful screening battery with both high sensitivity and specificity.

In contrast to the specialty clinic setting, when one practices within a general pediatric neurologic, neurosurgical, or rehabilitative setting, the etiologies and pathophysiologies of possible brain damage and the ages of the children often vary so widely that the clinician does not have the option of devising a sleek screening battery for a target population. If, in one's practice, one child has had a moderate head injury, the second has had a stroke, the third has partial complex seizures, and the next requires the assessment of the delayed effects of whole brain radiation, how does one go about developing a screening instrument?

In brief, if one's practice is devoted to a circumscribed clinical disorder, then Phase 1 and Phase 2 are possible and the decision-tree approach may generate a useful organizing principle for the assessment. However, if one's practice is less specialized, then, after Phase 1, one should go directly to Phase 3.

## Phase 3: the neuropsychological assessment

The child who has recently experienced an encephalopathic event may present almost any specific cognitive deficit, or none at all. Therefore one needs some sound clinical principles to organize the assessment and analysis of the accrued data. In this situation, one would do well to keep in mind the Second Rule of the Diagnostician (the one right after 'do no harm'): 'Cover your diagnostic derrière', that is, the 'rule-outs' are as important as the 'rule-ins'. All cognitive abilities must be assessed to some degree and the absence of cognitive disorders, as in the adult assessment, is every bit as critical to the understanding of the patient's neuropsychological status as are the positive findings. Therefore, at the very least, all the core battery tasks must be included and be supplemented by extensive follow-up assessment of all positive findings. There is no way to abbreviate the evaluation without increasing the probability of missing a positive finding. It is sometimes possible to use one's knowledge of the pathophysiology and recovery course of the etiologic event to organize one's examination. At times, such knowledge will allow one to gain a greater measure of confidence that a given neuropsychological process is rarely affected as a consequence of the target event and, therefore, might require a briefer screening assessment. One might also be better prepared to include a more extensive in-depth assessment of those processes known to be affected by the target event.

As the evaluation ensues, one must eventually come to a clinical decision as to when the evaluation procedures can be terminated. This decision is made when one determines that the possibility of missing a positive or negative finding has reached an acceptable level. That is, when (1) the probability of missing a finding is exceptionally slight given the etiology of the damage and the findings to date, and/or (2) the potential significance of the findings to the well-being or treatment of the patient is minimal. It is almost never appropriate to terminate the assessment when a *clinically significant* finding is still outstanding, independent of the amount of time the clinician expects to expend in the pursuit of the resolution of that question.

## Neuropsychological evaluation of the child with social–emotional disorders (Group IV)

Until very recently, a child whose difficulties were presumed to reflect social and/or emotional disorders would not necessarily be referred for neuropsychological assessment. However, those children who present with extremes of behavior are increasingly likely to be seen as demonstrating the early onset of genetic or biochemical disorders involving the central nervous system. Among those children, who are increasingly referred for neuropsychological assessment, are those whose family histories are contributing factors to symptom presentation, those whose social skills deficits are a prominent feature, and those whose impulsive or explosive behavior places them or those around them at risk. The diagnostic question involves the determination of which cognitive–affective factors are causal to the target aberrant behavior and thoughts, of which are concomitant features of the disorder, and of which are present but irrelevant (i.e. they represent cognitive deficit, they reflect central nervous system deficiencies, but they are not directly relevant to the chief complaint or treatment plan). There is little question, at this point in time, that the major psychiatric disorders that present in early childhood are of neurogenic etiology. Some psychiatric disorders with an early school age onset, such as Juvenile Onset Bipolar Disorder and Childhood Schizophrenia, are widely viewed as neurodevelopmental disorders. However, many psychiatric disorders with an early school age onset

are not uniformly viewed as the behavioral manifestations of biochemical and/or neurotransmitter-specific deficits. The hypothesis that the aberrant behavior is secondary to prior aberrant psychosocial experiences must always be entertained. However, for children with disorders of mood, social skills deficits, and disruptive behavior, the neuropsychological evaluation frequently results in findings that aid in both differential diagnostic considerations and treatment planning.

*Phase I: the clinical interview and review of records*

In most cases, the child with a social–emotional disorder has had a significant amount of testing and clinical assessment, either by school personnel or by a privately contacted professional, prior to the initial contact with the neuropsychologist. There are, therefore, generally a significant number of records that need to be reviewed prior to the initial interview. Rating scales that provide clinical behavioral data, such as the BASC and YBOCS, should be completed by the parents, in addition to the usual attentional rating scales. However, the most critical element at this phase is the attainment of an extensive description of the chief complaint, the history of the chief complaint, the developmental history of cognitive and motor processes, the present status and developmental history of psycho-social development, and, importantly, the family history and the history of significant family and individual events of psychological significance (e.g. deaths in the family or among close friends; divorce, separation, and their concomitant family discord and intense negative feelings; illness and separations; and other possible traumatic events). This is not a 30–45-minute endeavor, and it may take several hours to complete. At the end of this phase, the clinician should have a good idea of the atypical thoughts and behavior manifested by the child, of whether or not the symptomatology is venue-specific (i.e. at home but not in school, or in school but not at home), of the changes over time of symptoms (e.g. tics present at one time but absent later; separation anxiety dramatically present at one time but now manifested by different behaviors), of the level of the child's social success and wish for friends, and of external events which may foster or hinder the demonstration of social skills. We have found that, before the end of the interview with the parents, it is frequently a good idea to ask two questions: 'Does your child have any unusual habits?' and 'Is there anything else I should know?' One is rarely able to conclude the evaluation of a child with social–emotional issues after the clinical interview and review of records, primarily because it is highly unusual for one individual to have assessed the academic performance, neuropsychological status, and social–emotional development of the child. Usually, if these domains have been assessed at all, the separate examinations have been conducted serially over a lengthy period of time, so that it is difficult to make inferences about the relationships among the domains examined.

### Phase 2: the screening battery

At this level of clinical complexity, the screening battery is going to be insufficient either to answer the multiple differential diagnostic questions or to aid in treatment planning.

### Phase 3: the neuropsychological assessment

#### Core battery tests and instruments
The assessment procedures previously delineated for Children with Specific Learning Disorder (Group I) should be administered, including measures of general intellectual abilities, attention, perception, memory and learning, language, executive functions, constructional skills, motor skills, academic achievement, and social–emotional functioning. Unless there has been a significant intervening event, those core battery tests administered within the last year should not be given again. However, it is usually necessary to re-administer a sample of subtests representing the highs and lows of previous performance to assess patient (or perhaps examiner) reliability.

*Attention and arousal.* Many of the children with social–emotional disorders have had psychiatric consultation and may be taking psychotropic and/or stimulant medication. Whenever possible, therefore, it is usually prudent to include multiple administrations of a brief battery of attentional and motor speed tests (e.g. the CPT, Digit Span, Coding, Purdue Peg-

board, and Finger Tapping Test) to monitor quotidian and circadian modulation in attention and arousal.

*Executive processes.* Almost all of the most debilitating childhood psychiatric disorders diagnosed by DSM-IV criteria are associated in the research literature with neuropsychological deficits of one kind or another. Among the most common findings in children with dyscontrol symptomatology are executive skills deficits. One finds such deficits within the ADHD population, the social skills and relatedness deficit populations (e.g. high functioning autism and Asperger's syndrome), and the mood disorder population, especially those with Juvenile Onset Bipolar Disorder. It should be noted that executive skills deficits, similar to the manifest symptomatology of frontal circuitry deficits, do not constitute a single syndrome, i.e. there is not one cluster of deficits but rather several different clusters. The disorder may be confined to a verbal dyspraxia (manifested by fluency disorders and motor speech deficits), it may be expanded to include more widely distributed dyspraxias (similar to Walton's clumsy child syndrome, with its significant perseveration of motor activity and motor dyscontrol), it may be manifested by a more isolated ideational executive deficit (affecting the ability to monitor one's decisions, to determine whether or not the solution implemented is adequate, and, if not, to step back and derive an alternate solution), it may involve disinhibition of affect and an inflexibility in modulating affect as a function of social contingencies and feedback, or any combination of the above. The most commonly used measure of the ideational aspects of executive functioning is the Wisconsin Card Sorting Test which, unfortunately, has a significant drawback as an instrument for serial examination. It is not clear what measures may be used as alternative tasks. Perhaps the tower tasks assess some similar processes of decision-making, but not the shift in 'rule' nor the need to adapt to different external contingencies. It would seem that alternative measures with less troublesome practice effects need to be developed.

*Language processes.* Disorders in language, ranging from dysnomia to mixed aphasias, have been reported in children presenting with a wide variety of psychiatric disorders. The autistic spectrum disorders are among those most likely to impair the pragmatic use of language; they tend to be associated with significant impairment in relatedness, social skills, and judgment. Subtests of measures such as the CELF-3 may be useful adjuncts to the more traditional tests of comprehension, naming, sentence repetition, and expressive language. In addition, the CASL appears to contain reasonably good measures of pragmatic language, enabling the clinician to generate metrics to supplement the clinical description.

*Social–emotional development.* It is within the domain of social–emotional development that neuropsychology has demonstrated its most serious lack of creativity and diagnostic initiative. Without independent measures of social and emotional functioning for use in the assessment of a specific child, we are reduced to diagnosis by questionnaire. Certain inventories described above (Bar-On and Parker, 2000; Beck, Beck and Jolly, 2001) appear to be helpful in identifying key behavioral features and symptomatology.

At present, we generally augment questionnaires with the Rorschach and TAT. Laugh though you might, there is something eerie about a quiet ten year old boy's Rorschach response to Card II: 'It could be two people dancing, or two animals fighting with blood coming out, or a person with his guts coming out', suggesting that the boy's quiet inattention might reflect something other than an inattentive-type attention disorder. Similarly, TAT themes from one card to another, in which the resolution of conflict requires the protagonists to kill themselves, would require the examiner to inquire more fully as to suicidal ideation, actual plans, and the availability of the necessary implements. At this point, however, we have very few well validated instruments at our disposal for use with the child with relatedness and social awareness deficits.

## Future research

As of yet, we do not have any ecologically valid, well-normed measures of affective expression and social interactions of adults and children that would enable us to objectively observe and evaluate aspects of affect and social behavior in children. Are children with social skills deficits less adept at the identification of nonverbal expressions of emotions than are same-aged normal controls, or same-aged psychiatric patients without relatedness disorders? Do they demonstrate a relative deficit in the perception of affect of peers but not adults? Are there affect-specific deficits? For example, is the depressed child more likely to identify mood-congruent expression of affect? Conversely, do children with relatedness or social skills deficits have more difficulty communicating affect than do children with psychiatric disorders not affecting social skills, and/or non-psychiatrically affected children? Until we develop better measures of receptive and expressive communication of affect, as well as measures of what is presently considered social awareness, social confidence, and other processes that fall within the rubric of 'emotional intelligence', neuropsychology will have very little more to contribute to the neuropsychological study of the psychiatric patient.

Within those domains in which neuropsychology has a well-stocked armamentarium, there is a need to be increasingly precise about the sub-processes contributing to the final common behavior. Until recently, neuropsychological instruments were able to measure behavior more precisely than the brain sciences could gauge brain functioning. However, as fMRI dynamic contrast studies increase both spatial and temporal resolution, one can visualize increasingly precise changes in brain functioning. Unless there is a greater rate of progress in the measurement of neuropsychological behavior and changes in status, then direct measurement of neuropsychological behavior and changes in functioning will soon appear to be crude and imprecise compared to our growing ability to directly visualize brain functioning. It will be difficult, therefore, to correlate brain–behavior relationships in a clinically meaningful way.

In brief, the major challenges to the neuropsychological assessment of children lie in (1) the development of new neuropsychological concepts and new instruments for the assessment of social and emotional functioning, (2) research concerning the relationships among social awareness abilities, the spectrum of affective states, cognition, and behavior, and (3) more precise delineation and measurement of neuropsychological sub-processes recruited in the performance of the macro-processes of traditional neuropsychological domains.

# References

Adams W, Sheslow D: Wide Range Assessment of Memory and Learning. Wilmington, DE: Wide Range, Inc., 1990.

Aram DM, Ekelman BL: Cognitive profiles of children with early onset of unilateral lesions. Developmental Neuropsychology: 2(3); 155–172, 1986.

Barkley RA: Attention-deficit/hyperactivity disorder, self-regulation, and time: toward a more comprehensive theory. Journal of Developmental and Behavioral Pediatrics: 18(4); 271–279, 1997.

Bar-On R, Parker DA: BarOn Emotional Quotient, Inventory. North Tonawanda, NY: Multi-Health Systems, Inc., 2000.

Beck JS, Beck AT, Jolly J: Beck Youth Inventories of Emotional and Social Impairment. San Antonio, TX: The Psychological Corporation, 2001.

Beery KE: The Beery-Buktenica Developmental Test of Visual–Motor Integration, Administration, Scoring and Teaching Manual (4th ed). Cleveland, OH: Modern Curriculum Press, 1997.

Bender LA: A visual–motor gestalt test and its clinical use. American Orthopsychiatric Association Research Monographs, No. 3, 1938.

Benton AL: The Revised Visual Retention Test (4th ed.). New York: Psychological Corporation, 1974.

Benton AL, Hannay JH, Varney NR: Visual perception of line direction in patients with unilateral brain disease. Neurology: 25; 907–910, 1975.

Benton AL, Van Allen MW: Test of Facial Recognition. New York: Oxford University Press, 1983.

Berquin PC, Giedd JN, Jacobsen LK, Hamburger SD, Krain AL, Rapoport JL, Castellanos FX: Cerebellum in attention-deficit hyperactivity disorder: A morphometric MRI study. Neurology: 50(4); 1087–1093, 1998.

Bishop J, Knights RM, Stoddart C: Rey Auditory–Verbal Learning Test: Performance of English and French children aged 5–16. Clin. Neuropsychol.: 2(4); 133–140, 1990.

Blakeley RW: Screening Test for Developmental Apraxia of Speech. Tigard, OR: C.C. Publications, 1980.

Brown TE: Brown Attention-Deficit Disorder Scales for Children and Adolescents. San Antonio, TX: The Psychological Corporation, 2001.

Brown L, Sherbenor R, Dollar S: Test of Nonverbal Intelligence (TONI-2). Los Angeles, CA: Western Psychological Services, 1990.

Brownell R: Expressive One-Word Vocabulary Test — 2000 Edition. Itasca, IL: Riverside Publishing, 2000a.

Brownell R: Receptive One-Word Vocabulary Test — 2000 Edition. Itasca, IL: Riverside Publishing, 2000b.

Burgess PW, Alderman N, Evans JJ, Wilson BA, Emslie H, Shallice T: Modified six elements test. In Wilson BA, Alderman N, Burgess PW, Emslie H, Evans JJ (Eds), Behavioral Assessment of the Dysexecutive Syndrome. Bury St. Edmunds: Thames Valley Test Co. Ltd., 1996.

Burgess PW, Shallice T: Hayling Sentence Completion Test. Suffolk: Thames Valley Test Co. Ltd., 1997.

Buschke H: Two stages of learning by children and adults. Bull. Psychonom. Soc.: 2; 392–394, 1974.

Carrow-Woolfolk, E: Comprehensive Assessment of Spoken Language. Circle Pines, MN: American Guidance Service, Inc., 1999.

Chelune GJ, Baer RA: Developmental norms for the Wisconsin Card Sorting Test. Journal of Clinical and Experimental Neuropsychology: 8; 219–228, 1986.

Chelune GJ, Thompson LT: Evaluation of the general sensitivity of the Wisconsin Card Sorting Test among younger and older children. Developmental Neuropsychology: 3(1); 81–89, 1987.

Christensen AL: Luria's Neuropsychological Investigation. Copenhagen: Munksgaard, 1979.

Clarke AR, Barry RJ, McCarthy R, Selikowitz M: Age and sex effects in the EEG: Differences in two subtypes of attention-deficit/hyperactivity disorder. Clin. Neurophys.: 112(5); 815–826, 2001.

Clodfelter CJ, Dickson AL, Wilkes CN, Johnson RB: Alternate forms of the Selective Reminding Test for Children. Clin. Neuropsychol.: 1; 243–249, 1987.

Cohen M, Town P, Buff A: Neurodevelopmental differences in confrontational naming in children. Developmental Neuropsychology: 4(1); 75–81, 1988.

Conners CK: Conners' Parent Rating Scale-Revised. North Tonawanda, NY: Multi-Health Systems, Inc., 1997a.

Conners CK: Conners' Teacher Scale-Revised. North Tonawanda, NY: Multi-Health Systems, Inc., 1997b.

Conners K, Staff MHS: Conners' Continuous Performance Test II. North Tonawanda, NY: Multi-Health Systems Inc., 2000.

Conners CK, Wells K: Conners-Wells' Self-Report Scale. North Tonawanda, NY: Multi-Health Systems, Inc., 1997.

Costa LD, Scarola LM, Rapin I: Purdue Pegboard scores for grammar school children. Perceptual and Motor Skills: 18; 748, 1964.

Delis DC, Kaplan E, Kramer JH: Delis–Kaplan Executive Function System. San Antonio, TX: The Psychological Corporation, 2001.

Delis DC, Kramer JH, Kaplan E, Ober BA: California Verbal Learning Test-Children's Version. San Antonio, TX: The Psychological Corporation, 1994.

Denckla MB: Development of speed in repetitive and successive finger movements in normal children. Developmental Medicine and Child Neurology: 15(5); 635–645, 1973.

Denckla MB: Biological correlates of learning and attention: What is relevant to learning disability and attention-deficit hyperactivity disorder. Journal of Developmental and Behavioral Pediatrics 17(2); 114–119, 1996.

DiSimoni FD: The Token Test for Children. Boston, MA: Teaching Resources Corporation, 1978.

Fletcher JM, Miner ME, Ewing-Cobbs L: Age and recovery from head injury in children: Developmental issues. In Levin HS, Grafman J, Eisenberg HM (Eds), Neurobehavioral Recovery from Head Injury. New York: Oxford University Press, 1987.

Fridlund AJ, Delis DC: CVLT-C Scoring Assistant with Report Writer. San Antonio, TX: The Psychological Corporation, 1998.

Gaddes WH, Crockett DJ: The Spreen–Benton Aphasia Tests: Normative data as a measure of normal language development. Brain and Language: 2; 257–280, 1975.

Gansler DA, Fucetola R, Krengel M, Stestson S, Zimering R, Makary C: Are there cognitive subtypes in adult attention deficit/hyperactivity disorder? Journal of Nervous and Mental Disease: 186(12); 776–781, 1998.

Gardner MF: 1981: Expressive One-Word Picture Vocabulary Test. Novato, CA: Academic Therapy, 1981.

Gardner RA, Broman M: The Purdue Pegboard: Normative data on 1334 schoolchildren. Journal of Clinical Child Psychology: 8; 156–162, 1979.

Golden JC: Stroop Color and Word Test. Chicago, IL: Stoelting, 1978.

Goldman R, Fristoe M, Woodstock RW: Auditory Skills Battery. Circle Pines, MN: American Guidance Service, 1976.

Goodenough FL, Harris DB: Goodenough–Harris Drawing Test. New York: Psychological Corporation, 1963.

Goodman WK, Price LH, Rasmussen SA, Mazure C, Delgado P, Heninger GR, Charney DS: The Yale–Brown Obsessive–Compulsive Scale (Y-BOCS), Part II: Validity. Archives of General Psychiatry: 46; 1012–1016, 1989a.

Goodman WK, Price LH, Rasmussen SA, Mazure C, Fleischmann RL, Hill CL, Heninger GR, Charney DS: The Yale–Brown Obsessive–Compulsive Scale (Y-BOCS), Part I: Development, use and reliability. Archives of General Psychiatry: 46; 1012–1016, 1989b.

Gordon M: Microprocessor-based assessment of Attention Deficit Disorders. Psychopharm. Bull.: 22; 288–290, 1986.

Grant DA, Berg EA: A behavioral analysis of degree of impairment and ease of shifting to new responses in a Weigl-type card sorting problem. Journal of Experimental Psychology: 39; 404–411, 1948.

Greenberg L, Leark RA, Dupuy TR, Clifford MS, Corman CL, Kindschi DL, Cenedela M: Test of Variables of Attention. Los Alamitos, CA: Universal Attention Disorders, Inc., 1998a.

Greenberg L, Leark RA, Dupuy TR, Clifford MS, Corman CL, Kindschi DL, Cenedela M: Test of Variables of Attention — Auditory. Los Alamitos, CA: Universal Attention Disorders, Inc., 1998b.

Greenblatt E, Mattis S, Trade VP: Nature and prevalence of learning disabilities in a child psychiatric population. Developmental Neuropsychology: 6(2); 71–83, 1990.

Guy W: Physical and neurological examination for soft signs (PANESS). In Guy W (Ed), ECDEU Assessment Manual for Psychopharmacology. Rockville, MD: National Institute of Mental Health, 1976.

Halperin JM, Healy JM, Zeitschick E, Ludman WL, Weinstein L: Developmental aspects of linguistic and mnestic abilities in normal children. Journal of Clinical and Experimental Neuropsychology: 11; 518–528, 1989.

Halperin JM, Wolf LE, Pascualvaca DM, Newcorn JH, Healey JM, O'Brien JD, Morganstein AM, Young JF: Differential assessment of attention and impulsivity in children. Journal of the American Academy of Child and Adolescent Psychiatry: 27(3); 326–329, 1988.

Hammill DD, Larsen SC: Test of Written Language (3rd ed.). Austin, TX: Pro-ed., 1996.

Heaton RK: Wisconsin Card Sorting Test Manual. Odessa, FL: Psychological Assessment Resources, 1981.

Heaton RK, Staff PAR: Wisconsin Card Sorting Test: Computer Version 3. Odessa, FL: Psychological Assessment Resources, Inc., 1999.

Hecaen H: Acquired aphasia in children: revised. Neuropsychologia: 21; 581–587, 1983.

Hesslinger B, Thiel T, Tebartz van Elst L, Hennig F, Ebert D: Attention-deficit disorder in adults with and without hyperactivity: Where is the difference? A study in humans using short echo (1) H-magnetic resonance spectroscopy. Neurosciences Letter: 18; 304(1–2); 117–119, 2001.

Hood LJ, Berlin CI: Central auditory function and evaluation of auditory processing disorders. In Segalowitz SJ, Rapin I (Eds), Child Neuropsychology, Handbook of Neuropsychology, 2nd Edition, vol. 8, part II. Amsterdam: Elsevier, chapter 19, 2003.

Jantzen K, Mattis S: Dyslexia and graphomotor dyscoordination. J. Educ. Neuropsychol.: 4(1); 1–13, 1986.

Kaplan EF, Goodglass H, Weintraub S: The Boston Naming Test. Boston, MA: Kaplan and Goodglass, 1978.

Kaplan EF, Goodglass H, Weintraub S: The Boston Naming Test (2nd ed.). Philadelphia, PA: Lea and Febiger, 1983.

Kaufman AS, Kaufman NL: K-ABC: Kaufman Assessment Battery for Children. Circle Pines, MN: American Guidance Service, 1983.

Keith RW: Auditory Continuous Performance Test. San Antonio, TX: The Psychological Corporation, 1994.

Kinsbourne M, Warrington EK: A study of finger agnosia. Brain: 85; 47–66, 1962.

Klonoff H, Low M: Disordered brain function in young children and early adults: neuropsychological and electroencephalographic correlates. In Reitan RM, Davison LA (Eds), Clinical Neuropsychology: Current Status and Applications. Washington, DC: Winston and Sons, 1974.

Koppitz EM: The Bender Gestalt Test of Young Children. New York: Grune and Stratton, 1963.

Levin HS, Ewing-Cobbs L, Eisenberg HM: Neurobehavioral outcome of pediatric head injury. In Broman SH, Michel ME (Eds), Traumatic Head Injury in Children. New York: Oxford University Press, 1995.

Lezak MD: Neuropsychological Assessment (3rd ed.). New York: Oxford University Press, 1995.

Lindamood P, Bell N, Lindamood P: Sensory-cognitive factors in the controversy over reading instruction. Journal of Developmental and Learning Disorders: 1(1); 143–182, 1997.

Lindamood P, Bell N, Lindamood P: Issues in phonological awareness assessment. Annals of Dyslexia: 42; 242–259, 1992.

Lockwood KA, Marcotte AC, Stern C: Differentiation of attention-deficit/hyperactivity disorder subtypes: Application of a neuropsychological model of attention. Journal of Clinical and Experimental Neuropsychology: 23(3); 317–330, 2001.

Luria AR: Human Brain and Psychological Processes. New York: Harper and Row, 1966.

MacGinite WH, MacGinite RK, Maria K, Dreyer LG: Gates–MacGinite Reading Tests. Itaska, IL: Riverside Publishing, 2000.

Mattis S, French JH, Rapin I: Dyslexia in children and young adults: Three independent neuropsychological syndromes. Developmental Medicine and Child Neurology: 17; 150–163, 1975.

Meyers JE, Meyers KR: Rey Complex Figure Test and Recognition Trial. Odessa, FL: Psychological Assessment Resources, 1995.

Mostofsky SH, Reiss AL, Lockhart P, Denckla MB: Evaluation of cerebellar size in attention-deficit hyperactivity disorder. Journal of Child Neurology: (9); 434–439, 1998.

Murray HA: Explorations in Personality. NY: Oxford University Press, 1938.

Naglieri JA, McNeish TJ, Bardos AN: Draw a Person: Screening Procedure for Emotional Disturbance. Austin, TX: Pro-ed., 1991.

Osterreith PA: Le test de copie d'une figure complexe. Arch. Psychol. (France): 31; 206–356, 1944.

Owen AM, Downes JJ, Sahakian BJ, Polkey CE, Robbins TW: Planning and spatial working memory deficits following frontal lobe lesions in man. Neuropsychologia: (28); 1021–1034, 1990.

Pennington BF, Groissir D, Welsh MC: Contrasting cognitive deficits in attention deficit hyperactivity disorder versus reading disability. Dev. Psych.: (29); 511–523, 1993.

Phelps-Terasaki D, Phelps-Gunn T: Test of Pragmatic Language. Austin, TX: Pro-ed., 1992.

Purdue Research Foundation: Examiner's Manual for the Purdue Pegboard. Chicago, IL: Science Research Associates, 1948.

Raven JC: Progressive Matrices: A Perceptual Test of Intelligence: Individual Form. London: H.K. Lewis, 1938.

Raven JC: Colored Progressive Matrices Sets A, Ab, B. London: H.K. Lewis, 1947.

Raven JC: Guide to Using the Raven Coloured Progressive Matrices. London: H.K. Lewis, 1965.

Reitan RM: Manual for Administration of Neuropsychological Test Batteries for Adults and Children. Tuscon, AZ: Reitan Neuropsychological Laboratory, 1979.

Reitan RM, Davison LA: Clinical Neuropsychology: Current Status and Applications. New York: John Wiley and Sons, 1974.

Reynolds CR, Kamphaus RW: Behavioral Assessment System for Children. Circle Pines, MN: American Guidance Service, 1992.

Richardson E, DiBenedetto B: The Decoding Skills Test. Parkton, MD: York Press, 1985.

Rorschach H: Psychodiagnostics: A Diagnostic Test Based on Perception (Translated by Lemkau P and Kronenburg B). Berne: Huber, 1942.

Rosvold HE, Mirsky AT, Sarason I, Bronsome ED, Beck LH: A Continuous Performance Test of brain damage. J. Consult. Psychol.: 20; 343–350, 1956.

Rourke BP: The syndrome of Nonverbal Learning Disabilities: Developmental manifestations in neurological disease, disorder, and dysfunction. Clin. Neuropsychol.: 2(4); 293–330, 1988.

Rourke BP: Nonverbal Learning Disabilities: The Syndrome and the Model. New York: Guilford Press, 1989.

Said JA, Shores A, Batchelor J, Thomas D, Fahey P: The Children's Auditory–Verbal Selective Reminding Test: Equivalence and test–retest reliability of two forms with boys and girls. Developmental Neuropsychology: 6(3); 225–230, 1990.

Schmidt M: Rey Auditory Verbal Learning Test: A Handbook. Los Angeles, CA: Western Psychological Services, 1998.

Seashore CE, Lewis D, Saetveit DL: Seashore Measures of Musical Talents (rev. ed.). New York: Psychological Corporation, 1960.

Simon HA: The functional equivalence of problem solving skills. Cognitive Psychology: 7; 268–288, 1975.

Spreen O: The relationship between learning disabilities, emotional disorders and neuropsychology: some results and observations. Journal of Clinical and Experimental Neuropsychology: 11(1); 117–140, 1989.

Spreen O, Benton AL: Neurosensory Center Comprehensive Examination for Aphasia. Victoria: University of Victoria, Neuropsychology Laboratory, 1969.

Spreen O, Benton AL: Neurosensory Center Comprehensive Examination for Aphasia. Victoria: University of Victoria, Neuropsychology Laboratory, 1977.

Spreen O, Strauss E: A Compendium of Neuropsychological Tests (2nd ed.). New York: Oxford University Press, 1998.

Taylor HG: Childhood sequelae of early neurological disorders: A contemporary perspective. Developmental Neuropsychology: 3(2); 153–164, 1987.

The Psychological Corporation: The Wechsler Individual Achievement Test (2nd ed.). San Antonio, TX: The Psychological Corporation, 2001.

Thorndike RL, Hagen EP, Sattler JM: Stanford–Binet Intelligence Scale (4th ed.). Chicago, IL: Riverside Publishing Company, 1986.

Torgesen JK, Mathes PG: Basic Guide to Understanding, Assessing and Teaching Phonological Awareness. Austin, TX: Pro-ed., 2000.

Trommer BC, Hoeppner JB, Lorber R, Amstrong KJ: The Go–No-Go paradigm in attention deficit disorder. Annals of Neurology: 24; 60–614, 1988.

Waber DP, Holmes JM: Assessing children's copy productions of the Rey–Osterreith Complex Figure. Journal of Clinical and Experimental Neuropsychology: 7; 264–280, 1985.

Waber DP, Holmes JM: Assessing children's memory productions of the Rey–Osterreith Complex Figure. Journal of Clinical and Experimental Neuropsychology: 8; 563–580, 1986.

Wechsler D: Wechsler Intelligence Scale for Children (3rd ed.). San Antonio, TX: The Psychological Corporation, 1991.

Werry JS, Aman MG: The reliability and diagnostic validity of the physical and neurological examination for soft signs (PANESS). J. Autism Child. Schizophr.: 6; 253–262, 1976.

Wiederholt JL, Bryant BR: Gray Oral Reading Test (4th ed.). Itasca, IL: Riverside Publishing, 2001.

Wiig EH, Secord WA, Secord W: Clinical Evaluation of Language Fundamentals (3rd ed.). San Antonio, TX: The Psychological Corporation, 1995.

Wilkinson GS: Wide Range Achievement Test (3rd ed.). Wilmington, DE: Wide Range Inc., 1993.

Woodcock RW, McGrew KS, Mather N: Woodcock–Johnson III Tests of Achievement. Itasca, IL: Riverside Publishing, 2001a.

Woodcock RW, McGrew KS, Mather N: Woodcock–Johnson III Tests of Cognitive Abilities. Itaska, IL: Riverside Publishing, 2001b.

CHAPTER 13

# Behavioral fluctuations and the development of manual asymmetries in infancy: contributions of the dynamic systems approach

Daniela Corbetta [a],* and Esther Thelen [b]

[a] *Department of Health and Kinesiology, and Department of Psychological Sciences, Purdue University, Lambert Fieldhouse, 800 West Stadium Avenue, West Lafayette, IN 47907-2046, USA*
[b] *Department of Psychology, Indiana University, 1101 E 10th Street, Bloomington, IN 47405, USA*

## Introduction

The brain is endowed with striking functional asymmetries. These asymmetries are manifest in multiple behavioral lateralities. Some are obvious, such as preferring to use the right arm or right leg for tasks such as writing and kicking. Others, less obvious, but easily evidenced through neuropsychological testing, reveal distinct aptitudes between right and left hemispaces, such as a right ear or right eye advantage for processing verbal information, versus a left ear, left eye, and left hand advantage for processing music, recognizing faces, or identifying objects by touch, respectively (see Corballis and Beale, 1984; Hellige, 1993; Springer and Deutsch, 1989, for reviews).

Brain and behavioral asymmetries have been described since the 18th century (Marshall and Magoun, 1998). Since then, they have become an undeniable and fundamental aspect of the neuropsychological organization of the human brain. However, the question of whether these asymmetries are inborn or acquired during the first years of life has remained a continuous and vivid debate for many decades. Still today, we do not know what makes a person prefer to use one hand for certain tasks more than the other, or, what makes a person more efficient at processing some information with one hemisphere more than the other.

In this chapter, we critically reappraise some of the literature that addressed the origins of brain and behavioral asymmetries. We focus on the development of manual asymmetries and, in particular, review infant studies which asked about the early forms and developmental roots of human manual asymmetries. In our survey, we show that researchers initially sought to identify whether functional asymmetries were present at birth. Then, researchers studied how these early asymmetries predicted later hand preference and developed during the first years of life. As we will see, most researchers in this area explained their findings by adopting one of two opposing theoretical views. Some stressed the role of experience and environment in the emergence and formation of manual asymmetries. Others, in contrast, advocated biologically preformed asymmetries from early in life.

In this chapter, we identify problems and inadequacies with both of these views and present an alternative, contemporary theory inspired by the dynamic systems perspective. We argue that the development of functional manual asymmetries is not simply the result of a single genetic or environmental factor.

---

* Corresponding author. E-mail: dcorbet@purdue.edu

Rather, manual asymmetries emerge as the product of complex processes that involve the continuous and intertwined reorganization of multiple biological and experiential factors that change and evolve as infants grow. To support our claims, we present evidence from our own research laboratories. In conclusion, we briefly expand our argument to functional asymmetries in other domains, such as language and face processing, to illustrate that both cognitive and perceptual-motor functional asymmetries may result from similarly complex developmental processes.

## Newborns' spontaneous behavioral asymmetries: searching for the origins of human handedness

There are two undisputed facts about human handedness. The first one is that an overwhelming majority of people, across many cultures, display a strong dextral bias to perform tasks such as writing, throwing, or hammering. The second one is that this strong dextral population bias is unique to humans and has not been consistently reported in other species, nor consistently observed in nonhuman primates (see for example, Corballis, 1991; MacNeilage, Studdert-Kennedy and Lindblom, 1987; Warren, 1980).

This striking and unique phenomenon has stimulated tremendous scientific curiosity about the origins of human brain organization and raised many questions about how humans develop such strong lateral biases. As a result, many diverse proposals about the origins of human handedness have been offered. Nonetheless, all these proposals boil down to one fundamental issue: the well-known nature/nurture debate. In the last two decades especially, there have been many studies asking whether handedness is inherited or influenced by the environment (see for example, Carter-Saltzman, 1980; Laland, Kumm, Van Horn and Feldman, 1995; Longstreth, 1980; Orlebeke, Knol, Koopmans et al., 1996; Tambs, Magnus and Berg, 1987, to cite a few). Some authors have adopted an extreme position in this debate, favoring either a nature or a nurture account. On the nature side are accounts based on genetic models (see for example, Annett, 1972, 1985; Levy and Nagylaki, 1972; McManus, 1985). Nurture accounts, on the other hand, have attempted to link the origins of human handedness to various factors such as biased social environments (Harkins and

Michel, 1988; Harkins and Uzgiris, 1991; Provins, 1997), asymmetrical in-utero position of the fetus (Michel and Goodwin, 1979; Previc, 1991), or biased sensory-motor experience (Coryell and Michel, 1978; Harkins and Michel, 1988; Provins, 1997).

Infant researchers have been active participants in this nature/nurture debate. One approach has been to look for evidence of asymmetry in the spontaneous movements of newborn and young infants. These researchers reasoned that if behavioral asymmetries could be found in newborns, it would indicate that the direction of handedness and hemispheric specialization is already established at birth. If, instead, asymmetries were not seen in newborns, it would indicate that hand preference and hemispheric specialization develop progressively through infancy and early childhood (Lenneberg, 1967).

Indeed, scientists have been very successful at identifying consistent behavioral asymmetries in newborns that could be linked to both later hand preference and the population specific dextral bias. In particular, they reported rightward biases in spontaneous head orientation (Coryell, 1985; Coryell and Michel, 1978; Gesell, 1938; Harris and Fitzgerald, 1983; Hopkins, Lems, Wulfften-Palthe et al., 1990; Michel, 1981; Michel and Harkins, 1986; Turkewitz, Gordon and Birch, 1965; Viviani, Turkewitz and Karp, 1978), in neonatal reflexes (Trehub, Corter and Shosenberg, 1983), in hand closure (Cobb, Goodwin and Saelens, 1966), and grasping abilities (Caplan and Kinsbourne, 1976; Hawn and Harris, 1983).

But do these early asymmetries in spontaneous behavior truly correspond to the direction of later hand preference? Studies on newborns' spontaneous head orientation have been particularly successful in addressing this issue (Coryell, 1985; Coryell and Michel, 1978; Michel, 1981; Viviani et al., 1978). These studies showed that most newborns prefer to rotate their heads to the right, and they also demonstrated that for most infants this preferred head orientation corresponded to the direction of later handedness. However, interpretations of the processes underlying this match between newborns' head orientation and later hand preference differed quite dramatically. Some studies claimed that these lateral biases were the result of a progressively stronger right-biased visuo-motor experience during early development (Coryell and Michel, 1978; Viviani et al., 1978). Others interpreted the same data as revealing an underlying genetically based right shift (Annett, 1972, 1985; Coryell, 1985).

Here is how each line of argument was supported. The visuo-motor experience interpretation, based on Gesell and Ames' (1947) original proposal, posited that because newborns rotate their head to one side when in supine and adopt an asymmetrical tonic reflex, they end up looking more at the one hand that is located in the visual field on that same side. Because infants adopt this asymmetrical posture, they increase their chances of perceiving the self-produced movements of the seen ipsilateral hand. This presumably reinforces lateral eye–hand connections, and increases the likelihood that infants will prefer to use that hand more than the other in the future.

The genetic explanation, on the other hand, relied on the fact that the relation between head orientation and later hand preference correlates highly when infants prefer to turn their head to the right, but does not correlate as strongly when infants prefer to turn their head to the left. Such findings support the predictions of Annett's right-shift model stipulating that a right-shift gene may be responsible for the right bias, and if this right-shift gene is missing, then chances of becoming right- or left-handed are equal (Annett, 1985).

## The discontinuous development of newborns' manual asymmetries

That newborns come into the world with distinct lateral biases is now well established. Lateral biases were identified in very young infants in other domains as well, such as in language processing (Bates, 1999a; Molfese and Molfese, 1979), non-speech stimulus processing (Hahn, 1987; Molfese and Molfese, 1980), or face perception (De Schonen, Gil de Diaz and Mathivet, 1986; De Schonen and Mathivet, 1990). But the question of how these early biases develop later into established functional hemispheric asymmetries still remains open to debate. Do these newborn spontaneous asymmetries constitute a sufficient substrate to form established and directional functional asymmetries later in life? Beyond the correlational studies reported above, do

newborns' lateral biases remain age-invariant or do they change as infants grow older? When we begin to ask the question of the developmental continuity between behavioral events occurring at distinct times, we discover that the links and processes between these events are not always straightforward. Moreover, explanations based on either a nature or nurture assumption become largely unsatisfactory. Let us define more concretely where the problem lies by returning to the development of hand preference.

One puzzling issue regarding the development of spontaneous head orientation and the establishment of later hand preference is that there is no real continuous and logical developmental progression between the two behaviors. Regardless of whether one favors a genetic or experience-related explanation, one should expect that these early preferred biases develop either into stable and consistent asymmetries, or into increasingly greater asymmetries, such as using one hand progressively more than the other. But longitudinal reports which have followed the development of head orientation and hand preference during infancy have shown that this is not what happens. Rather, they pointed out the highly discontinuous and fluctuating developmental nature of these early lateral biases.

First, a longitudinal study from Harris and Fitzgerald (1983) which tracked changes in newborns' supine spontaneous head orientation during the first 3 months of life, revealed that the initial preferred head orientations were not maintained consistently throughout the 3 months of observations. Harris and Fitzgerald (1983) reported that some infants shifted their head to the right, then to the left alternately each month, and many infants revealed a decline in preferred lateral head orientation, showing an increased preference for adopting a midline position as they became older. Recently, two other longitudinal studies replicated these findings and similarly reported that whether in supine or seated, infants increasingly prefer to adopt a midline head position during the weeks preceding the onset of reaching (Hopkins et al., 1990; Spencer, Vereijken, Diedrich and Thelen, 2000). If this period preceding the onset of reaching is critical for strengthening connections between eye and hand coordination, how do these connections become lateralized when infants do not maintain a consistent lateral head orientation?

Other studies that tracked changes in infant reaching and object manipulation during the first years of life also demonstrated inconsistent lateral preferences in infants (Carlson and Harris, 1985; Corbetta and Thelen, 1999; Gesell and Ames, 1947; Provins, Dalziel and Higginbottom, 1987; Ramsay, 1984, 1985a,b; Ramsay and Willis, 1984; Young, 1977). These studies reported very unstable and changing patterns of hand use in infants, with highly fluctuating and individually defined developmental profiles. For example, at any given week or month, some infants used mostly their right hand to reach for an object presented at midline. But the following week or month, the same infants would use their left hand to reach for the same object. Moreover, fluctuations in right- versus left-hand use were reported to be combined with fluctuations in one- versus two-handed reaching, as if lateral biases were alternately appearing and disappearing at different developmental periods (Corbetta and Thelen, 1996; Corbetta and Thelen, 1999; Fagard and Pezé, 1997; Gesell and Ames, 1947). Finally, some studies pointed out that these fluctuations in the direction of hand preference continued until later in childhood (Gesell and Ames, 1947). Indeed, according to some authors the direction of hand preference can only be assessed with certainty from the age of 3 years old (McManus, Sik, Cole et al., 1988).

These findings clearly reveal that hand preference does not strengthen progressively as a function of time, nor does it show a consistent underlying right shift. Instead manual lateral preferences fluctuate, revert, and change abruptly many times throughout the first 3 years of life before settling into a defined and preferred direction. This neither strictly supports a nature nor a nurture account. What then are the processes underlying these developmental changes? And how do lateral biases arise from such a fluctuating developmental picture? While it is clear that infants display identifiable behavioral asymmetries from the first days of life, the mechanisms linking these early asymmetries to later functional lateralization still remain highly unclear.

One possible answer to this developmental puzzle — one that has not been much explored — might be that these successive shifts and fluctuations in hand preference occur as a result of other developing skills. In the rest of this chapter, we expand on these

ideas by showing: (1) that early instabilities in lateral preferences reflect successive cognitive, sensory, and motor reorganizations as infants develop a wide array of new skills, and (2), that these reorganizations are not preset nor the result of preprogrammed developmental factors, but rather the emergent property of combined biological, sensory-motor, and environmental factors that change and interact with each other as infants grow and develop. In the following sections we present the main theoretical foundations that guided our interpretation, followed by supporting data from our research laboratories.

## Developmental changes are multileveled and multirelational

During the first 3 years of life, infants and children acquire a vast number of adaptive skills. These skills range from learning to control posture, to developing eye–hand coordination, manipulating objects, locomoting, communicating, first with gestures, then with language, and apprehending the basic social rules and physical laws that govern varied cultural and environmental settings. The development of each of these fundamental skills has been studied in exquisite details. Typically, researchers have focused only on one of these different sensory-motor, cognitive, or social areas. Such specialization has led to great advances. The drawback is that it lacked providing a more comprehensive picture of development. More fundamentally, specialization has prevented scientists from understanding how a child's developing brain acquires the ability not only to master all these skills in such a short time, but also to integrate them together. This question of skill integration is central to brain development and we believe it to be closely related to the developmental discontinuities and fluctuations of lateralization of functions that we discussed so far. It is very possible indeed that the lateralization of functions, their developmental stabilization, and the emergence of hand preference proceed along with the development and integration of these multiple early skills. But the only way to verify such account would be to study how these different skills co-evolve during early development.

Although this has been an underrepresented approach in developmental research, some studies have investigated developmental links between different areas of study. For instance, certain studies have tried to assess how language, handedness, and object manipulation develop and lateralize in relation to each other. In particular, a series of studies from Ramsay (Ramsay, 1980a,b, 1984, 1985a; Ramsay, Campos and Fenson, 1979) have shown that changing patterns in handedness were related to specific milestones in speech development. Interestingly, Ramsay found that early handedness successively emerged and declined as infants began to produce duplicate babbling around 7–9 months, then, when they produced their first words around 12–14 months, and again when they formed their first sentences around 20 months old. Similarly, Bates, O'Connell, Vaid et al. (1986) found that strength in hand preference changed between 13 and 28 months old as infants solved novel linguistic problems. In particular, Bates et al. (1986) observed that the strength of hand preference declined around 20 months old when language emerged. Together, these studies revealed that early hand preference did not fluctuate randomly, but appeared and disappeared as infants learned and developed new cognitive skills.

Similar interactions between developmental domains were observed in other areas of study. For example, some research investigated how patterns of upper arm interlimb coordination changed as infants achieved new motor milestones such as sitting or crawling on hands and knees. In particular, Rochat (1992) and Goldfield (1993) found that both the mastery of sitting and the emergence of crawling reduced the rate of initial bilateral two-handed responses in infant reaching and facilitated the formation of one-handed responses. In other areas, involving more specifically infants' perceptual-motor and cognitive skills, researchers found that the emergence of new forms of locomotion (i.e. the use of walkers, crawling, or walking) had a significant impact on infants' understanding of spatial layouts and object locations (Adolph, 1997; Bertenthal, Campos and Barrett, 1984; Kermoian and Campos, 1988).

Thus, when scientists have studied multiple behaviors at once, they discovered that changes and progresses in the different domains were not independent from each other. Rather, these domains influenced each other in various and non-linear ways. In particular, sudden and abrupt changes, say, in lat-erality, motor patterning, and/or cognitive abilities appeared to be the product of changes and learning processes taking place in other areas of development. Moreover, these studies suggested that these developmental changes are complex and multicausal. For example, learning to crawl has an impact on laterality, but also on spatial understanding. Likewise, changes in laterality are affected by learning to sit and crawl, but also by learning to talk. In fact, these findings contrast quite dramatically from the nature or nurture views reviewed above that propose a single cause explanation to hand preference, or offer linear developmental mechanisms. When several behaviors are viewed at once, development is multileveled, multirelational, and highly non-linear (Thelen, 1986).

## A dynamic systems account of the development of hand preference

We believe that the non-linear and fluctuating development of hand preference is the product of such multileveled and multirelational developmental processes. Hand preference shifts during the first years of life because it is sensitive to important developmental changes that occur in other cognitive, perceptual and motor domains. However, before we expand and support this idea, we review the major theoretical premises that underlie it.

Dynamic systems theory is the framework that has emerged over the last two decades to study such nonlinear and multiple causal phenomena. Dynamic systems theory has been particularly successful for understanding many different aspects of development, including brain and behavioral development (Fischer and Rose, 1994), general developmental theory (Van Geert, 1994, 1998), and infant action and cognition (Smith and Thelen, 1993; Thelen and Smith, 1994, 1997; Thelen and Ulrich, 1991). Here, we briefly summarize the main tenets of that theoretical framework, and refer the reader to the above-mentioned literature for more complete accounts and applications of this approach.

Dynamic systems offer a general theory of change. More specifically, dynamic systems propose a framework to comprehend and capture the processes underlying the transitions occurring in any systems (whether biological or physical) when shifting from one mode of functioning to another mode of functioning.

One fundamental assumption of this framework is that behavior and change arise and *self-organize* from a complex web of interactions between an ensemble of contributing components. These components can be any elements defining the organism and the environment in which the organism resides. Precisely because these patterns of interaction between components are complex, it is impossible to establish a hierarchical order or privileged status to one or another of these components. For example, a maturing brain or a specific gene could not be considered more important than the level of experience, energetic status, or social environment that defines and interacts with the behavioral characteristics of an organism at a given point in time. Moreover, that behavior *self-organizes* also means that no pre-existing structure or plan contains the instructions of how the different components will successively be reassembled at different points in time. Therefore, according to dynamic systems, shifts in behavioral patterning, such as shifts in hand preference, for example, can neither be viewed as result of a single factor nor considered as the expression of a developmental plan.

A second fundamental assumption of dynamic systems is that patterns of change can only be understood as a function of time. Time reflects the history of a system and its transitions from one functional state to another. Any behavioral configuration at a given point in time is the result of previous pattern configurations and, at the same time, contributes to the formation of future pattern configurations. Therefore, capturing and understanding the processes underlying behavioral changes in a system can only be performed by tracking behavior as a function of continuous time scales.

Finally, directly linked to the assumption that patterns self-organize and form from complex interactions between multiple elements, change can arise from any modification that can occur in one or more of the contributing components. Such change can affect the dynamics of interaction between components and alter the stability of the behavior. Stability and instability, which can be inferred from the characteristics of variability of the behavior, are used as the metric of change. A highly variable behavior reflects unstable underlying dynamics, and expresses

that change, reassembly, or reorganization between components may be taking place. On the contrary, a consistent behavior that displays little variability reveals that its underlying dynamics are stable and no reorganizations or reassembly between components are likely to take place.

If we apply these dynamic systems concepts to the development of hand preference, we can draw the following conclusions: (1) that early unstable hand preference may emerge as one or more components change as infants grow and develop new skills; (2) and that later hand preference may become more stable, because these component changes become more subtle or only involve a fine-tuning within already existing dynamics. Important component changes may be linked to many fundamental physical, motor, and cognitive events that occur especially during the first 3 years of life, a time of rapid rate of physical and neural growth. During these years, infants gain the foundations of most lifelong fundamental skills, such as sitting, walking, and communicating with words. Any dramatic behavioral change may have tremendous potentials to modify the functional outcomes of the system at different points in time. Hand preference may be one functional outcome that may be affected by changes in other concurrent developing skills. Likewise, hand preference may stabilize and consolidate after 3 years because by that time most fundamental skills and component changes have already taken place. Indeed, after 3 years growth rate declines significantly and fundamental skills mainly undergo fine-tuning rather than complete and novel reorganizations.

For example, we mentioned earlier studies that found a decline in hand preference during the periods in which new language skills emerged (Bates et al., 1986; Ramsay, 1980a,b, 1984, 1985a). A transition in language development must reflect an important change in previously existing dynamics between components. Thus, the ensemble of existing skills must reassemble to *integrate* the newly emerging language skills. As argued by these authors, emerging language capabilities which are controlled by the left hemisphere may temporarily compete with other left hemisphere functions involving, for example, arm control. But, other newly emerging skills, not necessarily related to language development, may also disrupt hand preference. In our laboratories we have explored how the emergence of specific motor milestones such as developing arm control, sitting, crawling and walking may similarly affect the stability of infants' preferred manual biases. We report our findings in the following sections.

## Change in reaching control, posture, locomotion, and hand preference

We discuss first an extensive longitudinal study on infant reaching that we and many collaborators designed from an explicit dynamic systems approach. The purpose of this study was to map out multiple reaching behavioral components as a function of time. Such a dense, multileveled longitudinal design enabled us to identify periods of stability and change between components and identify specific developmental transitions in response patterns. Then, we used these observations to generate hypotheses about how the system reorganized during these specific developmental transitions. These hypotheses were then tested further in follow-up studies, which we will report in the next sections.

In this first longitudinal study, we mapped multiple reaching behavioral components by tracking changes in arm control and trajectory formation (Thelen et al., 1993, 1996), in interlimb coordination and laterality (Corbetta and Thelen, 1996, 1999), in muscle patterns (Spencer and Thelen, 2000) and in posture (Spencer et al., 2000) in four infants followed weekly from 3 to 30 weeks old and then every other week until 52 weeks old. Moreover, we compared how goal-oriented patterns of reaching related to patterns of spontaneous upper arm activity. This allowed us to compare preferred patterns of reaching at different developmental periods to corresponding underlying coordination tendencies or general pervasive biases (Corbetta and Thelen, 1996, 1999; Thelen et al., 1993, 1996). In terms of hand preference, we asked about the impact of arm control development and postural transitions on the lateral stability of reaching during the first year. We addressed the following questions. Does the emergence of increased arm control later in the first year facilitate the stabilization of hand preference? Do the successive transitions to sitting and crawling, which were found by previous studies to disrupt bimanual coupling, contribute to increase lateral stability? And

do lateral biases and fluctuations in reaching reflect generalized preferred lateral tendencies and shifts in spontaneous upper arm activity?

This study revealed that all four infants displayed more stable and better controlled reaching patterns in the second half of the first year (Thelen et al., 1996). Despite this overall improvement in arm control, however, infants continued to display fluctuating patterns of interlimb activity and unstable lateral biases (Corbetta and Thelen, 1996, 1999). Periods of one-handed reaching alternated with periods of two-handed reaching, and all four infants displayed an early period of right-hand preference followed by a period of no preferred biases in reaching. We found indeed that lateral biases were more consistent during the weeks following reach onset than during the second half of the first year, suggesting that improvement in arm control did not contribute substantially to the formation of stable lateral preferences. Finally, the analysis of patterns of spontaneous upper arm activity confirmed that these patterns of fluctuation in interlimb coordination and lateral biases were neither specific to goal-oriented reaching nor dependent on arm control, but seemed rather linked to general and pervasive tendencies of the system. Indeed, patterns of spontaneous upper arm activity which were not performed to meet specific task demands also shifted and fluctuated in a fashion that was similar to that seen in reaching (Corbetta and Thelen, 1996, 1999).

Fig. 1 illustrates these developmental trends in reaching in one of these four infants, NQ, who first attained the target successfully at 12 weeks old. The two top graphs of Fig. 1 report the average weekly changes in the straightness of the trajectory (graph A) and the number of movement units (graph B) performed by the hand that first contacted the target. The straightness index was calculated by dividing the actual trajectory length covered by the hand from reach start to toy contact by the length corresponding to the straight distance between hand position at reach start and hand position at reach contact. The resulting numbers, which varied between 0 and 1, were then normalized using Fisher's $z$-score transform. We determined the number of movement units by summing the number of velocity peaks performed during each reaching movement toward the target. Movement units represent a good index of arm control since they reflect the number of directional changes

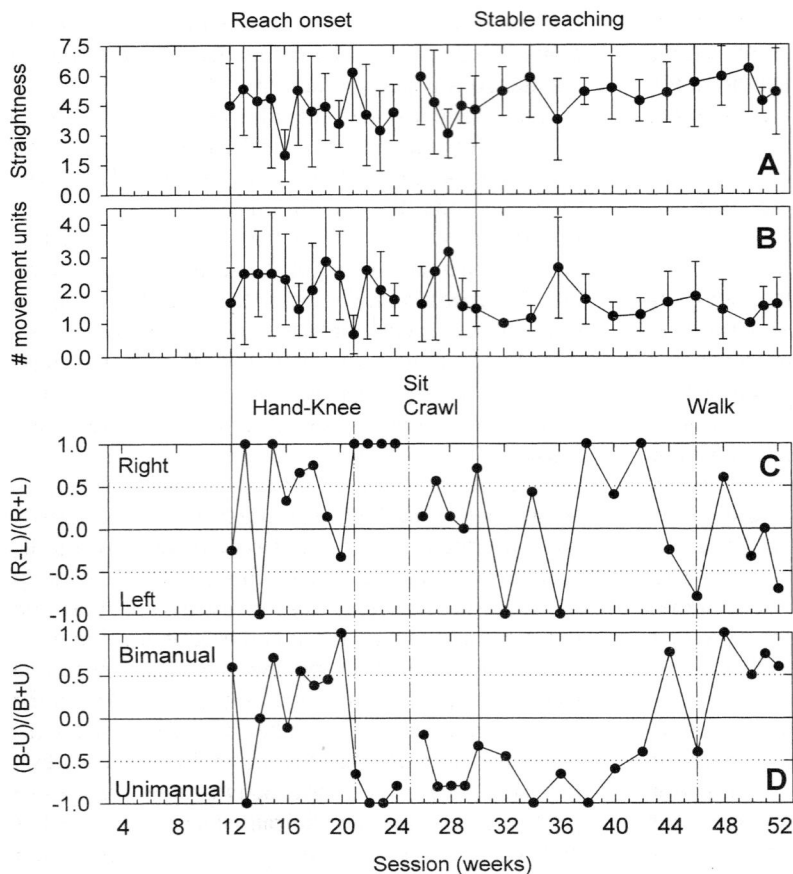

Fig. 1. Developmental change in reaching trajectory, hand use, and interlimb coordination in one infant, NQ, who was followed longitudinally from 3 to 52 weeks old. (A) Straightness of the reaching trajectory (mean and standard deviation) by week. (B) Number of movement units (mean and standard deviation) of the reaching hand path by week. (C) Hand used for reaching by week. (D) Pattern of interlimb coordination in reaching by week.

performed during the reaching trajectory (cf. Von Hofsten, 1991). In graph A, a higher index means that the trajectory is straighter. In graph B, a lower number of movement units means that less trajectory corrections were performed before attaining the target. Both graphs reveal two distinct developmental periods. During a first period following reach onset, both data curves fluctuate greatly revealing that early reaching trajectories were not consistently straight or smooth. The higher standard error bars around the means characteristic of this early period also reveal that reaching patterns were highly variable from trial to trial. From week 30, however, both curves display a more stable pattern over time with straighter trajectories, less movement units, and smaller error bars

around the means. This second more stable period indicates that, from week 30, NQ developed better arm control. We observed similar transitions in the other three infants (Thelen et al., 1996).

This increased arm control did not coincide, however, with greater stability in hand preference (Corbetta and Thelen, 1999). Graph C in Fig. 1 reports shifts in hand use for the same arm that contacted the target first. Hand use was indexed as the number of first right-hand toy contacts minus the number of first left-hand toy contacts, divided by the total number of toy contacts. This led to a value that varied from +1 to −1. A value of +1 meant that on those sessions NQ always contacted the toy with his right hand first and a value of −1 meant that on those sessions NQ always contacted the toy with his left hand first. Values in between meant that NQ reached the toy with either the right or left hand first; however, sometimes the right hand contacted the toy first more often (positive values), sometimes the left hand contacted the toy first more often (negative values), or sometimes both hands contacted the toy first the same number of times (zero value). Graph C reveals that during the first period following reach onset, NQ tended to contact the toys more often with his right hand first, although this rightward bias was quite unstable over time. After week 30, however, when his reaching skills became more stable, this right-handed bias disappeared. Indeed, when we averaged the hand preference index over these two developmental periods we found that during the first period, from week 12 to week 29, NQ's laterality index was of 0.420, while during the second period, from week 30 to week 52, NQ's hand preference index dropped to 0.004 revealing indeed that no lateral tendencies predominated in reaching during this second developmental period. In sum, lateral preferences became more unstable with improved reaching.

If improvement in arm control does not have a significant and lasting impact on the formation of stable lateral biases in reaching, what can account for the observed earlier right biased tendencies and their later disappearance? One possibility is that changes in lateral biases are not specifically linked to the formation of goal-oriented acts per se, but are rather sensitive to more general and pervasive component changes in the organism. This was suggested by the upper arm patterns observed in non-reaching movements. Indeed, when we analyzed NQ's self-generated, and freely performed spontaneous upper arm movements produced before and after reaching, we found shifts and fluctuations in lateral activity between arms that were similar to the lateral shifts observed in reaching. This was a consistent finding for all four infants. Interestingly, these spontaneous, self-generated movements were not performed as a function of goal and therefore did not respond to any particular task constraints or arm control requirement, nonetheless they revealed lateral shifts. This particular result strongly suggested that transitions and fluctuations in laterality were not specific to reaching but seemed more related to general and pervasive component changes in the system.

What are then these general and pervasive component changes in the system? One likely candidate is posture. The possibility that lateral changes in manual activity may be linked to changes in postural milestones has been considered before. We mentioned earlier that studies by Rochat (1992) and Goldfield (1993) found that the emergence of self-sitting and hands-and-knees crawling both acted to uncouple infants' initial bilateral tendencies and favored the emergence of lateral responses. Fig. 1 shows indeed that shifts in manual lateral patterning (graph C), and coupling between limbs (graph D) occurred around times when NQ developed new postural milestones such as sitting, crawling and walking.

Graph D, in particular, reports NQ's fluctuations in interlimb coupling between periods of bilateral reaching, when both arms were extended toward the target, and periods of unilateral reaching, when only one arm was extended toward the target (Corbetta and Thelen, 1996). A similar frequency index to the hand preference index was used to compute and report interlimb coordination as a function of the weekly sessions. Here, a positive index value indicates that NQ tended to reach more bimanualy, while a negative index value indicates that NQ tended to reach more unimanualy. Graph D in Fig. 1 shows that NQ had two bimanual periods, one right after the onset of reaching and another one at the end of the first year. In between, he primarily used one hand for reaching, but this unilateral reaching never matched consistent preferred hand use, except during 4 weeks, from week 21 to week 24, when NQ began reaching consistently with one hand.

In agreement with Rochat (1992) and Goldfield (1993), our data also show that these transitions in reaching coordination and lateral biases matched transitions in the development of new postural milestones. First, NQ's initial bimanual period disappeared when he began to adopt a hands-and-knees posture (Corbetta and Thelen, 1999). Then, NQ's right-handed tendency, that seemed to have stabilized after the disappearance of the first bimanual period, dissipated completely when NQ began to crawl on four limbs and sit alone (Corbetta and Thelen, 1999). Moreover, NQ returned to two-handed reaching when he began walking upright (Thelen and Smith, 1994). Therefore, these data seem consistent with the idea that successive shifts in posture and its control coincide with changes in the organization of the upper arm system. These data even suggest that some postural configurations may strengthen or weaken coupling tendencies between arms, by facilitating or hindering the expression of stable lateral preferences at certain developmental periods. We observed similar disruptions in lateral tendencies with the onset of crawling in the other infants (Corbetta and Thelen, 1999).

This first descriptive longitudinal study on reaching pointed to different factors that could affect transitions and stability in hand preference during the first year. In particular, it revealed that improvement in arm control may not play a substantial role in stabilizing hand preference and confirmed that posture may be a potential changing component that may affect lateral stability. However, our results were seriously limited by the small sample. With just these individual observations, we were not able to assert whether the observed developmental trends and shifts between components were truly representative of major developmental pathways common to most infants. The next step therefore was to reexamine the observed relationships between arm control, posture, and the stability of manual laterality with a larger sample. In the next section, we present two follow-up studies, still in progress, that were designed to reassess (1) the role of arm control on the stability of hand preference, (2) the decline of preferred lateral biases later in the first year, and (3) the respective postural influence of crawling and walking onsets on shifting patterns of hand preference.

## Arm control and hand preference

The fact that increase in arm control did not help stabilize hand preference later in the first year was puzzling and counterintuitive. Thus, we decided to investigate this issue further with a group of 12 infants that we followed every week from the age of 6.5 to about 8–9 months, that is, during the critical period when infants develop better control of their arms. In this study, however, we used a different task: a task that involved a complementary bimanual activity and division of labor. From the onset of the study, infants were invited to retrieve an attractive, symmetrically shaped rattle hidden in a box with a lid.

To achieve the task successfully, infants had to learn to coordinate and sequence their arms appropriately. That is, they had to learn to open the lid of the box with one or two hands, then hold the lid open with one hand while retrieving the toy from the box using the other hand. Previous studies using similar variations of this task demonstrated that, before the end of the first year, infants have difficulties in retrieving the toy from the box because they cannot sequence and time their arms appropriately to achieve this task (Bruner, 1970; Fagard and Pezé, 1997). Therefore, this task presented an adequate challenge to assess whether early coordination difficulties would alter the stability of hand preference and division of labor, and whether the progressive learning and consolidation of efficient coordination patterns would stabilize preferred hand use for opening the box, holding the lid, and retrieving the toy.

In order to track progress in bimanual coordination and change in hand preference as a function of time, we followed infants every week until they were able to perform stable coordination patterns with good sequencing and timing between arms. That is, infants did not hesitate between movement phases, they did not shift hand use in the process, and did not show interference between movements such as releasing the lid before having completely pulled the toy out of the box. Infants performed 6 trials per week. We ended our longitudinal observations when infants were able to perform stable and well timed coordination patterns on 5 out of 6 trials for 3 weeks in a row.

All infants began to successfully retrieve the toy from the box within their 3rd to 6th visit to the laboratory. Movements at first were poorly coordinated. Infants either attempted to use one hand to solve the task or displayed many timing problems between arm movements when using both arms in a complementary fashion. Remarkably, however, coordination difficulty did not seem to affect stability or instability in hand use for holding the lid and retrieving the toy. Seven out of the 12 infants displayed outstandingly stable division of labor throughout the successive weeks of testing. Despite initially struggling with the task, they consistently used the same hand for holding the lid or retrieving the toy. Five infants never revealed stable hand use throughout the study although they learned to coordinate their arms better. In either case, progress in bimanual coordination did not affect individually defined stable or unstable division of labor.

Fig. 2 shows two exemplars of representative infants with stable (EH two top graphs) and unstable (CS two bottom graphs) division of labor. These graphs illustrate bimanual performance, from the onset of the study until these infants were able to perform bimanual complementary patterns with good timing 5 out of 6 trials for 3 weeks in a row (our set criterion to end our longitudinal observations). For each example, the bar graphs report the percentage of the different retrieval strategies used every week according to four categories of behavior (failure, unimanual strategy, bimanual complementary strategy with poor timing, and bimanual complementary strategy with good timing). The line graphs underneath each bar graph show the corresponding patterns of preferred hand use for the different movement phases (opening, holding, and retrieving) from the week infants were able to retrieve the toy at least 50% of the trials. These data are reported using the same lateral index described before, where negative values represent a greater left-hand use and positive values represent a greater right-hand use.

Infant EH (top graphs) began to open and hold the lid of the box with her left hand and retrieved the toy with the right hand from week 3. Although there was some movement fluctuation in lid opening (sometimes EH used two hands for opening), both holding and retrieving phases of the movement were astonishingly consistent from week to week. Infant CS (bottom graphs), in contrast, displayed more variable hand use. CS began to retrieve the toy from the box successfully from week 5. During that first week, CS showed stable division of labor in hand use for holding and retrieving, but this stability was not maintained during the following weeks. CS displayed no hand preference for opening the lid, and although he showed an overall tendency to hold the lid with the right hand and retrieve the toy with the left hand, this division of labor was fluctuating over developmental time. Regardless of these differences in hand use stability, whether infants showed extremely consistent division of labor throughout the study (infant EH) or showed weaker division of labor (infant CS), this overall stability or instability in division of labor was not affected by progress

in bimanual coordination. Both examples reveal that during the last 3 weeks, when infants were able to perform well timed coordination patterns to solve this task, progress in bimanual coordination and control did not significantly affect infants' inherent stability or instability in hand use. This was a consistent finding in all 12 infants. In other words, this study confirmed our previous observations that progress in arm control does not contribute substantially to the formation and stabilization of hand preference.

## Do preferred lateral biases become more variable later in the first year?

A second puzzling result from our first longitudinal study on reaching was the decline of the early lateral biases in the last part of the first year. As illustrated in Fig. 1, NQ's hand use seemed to fluctuate more during the second part of the first year, revealing much greater variability in hand use as a function of time than after the onset of reaching. This result too seemed at first counterintuitive, thus we again decided to examine this developmental trend with a larger group of infants to see if we could replicate this finding. To do so, we compared the object retrieval data obtained with the twelve 6.5 to 8–9 months old infants reported above with object retrieval data obtained with another group of older infants that we followed longitudinally from 8 to 12–13 months old. This older group included ten infants. They were tested similarly to the younger group, with an identical box and object retrieval task, and also observed over time in weekly sessions. Variability in preferred hand use was determined for each movement phase (opening, holding, and retrieving) by averaging the weekly laterality indexes over the total number of visits to our laboratory (when infants were able to retrieve the toy) and by computing the standard deviation.

These data are reported in Fig. 3 for each infant as a function of movement phase and longitudinal group. As reported earlier, seven infants in the younger group (left panel) displayed remarkable stability in hand use for holding and retrieving from the time they were able to find the toy in the box. As a result, these infants displayed no or little hand use variability for holding the lid and retrieving the toy from

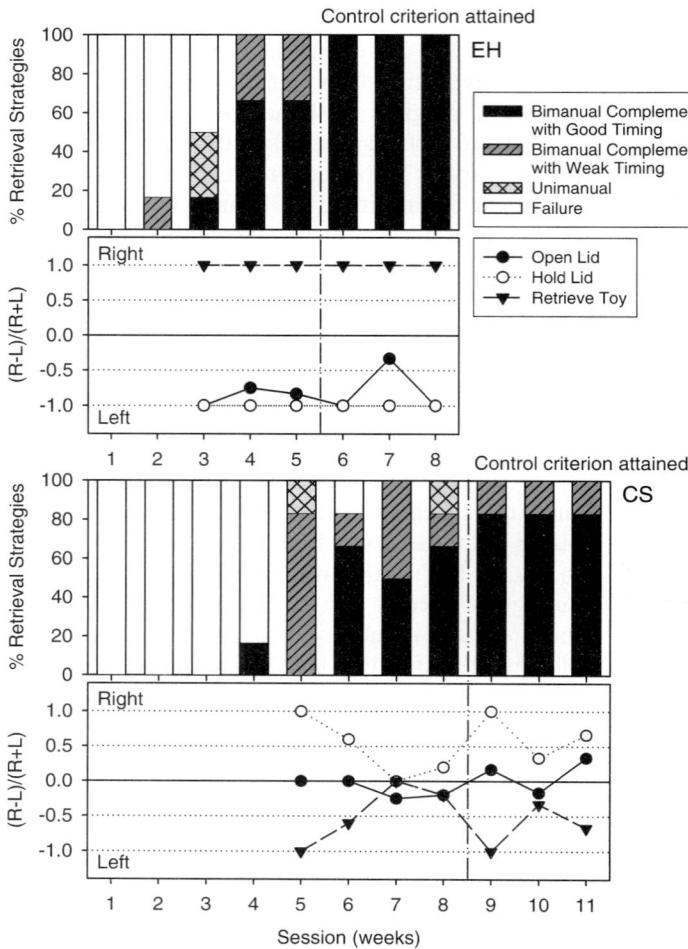

Fig. 2. Exemplars of developmentally stable (two top graphs) and developmentally unstable (two bottom graphs) patterns of division of labor in two young infants, EH and CS, while learning to solve the object retrieval task across consecutive weekly sessions. Each bar graph reports the rate of success and type of bimanual patterns used to retrieve the toy from the box for each infant as a function of the weekly sessions. The line graphs underneath the bar graphs report which hand was used by each infant for opening the box, holding the lid, and retrieving the toy during the same developmental period.

the box (infants AC, CB, DK, EH, GW, JB, and KH). The other five infants (AD, CS, DF, SK, and WC) revealed more variable hand use. In the older group, all ten infants displayed variable hand use for all three movement phases (right panel). We performed three unpaired $t$-tests on the data corresponding to each movement phase to compare performance between groups. These tests were all significant, confirming thus that the older group displayed more variable hand use over time than the younger group (unpaired $t$-tests: opening, $t(20) = 2.65$, $p < 0.01$; hold-

ing, $t(20) = 2.81$, $p < 0.01$; retrieving, $t(20) = 3.86$, $p < 0.0009$).

These group differences in hand use variability were obvious from the observation of individual performance. Fig. 4 presents two exemplars of variable hand use in two infants (EG and CO) of the older developmental group. Compared to EH's and CS's hand use in Fig. 2, EG and CO clearly revealed more variable patterns over time. Moreover, like NQ in Fig. 1, EG and CO frequently shifted hand use either week after week (EG), or by bouts (CO). CO even

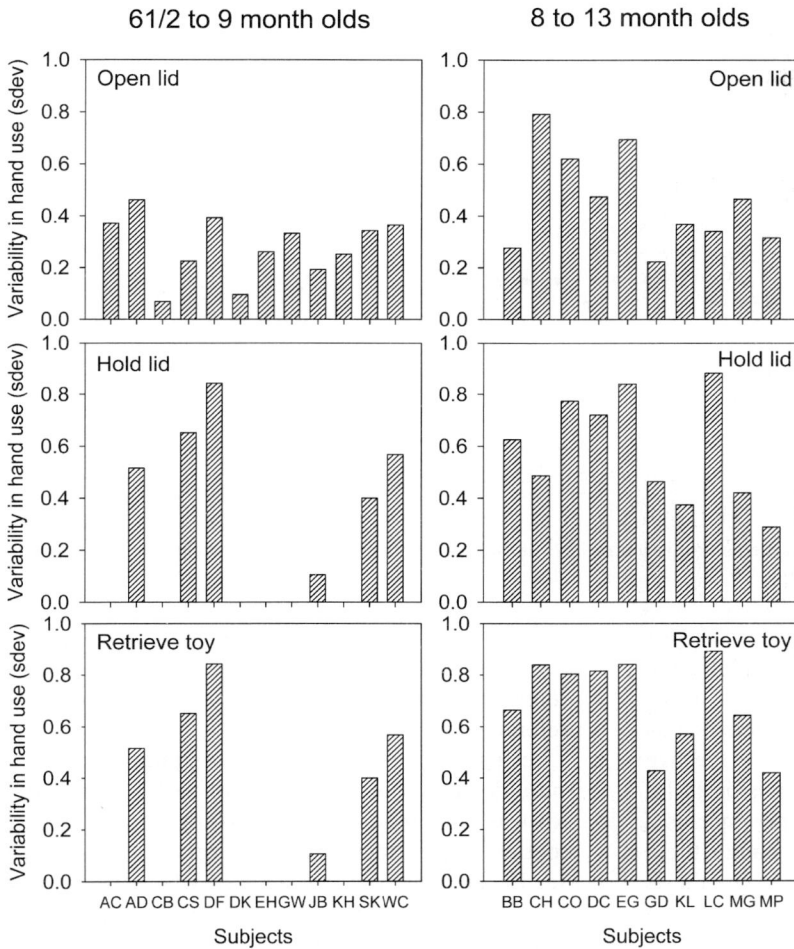

Fig. 3. Individual developmental variability in hand use for opening the box, holding the lid, and retrieving the toy for the younger (left panels) and older (right panel) group of infants while learning to solve the object retrieval task.

traversed a period, from week 5 to week 11, where she opened and retrieved the toy unimanually, with her right hand, without using the left. Therefore, these data confirmed that lateral biases tend to dissipate at the end of the first year. In the older group, patterns of hand use were unstable and preferred lateral tendencies were impossible to discern.

## What is the relative impact of crawling and walking on the destabilization of hand preference?

The last question that arose from our initial longitudinal study concerned the respective influence of the emergence of crawling and walking on shifting patterns of hand preference. In the first year longitudinal study on reaching, we found that the decline of NQ's initial lateral rightward bias occurred when NQ began to sit and crawl on hand and knees. Moreover, that first study revealed that later, when NQ began to walk, he also returned to two-handed reaching. Can we find the same relationship in the two groups of infants that we tested in the object retrieval task?

Our results were quite intriguing. First consider the younger group. In the younger group (6.5 to 8–9 months), four infants never crawled and eight began to crawl before completion of the study. When we sorted these 12 infants into two groups, the

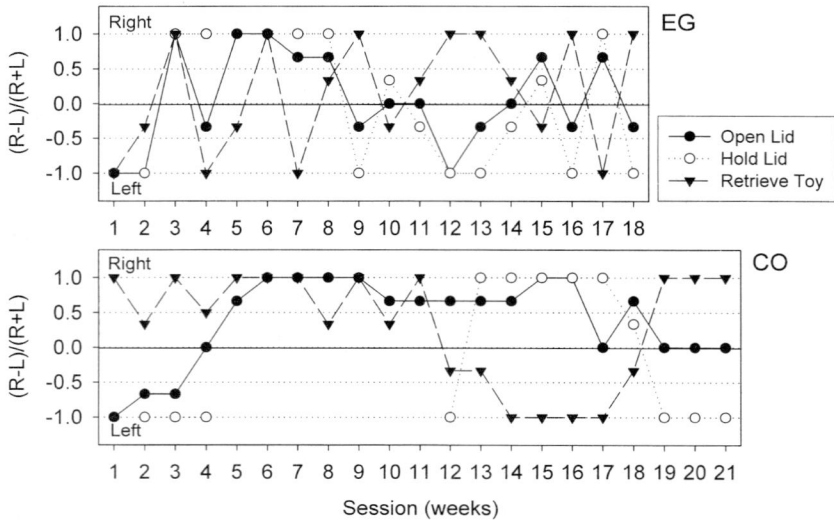

Fig. 4. Exemplars of developmentally unstable patterns of division of labor in two older infants, EG and CO, while solving the object retrieval task during consecutive weekly sessions.

one showing stable division of labor versus the one showing unstable division of labor, we found that the seven infants who displayed stable division of labor averaged only 2.2 weeks of crawling experience as a group before completing the study, while the five other remaining infants with unstable division of labor averaged 7.8 weeks of crawling experience as a group before completing the study. Although these differences between groups support the hypothesis that the emergence of crawling may play a role in disrupting the stability of hand preference, this link between crawling and stability of hand preference is not so direct. Indeed, disruption in hand preference did not occur exactly when infants began to crawl. Remember that we mentioned earlier that infants, who displayed stable division of labor between hands throughout the study, continued to maintain the same stable division of labor during the last sessions. In this group, stability was maintained even when infants began to crawl. For example, EH in Fig. 2 maintained stable division of labor despite beginning to crawl on hands and knees 3 weeks before completion of the study. Infants in the unstable group, on the contrary, began to crawl either before or at the time they began to solve the object retrieval task. Therefore, these data suggest that the emergence of crawling alone does not suffice to alter stability in hand preference. Rather, extended

crawling experience may better explain these differences between infants who maintained stable hand preference and those who displayed unstable hand preference.

Let us now consider the older group of infants. The older group of ten infants (8 to 12–13 months old) was composed only of crawling infants and, as reported above, they displayed very variable hand use. Because we did not witness when they began to crawl, it was difficult to estimate exactly how many weeks of crawling experience each one of them had at the time they entered the study. But certainly, throughout the study, all of them continued to crawl and develop many skills beyond crawling that involved different levels of postural control. In particular, in our laboratory, we observed them performing skills such as pulling up on furniture, cruising upright along furniture, going back down on their four limbs, pushing a cart while upright, and performing their first independent steps. This level of postural and whole body mobility contrasts enormously with what young sitters or just beginning crawlers can do. As infants develop these new and broad locomotor skills, they also learn to use their hands in new ways, not only for manipulating objects, but also for assisting and controlling their own body as they move and change orientation in their environment. In that sense, the last part of the first year is indeed a period of great postural instability, where infants constantly develop new ways to use and move their body around to achieve new goals. It is plausible that one reason why lateral biases become so unstable and shift so much during the end of the first year is because infants undergo continuous postural reorganizations as they go from a mainly sitting position toward adopting an upright posture. All the data that we have shown so far are consistent with such an interpretation. For instance, if we briefly return to Fig. 1, we see that NQ displayed a rightward bias early when sitting with support or lying were the predominant postures of that developmental period. His rightward bias decreased when he began to crawl and sit alone, but great fluctuations in hand use, with dramatic shifts from right- to left-hand use did not occur until a few weeks later when NQ was indeed able to use his body do much more than crawling. What happens when infants begin to walk? Do infants show a return to two-handed behavior as did NQ? And do infants resume a stable hand preference afterward, since no more fundamental postural transition occur further in development?

The data from the older group of infants were part of a study that was designed to assess the impact of the emergence of walking on the return to two-handed reaching at the end of the first year (Corbetta and Bojczyk, 2002). For that purpose, these infants were followed longitudinally every week until they began to walk and thereafter for a couple of months until they acquired a relatively stable gait pattern. As we reported already, these infants were tested in the object retrieval task, but they were also asked to reach for objects of different sizes. Before the onset of upright locomotion, infants used one-handed patterns for reaching for small objects and two-handed patterns for reaching for large objects. They also used bimanual complementary patterns to retrieve the toy from the box although division of labor between hands was unstable. When they began to walk independently, however, these behaviors changed. Infants significantly increased their rate of two-handed responses for reaching and for opening the lid during object retrieval. Fig. 5 displays exemplars of weekly data from three infants, CH, MP, and EG, for 7 weeks preceding and 7 weeks following the emergence of independent locomotion.

These exemplars compare the percentage of bimanual responses for reaching for small objects (CH and MP, line graphs, left panel) and lid opening (CH and EG, line graphs, right panel) to the number of independent steps (corresponding bar graphs) performed during the same weekly sessions. These exemplars show that before the onset of upright locomotion, all three infants used primarily one hand for reaching for small objects and for opening the lid of the box. Following the onset of upright locomotion, however, they significantly increased their rate of two-handed responses while reaching for the same small objects and opening the same box. This increase in two-handedness was significant for the group for both reaching and lid opening.

These findings confirmed the hypothesis that arm coupling increases around the end of the first year when infants begin to walk upright without support. Moreover, our results revealed that this change in the lateral organization of the upper limbs was not a task-specific effect, but a general and pervasive effect that was observed consistently across motor tasks, and even though infants displayed competent behaviors before learning to walk. How long did this increase in coupling last? The exemplars presented in Fig. 5 show that the intensity and the extent of this increase in bimanual coupling varied enormously from child to child. Some infants maintained this two-handed patterning in reaching for as little as 4 weeks (i.e. MP), while others had an increase in two-handed reaching lasting up to 9 weeks following the onset of upright locomotion (i.e. CH). Regardless of its duration, however, this increase in two-handed reaching almost always occurred during the weeks immediately following the onset of independent locomotion, when infants typically walked holding their arms above waist level and when their balance control was the most precarious. Two-handed reaching declined when infants began to show better balance control and managed to walk holding their arms at or below waist level. However, we could not assess whether this decline in coupling matched the resurgence of stable lateral preference in hand use. We did not follow these infants long enough afterward to be able to address that question. Nonetheless, the fact that early lateral biases disappeared as locomotor skills emerged and posture reorganized, let us presume that after infants have

## Reaching for Small Objects

## Lid Opening

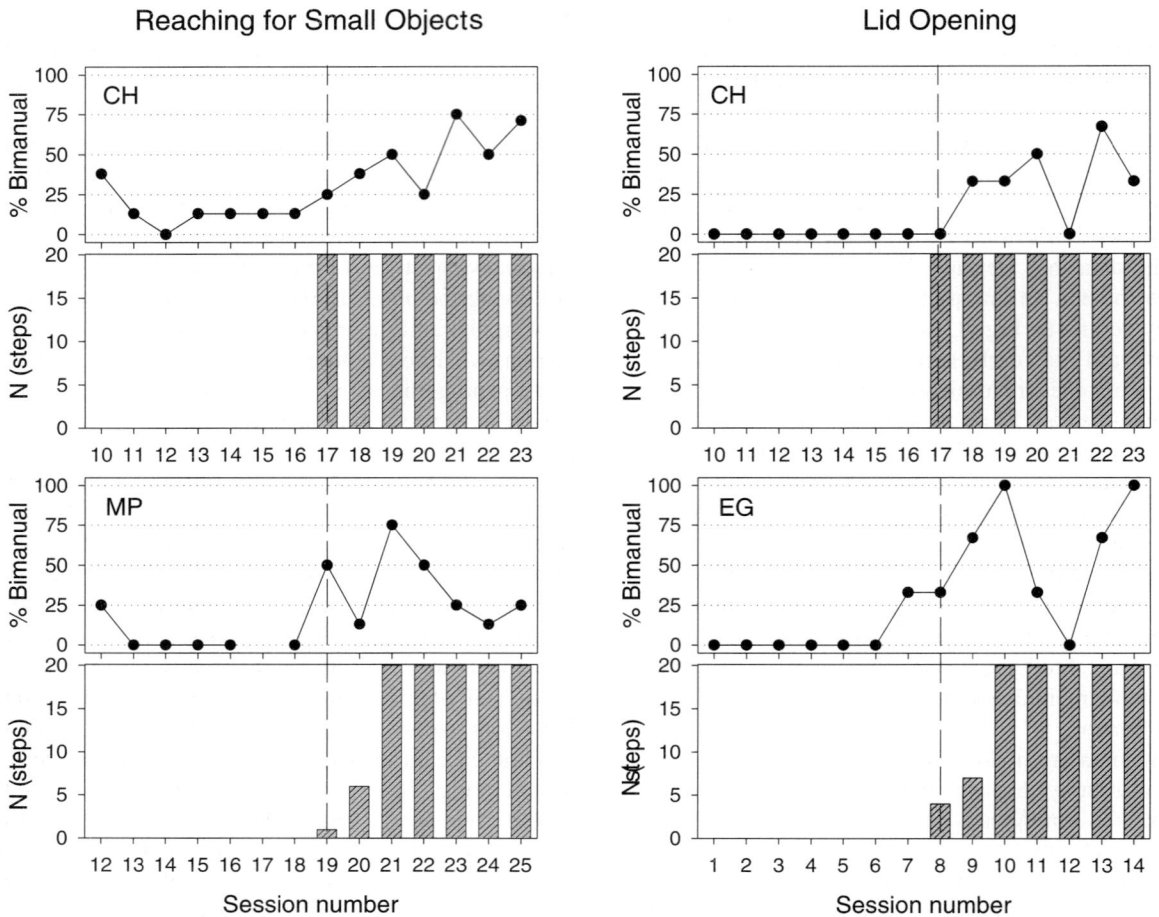

Fig. 5. Change in the percent of bimanual responses (line graphs) for reaching for small objects (left panel) and opening the lid of the box (right panel) in three infants, MP, CH, and EG, during 7 weeks prior to the emergence of upright locomotion and 7 weeks following the onset of upright locomotion (bar graphs). The bar graphs represent the number of independent steps that infants performed each weeks before and after beginning to walk.

mastered upright locomotion and undergo lesser postural reorganizations, hand preference should become stable again. Two studies, one from Ramsay and Weber (1986) and a recent one from Fagard and Marks (2000), report findings that are consistent with our predictions. Both studies found greater hand role differentiation in bimanual tasks in infants aged between 17 and 36 months old. Before 17 months old, Ramsay and Weber (1986) found that infants often used undifferentiated two-handed responses, and Fagard and Marks (2000) reported that manual laterality increased steadily between 18 and 36 months old.

## Conclusions

It is clear from the literature we surveyed and the work we presented that the development of manual asymmetries and hand preference in infancy does not follow a gradual or stable course over time. The fact that preferred hand use fluctuates in the first year of life suggests that hand preference is not strongly established from early in development but forms and develops in rather erratic ways in conjunction with the development of other fundamental skills. In this chapter, we followed a dynamic systems approach to illustrate how screening multiple behavioral components at a time provided a different account of the processes underlying the development and formation of infants' manual laterality and interlimb coordination. Clearly, the studies we presented revealed that shifts in interlimb patterning and manual laterality were not simply the result of one single factor, but rather reflected the pervasive behavioral reorganization of the system in response to multiple changing components. We illustrated how successive changes in posture entailed changes in hand use. But, as we pointed out, posture is not the only changing component. Many other components develop and change in the course of the first year of life. Other researchers, for example, have shown that the formation of preferred hand use can also be temporarily altered by the emergence of new milestones in language development (i.e. Bates et al., 1986; Ramsay, 1980a,b, 1984, 1985a).

Overall, the main message conveyed by all this work is that developmental change may not be prescribed, nor lateral asymmetries rigidly predefined. Early asymmetries present in newborns' responses may reflect the existence of preferred initial biases in the system, but these biases may be weak and extremely sensitive to perturbations that could arise from sudden changes in both the organism and the environment. In this view, biology and environment work together and interact continuously with each other. And, behavioral forms and developmental change might take place and evolve as the result of a dynamic and continuous process of modifications and alterations of current abilities as infants grow and learn new skills as a function of time. The development of hand preference and lateral asymmetries may be no exception to that process; they may follow the same dynamic reorganizational principles.

The view that brain and behavioral asymmetries form as the result of continuous, dynamic, and multiple interactive processes has recently been increasingly adopted by scientists in various areas of study (see for example, Bates, 1999a,b; Johnson, 1997, 1999; Stiles, 1998). These authors agree that functional specialization is not innate or already set from early in life, but forms as a result of increasing experience and biological adaptation. They recognize that functional asymmetries exist from early in development, but they also stress the fact that the site or location of where these functions develop later in life

may change. For example, Bates (1999a,b) and Stiles (1998) report evidence that the right hemisphere can develop an advantage for processing language after injury to the left hemisphere, notwithstanding the fact that the left hemisphere initially revealed an advantage for processing speech stimuli. Provins (1997) similarly stresses the fact that hand preference may shift to the non-preferred arm after injury or loss of the preferred arm, despite initial perceptual-motor biases in favor of the preferred arm. Finally, other authors stress the multicausal origins of functional specialization. A recent report from De Schonen, Mancini and Liegeois (1998) argues that regular exposure to faces alone does not suffice to develop hemispheric specialization for face processing, and that multiple events may rather lead to the development of a right-hemispheric advantage for face processing. Therefore, the fact that newborns show a series of lateral predispositions, such as preferring to turn their head to the right or showing greater responses to speech stimuli with their left hemisphere, may not necessarily be indicative of the formation of later brain organization. Hellige (1993) used the term of 'snowball mechanism' to convey the idea that small initial asymmetries depend on a series of inputs and events that occur as a function of time in order to form larger asymmetries, and that this process is tightly linked to the activities that each hemisphere assumes respectively and consecutively throughout life span. Here again, biology, behavior and environment are bound together in the time dimension.

Scientists have been asking for many generations what makes a person prefer to use one hand for certain tasks more than the other, or, what makes a person more efficient at processing some information with one hemisphere more than the other. It seems to us that the answer to that question may lies in the developmental processes that take place throughout people's life span.

## References

Adolph KE: Learning in the development of infant locomotion. Monographs of the Society for Research in Child Development: 62; 1–139 (Serial No. 251), 1997.

Annett M: The distribution of manual asymmetry. British Journal of Psychology: 63; 343–358, 1972.

Annett M: Left, Right, Hand and Brain: The Right Shift Theory. Hillsdale, NJ: Erlbaum, 1985.

Bates E: Language and the infant brain. Journal of Communication Disorders: 32; 195–205, 1999a.

Bates E: Plasticity, localization, and language development. In Broman SH, Fletcher JM (Eds), The Changing Nervous System: Neurobehavioral Consequences of Early Brain Disorders. New York, NY: Oxford University Press, pp. 214–253, 1999b.

Bates E, O'Connell B, Vaid J, Sledge P, Oakes L: Language and hand preference in early development. Developmental Neuropsychology: 2; 1–15, 1986.

Bertenthal BI, Campos JJ, Barrett K: Self-produced locomotion: An organizer of emotional, cognitive and social development in infancy. In Emde R, Harmon R (Eds), Continuities and Discontinuities in Development. New York, NY: Plenum, pp. 175–210, 1984.

Bruner JS: The growth and structure of skill. In Connolly K (Ed), Mechanisms of Motor Skill Development. New York, NY: Academic Press, pp. 63–92, 1970.

Caplan PJ, Kinsbourne M: Baby drops the rattle: Asymmetry of duration of grasp by infants. Child Development: 47; 532–534, 1976.

Carlson DF, Harris LJ: Development of the infant's hand preference for visually directed reaching: Preliminary report of a longitudinal study. Infant Mental Health Journal: 6; 158–172, 1985.

Carter-Saltzman L: Biological and sociocultural effects on handedness: Comparison between biological and adoptive families. Science: 209; 1263–1265, 1980.

Cobb K, Goodwin R, Saelens E: Spontaneous hand positions of newborn infants. The Journal of Genetic Psychology: 108; 225–237, 1966.

Corballis MC: The Lopsided Ape: Evolution of the Generative Mind. New York, NY: Oxford University Press, 1991.

Corballis MC, Beale IL: The Ambivalent Mind: The Neuropsychology of Left and Right. Chicago, IL: Nelson-Hall, 1984.

Corbetta D, Bojczyk KE: Infants return to two-handed reaching when they are learning to walk. Journal of Motor Behavior: 34; 83–95, 2002.

Corbetta D, Thelen E: The developmental origins of bimanual coordination: A dynamic perspective. Journal of Experimental Psychology: Human Perception and Performance: 22; 502–522, 1996.

Corbetta D, Thelen E: Lateral biases and fluctuations in infants' spontaneous arm movements and reaching. Developmental Psychobiology: 34; 237–255, 1999.

Coryell J: Infant rightward asymmetries predict right-handedness in childhood. Neuropsychologia: 23; 269–271, 1985.

Coryell J, Michel GF: How supine postural preferences of infants can contribute toward the development of handedness. Infant Behavior and Development: 1; 245–257, 1978.

De Schonen S, Gil de Diaz M, Mathivet E: Hemispheric asymmetry in face processing in infancy. In Ellis HD, Jeeves MA, Newcombe F, Young A (Eds), Aspects of Face Processing. Dordrecht: Martinus Nijhoff, pp. 199–208, 1986.

De Schonen S, Mancini J, Liegeois F: About functional cortical specialization: The development of face recognition. In Simion

F, Butterworth G (Eds), The Development of Sensory, Motor, and Cognitive Capacities in Early Infancy: From Perception to Cognition. Hove: Erlbaum, pp. 103–120, 1998.

De Schonen S, Mathivet E: Hemispheric asymmetry in a face discrimination task in infants. Child Development: 61; 1192–1205, 1990.

Fagard J, Marks A: Unimanual and bimanual tasks and the assessment of handedness in toddlers. Developmental Science: 3; 137–147, 2000.

Fagard J, Pezé A: Age changes in interlimb coupling and the development of bimanual coordination. Journal of Motor Behavior: 29; 199–208, 1997.

Fischer KW, Rose SP: Dynamic development of coordination of components in brain and behavior: A framework for theory and research. In Dawson G, Fischer KW (Eds), Human Behavior and the Developing Brain. New York, NY: Guildford Press, pp. 3–66, 1994.

Gesell A: The tonic neck reflex in the human infant: Its morphogenetic and clinical significance. Journal of Pediatrics: 13; 455–464, 1938.

Gesell A, Ames LB: The development of handedness. Journal of Genetic Psychology: 70; 155–175, 1947.

Goldfield E: Dynamic systems in development: Action systems. In Smith LB, Thelen E (Eds), A Dynamic Systems Approach to Development: Applications. Cambridge, MA: MIT Press, pp. 51–70, 1993.

Hahn WK: Cerebral lateralization of function: From infancy through childhood. Psychological Bulletin: 101; 376–392, 1987.

Harkins DA, Michel GF: Evidence for a maternal effect on infant hand-use preferences. Developmental Psychobiology: 21; 535–541, 1988.

Harkins DA, Uzgiris IC: Hand-use matching between mothers and infants during the first year. Infant Behavior and Development: 14; 289–298, 1991.

Harris LJ, Fitzgerald HE: Postural orientation in human infants: Changes from birth to three months. In Young G, Segalowitz SJ, Corter CM, Trehub SE (Eds), Manual Specialization and the Developing Brain. New York, NY: Academic Press, pp. 285–305, 1983.

Hawn PR, Harris LJ: Hand differences in grasp duration and reaching in two- and five-month old infants. In Young G, Segalowitz SJ, Corter CM, Trehub SE (Eds), Manual Specialization and the Developing Brain. New York, NY: Academic Press, pp. 331–348, 1983.

Hellige JB: Hemispheric asymmetry: What's right and what's left. Cambridge, MA: Harvard University Press, 1993.

Hopkins B, Lems YL, Wulfften-Palthe T, van Hoeksma J, Kardaun O, Butterworth G: Development of head position preference during early infancy: A longitudinal study in the daily life situation. Developmental Psychobiology: 23; 39–53, 1990.

Johnson MH: Developmental Cognitive Neuropsychology. Oxford: Blackwell, 1997.

Johnson MH: Cortical plasticity in normal and abnormal cognitive development: Evidence and working hypotheses. Development and Psychopathology: 11; 419–437, 1999.

Kermoian R, Campos JJ: Locomotor experience: A facilitator of spatial cognitive development. Child Development: 59; 908–917, 1988.

Laland KN, Kumm J, Van Horn JD, Feldman MW: A gene-culture model of human handedness. Behavior Genetics: 25; 433–445, 1995.

Lenneberg EH: Biological Foundations of Language. New York, NY: Wiley, 1967.

Levy J, Nagylaki TA: A model for the genetics of handedness. Genetics: 72; 117–128, 1972.

Longstreth LE: Human handedness: More evidence for genetic involvement. The Journal of Genetic Psychology: 137; 275–283, 1980.

MacNeilage PF, Studdert-Kennedy MG, Lindblom B: Primate handedness reconsidered. Behavioral and Brain Sciences: 10; 247–303, 1987.

Marshall LH, Magoun HW: Discoveries in the human brain: Neuroscience prehistory, brain structure, and function. Totowa, NJ: Humana Press, 1998.

McManus IC: Handedness, language dominance and aphasia: A genetic model. Psychological Medicine — Monograph Supplement: 8; 1–40, 1985.

McManus IC, Sik G, Cole DR, Mellon AF, Wong J, Kloss J: The development of handedness in children. British Journal of Developmental Psychology: 6; 257–273, 1988.

Michel GF: Right handedness: A consequence of infant supine head-orientation preference? Science: 212; 685–687, 1981.

Michel GF, Goodwin R: Intrauterine birth position predicts newborn supine head position preferences. Infant Behavior and Development: 2; 29–38, 1979.

Michel GF, Harkins DA: Postural and lateral asymmetries in the ontogeny of handedness during infancy. Developmental Psychobiology: 19; 247–258, 1986.

Molfese DL, Molfese VJ: Hemisphere and stimulus differences as reflected in the cortical responses of newborn infants to speech stimuli. Developmental Psychology: 15; 505–511, 1979.

Molfese DL, Molfese VJ: Cortical responses of preterm infants to phonetic and non-phonetic speech stimuli. Developmental Psychology: 16; 574–581, 1980.

Orlebeke JF, Knol DL, Koopmans JR, Boosma DL, Bleker OP: Left-handedness in twins: Genes or environment? Cortex: 32; 479–490, 1996.

Previc FH: A general theory concerning the prenatal origins of cerebral lateralization in humans. Psychological Review: 98; 299–334, 1991.

Provins KA: Handedness and speech: A critical re-appraisal of the role of genetic and environmental factors in the cerebral lateralization of function. Psychological Review: 104; 554–571, 1997.

Provins KA, Dalziel FR, Higginbottom G: Asymmetrical hand usage in infancy: An ethological approach. Infant Behavior and Development: 10; 165–172, 1987.

Ramsay DS: Beginnings of bimanual handedness and speech in infants. Infant Behavior and Development: 3; 67–77, 1980a.

Ramsay DS: Onset of unimanual handedness in infants. Infant Behavior and Development: 3; 377–385, 1980b.

Ramsay DS: Onset of duplicated syllable babbling and unimanual handedness in infancy: Evidence for the developmental change in hemispheric specialization? Developmental Psychology: 20; 64–71, 1984.

Ramsay DS: Fluctuations in unimanual hand preference in infants following the onset of duplicated syllable babbling. Developmental Psychology: 21; 318–324, 1985a.

Ramsay DS: Infants' block banging at midline: Evidence for Gesell's principle of 'reciprocal interweaving' in development. British Journal of Developmental Psychology: 3; 335–343, 1985b.

Ramsay DS, Campos JJ, Fenson L: Onset of bimanual handedness in infants. Infant Behavior and Development: 2; 69–76, 1979.

Ramsay DS, Weber SL: Infants' hand preference in a task involving complementary roles for the two hands. Child Development: 57; 300–307, 1986.

Ramsay DS, Willis MP: Organization and lateralization of reaching in infants: An extension of Bresson et al. Neuropsychologia: 22; 639–641, 1984.

Rochat P: Self-sitting and reaching in 5- to 8-month-old infants: The impact of posture and its development on early eye–hand coordination. Journal of Motor Behavior: 24; 210–220, 1992.

Rochat P, Bullinger A: Posture and functional action in infancy. In Vyt A, Bloch H, Bornstein MH (Eds), Early Child Development in the French Tradition. Hillsdale, NJ: Lawrence Erlbaum, pp. 15–34, 1994.

Smith LB, Thelen E: A Dynamic Systems Approach to Development: Applications. Cambridge, MA: MIT Press, 1993.

Spencer JP, Thelen E: Spatially specific changes in infants' muscle co-activity as they learn to reach. Infancy: 1; 275–302, 2000.

Spencer JP, Vereijken B, Diedrich FJ, Thelen E: Posture and the emergence of manual skills. Developmental Science: 3; 216–233, 2000.

Springer SP, Deutsch G: Left brain, right brain. New York, NY: Freeman, 1989.

Stiles J: The effects of early focal brain injury on lateralization of cognitive function. Current Directions in Psychological Sciences: 7; 21–26, 1998.

Tambs K, Magnus P, Berg K: Left-handedness in twin families: Support of an environmental hypothesis. Perceptual and Motor Skills: 64; 155–170, 1987.

Thelen E: Development of coordinated movement: Implications for early human development. In Wade MG, Whiting HTA (Eds), Motor Development in Children: Aspects of Coordination and Control. Dordrecht: Martinus Nijhoff, pp. 107–124, 1986.

Thelen E, Smith LB: A Dynamic Systems Approach to the Development of Cognition and Action. Cambridge, MA: MIT Press, 1994.

Thelen E, Smith LB: Dynamic systems theories. In Lerner RM (Ed), Theoretical Models of Human Development. Volume 1 of the Handbook of Child Psychology, 5th ed. Editor-in-chief: William Damon. New York, NY: Wiley, pp. 563–634, 1997.

Thelen E, Ulrich BD: Hidden skills. Monographs of the Society for Research in Child Development: 56; (Serial No. 223), 1991.

Thelen E, Corbetta D, Kamm K, Spencer JP, Schneider K, Zernicke RF: The transition to reaching: Mapping intension and intrinsic dynamics. Child Development: 64; 1058–1098, 1993.

Thelen E, Corbetta D, Spencer J: Development of reaching during the first year: Role of movement speed. Journal of Experimental Psychology: Human Perception and Performance: 22; 1059–1076, 1996.

Trehub SE, Corter CM, Shosenberg N: Neonatal reflexes: A search for lateral asymmetries. In Young G, Segalowitz SJ, Corter CM, Trehub SE (Eds), Manual Specialization and the Developing Brain. New York, NY: Academic Press, pp. 257–274, 1983.

Turkewitz G, Gordon EW, Birch HG: Head turning in the human neonate: Spontaneous patterns. Journal of Genetic Psychology: 107; 143–148, 1965.

Van Geert P: Dynamic systems and development. Change be-tween complexity and chaos. New York, NY: Harverster Wheatsheaf, 1994.

Van Geert P: A dynamic systems model of basic developmental mechanism: Piaget, Vygotsky, and beyond. Psychological Review: 105; 634–677, 1998.

Viviani J, Turkewitz G, Karp E: A relationship between laterality of functioning at 2 days and 7 years of age. Bulletin of Psychonomic Society: 12; 189–192, 1978.

Von Hofsten C: Structuring of early reaching movements: A longitudinal study. Journal of Motor Behavior: 23; 280–292, 1991.

Warren JM: Handedness and laterality in humans and other animals. Physiological Psychology: 8; 351–359, 1980.

Young G: Manual specialization in infancy: Implications for lateralization of brain function. In Segalowitz S, Gruber F (Eds), Language Development and Neurological Theory. New York, NY: Academic Press, pp. 289–311, 1977.

CHAPTER 14

# Human handedness: a biological perspective

Ronald A. Yeo [a,*], Robert J. Thoma [b] and Steven W. Gangestad [a]

[a] *Department of Psychology, Logan Hall, University of New Mexico, Albuquerque, NM 87131-1161, USA*
[b] *Department of Psychiatry, Albuquerque Veterans Administration Medical Center, Albuquerque, NM, USA*

## Introduction

The tendency toward right-handedness in humans has been the focus of intense interest since the inception of neuropsychology (Harris, 1992). Like language, the other most obviously lateralized function of our brain, the extent of right-handedness in humans has been thought to represent something unique about our species. Hence, study of the origins and significance of handedness might provide fundamental insights into human nature. Equally important is developing an understanding of the origins of individual variation in handedness. Indeed, the two issues are inextricably linked. Any possible adaptive significance of right-handedness (or more fundamental correlate) must be considered in the context of phenotypic variability, upon which natural selection acts.

In this chapter we attempt to provide an account of handedness from a biological perspective, an approach that we believe is most apt to help us understand what makes human brains unique. A biological perspective can be justified by the observations that variation in handedness is likely influenced by genetic factors (McManus and Bryden, 1992), that the phenomenon of right-handedness is pretty much invariant across cultures (Connolly and Bishop, 1992) and generations (Coren and Porac, 1977), and that manual asymmetry appears before birth (Hepper, Shahidullah and White, 1991). It should be noted

that a biological approach does not exclude systematic analysis of environmental influences, in the same way that biological analyses of language development need specify the nature and timing of important environmental influences (e.g., Pinker, 1994).

There are three major aspects to the biological approach adopted here. First, we approach handedness from the perspective of ontogeny. Neural development is the playing field on which nature and nurture interact. A developmental perspective of the temporal dynamics of phenotypic variation can also constrain our theories of causal influences on variation. Second, we attempt to understand the mechanisms whereby individual variation in hand preference and skill are instantiated. That is, what is the neural substrate for differences in handedness and how does it emerge? Finally, we shall investigate the evolutionary–genetic underpinnings of handedness. This entails two sorts of questions, concerning issues of both phylogeny and of the selection factors maintaining current genetic diversity.

The scientific literature on handedness is immense, reflecting both its enduring interest and ease of measurement. It is far too great to be reviewed in a single chapter. There are several recent comprehensive reviews on handedness and cerebral lateralization (Harris, 1992), the genetics of handedness (McManus and Bryden, 1992), and evolutionary perspectives (Corballis, 1997). Though our perspectives differ on some issues, we will attempt to build upon these excellent reviews, emphasizing new data.

A few words on the assessment of handedness are necessary. There are two major expressions of

---

* Corresponding author. E-mail: ryeo@unm.edu

handedness to consider, i.e., the preferred hand used for various tasks, and the relative difference in hand skill for a given task. Correlations between preference and performance asymmetry measures are generally significant, though the magnitude of the relationship varies across tasks and is diminished when left- and right-handers are examined separately (Provins and Magliaro, 1993). Preference inventories are the most common means to assess handedness. These vary greatly in length, but the shorter, more common versions generally yield a J-shaped distribution (Bishop, 1990). Preference for writing hand is generally acknowledged to be influenced more by social pressures than other activities. There are many different types of tasks used to assess relative hand skill, with the most important dimension of difference probably being task complexity (Bryden, Roy and Bryden, 1998). Performance measures are distributed with much less skew than preference measures (and may be normally distributed), because individuals who consistently prefer their right hands vary considerably in relative hand performance. Hence, performance measures do a much better job of distinguishing extreme from moderate right-handedness.

The choice of preference vs. performance measures depends on both practical and theoretical concerns. Ease of administration makes preference inventories the most common measure for large-scale studies. They are most appropriate for theories positing a categorical phenotype (McManus, 1985) and least for theories emphasizing continuously distributed phenotypes (e.g., Annett, 1985; Yeo and Gangestad, 1993). In general, preference inventories are less satisfactory than performance measures in distinguishing the direction from the degree of handedness, a potentially important issue in genetic analyses.

## The nature and ontogeny of the phenotype

Three different types of asymmetry in organisms have been described (Palmer and Strobeck, 1986). *Directional asymmetry* exists at the population level due to organismic 'design' for asymmetry. The asymmetrical design of the human heart is an example of directional asymmetry. *Antisymmetry* refers to the situation where individuals have different de-

signs for asymmetry, with some having the left side of a trait larger than the right, others the reverse. Antisymmetry may result in a bimodal distribution. *Fluctuating asymmetry* (FA) refers to deviation from symmetry for a trait, not due to developmental design for asymmetry. FA reflects the lack of precise control over the development of a trait in the face of such potential perturbations as mutations or pathogens, resulting in departure from developmental design for symmetry. For example, left and right human ears tend to be symmetrical. The fact that some individuals have larger right ears and some larger left ears is due to imprecise expression of developmental design, not because some individuals' genomes possess 'design' for ear asymmetry. In contrast, the fact that most people tend to be more skilled with the right than the left hand, a directional asymmetry, is probably the result of design, not developmental error. Palmer (1996) conducted a phylogenetic analysis of the manner by which directional asymmetries evolve and found that directional asymmetry tends to evolve from changes in the larval states of ancestral symmetric forms. While not ruling out a role for later environmental influences, this pattern suggests that, more often than not, internal cytogenic factors are important for the development of functional asymmetries.

Consistent with Palmer's analysis, much direct and indirect evidence indicates that the asymmetries associated with handedness emerge early in development. Direct evidence suggests that motoric asymmetries can be observed early in fetal development. Indirect evidence links variation in handedness with variation in other physical features determined early in development. However, relatively few studies provide a longitudinal perspective, limiting conclusions regarding the temporal stability of the laterality of expressions of handedness.

Ultrasound studies of human fetuses reveal marked manual asymmetries. In one study 274 fetuses were observed sucking their thumb and 92% demonstrated right-side thumb sucking (Hepper et al., 1991). Of those between 12 and 15 weeks gestational age, 87.5% sucked their right thumb, demonstrating the very early emergence of lateral preference. In a subsample of 20 fetuses studied on 3 separate occasions, lateral preference was found to be quite stable. In another study, three-quarters of 72 fetuses observed at 10 weeks gestational age showed more frequent right- than left-arm movement, whereas 12.5% showed more frequent left-arm use, and 12.5% equal arm use (Hepper, McCartney and Shannon, 1998). A much smaller number of fetuses ($N = 17$) were observed on 6 occasions between 12 and 27 weeks gestational age and more frequent right arm activity was seen at each time point (McCartney and Hepper, 1999). It was also noted that arm movements (both left and right) declined in frequency from 21 to 27 weeks. Though it is not known whether these very early asymmetries predict subsequent handedness in childhood or adulthood, right-thumb sucking is associated with a preference for right-side head turning shortly after birth (Hepper et al., 1991), which predicts hand preference at 18 months of age (Michel and Harkins, 1986).

Fetal growth rate appears to be related to adult handedness. An indirect way to investigate fetal growth rate is through measurement of dermatoglyphics. The genesis of dermatoglyphic features occurs in the 6th week of gestation and the final pattern is set by the 19th week (Mulvihill and Smith, 1969). Many studies have found that left- and right-handers show different patterns of dermatoglyphic features, though the magnitude of the effects are rather small (e.g., Coren, 1994; Cummins, 1940; Jantz, Fohl and Zahler, 1979; Newman, 1934; Rife, 1955). In one of the two largest studies, Rife (1955) reported that "*individual* bilateral asymmetry is greater while *group* asymmetry is lesser among left-handers than right-handers" (p. 177). That is, the left and right hands of left-handers were more different from each other than the two hands of right-handers, but greater systematic, directional asymmetries were evident in right-handers. As variation in dermal patterns reflects variation in growth rates (Mulvihill and Smith, 1969), Rife's data suggest greater lateral variation in growth rates for left- than right-handers. Coren (1994) noted that the pattern of dermatoglyphic features in the fingerprints of left-handers resembled the 'simplified' patterns seen in individuals with Down's syndrome. As Down's syndrome is associated with slower prenatal growth rates, Coren's observation raises the possibility that left-handedness in utero might also be linked with slower growth rates.

Reports of a greater number of minor physical anomalies (MPAs) in left-handers also indicate an association of handedness with variations in early growth rate (O'Callaghan, Burn, Mohay et al., 1993; Yeo, Gangestad and Daniel, 1993; Yeo, Gangestad, Thoma et al., 1997a). MPAs are most commonly assessed with the Waldrop and Halverson scale (Waldrop and Halverson, 1971; Waldrop, Halverson and Shetterly, 1989), which assesses various features of the face, head, hands, and body that reflect slowed or disrupted prenatal development, typically occurring in the first or early second trimester. An example is wide-spaced eyes (hypertelorism). At a particular point in prenatal development the eyes migrate toward each other; if development is slowed at this point the eyes forever remain wide-spaced. In human brains, asymmetry of the planum temporale is established by 15 weeks or so gestational age (Chi, Dooling and Gilles, 1977), and atypical planum asymmetries are often observed in adult left-handers (e.g., Steinmetz, Volkmann, Janke and Freunde, 1991). These links between variations in handedness and physical features determined during gestation draw attention to the importance of prenatal influences on the phenotype of adult handedness.

The development of handedness in infants and young children has been the subject of a great deal of research. Many studies provide evidence for some type of rightward bias from early infancy on, but the emergence of relatively stable hand preference at age three or so is preceded by a complex and sometimes fluctuating pattern of development (McManus, Sik, Cole et al., 1988). Michel (1998) describes right-hand reaching preference throughout the first year in approximately 50% of infants, with about 25% of infants showing left-hand or no preference. A slightly stronger right-hand preference for manipulation is observed during this same time period. In contrast, for bimanual object manipulation in which the preferred hand 'explores' and the non-preferred hand 'holds', no lateral preference is typically observed until the end of the first year. Forty-six percent of infants showed longitudinally stable preferences for the right hand for reaching and manipulation at 7, 9, 11, and 13 months of age, whereas 18% showed stable left preferences, and 36% did not exhibit stable hand preferences. Though clearly demonstrating an early right-hand bias for reaching, these studies reveal less striking laterality than Hepper's prenatal studies, in which the proportions of right-handedness more closely approximate adult figures.

More fine-grained analyses of developmental changes in handedness in individual infants reveal notable fluctuations in asymmetry. A recent study by Corbetta and Thelen, 1999 (see also Corbetta and Thelan, 2002, this volume) demonstrates this very clearly. Four infants were studied weekly through the first year of life with sophisticated kinematic techniques, providing measures of preference in both reaching and non-reaching movements. Striking temporal variability in asymmetries was noted, though overall, each infant showed some degree of right-hand preference. Further, at three and one-half years of age each child was found to demonstrate a fairly consistent right-hand preference for object use. The authors favor a 'dynamic systems' interpretation of these data, asserting that "developmental shifts in lateral biases may be influenced by postural shifts as infants learn to sit, crawl and walk" (p. 253). The emergence of these other motor skills forces the reorganization of lateral skills more than once in the first year of life.

The degree of right-hand superiority observed on manual tasks such as peg moving appears to be relatively stable after three years of age (Annett, 1998). Thus, despite many additional years of preferred hand use, adults and older children show the same degree of performance asymmetry. Hand preference, however, seems to show a different developmental course. Harris (1992) reviewed several studies demonstrating that the incidence of 'ambiguous' handedness (children with inconsistent hand preference) decreased during childhood, in association with an increase in right-hand preference.

Despite its apparent early prenatal roots, the complex manner in which the phenotype of handedness unfolds is indeed probably best characterized as a dynamic process (Corbetta and Thelen, 1999). In this sense it can be clearly distinguished from other physical traits influenced by early developmental processes, such as dermatoglyphics and MPAs. In contrast to these 'fossil relics' of prenatal events, handedness is an evolving phenotype, at least through the early childhood years. Our challenge is to understand at which time points genetic and/or environmental influences affect specific aspects of this dynamical process.

Thus far we have discussed the phenotype of handedness as having two correlated dimensions, i.e., preference, and performance asymmetry. There is much evidence, however, that in adults the phenotype may be more complex. Peters (1990) demonstrated that different patterns of preference emerge in consistent left-handers (those with a marked and stable preference for the left hand across tasks) vs. inconsistent left-handers (those who prefer their left hand for some tasks and their right for others). While both groups write with their left hand and demonstrate greater left-hand skill on the Purdue Pegboard test, the inconsistent left-handers are stronger in their right hand, prefer to throw with their right hand (and, not surprisingly, throw better with it). Thus, asymmetries for skills that require fine-motor control appear dissociable from those involving strength and whole arm movements. Support for this notion also emerged from cluster analysis of questionnaire data (Peters and Murphy, 1993). As will be discussed below, these results may pose a challenge for single-gene theories of handedness.

Among adults several cross-sectional studies have demonstrated an increase in right-hand preference with advancing age (Coren and Halpern, 1991). This trend may in part reflect a cohort effect rather than an age effect, due to somewhat reduced social pressure against left-handedness in recent years. What is unclear, however, is whether this is the only factor involved. McManus (2000) has suggested that actual gene frequencies may be changing, such that alleles favoring left-handedness are becoming more common. Rarely, some individuals switch from left- to right-handedness with advancing age, though this effect does not fully account for the reduced incidence of left-handedness with age (Hugdahl, Satz, Mitrushina and Miller, 1993). Ellis et al. (1998) attempted to discriminate hand preference items that were more apt to be the subject of social pressure (e.g., writing hand) from those less so (e.g., throwing) and found that even with the elimination of the former, age-related increases in right-hand preference were still observed. Halpern and Coren (1991) speculate that left-handers may be more prone to premature mortality, though Harris (1993) has vigorously disputed this notion.

## Brain mechanisms underlying asymmetry of hand skill and preference

In this section, we discuss evidence regarding the neural substrates of handedness. Numerous anatomic asymmetries are correlated with variations in handedness, though only some of these likely represent the its anatomic substrates. Some asymmetries linked with handedness, by virtue of their anatomic location, are unlikely to relate directly to motor skills. Most prominent among these are asymmetries of the planum temporale and frontal and occipital petalia. Beaton (1997) recently provided a critical analysis of studies relating variation in planum asymmetry to handedness. He concluded that "it appears that handedness and planum temporale asymmetry are related in some way, but the exact nature of the relationship is obscure" (p. 271). Further, results across studies "raise the possibility that any differences in magnitude of planum asymmetry is related not so much to the direction as to the degree of handedness" (p. 271). LeMay (1976, 1977) drew attention to the tendency for humans to have relatively longer and wider right anterior cortices and relatively longer and wider left posterior cortices (petalia). These patterns may be attenuated or reversed in left-handers. Bear and colleagues (Bear, Schiff, Saver et al., 1976) found that left-handers had atypical posterior but normal anterior asymmetries, while another study (Koff, Naeser, Pieniadz et al., 1986) observed no handedness differences.

The same pattern of asymmetries noted for cortical petalia have been identified in the cerebellum, and these too appeared to be attenuated in left-handers (Snyder, Bilder, Wu et al., 1995). However, since the cerebellum projects ipsilaterally, in contrast to the cortex, the fact that the same asymmetries are noted at different levels of the neuraxis raises concern about whether these cerebellar asymmetries are part of the anatomic substrate for asymmetric hand skill or preference. Perhaps, a greater incidence of atypical cortical and cerebellar 'tourque' in left-handers reflects the fact that left-handers are more apt to demonstrate minor neural anomalies analogous to the demonstrated greater incidence of MPAs.

Differences between left- and right-handers in callosal anatomy are also probably unrelated in any direct way to motor skills. Dreisen and Raz (1995) conducted a meta-analysis (7 studies) of handedness effects on the area of the corpus callosum; left-handers had slight larger callosa. However, the largest study to date ($N = 120$) found no relation between handedness and callosal area (Steinmetz, Staiger, Schlaug et al., 1995). Burke and Yeo (1994) noted that in a large sample of elderly individuals greater right-hand preference (as defined by the 55-item scale developed by Healy, Liederman and Geschwind, 1986) predicted greater posterior callosal area in men and less total callosal area in women. A more recent study (Moffatt, Hampson and Lee, 1998) found greater callosal area in left-handed men with presumed right hemisphere language dominance than left-handed men with presumed left hemisphere language dominance or right-handed men (women were not studied).

Variations in the sensorimotor cortex and its connections are probably of greater relevance for individual variation in handedness. Different regions may contribute to distinct aspects of the phenotype. Handedness is evident in several aspects of motor skill, including fine-motor control for independent finger movements, control for grasping and manipulating objects, and throwing and targeting. Each of these functions is controlled by different aspects of the motor system, with more distal finger movements controlled primarily by corticospinal tracts originating in Brodmann area 4. However, movements involving the arm and trunk receive indirect cortical control through occipito-temporal and frontal connections to subcortical nuclei of the lateral and ventromedial systems (Kolb and Whishaw, 1996). Thus, the degree to which different cortical asymmetries underlie handedness depends on the specific function discussed. On the basis of lesion studies, Jakobson and Goodale (1994) argue that visually guided reaching and grasping movements require information that must undergo processing within the dorsal cortical stream of visual projections. Initial integration takes place in posterior parietal cortex and later in frontal cortical areas. Asymmetries identified in motor systems relevant to handedness probably represent only a subset of the diverse regions involved in hand and arm movements.

Asymmetrical function related to handedness has been documented in both subcortical motor areas as well as in spinal and distal motor control pathways.

The corticospinal tract is the largest descending fiber tract from the brain (Ghez, 1991). At the junction of the medulla and the spinal cord most of these fibers cross the midline and descend in the contralateral ventral column of the spinal cord. Approximately 10–15% of these fibers descend on the ipsilateral side (Nyberg-Hansen and Rinvik, 1963). Although prominent asymmetries of the corticospinal tract have been reported, they are not related to handedness (Kertesz and Geschwind, 1971; Nathan, Smith and Deacon, 1990). However, cellular morphological asymmetry may exist in the spinal cord. In segments of the spinal cord innervating the arms and hand, larger motorneuron perikaryas were observed on the right side, perhaps representing a cellular-level precursor to handedness (Melsbach, Wohlschlager, Speiss and Gunturnkun, 1996).

Quantitative postmortem and magnetic resonance imaging (MRI) analyses have examined the symmetry of those portions of the motor cortex that probably contribute to asymmetric hand skill. The relevant part of the motor cortex for the hand is a 'knob' on the precentral gyrus (Fig. 1; Yousry, Schmid, Alkadhi et al., 1997). An anatomical asymmetry in this region favoring the left hemisphere was described in one postmortem study (White, Lucas, Richards and Purves, 1994), but no significant anatomical asymmetries were noted subsequently in a larger sample (White, Andrews, Hulette et al., 1997). However, a recent quantitative MRI study of both left- and right-handers revealed that the depth of the central sulcus was greater in the hemisphere contralateral to the dominant hand (Amunts, Schlaug, Schleicher et al., 1996).

Functional blood flow studies have examined contralateral vs. ipsilateral activation during fine-motor control. For simple, repetitive finger movements, pre- and post-central gyrus (i.e., Grafton, Mazziotta, Woods and Phelps, 1992), lateral premotor cortex (Freund, 1987; Kawashima et al., 1994; Roland, Larsen, Lassen and Skinhoj, 1980), supplementary motor cortex (Rao et al., 1993; Roland et al., 1980), and parietal cortex (Mattay, Callicott, Bertolino et al., 1998) activations occur primarily in the hemisphere contralateral to movement (Halsey et al., 1979; Kawashima et al., 1994). Grafton, Fagg, Woods and Arbib (1996) showed greater cuneate and dorsal occipital cortex activation than ventral or temporal activation during both pointing and grasping. The left parietal operculum was recruited during grasping but not pointing with the contralateral hand. These results demonstrate that a wide network of brain regions are involved in the set of tasks for which preference and skill asymmetries are observed.

Functional neuroimaging studies have produced more consistent results than anatomic studies re-

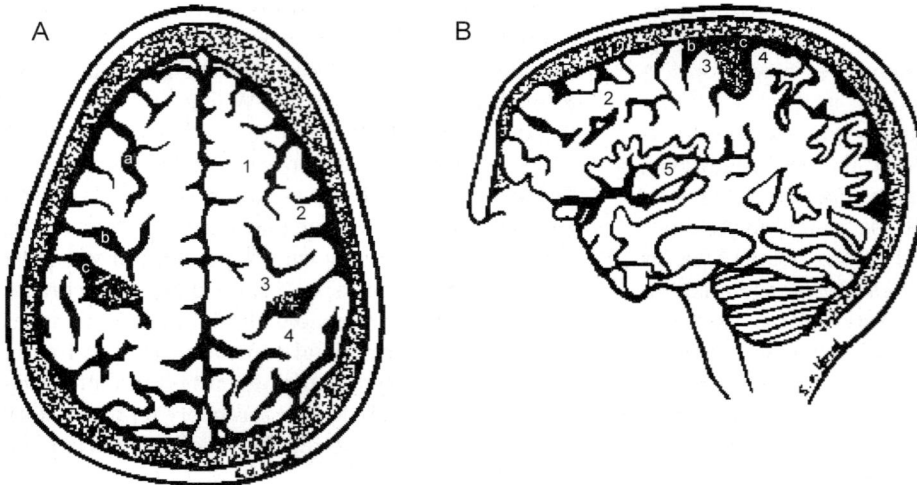

Fig. 1. Schematic drawing of the precentral knob (c, shaded) identified by Yousry et al. (1997) as the region controlling motor hand function. Other landmarks: 1, superior frontal gyrus; 2, middle frontal gyrus; 3, precentral gyrus; 4, postcentral gyrus; 5, posterior part of the insula (from Yousry et al., 1997, p. 151).

garding asymmetries possibly related to handedness. In the first fMRI study comparing right- and left-handers (Kim, Ashe, Hendrich et al., 1993) a sequential thumb to finger touching task was used. Right motor cortex activation was seen with left-hand finger movements in both left- and right-handers. Left motor cortex activation was observed with both ipsilateral and contralateral finger movements, though the extent of ipsilateral activation was greater in right-handers. Another recent fMRI study also demonstrated greater activation in the primary motor cortex contralateral to the dominant hand than the non-dominant hand (Dassonville, Zhu, Ugurbil et al., 1997). Further, the degree of asymmetry in motor cortex activation was correlated with degree of hand preference (determined from the Edinburgh Inventory) in a group of seven right-handers and six left-handers. Fig. 2 shows the difference observed between a 'moderate' and a 'strong' left-hander.

Precise temporal resolution of functional brain activity is possible in measurement of neuromagnetic activation of primary sensory–motor cortical regions (Lewine and Orrison, 1995). Neuromagnetic response prior to (primary motor cortex) and follow-ing (primary sensory cortex) movement is affected by handedness. A contralateral source dipole localizing to motor cortex has been shown for the dominant hand in both left- and right-handers, but bilateral activation is seen in each group for the non-dominant hand (Taniguchi, Yoshomine, Cheyne et al., 1998). Further, Volkmann, Schnitzler, Witte and Freund (1998) demonstrated larger functional cortical motor representation for the dominant hand in both left- and right-handed subjects. The asymmetry in size of the left and right motor representations (in five right-handed and five left-handed subjects) was highly correlated with degree of handedness. See Fig. 3 for differences between left- and right-handers. A similar MEG asymmetry for the somatosensory component of finger movement was documented by Thoma, Yeo, Gangestad et al. (2002). The size of the hand area of the sensorimotor region in each hemisphere was mapped by computing the distance between thumb and little fingers. The size of this sensorimotor region was greater for the dominant hand. Further, the asymmetry $(L - R)$ of these regions was positively correlated with asymmetry $(L - R)$ of hand skill on a pegboard task $(r = 0.80, p < 0.01)$,

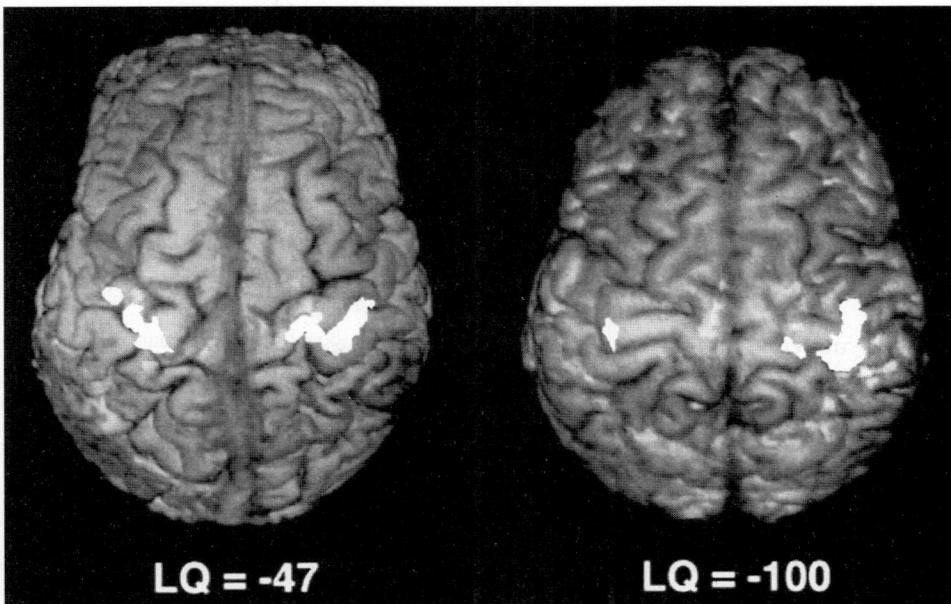

Fig. 2. Motor cortex fMRI activations identified during movement in two left-handed subjects identified by Dassonville et al. (1997). On the left is a moderate left-hander with a laterality quotient of −47 on the Edinburgh Inventory and on the right is a strong left-hander with a laterality quotient of −100 (from Dassonville et al., 1997, p. 14017).

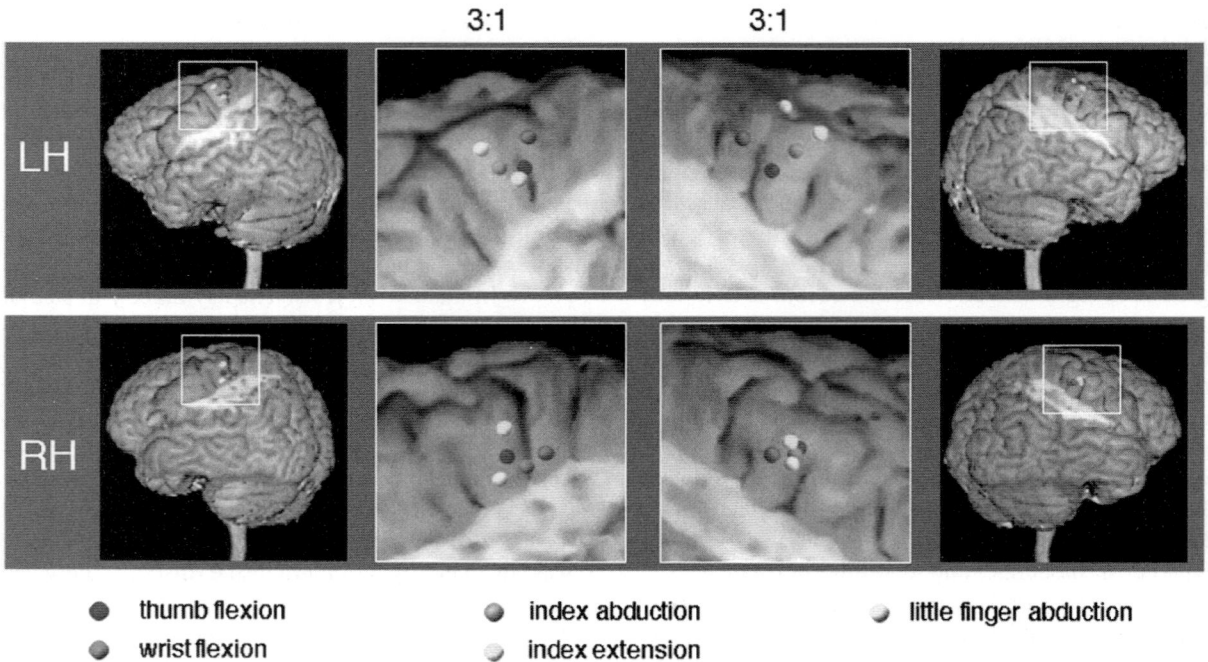

Fig. 3. Equivalent current dipole sources detected by magnetoencephalography for motor activity of various types of hand and finger movements. Source locations are superimposed on MRI images for anatomical localization. (Top panel) Dipole locations in a left-hander that spread over a relatively greater area in the right than left hemisphere. (Bottom panel) Dipole locations for a right-hander showing the opposite effect. (From Volkmann et al., 1998, p. 2152.)

suggesting that asymmetry in the neural substrate of hand skill is continuously distributed, rather than dichotomous. Similarly, mapping of cortical motor regions with transcranial magnetic stimulation has revealed right-handers have greater motor representation in the left hemisphere and left-handers greater representation in the right hemisphere (Triggs, Subramanium and Rossi, 1999).

## Embryonic establishment of asymmetries

The anatomic substrates of handedness thus emerge from a distributed network with asymmetric components most centrally involving fronto-parietal cortex. How is this asymmetric network established? Hepper and colleagues (Hepper et al., 1998) have raised a very important point. Motor asymmetries emerge at a point in development before the brain is able to control motor activity. Indeed, the human motor cortex is at a rather rudimentary stage of development at five months gestational age (Marin-Padilla,

1970). Hence, asymmetries in peripheral neural control are much more likely to be responsible for motoric asymmetries than are cortical or subcortical asymmetries. Prenatal motoric activity likely represents self-generated or 'autogenic' movements involving both excitatory and inhibitory neurons (Oppenheim and Reitzel, 1975). Hall and Oppenheim (1987) state:

Autogenic behavior constitutes a primary and fundamental feature of the earliest stages of ontogeny. Many of the complex species-typical motor action patterns that characterize the behavioral repertoire of adult animals (swimming, locomotion, flying, etc.) very likely represent the activation of neuronal circuitry that to a large extent has its origins in a basic neurobiological substrate laid down in the embryo and whose functional manifestation is reflected in spontaneous prenatal behavior (p. 96).

Thalamic and basal ganglia fibers from the internal capsule penetrate the developing cortex by two or three months gestational age (Poliakov, 1961) and the development of normal cortical laminae appears to depend upon the availability of prior inputs to the motor cortex (Marin-Padilla, 1970). The importance of patterned afferent activity for proper development of the visual system is well known (e.g., Wong, Sanes and Wong, 1998). For example, rhythmic waves of activity sweep across the retina providing patterned input to the lateral geniculate nucleus; the waves from the two retinas are uncorrelated. Based on the principle that 'neurons that fire together, wire together', this particular type of activity helps assure both retinotopic organization and neural segregation of thalamic and cortical inputs from each eye. In a similar way, prenatal movements of the upper limbs represent 'patterned activity', as opposed to noise, and asymmetric input to the developing thalamus might have consequences for development. Perhaps asymmetric embryonic upper limb activity leads to asymmetric thalamic and cortical development, ultimately contributing to the cortical asymmetries described in the previous section.

What produces this asymmetric peripheral activity? The best candidates at present are asymmetrically expressed molecules regulating cell proliferation, adhesion, and migration early in embryonic development (Varlet and Robertson, 1997). Though the manner in which the primary definition of the left–right axis is determined early in embryonic development is unknown, a cascade of recent studies provide evidence that many different molecules are expressed asymmetrically, in different embryonic locations and at different developmental stages. Of special interest is *lefty*, a member of the transforming growth factor-β (TGF-β) superfamily that is expressed in the mesoderm of the left lateral plate just prior to asymmetric heart development in mice (Meno, Saijoh, Fujii et al., 1996). It is also found only in the left half of the floorplate in the developing mid and hindbrain. Another molecule, *nodal*, has been found to be expressed more on the left edge of the notochord plate (Collignon, Varlet and Robertson, 1996). Variations in the lateral expression of these molecules accompany mutations affecting asymmetry of the viscera. Individuals homozygous for the *iv* gene have a 50% incidence of *situs inversus*, or a reversal of the laterality of the viscera, and *lefty* asymmetry is inverted in half of the homozygotes (Meno et al.,

1996). Individuals homozygous for the *inv* gene are nearly all characterized by *situs*, and *lefty* and *nodal* are expressed only on the right side (Meno et al., 1996). These results suggest that *lefty* and *nodal* may be downstream of the *iv* and *inv* genes.

Seven different gene products have been shown to have asymmetric expression in chick embryos and three in mouse embryos (Varlet and Robertson, 1997). Only *nodal* appears to be expressed in both chicks and mice, raising important questions regarding species differences in the precise means whereby asymmetry is established. Presumably, a similar or overlapping set of molecules is expressed asymmetrically in human embryos. Asymmetric molecular expression could conceivably lead to asymmetric motor activity through actions on peripheral neurons, though of course, this remains to be demonstrated.

## Prenatal influences on individual variation in handedness

A great many factors potentially affect the developing nervous system. These include infections, stress, and hormonal variation. Of these, hormonal influences have clearly been the subject of greatest scrutiny in the handedness literature. In a landmark paper, Geschwind and Galaburda (1985) suggested that higher prenatal testosterone levels slow the growth of the left hemisphere relative to the right, leading to, among many other things, a greater incidence of left-handedness. Galaburda (1990) offered a revised version of this hypothesis, i.e., greater testosterone leads to less neuronal pruning in the right hemisphere, and hence the relatively larger size of the right planum temporale. The Geschwind–Galaburda formulation spawned an immense body of research illuminating many issues in developmental neuropsychology, but not, in general, supporting either the original or the revised hypotheses on testosterone effects (see Bryden, McManus and Bulman-Fleming, 1994, and associated commentaries).

There are several ways to study the relationship between testosterone and handedness. Rodent models provide precise experimental control, but are of uncertain relevance as these species do not demonstrate directional handedness and the molecular determinants of asymmetry may differ from humans. In humans, hormone levels in second trimester amniotic fluid have been assessed and relationships with handedness examined at age 7 years (Grimshaw, Bryden and Finnegan, 1995). Among girls, greater testosterone levels predicted more right-handedness, whereas no relationship was observed in boys. Another research strategy involves analysis of handedness in opposite- and same-sex dizygotic twins. Females with a male co-twin are exposed to higher testosterone levels than females with a female cotwin; similarly, males with a male co-twin are exposed to higher testosterone levels than those with a female co-twin (Vom Sall and Bronson, 1978), and hence, each should exhibit an elevated incidence of left-handedness. A recent study (Elkadi, Nicholls and Clode, 1999) observed no such effects.

Two studies have found that females exposed to diethylstilbestrol (DES) in utero, a masculinizing hormone, demonstrated an increased incidence of left-handedness as adults (Schachter, 1994; Scheirs and Vingerhoets, 1995). One study found that congenital adrenal hyperplasia (CAH), a disorder associated with excess androgen levels, was associated with greater left-handedness (Nass, Baker, Virdis et al., 1987), but another (Baker and Erhardt, 1974) did not. Tan (as reviewed in Bryden et al., 1994) has shown in several studies with rather small samples that greater serum testosterone levels might be associated with increased right-hand performance in men, but not women. Moffat and Hampson (1996) found that left-handers had lower salivary testosterone, but this effect was not replicated in a more recent study (Moffat and Hampson, 2000). Obviously, it is difficult to draw firm conclusions regarding testosterone levels and handedness, but the extant studies do not support the Geschwind–Galaburda formulation.

'Season of birth' (or nine months earlier, 'season of conception') may serve as a proxy variable for several potentially important factors, as both the incidence of infections and hormone levels vary across seasons. A number of developmental disorders show seasonal effects. Schizophrenia appears to be associated with summer conceptions (late winter or early spring births; Torrey, Miller, Rawlings and Yolken, 1997a,b), while dyslexia occurs more often with early fall conceptions (Livingston, Adam and Bracha, 1993). Fall conception also increases risk for mental retardation and reading and arithmetic

disability (though not seizures, cerebral palsy, or articulation disorders; Liederman and Flannery, 1994). Fall conception may be associated with increased occurrence of infections during the late 1st trimester and the 2nd trimester. Because pineal activity, sex-hormone levels, and melatonin secretion vary seasonally, however, these factors may also contribute to seasonal effects on neurodevelopmental disorders (Liederman and Flannery, 1994).

A season of birth effect for handedness has not been demonstrated conclusively. Early studies of relatively small samples led to discrepant conclusions (Badian, 1983; Leviton and Kilty, 1979). A large-scale study of French men (Dellatolas, Curt and Lellouch (1991) found no relationship, but a subsequent re-analysis by Rogerson (1994), with further analyses of additional data sets, suggested that left-handers were somewhat more apt to be born in the months of March through July, and hence, be conceived during summer and early fall. A recent prospective study (Martin and Jones, 1999) confirmed these observations. Taken as a whole, it seems likely that season of conception is somehow weakly related to variation in nervous system development. It is not yet clear whether handedness is affected, and if so, in what manner.

## Perinatal and early postnatal influences on individual variation in handedness

The notion that perinatal birth trauma causes individual variation in handedness has a long history (Harris, 1992). No one seriously doubts that frank left hemisphere damage can lead to what has been termed 'pathological left-handedness'. Because more infants are predisposed to right- than left-handedness, the incidence of pathological left-handedness will be greater than that of pathological right-handedness. What is debated are two related issues. First, what is the incidence of pathological left-handedness? Second, is there any relationship between handedness and types of birth stress 'less serious' than frank left hemisphere damage? And if so, is the relationship correlational or causal?

Satz and colleagues (Orsini and Satz, 1986; Satz, 1972; Satz, Orsini, Saslow and Henry, 1985) have stated that pathological left-handedness is accompanied by left hemisphere injury, motor difficulties of the right hand, atypical lateralization for speech, and hypoplasia of the right foot. These criteria emerged from the study of specific clinical populations, however, and do not permit an estimate of the population incidence of pathologic left-handedness. Bishop (1984) reasoned that if pathologic handedness contributes more to left- than right-handedness, then the proportion of individuals with very poor motor skill in the non-preferred hand would be greater in left- than right-handers. She analyzed data from over 12,000 children in the National Child Development Study on two motor tasks: (1) a square marking test using writing implements, and (2) the time taken to transfer 20 matches from one box to another. The pattern expected under the hypothesis of pathologic left-handedness, i.e., a greater incidence of very poor performance with the non-preferred hand in left-handers, was observed only for the matchbox test. For this test, Bishop estimated that one in twenty left-handers might be considered pathologic. However, this probably is an overestimate of the true incidence, as there is no reason to expect pathologic handedness to emerge only for the matchbox test and not the square marking test. In any case, the vast majority of left-handers do not seem to suffer from early left hemisphere dysfunction, and thus, some other mechanism must be operating to produce left-handedness.

Is there a relationship between greater birth stress and left-handedness? The best answer emerges from a meta-analysis performed by Searleman, Porac and Coren (1989). They found no evidence that birth order is related to handedness, though birth order is a relevant marker for a variety of types of birth stressors. Advanced maternal age, multiple births, fast labor, slow labor, and breathing difficulties were also unrelated to handedness in both males and females. Among males, Rh incompatibility, low birth weight, prematurity, caesarian birth, and breech birth were each weakly related to handedness, accounting for less than one percent of the variance. No birth stress factors were predictive in females. More recent studies offer little to mitigate these conclusions, though some studies have found weak relationships between some measures of birth stress and handedness (e.g., Coren, 1995; McKeever, Suter and Rich, 1995). There may be a weak positive correlation between birth stress and left-handedness. It still remains to be demonstrated, however, that any such a relationship is causal, as it is possible that fetuses with some manner of mild or sub-clinical abnormality prior to birth are more prone to perinatal complications (Goodman, 1988), and evidence reviewed above reveals differences between left- and right-handers during fetal development.

Specific environmental influences on handedness during childhood have proven difficult to identify. Possibly, handedness is influenced by direct instruction or imitation from parents or sibs. A contrasting possibility is that postnatal non-biological environmental factors are of no relevance for individual variation in handedness. In behavior genetic studies, non-genetic influences are often conceptualized as falling into two broad classes. Those social and environmental factors that are shared by members of a given family are termed 'shared' influences and those unique to a given family member 'unique' factors. Scores of studies over the past two decades of virtually every imaginable psychological variable have revealed that unique factors are more important than shared (e.g., Plomin and Daniels, 1987). When shared effects are observed, they often diminish as children grow up. In the area of intelligence, for example, adoption studies have found that shared environmental effects are associated with 4–5% of the variance in IQ scores in younger non-biologically related siblings, but this diminishes to 0% by age 18 (Scarr, 1992).

The most straightforward way to estimate the relative importance of shared and unique environmental factors is through adoption studies. Adopting parents do not share the genetic make-up of their adopted children. Hence, resemblance between them would likely reflect shared effects, e.g., children being taught to use a certain hand for a given task or simply imitating their parents. The extent to which adopted-away children resemble their biological parents provides a measure of genetic influence. A very important adoption study by Carter-Saltzman (1980) sheds some light on these issues. Most centrally, offspring handedness was related to that of their biologic parents, not their adopting parents. If training or imitation of left-hand use were causally related to left-hand use in children, one would expect that adopting parents who were left-handed would have more adopted children who were left-handed. We can compare the incidence of right-handedness in adopted children with one left-handed parent (86%) vs. those with none (87%) in the Carter-Saltzman study. These data make a compelling case that parental influences within the home do not contribute to individual variation in handedness.

It is, of course, possible that unique environmental factors contribute to variations in handedness. However, the identification of 'unique' factors is more complex than for shared factors, and most statistical expressions of their importance conflate unique social influences (e.g., having a left-handed baseball coach) and non-directional genetic influence (Molenaar, Boorsma and Dolan, 1993), as discussed in greater detail below. There is indeed evidence that severe injuries to one arm or hand can shift handedness in a small proportion of individuals (Porac, 1995), but this sort of effect seems unlikely to help us understand the development of atypical handedness in the vast majority of individuals absent such trauma. In this regard it is also important to recall the impressive evidence for the stability of relative hand skill over the childhood and adult life span (Annett, 1998), data raising serious questions about the possible importance of postnatal unique environmental determinants.

## The genetics of handedness

Theories regarding the heritability of handedness date to the early part of this century (Harris, 1992), yet there still exists no consensus on whether there is indeed a genetic component (i.e., Provins, 1997) or, if there is, exactly what aspect of the phenotype is to be the focus of a genetic model. In the next two sections evidence for genetic influences on hand preference and relative hand skill are reviewed. Then, new data suggesting the importance of specific genes or chromosomes are discussed. Finally, genetic models of handedness are critically analyzed.

### Hand preference

Carter-Saltzman's (1980) adoption study suggested that genetic factors are important in explaining familial resemblance in handedness: adopted away offspring resembled their biological parents, not the parents who adopted them. It would seem a simple matter to apply the powerful techniques of behavior genetics research to provide estimates of the relative importance of genetic as well as shared and unique environmental sources of variance. However, no agreement about the magnitude of genetic influence has yet emerged and it is important to understand why.

One important problem is that the phenotype of handedness is age-dependent and multi-faceted. Do we wish to model the prenatal preference asymmetries, the dichotomous and socially influenced phenotype of writing hand, the continuous asymmetries of the putative cortical substrates of manual skill asymmetry, or the asymmetry of skill on peg moving tasks? Do we wish to model fine-motor skill asymmetries or strength/throwing asymmetries? Do we wish to model directional asymmetries or the extent of deviation from the population mean, which appears to be heritable in nonhuman species (e.g., Collins, 1985)? The obvious answer is that we would like to have behavior genetic analyses on all such aspects of handedness, but the vast majority of analyses have examined only the dichotomous variable of preferred writing hand. This data base is optimal for testing a genetic theory of handedness that posits two discrete categories of handedness (i.e., McManus and Bryden, 1992), adequate for testing a genetic theory that posits three different genotypes (Annett, 1985), and inadequate for testing a genetic theory that posits that the degree of atypicality, in either direction from the population mean, is heritable (Collins, 1985; Yeo and Gangestad, 1993).

Another difficulty inherent in studying the genetics of handedness is the questionable utility of using a twin design, the workhorse of contemporary behavior genetics. There have been several issues raised regarding twins, though, as is so typical in this field, consensus has proven elusive. Some have suggested an elevated incidence of left-handedness in twins (e.g., Davis and Annett, 1994) or in the parents of twins (Bocklage, 1981). Others have pointed out that some monozygotic twins are 'mirror images' of each other, down to the direction of hair whorls, a factor obviously complicating analyses of laterality. Some MZ twins are monochorionic, sharing the same fetal membranes (approximately 30%), while others are dichorionic, which tends to occur if egg splitting takes place in the first 72 hours after fertilization. A recent study found no evidence that chorion status influenced either the incidence of left-handedness or concordance among MZ twins (Carlier, Spitz, Vacher-Lavenu et al., 1996), but may have had limited power to detect such effects. In any case, the data emerging from twin studies do not appear to be consistent with the data emerging from family studies. In behavior genetic analyses of other traits, the conflation of home environment and genetic influences inherent in family studies would render them much less preferred as designs for genetic analyses than twin studies. If one assumes, however, that family environment contributes little to handedness (as suggested by Carter-Saltzman's adoption study), and twin studies have their own unique problems in the study of handedness (which may or may not be the case), family studies may provide the best data available.

One thing we know for sure: hand preference runs in families. In a recent meta-analysis McManus and Bryden (1992) reviewed the incidence of left-handedness (a categorical variable) across 72,600 individuals. When both parents were right-handed, 9.5% of their offspring were left-handed. When one parent was left-handed and the other right-handed 19.5% of offspring were left-handed. Interestingly, if the mother was left-handed 21.9% of offspring were left-handed, as opposed to 16.8% if the father was left-handed (the so-called 'maternal effect'). Finally, if both parents were left-handed, 26.1% of offspring were left-handed. These data can also be expressed as the ratio of two different odds, i.e., an 'odds ratio'. The ratio of one set of odds, the number of left-handed children born to parents in which at least one parent was left-handed divided by the number of right-handed children born to such parents, is divided by the ratio of another set of odds, the number of left-handed children born to two right-handed parents divided by the number of right-handed children born to such parents. This odds ratio is 2.08 for the McManus and Bryden meta-analysis and represents a quantitative expression of the greater tendency for left-handed children to be born to a set of parents with at least one left-hander than to two right-handed parents. These family patterns must be accounted for by any theory, environmental or genetic, that purports to account for individual variation in handedness.

An important new study has examined resemblance for hand preference in families from India and Canada (Bryden, Roy, McManus and Bulman-Fleming, 1997). These authors obtained data on preferred hand use for 10 activities in both children and their parents. They also attempted to evaluate (via odds ratios) heritability of the strength of handedness (irrespective of direction) and extremity of handedness, variables critical to certain genetic approaches described in detail below. In Canada, the odds of having a left-handed child given at least one left-handed parent are approximately twice as great as when both parents are right-handed, whereas in India the odds are three times as great. The heritability of the strength of hand preference, regardless of the direction of preference, was also significant in both countries, and the odds ratio was greater than for direction of preference. The effect was also much larger in India than Canada. Similar data were provided by Coren and Porac (1980), who found weak, though significant, correlations for the nondirectional degree of hand, eye, foot, and ear preference asymmetry among family members. They found no significant correlations for the direction of preferences. This same type of effect has also been demonstrated by Collins (1985) in mice: the degree of asymmetry, in either direction, proved heritable, but not the direction.

In a related analysis, Bryden et al. also examined the heritability of 'extremity', which is relevant to the developmental instability model of the genetics of handedness (Yeo and Gangestad, 1993; Yeo et al., 1997a). Hand preference scores were divided into quartiles, with the middle two being termed 'moderate' and the others 'extreme'. The ratio of the odds of (a) two parents, at least one of whom was extreme, having a child of extreme handedness, to (b) two parents without extreme handedness having a child of extreme handedness, was computed and found to be significant in the Indian sample but not the Canadian sample.

Two recent studies have summarized research conducted before 1990 on hand preferences of twins (Coren and Halpern, 1991; McManus and Bryden, 1992). Aggregating data across studies, they suggest that the overall rate of concordance for hand preference is nearly identical for monozygotic (MZ) and dizygotic (DZ) twins. A new study of preference patterns in 1700 adolescent twin pairs and their parents offered a variety of interesting observations (Orlebeke, Knol, Koopmans et al., 1996). In contrast to some studies (e.g., Davis and Annett, 1994), but consistent with others (McManus, 1980), left-handedness was not more common in twins than the general population. Calculation of odds ratios indicated a higher association of left-handedness in male MZ twins than male DZ twins; for females, a trend in the same direction was noted. Maternal handedness was associated with handedness of both male and female offspring, but paternal handedness influenced only the handedness of sons, raising the possibility of a Y-chromosome effect. Left-handedness was more common in firstborn than secondborn twins of both types, and among the firstborn, the incidence of left-handedness increased in proportion to the degree to which the secondborn twin was heavier than the first. The authors suggest that left-handedness "is associated with intra-uterine growth disturbances — for which a large intra-pair birth weight disparity is an indication — and that the first born twin could be more vulnerable when birth weight is lower than the second born" (p. 488).

This study provides an opportunity to compare heritability in twin vs. family studies. One can calculate an odds ratio limited to MZ and DZ twins and their parents. Re-analyzing the original data, the odds ratio is 1.31, notably less than the figure achieved across all children (2.08) in the McManus and Bryden meta-analysis or the figure one can compute from Carter-Saltzman's study of adopted children and their biologic parents (2.29). Factors determining of handedness in twins may thus be somewhat different than those important in non-twins. Hence, one should probably be cautious in generalizing conclusions emerging from studies of twins to the far more numerous non-twin population.

### Relative hand skill

Very few studies have examined heritability of relative hand skill. Annett (1978) observed no resemblance of left minus right peg moving speed among all combinations of family members (e.g., father–son, brother–sister) except for a very weak relationship between mothers and daughters. A computerized peg moving task allowing separate measures of

'transport time' (the time spent physically moving one peg to the next hole) and 'search time' (the time spent reaching to grasp the next peg) was used in a large study of children ($N = 1150$ children) and their parents (Curt, De Agostini, Maccario and Dellatolas, 1995). Transport time was more strongly related to hand preference and showed a greater degree of asymmetry. Maternal left-handedness predicted reduced rightward asymmetry of both measures in children, while only reduced asymmetry for search time was predicted by paternal left-handedness. Carlier and colleagues (Carlier, Beau, Marchand and Michel, 1994) examined sibling ($N = 46$ pairs) resemblance for Tapley and Bryden's (1985) dot-filling test and a computerized tapping test from which two measures were analyzed, the relative difference in speed between the two hands and the regularity of tapping (the ratio of the standard deviations in inter-tap interval between non-preferred and preferred hands). Sibling resemblance was found only for the dot-filling task.

Carlier et al. (1996) used the same performance measures from their sibling study in a separate study of twins. Asymmetry scores were only weakly inter-correlated and intra-class correlations were not higher in MZ than DZ twins. Jancke and Steinmetz (1995) examined 10 MZ twin pairs concordant for right-handedness and 10 MZ twin pairs discordant for handedness. Intra-class correlations in each group for the absolute degree of asymmetry (irrespective of direction) were not significant, though small sample size limited statistical power.

We explored the possibility that what is heritable is the extent to which an individual differs from the population-typical skill asymmetry (Gangestad and Yeo, 1994). In essence, we thought this might reflect the 'human version' of Collins' (1985) hypothesis that degree but not direction of asymmetry is heritable in mice, the only difference being that in humans the population mean is shifted from zero laterality towards greater right-hand skill. Using Annett's pegboard test (Annett, 1971) we determined for each subject the extent to which they deviated from the sample mean. We predicted that individuals with 'extreme' handedness, either greater left-hand skill or relatively greater-than-average right-hand skill, would be more apt to have parents they reported to be left-handed, as left-hand preference is more atypical than right. A significant curvilinear relationship was observed, so that individuals at either end of the distribution of relative (left minus right) hand skill were more apt to have left-handed parents, consistent with our hypothesis that extent of atypicality is heritable. Annett (1996) did not observe this relationship in a similar analysis, however, so the issue awaits additional data. The best way to test the idea is to explore correlations of atypicality in hand skill in both parents and children, rather than relying upon hand preference reports of the parents.

Comparing genetic studies of preference and performance, two observations might be made. First, as was noted across studies of genetic influence on preference, family studies provide somewhat more support for a genetic factor than twin studies. Second, there is less striking evidence for heritability of relative hand skill than hand preference. A possible reason for the latter is that preference measures aggregate responses across a number of tasks and hence provide a broader measure of handedness than a measure of relative hand skill from a single task. Perhaps, a composite measure of relative skill across a number of tasks would have a heritability more closely resembling that of preference measures. This would also render studies of the heritability of handedness more like studies of the heritability of intelligence, which rely upon assessment of composite skills.

*Attempts to identify specific genetic influences*

A genetic contribution to variation in handedness is fairly well established. The next step is to identify specific genetic influences, i.e., individual alleles or chromosomes, or broader genomic factors. In this exciting and rapidly developing area, several such specific influences have been suggested.

Yeo and Gangestad (1993) have attempted to link variations in handedness to broad genomic factors. They hypothesized that variation around the population mean for relative hand skill in humans (a directional asymmetry) reflects the same factors that determine variation around the population mean (zero) for other asymmetries characterized by fluctuating asymmetry (FA). There has been much research in diverse species as to the determinants of the magnitude of FA, and both genetic and environmental influences have been found (Markow, 1994; Møller and Swaddle, 1997). Genetic factors include mutation load, disruption of co-adapted gene complexes through sexual recombination, and possibly, polygenic homozygosity. Environmental factors include maternal physiologic stress, toxins, and pathogens. These environmental factors are most apt to influence developmental stability, i.e., the ability of an organism to faithfully execute its ontogenetic program for development, in susceptible genomes. The two major phenotypic expressions of developmental instability are the presence of morphologically phenodeviant traits, such as MPAs, and FA (Møller and Swaddle, 1997).

In three studies an overall index of developmental stability, comprised of MPAs (by definition, morphologically atypical traits) and FA of several body characteristics, was related to measures of hand preference and relative hand skill (Yeo et al., 1993, 1997a). The total MPA and FA scores were $z$-scored and combined to provide a total index of developmental instability. The group of subjects with left-hand preference had greater developmental instability than those with a right-hand preference. The relationship between relative hand skill and developmental instability is shown in Fig. 4. Two features are noteworthy. As one deviates from a moderate right-hand skill advantage, in either direction, developmental instability increases. Second, the value of relative hand performance associated with minimal developmental instability is very near the median value of relative hand skill. The theoretical implications of this observation are discussed in the next section. However, the association of markers of developmental instability with handedness suggests the importance of the known genetic and environmental underpinnings of developmental instability for individual variation in handedness. A summary measure of 'extremity' of physical characteristics (e.g., atypically wide or atypically narrow feet) was also related to atypical handedness (Yeo and Gangestad, 1993); such atypicality could reflect overall mutation load or polygenic homozygosity.

New data link FA with handedness in chimpanzees. In male chimpanzees, greater FA for testicle size (a trait under intense selection pressure in this primate species) is greater for non-right-handed than right-handed individuals. An even stronger

**Developmental Instability**

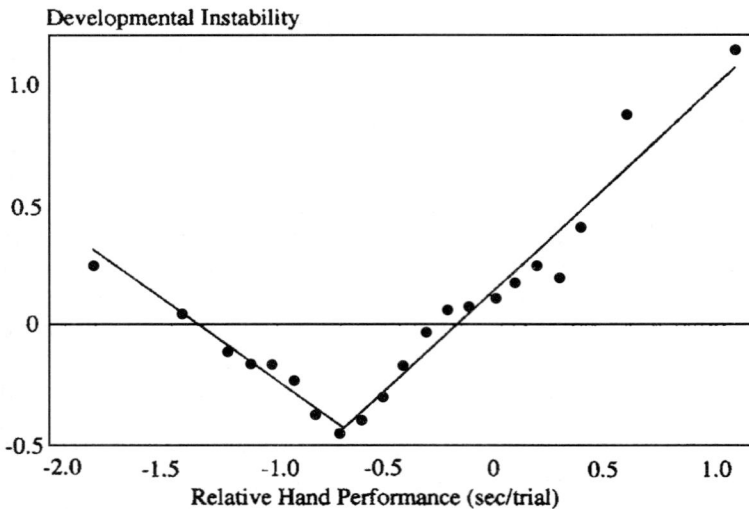

Fig. 4. Relationship between developmental instability and relative hand preference. The *y*-axis represents a composite measure of minor physical anomalies and fluctuating asymmetry and the *x*-axis represents relative hand skill on Annett's peg-moving test. Each subject's hand performance score ($N = 348$) was rounded to the nearest 0.1 s and averaged. Towards the ends of the distribution several intervals were combined so that each data point represented included at least nine subjects. Lines are best-fit regression lines. (From Yeo, Gangestad, Thoma et al., 1997a.)

effect was found when individuals with extreme handedness (in either direction) were compared to those with moderate handedness (Dahl, Hopkins and Pilcher, personal communication).

Left-hand preference has been linked with particular alleles in the human leukocyte antigen (HLA) system (Gangestad, Yeo, Shaw et al., 1996). This study was prompted by reports (reviewed in Bryden et al., 1994) that left-handedness was associated with autoimmune disorders of the thyroid (Grave's Disease and Hashimoto's thyroiditis), autoimmune disorders of the gut (celiac disease and Crohn's Disease) and systemic lupus erythematosus. Each of these disorders has been linked with the same set of HLA alleles on chromosome 6: A1, B8, and DR3. These alleles are in linkage disequilibrium and thus tend to aggregate within individuals. In a sample of 664 healthy adult blood donors, data were available for the A and B loci, though only a subset underwent DR typing. Individuals with left-hand preference were more apt to possess the B8 and DR3 alleles, as well as the A1/B8 haplotype. The manner in which these alleles, or others in which they are in linkage disequilibrium, are related to handedness is uncertain. One clue may be that the B8 allele and the A1/B8 haplotypes predicted fewer offspring by

that individual. We speculated that these alleles may adversely affect (or may be linked with other alleles that affect) either the mother's or the infant's immune response to pathogenic threats to fetal development and thereby influence developmental stability of the fetus, ultimately producing atypical handedness. In support of this view, maternal infections have been reported to increase fluctuating asymmetry in offspring (Livshits, Davadi, Kobylianski et al., 1988). Interestingly, the DR3 allele appears to be linked to a higher incidence of spontaneous abortion (Christiansen, Pedersen, Mathiesen et al., 1996).

Other recent studies point to a role for genes on the sex chromosomes. The Orlebeke et al. (1996) twin study described earlier raised the possibility of a gene or genes on the Y-chromosome related to hand preference. A recent study of five data sets providing information on the relatedness of almost 15,000 sibling pairs (Corballis, Lee, McManus and Crow, 1996) also suggested a sex chromosome locus. Same-sex sib pairs were about 10% more likely to be concordant for handedness than opposite-sex sib pairs. This is consistent with the possibility of a gene (or genes) on the sex chromosomes related to hand preference.

Corballis (1997) expressed skepticism about the existence of different alleles for handedness on the Y-chromosome. He demonstrated through modeling procedures that polymorphisms on the Y-chromosome were very unlikely to be maintained at a stable population incidence in males given even very minimal differences between the sexes in the fitness consequences associated with this gene. Thus, there may be other explanations for the weak same- vs. opposite-sex concordance effect. Perhaps XY and XX genotypes may occasion somewhat different prenatal growth dynamics, affecting handedness in consistently different ways. In this fashion, these genotypes may not only lead to slight sex differences in the incidence of left-handedness, but also differently moderate the developmental processes leading to handedness. More generally, Rice and Holland (1998) have shown that some genes 'work better' when in males, others when in females. As a result, same-sex sibs may share developmental stress more so than opposite-sex pairs. If developmental stress contributes to left-handedness (see Developmental Instability model, below) this could explain the difference in concordance rates across same- and opposite-sex sib pairs. This possibility represents more of a 'whole chromosome' or genomic influence than a single-gene effect.

Another recent study (Laval, Dann, Butler et al., 1998) investigated the possibility of an X-chromosome locus for both handedness and psychosis, reflecting the theory of Crow (1997) that a single gene may relate to both left-handedness and psychosis-proneness. In the group of families in which sibling pairs were affected by psychosis, a locus near the centromere was more apt to be shared by affected than non-affected male siblings, but not female siblings or mixed-sex sibships. In a second family sample in which a pair of brothers were left-handed, a locus in a similar region of the X-chromosome was associated with degree of left-handedness, but not left- vs. right-hand preference. These results are intriguing, but several questions remain. Why is the psychosis effect found only in male–male sibships, and does the observation regarding hand skill generalize to all types of sibships?

Based on a new set of family data, as well as re-analysis of existing data sets, McKeever (2000) has suggested X-linked transmission for hand preference. He noted that "left-handed mothers produce significantly more left-handed sons than daughters,

left-handed fathers produce significantly more left-handed daughters than sons, and left-handed fathers do not produce more left-handed sons than right-handed fathers" (p. 32). X-linkage would predict a much greater incidence of left-handedness in males than females, but the incidence of left-handedness in males is only 2% greater than the incidence for females. To account for the slight sex difference McKeever hypothesized that females may be more vulnerable to non-genetic causes of left-handedness, such as developmental instability or birth stress. To our knowledge, there is no empirical support for a greater incidence of developmental instability in females, and the meta-analysis of Searleman et al. (1989) found no evidence that perinatal stress affected handedness in females.

Much more research is necessary before one can conclude that specific genetic influences on handedness have been identified. Candidate factors include mutation load, polygenic homozygosity, specific HLA alleles, as well as genes on the sex chromosomes. Of course, these alternatives are not mutually exclusive.

*Genetic theories of handedness*

A variety of models have been proposed to explain the nature of genetic factors producing variation in human handedness. The first issue confronted by any genetic theory of handedness is the definition of the phenotype, in particular, the nature of the behavioral trait and whether it is a dichotomous or continuously distributed variable. There are many correlated dimensions to the trait of handedness, including preference, fine-motor skill and strength/throwing skill. Further, handedness is weakly correlated with a plethora of non-manual asymmetries, from ear and foot dominance to variation in almost any cognitive skill showing cerebral lateralization at a population level. As noted above, it is correlated with a wide variety of neuroanatomical asymmetries. What are the appropriate boundaries for a genetic theory of handedness? There is no doubt that phenotypic variation in the hand used for writing can be expressed as a dichotomous trait, and this probably well characterizes performance on many paper and pencil skill tests, such as that of Tapley and Bryden (1985). But all the other various manifestations of handedness, and all the other correlated anatomic and cognitive skill asymmetries, are continuously distributed.

A summary of the central components of genetic theories of handedness is provided in Table 1. The first major distinction among theories of handedness is between those that posit dichotomous vs. continuously distributed phenotypes. Of the major theories, Laland, Kumm, Van Horn and Feldman (1995) and McManus and Bryden (1992) are examples of the former, while Annett (1985) and Yeo and Gangestad (1993) are examples of the latter. In his model of handedness in mice, Collins (1985) also opts for a continuously distributed phenotype. A clear advantage to models of a dichotomous phenotype is that they can attempt to model the vast collection of data on familial resemblance for the one aspect of handedness that is dichotomous: writing hand. They risk, however, focusing too narrowly on a selected aspect of the phenotype.

The second major distinction among theories concerns whether the phenotype is best represented as skill or preference. There is a bit of the 'chicken or the egg' flavor to this issue, as one aspect of the phenotype may inevitably lead to the other. In this sense the choice may not be critical. Preference and skill asymmetry frequency distributions look quite different, though, as the former are typically J-shaped while the latter are closer to normal. Hence, skill asymmetries offer the possibility of achieving greater discrimination among phenotypes. For example, skill asymmetry distributions can distinguish among the vast proportion of the population who are self-described right-handers, while preference inventories are limited in this regard (and the shorter the inventory, the more limited they are). However, there are obviously limits on how many activities can be measured in an individual, so studies of hand preference have real practical benefits. Following Annett (1985), our inclination has been for skill measures, while Laland et al. (1995) and McManus and Bryden (1992) prefer to focus on preference, as does Collins (1985).

Two different phenomena must be explained: (1) the species-wide tendency toward right-handedness; and (2) individual variation. Annett (1985) and McManus and Bryden (1992) suggest that a single gene makes humans different from other species in terms of handedness and language dominance; allelic vari-

ation at this single locus accounts for all genetic variation in the population. Laland et al. (1995) and Yeo and Gangestad (1993) suggest that many genes, shared amongst all members of the species, contribute to making human asymmetry different from other animals, but these theories differ in how to account for individual variation. Let us turn to the models themselves. Annett's Right Shift Model (1985) and McManus and Bryden's (1992) model have been reviewed in detail several times (e.g., Annett, 1996; Corballis, 1997; McManus, 1985; McManus and Bryden, 1992). Hence, we shall devote a bit more consideration to the newer models of Laland et al. (1995) and Yeo and Gangestad (1993).

*Annett's Right Shift theory*

The best known genetic model of handedness is Marian Annett's Right Shift Model. Annett (1985) proposes that a certain allele, the right shift (or $rs^+$) allele, tends to slow right hemisphere development in utero, biasing brain growth so as to increase the probability of left hemisphere dominance for language and right-handedness. Another allele, the right shift minus ($rs^-$) allele, has no such biasing tendency. Annett has always argued for an element of 'chance' in the development of handedness, such that random factors act to influence the phenotype. However, the $rs^+$ gene accounts for about 50% of phenotypic variation (Gilger, 1995). In individuals with two copies of the $rs^-$ allele, chance factors along with environmental influences produce phenotypic variation. Genetic effects are additive (though in earlier versions of her model the $rs^+$ allele was dominant). Estimates of allele frequencies were derived from the proportion of individuals rendered aphasic after right hemisphere lesions ($rs^+ = 0.57$, $rs^- = 0.43$) and can be used to generate genotype frequencies ($rs^-$, $rs^- = 0.18$; $rs^+$, $rs^- = 0.49$; $rs^+$, $rs^+ = 0.32$). Two added assumptions concern sex differences and handedness in twins. Annett (1985) assumes that the $rs^+$ allele is expressed more strongly in women than men. This allows her to account for the slightly greater left-handedness evident in men. It also helps account for the maternal effect (though McManus and Bryden, 1992, point out that this detail of her model predicts a much smaller maternal effect than that which is observed). She also assumes that the $rs^+$

TABLE 1

Summary of major differences among theories of variation in handedness

| Issue | Annett | McManus and Bryden | Yeo and Gangestad | Laland et al. | Collins (in mice) |
|---|---|---|---|---|---|
| What is the fundamental phenotype? | continuously distributed skill differences | dichotomous preference differences | continuously distributed skill differences | dichotomous preference differences | continuously distributed preferences |
| What accounts for our species' right-handedness? | a single gene | a single gene | species-wide polygenes for asymmetry | species-wide polygenes for handedness | not relevant |
| What mechanisms account for individual differences? | allelic variation at a single locus | allelic variation at a major locus and a modifier locus | nondirectional genetic/environmental influences in development | non-genetic parental factors | nondirectional genetic/environmental influences in development |
| How do these mechanisms work? | $rs^+$ allele shifts dominance, $rs^-$ has null effect | D allele shifts dominance, C has null effect, M modifies D | affect prenatal developmental stability | not specified | not specified |
| How is genetic variation maintained? | heterozygote advantage for cognitive ability | unspecified heterozygote advantage | spontaneous mutation, recombination, gene–parasite co-evolution | not relevant | not specified |
| How is the sex difference explained? | the $rs^+$ allele is expressed more strongly in females | LH mothers are more apt to transmit C allele than LH males | not specified | not specified | not specified |
| How is the 'maternal' effect explained? | the $rs^+$ allele is expressed more strongly in females | the M allele is recessive, on X-chromosome | maternal genes influence both fetus and prenatal envt. | not specified | not specified |
| How is variation in other asymmetries explained? | genes affect language and handedness, others not specified | genes affect language and handedness, others not specified | the same genetic/environmental influences as for variation in handedness | not specified | not specified |

allele is expressed more strongly in singletons than twins.

Given these assumptions, Annett's model fairly successfully predicts patterns of familial resemblance regardless of sex (see McManus (1985) for a detailed analysis of the model's weaknesses). Another major feature of Annett's model is that it attempts to specify the selection forces maintaining gene frequencies at stable rates (Annett, 1985). The three different genotypes are hypothesized to be associated with different patterns of cognitive ability. The rs$^+$, rs$^+$ genotype is said to have relative weaknesses in spatial reasoning and mathematics, due to excessive handicapping of the right hemisphere early in development. The rs$^-$, rs$^-$ genotype is said to have weaknesses in phonological processing due to the lack of cerebral dominance for language. The heterozygote (rs$^+$, rs$^-$) genotype suffers neither of these disadvantages and is thus favored by natural selection. The alleged heterozygote advantage maintains genetic variability across generations because this genotype cannot breed true. A certain proportion of the offspring of two advantaged heterozygotes will inevitably be the disadvantaged rs$^+$, rs$^+$ and rs$^-$, rs$^-$ genotypes. The empirical support for the predicted associations of patterns of cognitive skill with handedness is mixed at best (see Annett, 1985; Cerone and McKeever, 1999; Corballis, 1997; McManus, Shergill and Bryden, 1993). We return to Annett's model after considering the related views of McManus and Bryden (1992).

*McManus and Bryden's theory*

McManus and Bryden (1992) offered a genetic model that, as does Annett's, proposes an autosomal locus with two possible alleles that work in additive fashion, the D (for dextral) and C (for chance) alleles. The DD genotype always produces right-handedness, whereas the CC genotype results in fluctuating asymmetry, with 50% left-handers and 50% right-handers. The DC genotype produces 25% left-handers and 75% right-handers. Gene frequencies were chosen to optimize the fit of the model to family handedness data. Twin data are accommodated by presuming that in the CC and DC genotypes the chance factors operate independently in each pair. There are three major differences between Annett's model and that of McManus and Bryden.

First, as noted above, McManus and Bryden posit two fundamental phenotypes, people with left- or right-hand preference. Second, chance factors operate only on the DC and CC genotypes, whereas for Annett they affect each of the three genotypes. Third, McManus and Bryden propose a modifier locus on the X-chromosome. The dominant M allele has no effect on laterality, whereas the recessive m allele renders the function of the D allele the same as the C allele. Since males have only one X-chromosome, the m allele is more apt to be expressed, accounting for the greater incidence of left-handedness in males as well as the maternal effect. Some manner of heterozygote advantage is presumed to account for the static equilibrium gene frequencies, but the nature of this advantage has not been specified.

Both of these models (as well as others described below) provide reasonably good fits to the family data. Klar (1996) has offered a similar model that also accounts well for much family data. Being able to fit accurately family data, however, does not mean that a model is correct (as is obvious given that *different* models fit the data well). A good fit of the model to the data indicates only that the model is not inconsistent with the data. Unless a specific gene is in fact found, there remains a rather 'ad hoc' quality to these models and their assumptions. Is it biologically reasonable to presume that a single gene distinguishes human from other primates in terms of language lateralization and handedness? As Gilger (1995, p. 546) stated, "with some 30% of our 75,000 or so structural genes playing specific roles in CNS development, a single gene alone being responsible for at least half the variability in cerebral dominance stretches the imagination." Further, we are aware of no other complex behavioral phenotype in normal humans that is determined by a single gene, so, if single-gene models of handedness are correct, they are certainly unique.

It must also be asked how well these models account for variation in other asymmetries than language dominance and handedness. Different cognitive asymmetries are essentially uncorrelated (Boles, 1991), as are different neuroanatomic asymmetries. Patterns of hand-clasping, arm-folding, and eye dominance each appear to run in families, suggesting a genetic component, and further, these are at best only weakly related to handedness (McManus and

Bryden, 1992). It appears difficult for single-gene models to account for the genetics of other aspects of laterality, which also seem to be characterized by a genetic component unique to humans. Also, how plausible is the notion that gene frequencies are maintained by heterozygote advantage? About half the human population is theoretically rendered less fit by possessing either of the homozygous genotypes. If two different alleles provide a substantial benefit that a single allele at the locus does not, one might expect that selection pressures would lead to the emergence of two different alleles existing at different loci, which might provide the benefits of heterozygosity without the cost. Or, one might expect the evolution of additional genes that otherwise moderate the deleterious effects of homozygosity at the locus. Although heterozygote advantage has been shown to account for genetic polymorphism responsible for phenotypic variation in a human trait (the famous example of sickle-cell anemia), such instances appear to be extremely rare.

There is evidence that left-handers have traits correlated with reduced fitness (Yeo and Gangestad, 1993) and also lower fecundity (Gangestad and Yeo, 1994; McManus and Bryden, 1992) than right-handers. Across 15,303 pairs of parents described in one study, two right-handed parents had an average of 2.84 births, compared to 2.56 when one parent was left-handed (McManus and Bryden, 1992). In a separate study, we estimated that left-handers would have 1.62 children by age 45 and right-handers 2.03 (Gangestad et al., 1994). While low fecundity today may result from a conscious decision to use contraception, a factor that may not have operated in ancestral times, there is evidence that the lower fecundity of left-handers is at least partly due to fertility problems. An epidemiological study found that left-handers were less likely to ever marry (Stellman, Wynder, DeRose and Muscat, 1997), suggesting that data from only married couples may underestimate the extent to which left-handers have fewer children. Perhaps consistent with this observation, homosexual men have a 34% greater chance of being left-handed than heterosexual men, and homosexual women have a 91% greater chance of being left-handed than heterosexual women (Lalumiere, Blanchard and Zucker, 2000). To our knowledge, no survival advantages associated with left-handedness have been reported that might offset these disadvantages.

*The developmental instability theory*

We have proposed that variation in human handedness is an outcome of developmental instability (DI) (Gangestad and Yeo, 1994; Gangestad et al., 1996; Yeo and Gangestad, 1993, 1998; Yeo et al., 1993, 1997a; see also Markow, 1992). Our approach was prompted by the dilemma posed above. If, as appears to be the case, left-handedness has a genetic component, how can it possibly be maintained at a steady incidence when it appears to be disadvantaged? The DI approach draws on a vast and expanding literature in evolutionary biology that began with an attempt to understand the causes and significance of fluctuating asymmetry (for recent reviews see Markow, 1994; Møller and Swaddle, 1997; Thornhill and Møller, 1997). DI refers to organisms' inability to express completely and accurately the species-specific plan for development. Slight departures from design caused by the random effects of mutations, pathogens, and toxins result in a less than perfect expression of the ontogenetic plan. Individual members of a species differ in their exposure to deleterious perturbations and/or their ability to resist their effects.

The DI model of handedness proposes that (1) population-typical right-handedness in humans is accounted for by a universal (or 'near-universal', see Yeo and Gangestad, 1993) developmental design culminating in moderate right-handedness, and (2) deviations from modal right-handedness result from developmental instability during early prenatal periods. We suggest that genetic effects on handedness do not result from variations in genes that code for lateralization, as is claimed by both Annett (1985) and McManus and Bryden (1992). Rather, they result from three sets of factors. First, broad genomic characteristics such as disruption of co-adapted gene complexes and polygenetic homozygosity can influence susceptibility to DI. Second, mutations can disrupt developmental processes. Third, pathogens can disrupt development and genes that affect susceptibility to pathogens may also affect DI. The DI approach is consistent with much of the genetic data cited above. In terms of preference, left-handedness is atypical and hence should be associated with greater DI, which it is (Yeo et al., 1993). In terms of hand skill, atypicality in either direction from the population mean should be associated with greater DI.

Though genetic influences clearly underlie DI, the genotype–phenotype relationship is complex and should be understood in terms of epigenetics. "Epigenetics or epigenetic control refers to the multiple genetic and non-genetic factors that influence or regulate gene activity during development" (Hall, 1998, p. 113–114). In their discussion of the developmental biology of FA, Klingenberg and Nijhout (1999) put it this way, "Heritable variation of FA is due to the genetically modulated expression of random noise that is itself independent of the genotype. There is therefore no clearcut dichotomy between genetic and environmental variation" (p. 373). They also note that nonlinear relationships between genetic or environmental influences and phenotype are ubiquitous in development. Molenaar and colleagues have referred to this influence on phenotype as a "third source of developmental differences" (Molenaar et al., 1993), along with environmental and genetic processes, and suggest "that variation in this epigenetic process. . . can be considered of chaotic origin" (p. 519). In standard biometrical models, this source of variance is captured under the 'unique' or 'within family' environmental variance term (Molenaar et al., 1993; Yeo, Gangestad and Turkheimer, 1995).

Two recent studies suggest that DI is associated with a genome less buffered from environmental perturbations. In a sample (120 total pairs) of 7-year-old MZ and DZ twins we used regression-based methods to fit genetic models for a variety of physical and behavioral phenotypes (Turkheimer, Wilkniss and Yeo, 1997). Children who demonstrated greater asymmetry between the hands on the Wallin Pegboard test showed lower levels of heritability for most physical and cognitive measures. Extreme left-handed and right-handed children appeared to contribute equally to this effect. Thus, environmental or epigenetic factors appear to be relatively more important for phenotypes with greater asymmetry in hand skill. This is consistent with the hypothesis that atypical hand skill asymmetry reflects DI; the genetic plan for development is less accurately expressed, resulting in greater environmental or epigenetic determination.

In another study, we examined individual differences as a function of DI in response to caffeine ingestion (Jung, Yeo and Gangestad, 2000). On verbal memory tasks, caffeine typically has a mild negative impact. We found that individuals with greater DI (MPAs, FA) had a greater decrement in verbal learning after caffeine ingestion. This again is consistent with the notion that markers of DI denote an individual less buffered from environmental perturbations. It might also help explain the observation that left-handers tend to be relatively sensitive to various drugs (Coren, 1998; Irwin, 1985).

The DI model can easily be extended to other cognitive and neuroanatomic asymmetries. Suppose that these various directional asymmetries, like handedness, are part of human nature, and thus, there are no individual differences in genes coding for such asymmetries. We differ only in how accurately the human plan for all these lateralities is expressed, which is determined largely by DI. In a recent study we demonstrated that DI is related to variation in the lateralization of a set of cognitive skills (Yeo et al., 1997a). Atypicality of lateralization was predicted by the same markers of DI used in our studies of handedness, but the direction of lateralization was not. For example, greater DI was thus associated with *both* left hemisphere dominance for judging facial affect (a task for which there is a population bias for moderate right dominance) and greater-than-typical right hemisphere dominance. Of some interest was the observation that the MPA component of our DI measure was more related to handedness, while the FA component was more related to cognitive lateralization. As MPAs are fixed before birth and FA can change over the life span (Thornhill and Gangestad, 1994), this suggests that the developmental influences on handedness are ontogenetically prior to those of cognitive lateralization.

If DI is related to atypicality of manual and cognitive asymmetries, one would expect it to be related to neuroanatomic asymmetries. In a recent study (Thoma et al., 2002) we examined the relation between body FA and a composite measure of atypical brain asymmetries (atypical planum temporale asymmetry, atypical cerebral hemisphere gray matter volume asymmetry, atypical cerebral white matter volume asymmetry, and atypical cerebral hemisphere volume asymmetry). After partialing out the effects of body size and sex, the composite measure of atypical brain asymmetry correlated with the composite measure of body FA (partial $r = 0.48$). This result has recently been replicated (Thoma, 1999). The same genetic and environmental factors thought to underlie FA of body characteristics (for a more detailed discussion see Yeo and Gangestad, 1998) produce variations from species-typical patterns of brain asymmetry. In a subset of individuals, we examined the relationship between a combined measure of brain and body FA (since these seem to reflect the same underlying developmental instability) and asymmetry of the size of the somatosensory region of the hand as determined by MEG (described earlier). This correlation was significant ($r = 0.63$), demonstrating that greater FA predicts greater asymmetry in an important aspect of the substrate of human handedness.

The DI model provides a straightforward account of why non-right-handedness is associated with many neurodevelopmental disorders (e.g., autism, schizophrenia, dyslexia, mental retardation; Coren, 1990). Each of these disorders also shows an elevated incidence of markers of DI (Yeo and Gangestad, 1993). Thus, what may be shared across these disorders is not any specific abnormality, but rather, a general susceptibility to developmental noise. Atypical handedness, FA, and MPAs by themselves obviously represent benign manifestations of DI. Their presence, however, denotes an individual who *may* be relatively vulnerable to the different and specific factors underlying each neurodevelopmental disorder (for a specific application of the DI approach to schizophrenia see Yeo, Gangestad, Edgar and Thoma, 1999). Similarly, the DI model may help account for the greater incidence of left-handedness in homosexual men and women (Lalumiere et al., 2000).

The DI model also provides a simple explanation for the greater influence of maternal than paternal handedness on offspring handedness (McManus and Bryden, 1992). The handedness of offspring is influenced not only by the degree of DI conferred by maternal and paternal genes, but also by the DI of the mother as the fetus develops. The DI of the mother, associated with her own handedness, therefore has an effect on the fetus's development that paternal DI does not have.

As we noted, one reason why we developed the DI model is because evidence shows that left-handedness is associated with lower fertility, yet left-handedness appears to be maintained at nearly the same level over time. Selection tends to remove deleterious alleles, which leads to the question of how left-handedness can be maintained in the population. The DI model provides an account consistent with evolutionary biology. Despite selection against deleterious alleles, variation in fitness-related traits can be maintained in at least four ways. First, mutations in DNA occur, most of which are deleterious. While selection tends to remove these mutations, it does not effectively remove all mutations in a single generation. At any given point in time, humans probably possess, on average, tens to hundreds of mildly deleterious mutations that will eventually be removed by selection, with substantial variation around the mean due to chance. Second, the selective environment does not remain constant. Rapid changes in the selective environment can maintain genetic variation in fitness. Key selective forces for long-lived organisms are pathogens, which themselves evolve and therefore change. Host–pathogen co-evolution can maintain genetic variability in host ability to resist pathogens, including the disease-resistance capabilities conferred by HLA alleles (Anderson and May, 1982). Recently, it has been suggested that toxins created by plants we eat may also co-evolve with our abilities to resist their effects and, hence, maintain genetic variation in our resistance of those effects (Von Schantz, Bensch, Grahn et al., 1999). Third, and relatedly, other co-evolutionary processes can maintain genetic variation in fitness (e.g., Rice and Holland, 1998). For example, conflict between the sexes or maternal–fetal conflict can result in continual change in selection pressures and hence maintain fitness (Haig, 1990). Sexually antagonistic genes (in which a given allele may not work equally well in males and females) is a related phenomenon. For periods of time, alleles that do not work extremely well in one sex or the other can be maintained in a population, leading to sustained variation in fitness within the sexes. Fourth, some genomic characteristics that do not breed true may help resist developmental perturbations. Heterozygosity may increase the ability of an organism to adapt to a variety of challenges to its fitness and, while heterozygosity at a single locus can be expected to have generally small effects on fitness (see discussion above), the aggregated effects of heterozygosity across the genome (polygenic heterozygosity) may be significant (though for recent evidence suggesting that its effects may be small, see Britton, 1996). Heterozygosity does not breed true, however, for an individual who is heterozygotic at many loci cannot pass on that characteristic to offspring. Genetic variation in developmental instability may be substantial (Gangestad and Thornhill, 1999; Pechenkina, Benfer, Vershoubskaya and Koslov, 2000).

The DI approach has generated many observations which cannot be accounted for in the genetic models of Annett (1985) or McManus and Bryden (1992), including the relationship shown in Fig. 3, evidence for the heritability of degree of handedness, the association with HLA alleles, and the association of atypical handedness with variations in growth and development. It also presents a plausible model of how genetic variation is maintained, despite the probable reduced fitness of left-handers. At present there is one major gap in the theory. Though DI has been shown to be heritable in a variety of species, we have yet to demonstrate in a convincing fashion that the degree of atypicality in handedness is heritable. Our observation (Gangestad and Yeo, 1994) that extreme right-handers (in terms of hand skill) have more left-handed parents (in terms of hand preference) was a step on the way, but Annett (1996) did not replicate this relationship. Given the fact that determination of handedness in twins may be under less genetic control than in singletons (reviewed above), the best sort of data would come from families given multiple tests of relative hand skill.

### The gene-culture model

Laland et al. (1995) have provided a novel model of human handedness. They first offer a quantitative analysis of how selection factors might direct gene frequencies in a genetic system based on the original McManus (1985) genetic model, which differs from McManus and Bryden (1992) in that no modifier locus is assumed. Laland et al. thus propose D and C alleles that act as described above, but they also propose that cultural (especially parental) biases can distort the genetic distribution to varying degrees. They assume that, prior to the introduction of the D

allele in the gene pool, genetic, cultural and environmental factors are assumed to be in equilibrium. The DD and CD have different fitness advantages over the CC genotype, and they state, "our parameterization reflects our goal to explore whether it might be possible to account for variation in handedness without assuming heterozygote advantage" (p. 437). Their analysis suggests that under these assumptions an equilibrium state will be reached and that "at this equilibrium, all genetic variation has been lost, (and) this final state is clearly not consistent with either of the leading genetic models of handedness" (p. 438). Their analysis does not exactly test the ability of the Annett and McManus models to predict gene frequencies, as it does not include a heterozygote advantage. It does, however, suggest that when one eliminates the alleged heterozygote advantage, for which no solid evidence exists, the models do not allow maintenance of genetic diversity producing variation in the direction of handedness.

Given this conclusion, Laland et al. develop their own model, a 'gene-culture' model. They derive estimates for the probability that offspring of right-handed parents become right-handed (a cultural effect) and the probability that individuals with the DD genotype become right-handed (a genetic effect) from a maximum-likelihood analysis of data from older family studies on the proportions of left-handed and right-handed children being born to different parent combinations (R × R, R × L, L × L). Their model thus includes a universal genetic effect as well as some type of parent–child influence leading to phenotypic similarity, presumably reflecting imitation or training. Formal analysis of this model indicates a good fit to 16 of the 17 family studies analyzed. Further, the model generates very low expectations for concordance rates among twin or sib pairs, and is consistent with the observed concordance rates across 13 of 14 studies. Laland et al. argue that it is plausible that all humans have the same genotype for handedness. In this regard it is consistent with one of the fundamental tenets of the DI model in that there is no individual variation among humans in the genetic plan for laterality.

### Critical comparisons

Let us consider the criteria by which genetic theories of handedness might be judged. Table 2 summa-

TABLE 2

Suggested criteria by which to judge theories of handedness

| | |
|---|---|
| 1. | Its ability to account for the different rates of left-handedness if offspring of R × R, R × L, and L × L parents. |
| 2. | Its ability to account for the observation that adopted away children resemble their biological parents, not those who adopt them. |
| 3. | Its ability to account for the minimal resemblances among pairs of siblings and MZ twins. |
| 4. | Its ability to account for evidence that degree of handedness may be heritable. |
| 5. | Its ability to account for the greater concordance of maternal and offspring handedness than paternal and offspring handedness. |
| 6. | Its ability to account for the sex differences in handedness. |
| 7. | Its ability to account for the fact that all human cultures are right-handed. |
| 8. | Its ability to account for the fact that there is nonetheless some variation in handedness across cultures. |
| 9. | Its ability to account for how the processes that underlie human handedness came into existence. |
| 10. | Its ability to account for the known correlates of handedness: other functional and anatomic lateralities, markers of variation in early growth rates, neurodevelopmental disorders. |
| 11. | Its ability to account for evidence of reduced fertility in left-handers. |
| 12. | Its ability to do all the above with minimal ad hoc assumptions, maximal parsimony and generalizability. |

rizes those suggested by Laland et al. (1995) and McManus (1985) and adds a few, hopefully uncontroversial, suggestions. Clearly, no theory is able to claim success on all measures, and better theories await more data. The major strength of Annett (1985) and McManus and Bryden (1991) is their ability to effectively model patterns of familial resemblance for hand preference. They cannot account for evidence that the degree of handedness may be heritable, nor can they account for recent data linking HLA alleles to left-handedness (Gangestad et al., 1996) or an X-chromosome gene to degree of handedness (Laval et al., 1998). Further, they cannot easily account for the correlates of handedness demonstrated in studies supporting the DI approach. Moreover, they have not provided convincing accounts of how the genetic variability is maintained. Heterozygote advantage is invoked, but not demonstrated. If, as these theories posit, a single gene has major effects on handedness, large linkage studies should detect them. No such major gene effect has yet turned up.

The gene-culture model of Laland et al. (1995) also effectively models the family data, and does so without invoking a hypothetical gene, unique to humans, that confers directional variation in brain asymmetry. But, it has two major flaws. It suggests that familial resemblance is all of sociocultural origin, an hypothesis at odds with the data on adopted children (Carter-Saltzman, 1980) and the observations that degree of handedness is heritable. It is also simply unable to account for many of the associations of handedness reviewed above.

The DI model shares the advantages of the gene-culture model, but is better able to account for the wealth of demonstrated correlates of handedness. We believe that the DI model is also the most parsimonious, in two different ways. First, no determinants of individual differences in asymmetry are invoked beyond those described in other species. The same factors that lead to FA in other species lead to variation in the extent of atypical hand or cerebral asymmetry in humans. What is different about our species, and what is shared by every member of our species, is a unique plan for neural development that culminates in our many asymmetries. Second, it is an approach that can be readily extended to asymmetries other than handedness, and it does not require the assumption of separate, multiple genetic determinants of individual differences in other asymmetric systems (e.g., hand clasping).

## An evolutionary perspective on handedness

At the beginning of this chapter we suggested that an understanding of handedness might provide some insights into human nature, into the nature of our brain and its unique skills. In this section we hope to fulfill this promise with analysis of an important implication of both the DI model and the gene-culture model. Each suggests that all humans share the same basic genetic plan that, among other things, culminates in the species-typical degree of right-handedness. If indeed the plan is universal, then it may well serve an adaptive function. That is, it may have been sufficiently adaptive in ancestral human environments that selection effectively eliminated designs for other phenotypes. Several questions emerge. When in the course of primate evolution did handedness first appear? Is the design *for* handedness, or for some more fundamental property of the nervous system? What exactly is the nature of the advantage provided by the design underlying handedness?

*Phylogenetic and historical considerations*

Important clues as to when handedness first appeared in the primate brain have emerged from recent studies of nonhuman primates. Let us now focus on chimpanzees, our closest relative among primates, with whom we share approximately 98% of our genetic material. Lateral biases are not evident in simple reaching tasks (e.g., Hopkins, 1995) or in tool use (Boesch, 1991; Marchant and McGrew, 1991). However, consistent right-hand biases have been described for bimanual feeding (Hopkins, 1994) and more complex manual tasks (e.g., Fagot and Vauclair, 1991). Thus, some directional tendencies toward handedness may be present in chimpanzees, but they demonstrate neither the degree of population asymmetry nor the broad cross-task preference seen in humans.

In this regard it is interesting to note that two recent studies have reported that there is a leftward asymmetry of the planum temporale in chimpanzees, equivalent in magnitude to that observed in humans (Gannon, Holloway, Broadfield and Braun, 1998; Hopkins, Marino, Rilling and MacGregor, 1998). Traditionally, the greater left planum size has been thought to represent part of the substrate for left hemisphere language dominance (e.g., Geschwind and Levitsky, 1968). Additionally, asymmetries in Broca's area analogous to those seen in humans have recently been reported to be present in three great ape species (Cantalupo and Hopkins, 2001). The emergence of these asymmetries in our close relatives suggests that the relevant selection pressures were unrelated to language. Thus striking cortical anatomic asymmetries likely emerged in a common ancestor at least five million years ago, prior to the development of either handedness or language. This is potentially an important clue as to the origin of our asymmetries, of which handedness is but one

functional example, suggesting that they may serve a rather general cognitive purpose, perhaps related to the organizational needs of large brains. Annett (1992) suggested that the $rs^+$ allele leads to both an asymmetric planum and asymmetry in the substrate for handedness; this now appears to be quite unlikely.

The increase in laterality seen in humans might, of course, not have been selected for directly. A recent comparative study (Rilling and Insel, 1998) demonstrated that the tremendous increase in brain size seen from the squirrel monkey (23 cm$^3$) to humans (1300 cm$^3$) has been accompanied by a decrease in the relative size of both the corpus callosum and the anterior commissure. That is, larger primate brains are characterized by relatively less functional hemispheric integration. The same trend is noted across cetacean species (Tarpley and Ridgway, 1994), suggesting that less connectedness, and greater hemispheric independence, may be a design feature consistently associated with greater brain volume. Rilling and Insel (1998) suggest that "lateralization of function may be an emergent property accompanying brain enlargement in primate evolution" (p. 1459).

Increased anatomic asymmetry also accompanies increases in brain volume within the primate line. Hopkins and Rilling (2000) analyzed MRI scans of 45 primates (5 New World Monkeys, 10 Old World monkeys, 4 lesser apes, 17 great apes, and 6 humans). Greater leftward asymmetry of petalia (especially occipital) predicted greater total brain size and smaller relative callosum size. Further, primate species with greater right-hand preference had smaller callosal area (relative to brain volume). Reanalysis of data from LeMay (1976) also suggests an association between brain size and brain asymmetry in primates. LeMay (1976) published data on several types of asymmetry in diverse primate species, though the number of brains examined for each species (except ours) was quite small. She provided information on the presence of asymmetry, either leftward or rightward, for these traits: the length of the cerebral hemispheres, the height of the Sylvian fissure, occipital petalia, and width of the occipital pole. We calculated the average number of asymmetries observed per individual in each species, regardless of the direction of asymmetry. Brain volume

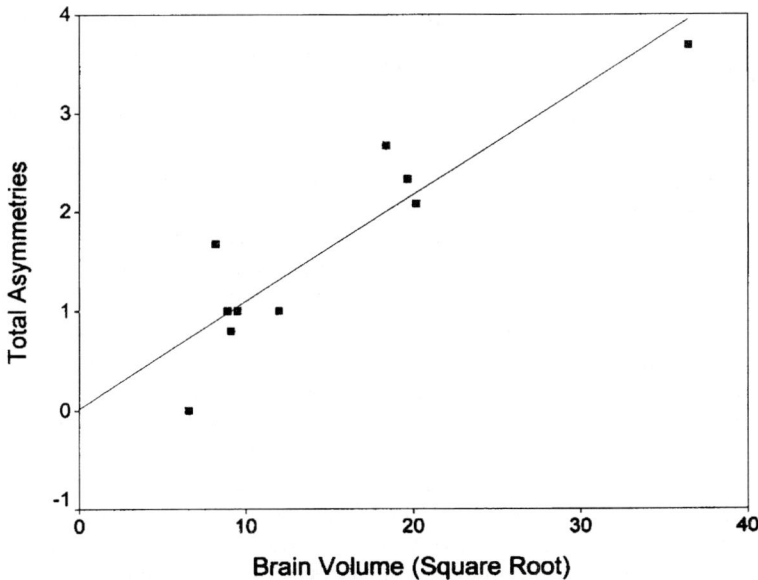

Fig. 5. Relationship between the square root of total brain volume and number of asymmetries determined by LeMay (1976) for 10 different primate species ($r = 0.91$, $p < 0.001$).

data were obtained from Rilling and Insel (1998) and Stephan, Baron and Frahm (1996). In order to minimize the impact of one outlier on brain volume, we computed the square root of brain volume and correlated this value with the overall measure of asymmetry. A strong relationship was observed across species, $r = 0.91$, $p < 0.001$, as shown in Fig. 5. It thus seems that in primates increases in brain volume are associated with greater asymmetry and less cortical connectivity. As larger brains are apt to be more intelligent (Jerison, 1982), asymmetry may be a design feature linked with intelligence.

Consistent with the new findings of anatomic asymmetries in other primates, and the suggestion that asymmetry may represent a design feature of large brains, handedness appears to have emerged quite early in the hominid line, along with large brains (Leakey, 1994). In an influential report Toth (1985) examined stone tool artifacts from *Homo habilis* made 1.4 to 1.9 million years ago. He concluded that the shape of stone flakes made in the process of producing stone tools indicates that they were likely made by right-handed individuals. Corballis (1991) cites other examples suggesting a very early emergence of right-handedness, including studies indicating greater evidence of wear on the right

side of stone tools. While these studies suggest a very early appearance of right-handedness, they are insufficient to establish whether the incidence of right-handedness was similar to current figures.

The genetic theories of Annett (1985) and McManus (1985) state that right-handedness emerged secondary to left hemisphere dominance for language, and hence, the order of the appearance of these two traits in our ancestors is of great interest. There has been much debate about exactly when human language first emerged, but it seems likely that modern language is of more recent origin than handedness. Bickerton (1990) has argued that a 'protolanguage', differing significantly from our own in grammatical and phonemic complexity, most likely emerged with *Homo erectus,* approximately 1.6 million years ago. Modern language is much more than social communication, providing for the development of a rich culture of ideas and knowledge, as well as serving as a vehicle for symbolism and abstract thought. Hence, many scholars have argued that the emergence of real language should be coincident with the emergence of the many products conferred by language (Leakey, 1994). As far as one can infer from the diversity and complexity of stone tools, there was no significant change from the time of *H. erectus* (1.4 million years ago) until approximately 100,000 years ago. The stone tool kits of *H. erectus* were remarkably stable over this time period. This suggests the absence of modern language, with its ability to record and communicate historical developments and thus facilitate technological improvement. White (1985) pointed to several developments in the Paleolithic period that might coincide with the functional emergence of modern language: artistic expression in cave art and body adornment, deliberate burial, a rapid increase in the rate of new tool development and the number of materials used for tools, increased size of communities, and regional variation in culture. Mellars (1998) recently stated, "It seems almost inconceivable to many workers that this explosion of explicitly symbolic behaviour could have been achieved without at least some associated shifts in the overall complexity, structure, or efficiency of language" (p. 184).

It thus seems that the emergence of handedness and important cerebral anatomic asymmetries antedate modern human language. If so, there are important implications for theories of the origins of handedness. The advantage associated with an asymmetrical brain, of which handedness is an obvious manifestation, would not be modern language, though one could argue that the early appearance of asymmetry was associated with the development of some protolanguage. The evidence reviewed above, however, persuades us that the human pattern of asymmetry serves a more general purpose than that of language. Along with most others (e.g., Annett, 1985; Corballis, 1997; McManus, 1985) we believe that neither right-handedness nor any other type of motor skill was the phenotype actively selected over eons of prehuman history. Rather, right-handedness is a by-product of selection pressures for other phenotypes. We suggest that the human pattern for the development of brain asymmetry represents a design facilitating the development of computational efficiency or intelligence (Yeo et al., 1997a).

*Asymmetry and adaptive brain design*

Let us assume that cortical function is massively parallel in architecture, and that, at best, only a vague 'protomap' exists to specify cortical localization of function (for a review see Elman, Bates,

Johnson et al., 1996). Genetic influences on cortical development are likely to code for rather broad 'self-organizing' strategies, rather than the fates of specific cells or cell assemblies. Whatever these strategies may be, they need to eventuate in a design that is efficient and flexible enough to work effectively across the broad range of environments in which humans may be expected to develop (e.g., an English or Japanese linguistic environment).

Some clues as to the design features allowing efficiency may be gleaned from the principles governing massively parallel computers. Marr (1976) noted that modularity (in the 'weak' sense) is an efficient design principle, for both brains and computers, allowing efficient 'debugging'. Nelson and Bower (1990) describe two fundamental sources of computational inefficiency in both parallel computers and brains. *Load imbalance* refers to "how uniformly the computational workload is distributed among the available processors. Since the speed of the parallel computation is limited by the speed of the slowest processor, unduly burdening even a single processor can dramatically deplete the overall performance (p. 404)." The second factor, *communication overhead*, is "the cost of communicating information between processors. . . primarily associated with the time–cost for exchanging information between processors [and] the physical space taken up by connections between processors (p. 404)."

Putting together the virtues of modularity and the costs of communication overhead and load imbalance, two principles of efficient cortical design emerge: (1) modules should be equally distributed across the two hemispheres (limiting load imbalance); and (2) modules that interact frequently should develop in close physical proximity (limiting communication overhead). This design cannot be hard-wired and, as with other aspects of cortical development, is likely achieved through a self-organizing developmental strategy. We suggest that the neurodevelopmental plan to implement these principles culminates in the modal pattern of human laterality. A specific pattern of hand or language dominance is not the goal of this plan, but a by-product. The mechanism to implement this plan is postulated to be an alternating sequence of asymmetric hemispheric growth rates. The best data for such a 'dialectic' pattern of development come from Thatcher's (1992) study of EEG changes across childhood, though there is also evidence for asymmetric prenatal growth rates of cortical gyri (Chi, Dooling and Gilles, 1977) and for asymmetric dendritic growth rates (Schiebel, Conrad, Perdue et al., 1990). As long as the duration of growth spurts are approximately equal for each hemisphere, this developmental plan distributes modules equally over the two hemispheres. This will minimize load imbalance. That portion of the cortex developing most rapidly at a given point in time will be maximally influenced by prevalent environmental inputs and behaviors, shaping patterns of cortical activity. Because the life skills to be learned through childhood are somewhat age-specific (e.g., language vs. peer relations), those modules related to a given set of skills are likely to develop in close physical proximity. This will minimize communication overhead.

Thatcher (1992) notes that only particular portions of each hemisphere may show a growth spurt during a given phase (e.g., right faster or left faster). Thus, the time frame during which a given asymmetry is established will differ according to the developmental trajectory of the specific cortical substrate. The direction of a given functional asymmetry is determined by the phase (i.e., which hemisphere is developing most rapidly). We assume that species-wide directional asymmetries reflect chance events in our distant phylogenetic history. That is, there is no computational advantage for the species-typical directional asymmetries, such as left hemisphere dominance for language, as compared to its mirror image.

This perspective suggests that the proposed universal neurodevelopmental dialectic, which culminates in typical cerebral lateralization, was selected as a means to ensure computational efficiency. Other strategies may well be more desirable in species for which postnatal adaptation to particular environmental circumstances is less important than in our own. Two predictions follow. First, greater lateralization of function across species should be associated with greater computational efficiency. This hypothesis is difficult to test directly, in large part because it is far from clear exactly how 'computational efficiency' should be operationalized for cross-species comparisons. Second, variations from typical brain asymmetry should predict lower computational efficiency within members of big-brained species. For the sake of simplicity, let us consider 'intelligence' as a proxy for computational efficiency.

Possession of this human pattern of growth would thus be more central to intelligence than specific directional variations in lateralization. An individual with hand and cognitive asymmetries exactly the opposite of the population norm nonetheless achieves a brain design limiting communication overhead and load imbalance due to developmentally asymmetric growth rates. In such a case, an early delay in growth likely led to a 'phase reversal' in the dialectic growth pattern, but modules still develop equally across the two hemispheres and functionally related modules are apt to be in the same hemisphere. Instead, it is the individual without this special growth pattern, i.e., one absent any directional asymmetries, who may suffer from cognitive inefficiency. In terms of handedness, it is the 'ambiguous' individual, with no real skill or preference difference across tasks, who should suffer cognitive difficulties. In this regard it is important to note that the various neurodevelopmental disorders often linked with variations in handedness are characterized more by an excess of individuals with ambiguous handedness than left-handedness per se. This is true for mental retardation (Grouios, Sakadami, Poderi and Alevriadou, 1999), schizophrenia (Orr, Cannon, Gilvarry et al., 1999), and dyslexia (Daniel, Naslund and Thoma, 1994). Further, Crow, Crow, Done and Leask (1998) demonstrated that relatively lower IQ was found at the point of 'hemispheric indecision', or left- equals right-hand skill, in normal individuals.

If DI leads to atypical lateralization, it should also lead to less efficient cognitive functioning. In support of this hypothesis, relatively greater body FA, which we have linked with atypical brain asymmetry, predicts lower fluid intelligence (Furlow, Armijo-Prewitt, Gangestad and Thornhill, 1997). Based on a mathematical model detailing the strength of association between FA and the underlying trait of developmental instability (Gangestad and Thornhill, 1999), 17 to 50% of the heritable variance in intelligence is related to DI. One might suspect that measures of atypical brain asymmetry would show an even stronger relationship with intelligence than body FA measures.

## Conclusions

Handedness, and related anatomic and functional brain asymmetries, represent attributes of humans that quantitatively distinguish us from other primates. A biological perspective of handedness may well hold promise for illuminating fundamental aspects of human nature and their evolutionary history. Yet there is much to learn, and the necessary empirical foundation is fraught with gaps and inconsistencies. Harris (1992) emphasized that progress in understanding handedness would depend upon additional analysis of the phenotype, larger sample sizes, technical developments in neuroimaging, and a closer look at causes of developmental changes. Significant progress has indeed followed from attention to these issues, yet each remains a relevant concern. Additionally, developments in evolutionary psychology and quantitative genetics will surely have an impact on the field in years to come.

## References

Amunts K, Schlaug G, Schleicher A, Steinmetz H, Dabringhaus A, Roland PE, Zilles K: Asymmetry in the human motor cortex and handedness. Neuroimage: 4; 216–222, 1996.

Anderson RM, May RM: Coevolution of hosts and parasites. Parasitology: 10; 97–140, 1982.

Annett M: A classification of hand preference by association analysis. British Journal of Psychology: 61; 303–321, 1971.

Annett M: Genetic and nongenetic influences on handedness. Behavior Genetics: 8; 227–249, 1978.

Annett M: Left, Right, Hand, and Brain: The Right Shift Theory. Hillsdale, NJ: Erlbaum, 1985.

Annett M: Parallels between the asymmetry of the planum temporale and of hand skill. Neuropsychologia: 30; 951–962, 1992.

Annett M: In defence of the right shift theory. Perceptual and Motor Skills: 82; 115–137, 1996.

Annett M: The stability of handedness. In Connolly KJ (Ed), The Psychobiology of the Hand. Cambridge: Cambridge University Press, pp. 63–76, 1998.

Badian NA: Birth order, maternal age, season of birth, and handedness. Cortex: 19; 451–463, 1983.

Baker SW, Erhardt AA: Prenatal androgen, intelligence, and cognitive sex differences. In Friedman RC, Richart R, Vande Wiele R (Eds), Sex Differences in Behavior. New York: Wiley, pp. 53–76, 1974.

Bear D, Schiff D, Saver J, Greenberg M, Freeman R: Quantitative analysis of cerebral asymmetries: Fronto-occipital correlation, sexual dimorphism, and association with handedness. Archives of Neurology: 43; 598–603, 1976.

Beaton AA: The relation of planum temporale asymmetry and morphology of the corpus callosum to handedness, gender, and dyslexia: A review of the evidence. Brain and Language: 60; 255–322, 1997.

Bickerton D: Language and Species. Chicago, IL: University of Chicago Press, 1990.

Bishop DVM: Using non-preferred hand skill to investigate pathological left-handedness in an unselected population. Developmental Medicine and Child Neurology: 26(2); 214–226, 1984.

Bishop DVM: Handedness and Developmental Disorders. Oxford: Blackwell Scientific Publishing, 1990.

Bocklage CE: On the distribution of nonrighthandedness among twins and their families. Acta Genetica Medical Gemellologica: 30; 167–187, 1981.

Boesch C: Handedness in wild chimpanzees. International Journal of Primatology: 12; 541–558, 1991.

Boles DB: Factor analysis and the cerebral hemispheres: Pilot study and parietal functions. Neuropsychologia: 29; 59–91, 1991.

Britton HB: Meta-analysis of the association between multilocus heterozygosity and fitness. Evolution: 50; 2158–2164, 1996.

Bryden MP, McManus IC, Bulman-Fleming MB: Evaluating the empirical support for the Geschwind–Behan–Galaburda model of cerebral lateralization. Brain and Cognition: 26; 103–167, 1994.

Bryden PJ, Roy EA, Bryden MP: Between task comparisons: Movement complexity affects the magnitude of manual asymmetries. Brain and Cognition: 27; 47–50, 1998.

Bryden MP, Roy EA, McManus IC, Bulman-Fleming MB: On the genetics and measurement of human handedness. Laterality: 2; 317–336, 1997.

Burke HL, Yeo RA: Systematic variation in callosal morphology: The effects of age, gender, hand preference, and anatomic asymmetry. Neuropsychology: 8; 563–571, 1994.

Cantalupo C, Hopkins WD: Asymmetric Broca's area in great apes. Nature: 414; 505, 2001.

Carlier M, Beau J, Marchand C, Michel F: Sibling resemblance in two manual laterality tasks. Neuropsychologia: 32; 741–746, 1994.

Carlier M, Spitz E, Vacher-Lavenu MC, Villeger P, Martin B, Michel F: Manual performance and laterality in twins of known chorion type. Behavior Genetics: 26; 409–417, 1996.

Carter-Saltzman L: Biological and socio-cultural effects on handedness: Comparison between biological and adoptive families. Science: 209; 1263–1265, 1980.

Cerone LJ, McKeever WF: Failure to support the right-shift theory's hypothesis of a 'heterozygote advantage' for cognitive abilities. British Journal of Psychology: 90; 109–123, 1999.

Chi JC, Dooling EC, Gilles FH: Gyral development of the human brain. Annals of Neurology: 1; 86–93, 1977.

Christiansen OB, Pedersen B, Mathiesen O, Husth M, Grunnet N: Maternal HLA class II alleles predispose to pregnancy losses in Danish women with recurrent abortions and their female relatives. American Journal of Reproductive Immunology: 35; 239–244, 1996.

Collignon J, Varlet I, Robertson EJ: Relationship between asymmetrical *nodal* expression and the direction of embryonic turning. Nature: 381; 155–158, 1996.

Collins RL: On the inheritance of the direction and degree of asymmetry. In Glick SD (Ed), Cerebral Lateralization in Nonhuman Species. New York: Academic Press, pp. 41–71, 1985.

Connolly KJ, Bishop DVM: The measurement of handedness: A cross-cultural comparison of samples from England and Papua New Guinea. Neuropsychologia: 30; 13–26, 1992.

Corballis MC: The Lopsided Ape. New York: Oxford University Press, 1991.

Corballis MC: The genetics and evolution of handedness. Psychological Bulletin: 104; 714–727, 1997.

Corballis MC, Lee K, McManus IC, Crow TJ: Location of the handedness gene on the X and Y chromosomes. American Journal of Medical Genetics (Neuropsychiatric Genetics): 67; 50–52, 1996.

Corbetta D, Thelen E: Lateral biases and fluctuations in infants' spontaneous arm movements and reaching. Developmental Psychobiology: 34; 237–255, 1999.

Corbetta D, Thelen E: Behavioral fluctuations and the development of manual asymmetries in infancy: contributions of the dynamic systems approach. In Segalowitz SJ, Rapin I (Eds), Child Neuropsychology, Handbook of Neuropsychology, 2nd Edition, vol. 8, part I. Amsterdam: Elsevier, pp. 311–330, 2002.

Coren S: Left-handedness. Behavioral Implications and Anomalies. New York: Elsevier, 1990.

Coren S: Are fingerprints a genetic marker for handedness? Behavior Genetics: 24; 141–148, 1994.

Coren S: Family patterns in handedness: Evidence for indirect inheritance mediated by birth stress. Behavior Genetics: 25; 517–524, 1995.

Coren S: Handedness as a marker for drug hypersensitivity. Laterality: 3; 161–172, 1998.

Coren S, Halpern DF: Left-handedness: A marker for decreased survival fitness. Psychological Bulletin: 109; 90–106, 1991.

Coren S, Porac C: Fifty centuries of right-handedness: The historical record. Science: 198; 631–632, 1977.

Coren S, Porac C: Family patterns in four dimensions of lateral preference. Behavior Genetic: 10; 333–348, 1980.

Crow TJ: Schizophrenia as a failure of hemispheric dominance for language. Trends in Neurosciences: 20; 339–343, 1997.

Crow TJ, Crow LR, Done DJ, Leask S: Relative hand skill predicts academic ability: Global deficits at the point of hemispheric indecision. Neuropsychologia: 36; 1275–1282, 1998.

Cummins H: Fingerprints correlated with handedness. American Journal of Physical Anthropology: 26; 151–166, 1940.

Curt F, De Agostini M, Maccario J, Dellatolas G: Parental hand preference and manual functional asymmetry in preschool children. Behavior Genetics: 25; 525–536, 1995.

Daniel WF, Naslund JC, Thoma RJ: Dyslexia in relation to handedness: A meta-analysis. Paper presented at the 1994 meeting of the International Neuropsychological Society, 1994.

Dassonville P, Zhu X, Ugurbil K, Seong-Gi K, Ashe J: Functional activation in motor cortex reflects the direction and degree of handedness. Proceedings of the National Academy of Science: 94; 14015–14018, 1997.

Davis A, Annett M: Handedness as a function of twinning, age, and sex. Cortex: 30; 105–111, 1994.

Dellatolas G, Curt F, Lellouch J: Birth order and month of birth are not related with handedness in a sample of 9,370 young men. Cortex: 27; 137–140, 1991.

Dreisen NR, Raz N: The influence of sex, age, and handedness on corpus callosum morphology: A meta-analysis. Psychobiology: 23; 240–247, 1995.

Elkadi S, Nicholls MER, Clode D: Handedness in opposite and same-sex dizygotic twins: Testing the testosterone hypothesis. Neuroreport: 10; 333–336, 1999.

Ellis SJ, Ellis PJ, Marshall E, Windridge C, Jones S: Is forced dextrality an explanation for the fall in the prevalence of sinistrality with age? A study in northern England. Journal of Epidemiology and Community Health: 52; 41–44, 1998.

Elman JL, Bates EA, Johnson MH, Karmiloff-Smith A, Parisi D, Plunkett K: Rethinking Innateness: A Connectionist Perspective on Development. Cambridge: Bradford, 1996.

Fagot J, Vauclair J: Manual laterality in nonhuman primates: A distinction between handedness and manual specialization. Psychological Bulletin: 109; 76–89, 1991.

Freund H: Abnormalities of motor behavior after cortical lesions in humans. In: Mountcastle V (Ed), Handbook of Physiology, (5), Neurophysiology: Higher Functions of the Brain, Part 2. Washington, DC: American Physiological Society, pp. 763–810, 1987.

Furlow FB, Armijo-Prewitt T, Gangestad SW, Thornhill R: Fluctuating asymmetry and psychometric intelligence. Proceedings of the Royal Society, London B: 264; 823–830, 1997.

Galaburda AM: The testosterone hypothesis: Assessment since Geschwind and Behan, 1982. Annals of Dyslexia: 40; 18–37, 1990.

Gangestad SW, Thornhill R: Individual differences in developmental precision and fluctuating asymmetry: a model and its implications. Journal of Evolutionary Biology: 12; 402–416, 1999.

Gangestad SW, Yeo RA: Parental handedness and relative hand skill: A test of the developmental instability hypothesis. Neuropsychology: 8; 572–578, 1994.

Gangestad SW, Yeo RA, Shaw PK, Thoma R, Daniel WF, Korthank A: Human leukocyte antigens and hand preference: Preliminary observations. Neuropsychology: 10; 423–428, 1996.

Gannon PJ, Holloway RL, Broadfield DC, Braun AR: Asymmetry of chimpanzee planum temporale: humanlike pattern of Wernicke's brain language area homolog. Science: 279; 220–222, 1998.

Geschwind N, Galaburda AM: Cerebral lateralization: Biological mechanisms, associations, and pathology: I. A hypothesis and program for research. Archives of Neurology: 42; 428–459, 1985.

Geschwind N, Levitsky W: Human brain: Left–right asymmetries in temporal speech region. Science: 161; 186–187, 1968.

Ghez C: The control of movement. In Kandel E, Schwartz J, Jessell T (Eds), Principles of Neural Science. Norwalk, CT: Appleton and Lange, 1991.

Gilger JW: The right-shift theory of handedness and cerebral dominance: Goodness of fit and evolution. Current Psychology of Cognition: 14; 543–549, 1995.

Goodman R: Are complications of pregnancy and birth causes of schizophrenia? Developmental Medicine and Child Neurology: 30; 59–67, 1988.

Grafton ST, Fagg AH, Woods RPM, Arbib MA: Functional anatomy of pointing and grasping in humans. Cerebral Cortex: 6; 226–237, 1996.

Grafton ST, Mazziotta J, Woods R, Phelps M: Human functional anatomy of visually guided finger movements. Brain: 115; 565–587, 1992.

Grimshaw GM, Bryden MP, Finnegan JK: Relations between testosterone and cerebral lateralization in children. Neuropsychology: 9; 68–79, 1995.

Grouios G, Sakadami N, Poderi A, Alevriadou A: Excess of nonright-handedness among individuals with intellectual disability: Experimental and possible explanations. Journal of Intellectual Disability Research: 43; 306–313, 1999.

Haig D: Brood reduction and optimal parental investment when offspring differ in quality. American Naturalist: 136; 550–556, 1990.

Hall BK: Evolutionary developmental biology. London: Chapman and Hall, 1998.

Hall WG, Oppenheim RW: Developmental psychobiology: Prenatal, perinatal, and early postnatal aspects of behavioral development. Annual Review of Psychology: 38; 91–128, 1987.

Halpern DF, Coren S: Handedness and life-span. New England Journal of Medicine: 324(14); 998, 1991.

Halsey JH, Blauenstein UW, Wilson FM, Wills EH: Regional cerebral blood flow comparison of right and left hand movement. Neurology: 29; 21–28, 1979.

Harris LJ: Left-handedness. In Rapin I, Segalowitz SJ (Eds), Handbook of Neuropsychology, Vol. 6. Child Neuropsychology. New York: Elsevier, pp. 145–208, 1992.

Harris LJ: Left-handedness and life span: Reply. Psychological Bulletin: 114; 242–247, 1993.

Healy JM, Liederman J, Geschwind N: Handedness is not a unidimensional trait. Cortex: 22; 33–53, 1986.

Hepper PG, Shahidullah S, White R: Handedness in the human fetus. Neuropsychologia: 28; 1107–1111, 1991.

Hepper PG, McCartney GR, Shannon EA: Lateralized behaviour in first trimester human foetuses. Neuropsychologia: 36; 531–534, 1998.

Hopkins WD: Hand preferences for bimanual feeding in 140 captive chimpanzees (Pan troglodytes): Rearing and ontogenetic factors. Developmental Psychobiology: 27; 395–407, 1994.

Hopkins WD: Hand preference for a coordinated bimanual task in 110 chimpanzees (Pan troglodytes): Cross-sectional analysis. Journal of Comparative Psychology: 109; 291–297, 1995.

Hopkins WD, Marino L, Rilling JK, MacGregor LA: Planum temporale asymmetries in great apes as revealed by magnetic resonance imaging (MRI). Neuroreport: 9; 2913–2918, 1998.

Hopkins WD, Rilling JK: A comparative MRI study of the relationship between neuroanatomical asymmetry and interhemispheric connectivity in primates: Implications for the evolution of functional asymmetries. Behavioral Neuroscience: 114; 739–748, 2000.

Hugdahl K, Satz P, Mitrushina M, Miller E: Incidence of left-handedness in young and old individuals. Journal of Clinical and Experimental Neuropsychology: 15; 26, 1993.

Irwin P: Greater brain response of left-handers to drugs. Neuropsychologia: 23; 61–67, 1985.

Jakobson L, Goodale M: The neural substrates of visually guided prehension: The effects of focal brain damage. Advances in Psychology: 105; 199–214, 1994.

Jancke L, Steinmetz K: Hand motor asymmetry and degree of asymmetry in monozygotic twins. Cortex: 31; 779–785, 1995.

Jantz RL, Fohl FH, Zahler JW: Finger ridge-counts and handedness. Human Biology: 51; 91–99, 1979.

Jerison HJ: The evolution of biological intelligence. In Sternberg RJ (Ed), Handbook of human intelligence. Cambridge: Cambridge University Press, pp. 723–791, 1982.

Jung R, Yeo RA, Gangestad SW: Developmental instability predicts individual variation in verbal memory skill following caffeine ingestion. Neuropsychiatry, Neuropsychology, and Behavioral Neurology: 13; 195–198, 2000.

Kawashima R, Roland P, O'Sullivan B: Activity in the human primary motor cortex related to ipsilateral hand movements. Brain Research: 663; 251–256, 1994.

Kertesz A, Geschwind N: Patterns of pyramidal decussation and their relationship to handedness. Archives of Neurology: 24; 326–332, 1971.

Kim SG, Ashe J, Hendrich K, Ellerman JM, Merkle H, Urgurbil K, Georgopulos AP: Functional magnetic resonance imaging of motor cortex: Hemispheric asymmetry and handedness. Science: 261; 615–617, 1993.

Klar AJS: A single locus, RGHT, specifies preferences for hand utilization in humans. Cold Spring Harbor Symposia on Quantitative Biology: 61, 59–65, 1996.

Klingenberg CP, Nijhout HF: Genetics of fluctuating asymmetry: A developmental model of developmental instability. Evolution: 53; 358–375, 1999.

Koff E, Naeser MA, Pieniadz JM, Foundas AL, Levine HL: Computed tomographic scan hemispheric asymmetries in right- and left-handed male and female subjects. Archives of Neurology: 43; 487–491, 1986.

Kolb B, Whishaw IQ: Fundamentals of Human Neuropsychology, 4th ed. New York: Freeman Worth, 1996.

Laland KN, Kumm J, Van Horn JD, Feldman MW: A gene-culture model of human handedness. Behavior Genetics: 25; 433–445, 1995.

Lalumiere ML, Blanchard R, Zucker KJ: Sexual orientation and handedness in men and women: A meta-analysis. Psychological Bulletin: 126; 575–592, 2000.

Laval SH, Dann JC, Butler RJ, Loftus J, Rue J, Leask SJ, Bass N, Comazzi M, Vita A, Nanko S, Shaw S, Peterson P, Shields G, Smith AB, Stewart J, DeLisi L, Crow TJ: Evidence for linkage to psychosis and cerebral asymmetry (relative hand skill) on the X chromosome. American Journal of Medical Genetics (Neuropsychiatric Genetics): 81; 420–427, 1998.

Leakey R: The Origin of Humankind. New York: Basic Books, 1994.

LeMay M: Morphological asymmetries of modern man, fossil man, and nonhuman primate. Annals of the New York Academy of Sciences: 280; 349–366, 1976.

LeMay M: Asymmetries of the skull and handedness: Phrenology revisited. Journal of the Neurological Sciences: 32; 243–253, 1977.

Leviton A, Kilty T: Seasonal variation in the birth of left-handed schoolgirls. Archives of Neurology: 35; 115–116, 1979.

Lewine J, Orrison WW: Magnetoencephalography and magnetic source imaging. In Orrison WW, Lewine J, Sanders J, Hartshorne M (Eds), Functional Brain Imaging. St Louis: Mosby, 1995.

Liederman J, Flannery KA: Fall conception increases the risk for neurodevelopmental disorder in offspring. Journal of Clinical and Experimental Neuropsychology: 16; 754–768, 1994.

Livingston R, Adam BS, Bracha HS: Season of birth and neurodevelopmental disorders: Summer birth is associated with dyslexia. Journal of the American Academy of Child and Adolescent Psychiatry: 32; 612–616, 1993.

Livshits G, Davadi L, Kobylianski E, Ben-Amitai D, Levi Y, Merlob P: Decreased developmental stability as assessed by fluctuating asymmetry of morphometric traits in preterm infants. American Journal of Medical Genetics: 29; 779–805, 1988.

Marchant LF, McGrew WC: Laterality of function in apes: A meta-analysis of methods. Journal of Human Evolution: 21; 425–438, 1991.

Marin-Padilla M: Prenatal and early postnatal ontogenesis of the human motor cortex: A golgi study. I. The sequential development of the cortical layers. Brain Research: 23; 167–183, 1970.

Markow TA: Human handedness and the concept of developmental instability. Genetica: 87; 87–94, 1992.

Markow TA: Developmental Instability: Its Origins and Evolutionary Implications. Dordrecht: Kluwer, 1994.

Marr D: Early processing of visual information. Philosophical Transactions of the Royal Society of London Biological Sciences: 290; 483–524, 1976.

Martin M, Jones GV: Handedness and season of birth: A gender-invariant relation. Cortex: 35; 123–128, 1999.

Mattay V, Callicott J, Bertolino A, Santha A, Van Horn J, Tallent K, Frank J, Weinberger D: Hemispheric control of motor function: A whole brain echo planar fMRI study. Psychiatry Research: Neuroimaging: 83; 7–22, 1998.

McCartney G, Hepper P: Development of lateralized behavior in the human fetus from 12 to 27 weeks gestation. Developmental Medicine and Child Neurology: 41; 83–86, 1999.

McKeever WF: A new family handedness sample with findings consistent with X-linked transmission. British Journal of Psychology: 91; 21–39, 2000.

McKeever WF, Suter PJ, Rich DA: Maternal age and parity correlates of handedness: Gender, but no parental handedness modulation of effects. Cortex: 31; 543–553, 1995.

McManus IC: Handedness in twins: A critical review. Neuropsychologia: 18; 347–355, 1980.

McManus IC: Handedness, language dominance, and aphasia: A genetic model. Psychological Medicine (Monograph Supplement 8). Cambridge: Cambridge University Press, 1985.

McManus IC: Cultural and historical differences in the incidence of left-handedness are due to differences in gene frequency, not social pressure. Paper presented at the annual meeting of the International Neuropsychological Society, Denver, CO, 2000.

McManus IC, Bryden MP: The genetics of handedness, cerebral dominance, and lateralization. In Rapin I, Segalowitz S (Eds), Handbook of Neuropsychology: Sect. 10, Developmental Neuropsychology. Amsterdam: Elsevier, pp. 115–144, 1992.

McManus IC, Shergill S, Bryden MP: Annett's theory that individuals heterozygous for the right shift gene are intellectually advantaged: Theoretical and empirical problems. British Journal of Psychology: 84; 517–537, 1993.

McManus IC, Sik G, Cole DR, Mellon AF, Wong J, Kloss J: The development of handedness in children. British Journal of Developmental Psychology: 6; 257–273, 1988.

Mellars P: The emergence of biologically modern populations in Europe: A social and cognitive 'revolution?' In Runciman WG, Smith JM, Dunbar RIM (Eds), Evolution of social behavior patterns in primates and man. Oxford: Oxford University Press, pp. 179–201, 1998.

Melsbach G, Wohlschlager A, Speiss M, Gunturnkun O: Morphological asymmetries of motor neurons innervating upper extremities: Clues to the anatomical foundations of handedness. International Journal of Neuroscience: 86(3–4); 217–224, 1996.

Meno C, Siajoh Y, Fujii H, Ikeda M, Yokoyama T, Yokoyama M, Toyoda Y, Hamada H: Left–right asymmetric expression of TGF-B family member *lefty* in mouse embryos. Nature: 381; 151–155, 1996.

Michel G: A lateral bias in the neuropsychological functioning of human infants. Developmental Neuropsychology: 14; 495–518, 1998.

Michel G, Harkins DA: Postural and lateral asymmetries in the ontogeny of handedness. Developmental Psychobiology: 19; 247–258, 1986.

Moffat SD, Hampson E: Salivary testosterone levels in left and right-handed adults. Neuropsychologia: 34; 225–233, 1996.

Moffat SD, Hampson E: Salivary testosterone concentrations in left-handers: An association with cerebral language lateralization? Neuropsychology: 14; 71–81, 2000.

Moffatt SD, Hampson E, Lee DH: Morphology of the planum temporale and corpus callosum in left-handers with evidence of left and right speech representation. Brain: 121; 2639–2379, 1998.

Molenaar PCM, Boomsma DJ, Dolan CV: A third source of developmental differences. Behavior Genetics: 23; 519–524, 1993.

Møller AP, Swaddle JP: Asymmetry, developmental stability and evolution. Oxford: Oxford University Press, 1997.

Mulvihill JJ, Smith DW: The genesis of dermatoglyphics. The Journal of Pediatrics: 75; 579–589, 1969.

Nass R, Baker S, Virdis R, Balsamo A, Cacciari E, Loche A, Dumic M, New M: Hormones and handedness: Left-hand bias in female congenital adrenal-hyperplasia patients. Neurology: 37; 711–715, 1987.

Nathan PW, Smith MC, Deacon P: The corticospinal tracts in man. Course and location of fibres at different segmental levels. Brain: 303–324, 1990.

Nelson ME, Bower JM: Brain maps and parallel computers. Trends in Neurosciences: 13; 403–409, 1990.

Newman HH: Dematoglyphics and the problem of handedness. American Journal of Anatomy: 55; 277–322, 1934.

Nyberg-Hansen R, Rinvik E: Some comments on the pyramidal tract with special reference to its individual variations in man. Neurologica Scandinavica: 39; 1–30, 1963.

O'Callaghan MJ, Burn YR, Mohay HA, Rogers Y, Tudehope DJ: Handedness in extremely low birth weight infants: Aetiology and relationship to intellectual abilities, motor performance, and behavior at four and six years. Cortex: 29; 617–627, 1993.

Oppenheim RW, Reitzel J: Ontogeny of behavioral sensitivity to strychnine in the chick embryo. Evidence for the early onset of CNS inhibition. Brain, Behavior, and Evolution: 11; 130–159, 1975.

Orlebeke JF, Knol DL, Koopmans JR, Boomsma DI, Bleker OP: Left-handedness in twins: Genes or environment. Cortex: 32; 479–490, 1996.

Orr KGD, Cannon M, Gilvarry CM, Jones PB, Murray RM: Schizophrenic patients and their first-degree relatives show an excess of mixed handedness. Schizophrenia Research: 39; 167–176, 1999.

Orsini DL, Satz P: A syndrome of pathological left-handedness. Archives of Neurology: 43; 333–337, 1986.

Palmer AR: From symmetry to asymmetry: Phylogenetic patterns of asymmetry variation in animals and their evolutionary significance. Proceedings of the National Academy of Sciences: 93; 14279–14286, 1996.

Palmer AR, Strobeck C: Fluctuating asymmetry: Measurement, analysis, patterns. Annual Review of Systematics: 17; 391–421, 1986.

Pechenkina EA, Benfer RA, Vershoubskaya GG, Koslov AI: Genetic and environmental influence on the asymmetry of dermatoglyphic traits. American Journal of Physical Anthropology: 111; 531–543, 2000.

Peters M: Subclassification of non-pathological left-handers poses problems for theories of handedness. Neuropsychologia: 28; 279–289, 1990.

Peters M, Murphy K: Factor analyses of pooled hand questionnaire data are of questionable value. Cortex: 29; 305–314, 1993.

Pinker S: The Language Instinct. New York: Harper-Collins, 1994.

Plomin R, Daniels D: Why are children in the same family so different from each other? Behavioral and Brain Sciences: 10; 1–16, 1987.

Poliakov GI: Some results of research into the development of the neuronal structure of the cortical ends of the analysers in man. Journal of Comparative Neurology: 117; 197–212, 1961.

Porac C: Genetic vs. environmental contributions to human hand-edness: Insights gained from studying individuals with unilateral hand injuries. Behavior Genetics: 25; 447–455, 1995.

Provins KA: Handedness and speech: A critical reappraisal of the role of genetic and environmental factors in the cerebral lateralization of function. Psychological Review: 104; 554–571, 1997.

Provins KA, Magliaro J: The measurement of handedness by preference and performance tests. Brain and Cognition: 22; 171–181, 1993.

Rao S, Binder J, Bandettini P, Hammeke T, Yetkin F, Jesmanowicz A, Lisk L, Morris G, Mueller W, Estkowski R, Wong E, Haughton V, Hyde J: Functional magnetic resonance imaging of complex human movements. Neurology: 43; 2311–2318, 1993.

Rice WR, Holland B: The enemies within: intergenomic conflict, interlocus contest evolution (ICE), and the intraspecific Red Queen. Behavioral Ecology and Sociobiology: 41; 1–10, 1998.

Rife DC: Hand prints and handedness. American Journal of Human Genetics: 7; 170–179, 1955.

Rilling JK, Insel TR: Differential expansion of neural projection systems in primate brain evolution. Neuroreport: 10; 1453–1459, 1998.

Rogerson PA: On the relationship between handedness and season of birth for men. Perceptual and Motor Skills: 79; 499–506, 1994.

Roland P, Larsen B, Lassen N, Skinhoj E: Supplementary motor area and other cortical areas in organization of voluntary movements in man. Journal of Neurophysiology: 43; 118–136, 1980.

Satz P, Orsini DL, Saslow E, Henry R: The pathological left-handedness syndrome. Brain and Cognition: 4(1); 27–46, 1985.

Scarr S: Developmental theories for the 1990's: Development and individual differences. Child Development: 63(1); 1–19, 1992.

Schachter SC: Handedness in women with intrauaterine exposure to diethylstibestrol. Neuropsychologia: 32(5); 619–623, 1994.

Scheirs JGM, Vingerhoets AJJM: Handedness and other laterality indexes in women prenatally exposed to DES. Journal of Clinical and Experimental Neuropsychology: 17; 725–730, 1995.

Schiebel AB, Conrad T, Perdue S, Tomiyasu U, Wechsler A: A quantitative study of dendritic complexity in selected areas of the human cerebral cortex. Brain and Cognition: 12; 85–101, 1990.

Searleman A, Porac C, Coren S: Relationship between birth order, birth stress, and lateral preferences: A critical review. Psychological Bulletin: 105; 397–408, 1989.

Snyder PJ, Bilder RM, Wu H, Bogerts B, Lieberman JA: Cerebellar volume asymmetries are related to handedness: A quantitative MRI study. Neuropsychologia: 33; 407–419, 1995.

Steinmetz H, Staiger JF, Schlaug G, Huang YX, Jancke L: Corpus callosum and brain volume in women and men. Neuroreport: 6; 1002–1004, 1995.

Steinmetz H, Volkmann J, Janke L, Freunde H: Anatomical left–right asymmetry of language related temporal cortex is different in left- and right-handers. Annals of Neurology: 29; 315–319, 1991.

Stellman SD, Wynder EL, DeRose DJ, Muscat JE: The epidemiology of left-handedness in a hospital population. Annals of Epidemiology: 7; 167–171, 1997.

Stephan H, Baron G, Frahm HD: Comparative size of brains and brain components. In Stklis HD, Erwin J (Eds), Comparative Primate Biology, Vol. 4: Neurosciences. New York: Alan R. Liss, pp. 1–38, 1996.

Taniguchi M, Yoshomine T, Cheyne D, Kato A, Kihara T, Ninomiya H, Hirata M, Hirabuki N, Nakamura H, Hayakawa T: Neuromagnetic fields preceding unilateral movements in dextrals and sinistrals. Neuroreport: 9; 1497–1502, 1998.

Tapley SM, Bryden MP: A group test for the assessment of performance between the two hands. Neuropsychologia: 23; 215–221, 1985.

Tarpley RJ, Ridgway SH: Corpus callosum size in delphinid cetaceans. Brain, Behavior, and Evolution: 44; 156–165, 1994.

Thatcher RW: Cyclic cortical reorganization during early childhood. Brain and Cognition: 20; 24–50, 1992.

Thoma R: An investigation of the expression of developmental instability in human behavioral and brain functioning. Unpublished Doctoral Dissertation, University of New Mexico, 1999.

Thoma R, Yeo RA, Gangestad SW, Lewine JD, Davis J: Fluctuating asymmetry and the human brain. Laterality: 7; 45–58, 2002.

Thornhill R, Gangestad SW: Human fluctuating asymmetry and sexual behavior. Psychological Science: 5; 297–302, 1994.

Thornhill R, Møller AP: Developmental stability, disease, and medicine. Biological Reviews of the Cambridge Philosophical Society: 72; 497–548, 1997.

Torrey EF, Miller J, Rawlings R, Yolken RH: Seasonality of births in schizophrenia and bipolar disorder: A review of the literature. Schizophrenia Research: 24; 260, 1997a.

Torrey EF, Miller J, Rawlings R, Yolken RH: Seasonality of births in schizophrenia and bipolar disorder: A review of the literature. Schizophrenia Research: 28; 1–38, 1997b.

Toth N: Archeological evidence for preferential right-handedness in the lower and middle Pleistocene and its possible implications. Journal of Human Evolution: 14; 607–614, 1985.

Triggs WJ, Subramanium B, Rossi F: Hand preference and transcranial magnetic stimulation asymmetry of cortical motor representation. Brain Research: 835; 324–329, 1999.

Turkheimer E, Wilkniss S, Yeo RA: Extreme handedness, developmental instability, and the heritability of behavior. Paper presented at the 1997 meeting of the American Society of Medical Genetics, 1997.

Varlet I, Robertson EJ: Left–right asymmetry in vertebrates. Current Opinion in Genetics and Development: 7; 519–523, 1997.

Volkmann J, Schnitzler A, Witte OW, Freund HJ: Handedness and asymmetry of the hand representation in human motor cortex. Journal of Neurophysiology: 79; 2149–2154, 1998.

Vom Sall FS, Bronson FH: In utero proximity of female mouse fetuses to males: Effect on reproductive performance during later life. Biology of Reproduction: 19; 842–853, 1978.

Von Schantz T, Bensch S, Grahn M, Hasselquist D, Wittzell H: Good genes, oxidative stress and condition-dependent sexual signals. Proceedings of the Royal Society of London Series B: Biological Sciences: 266; 1–12, 1999.

Waldrop MF, Halverson CF: Minor physical anomalies and hyperactive behavior in children. In Helmuth IJ (Ed), Exceptional Infant: Studies in Abnormality. New York: Bruner–Mazel, pp. 343–380, 1971.

Waldrop MF, Halverson CF, Shetterly K: Manual for Assessing Minor Physical Anomalies (rev. ed.). Unpublished manuscript, University of Georgia, Athens, 1989.

White LE, Andrews TJ, Hulette C, Richards A, Groelle M, Paydarfar J, Purves D: Structure of the human somatosensory system 2. Lateral asymmetry. Cerebral Cortex: 7; 31–47, 1997.

White LE, Lucas G, Richards A, Purves D: Cerebral asymmetry and handedness. Nature: 368; 197–198, 1994.

White R: Thoughts on social relationships and language in human evolution. Journal of Social and Personal Relationships: 2; 95–115, 1985.

Wong WT, Sanes JR, Wong ROL: Developmentally regulated spontaneous activity in the embryonic chick retina. Journal of Neuroscience: 18; 8839–8852, 1998.

Yeo RA, Gangestad SW: Developmental origins of variation in human hand preference. Genetica: 89; 281–296, 1993.

Yeo RA, Gangestad SW: Developmental instability and phenotypic variation in neural organization. In Raz N (Ed), Development, Exceptionality, and Pathology as Models for Cognitive Neuroscience. Amsterdam: Elsevier, 1998.

Yeo RA, Gangestad SW, Edgar C, Thoma R: The evolutionary–genetic underpinnings of schizophrenia: The Developmental Instability model. Schizophrenia Research: 39; 197–206, 1999.

Yeo RA, Gangestad SW, Daniel WF: Hand preference and developmental instability. Psychobiology: 21; 161–168, 1993.

Yeo RA, Gangestad SW, Thoma RA, Shaw P, Repa K: Developmental instability and cerebral lateralization. Neuropsychology: 11; 552–561, 1997a.

Yeo RA, Gangestad SW, Turkheimer E: Non-directional genetic influences on development. Paper presented at the 1995 meeting of the Society for Research in Child Development, Cincinnati, OH, 1995.

Yeo RA, Hodde-Vargas J, Hendren RL, Vargas LA, Brooks WM, Ford C: Brain abnormalities in schizophrenia-spectrum children: Implications for the etiology of adult schizophrenia. Psychiatric Research Neuroimaging: 76; 1–13, 1997b.

Yousry TA, Schmid UD, Alkadhi H, Schmidt D, Peraud A, Buettner A, Winkler P: Localization of the motor hand area to a knob on the precentral gyrus. Brain: 120; 141–157, 1997.

CHAPTER 15

# Motor soft signs and development

## Ruthmary K. Deuel [*]

*Department of Neurology, Saint Louis University Health Sciences, 3635 Vista at Grand Boulevard, P.O. Box 15250,
St. Louis, MO 63110-0250, USA*

## Introduction

During the past two decades major shifts have occurred in concepts of motor system organization. The shifts in models of motor system function have come in concert with new neurophysiological techniques, such as functional imaging and magnetic brain stimulation, that allow direct observation of brain activity in alert humans performing integrative functions, including complex motor acts. Although normal development of motor skills and behaviors has only partially been addressed by these methods, the non-invasive nature of the new techniques opens the door to much investigation. Non-invasive functional studies should allow new understanding of motor development, and a better understanding of the impact, and better remediation or even prevention, of motor execution deficits that often accompany motor soft signs.

Intelligence may be defined for the purposes of the present topic as manifest in purposive acts that influence the environment to the advantage of the actor. Children whose purposive acts are ineffectual in influencing their environments in an age-appropriate fashion are often seen as 'slow' and 'unintelligent'. Sometimes they are even held guilty of carelessness, inattention, or deliberate oppositional refusal to perform, and this reputation may result in marked and life-long adverse effects on their self-esteem (Hol-

lander et al., 1991; Shaw, Levine and Belfer, 1992). For children who manifest motor soft signs in the earliest years, preventing destruction of self-esteem by early remediation of motor developmental abnormalities would be ideal. Although this is seldom possible at the present time, given new concepts of motor system function and new techniques to specify and quantify motor abnormalities, such prevention of long-term ill effects may soon become feasible.

The present review will provide descriptions and definitions of the most readily documented and significant motor soft signs. Clinical evaluation and differential diagnostic considerations for each, and their place in currently used clinical nosologies will be discussed. Changing concepts of motor system organization, learning and performance will be described with reference to some experimental evidence. Finally, speculations about motor system development and the future direction of diagnosis and treatment of developmental motor learning and performance deficits will be made.

## Motor soft signs

By the 1930s there was general recognition within the medical community of children with learning and attention deficits (cognitive abnormalities), in the absence of other medical or neurological disease (Clements, 1966; Gesell and Amatruda, 1947; Orten, 1925). Since then, there has been a great deal of systematic study of children's cognitive development, and some more limited study of sensory and motor capacities, both in normal children and those who ap-

[*] Tel.: +1 (314) 268-4105; Fax: +1 (314) 268-6411;
E-mail: deuelr@slucare1.sluh.edu

pear to have learning and attention deficits. Samuel Orten, a neurologist, was the first to point out (Orten, 1925) that children with dyslexia (now designated a 'specific learning disability') may also demonstrate neurological physical examination findings. He spoke of "that mild motor incoordinate type". Later other neurologists christened as 'soft signs' the mildly slowed or clumsy fine (and sometimes gross) motor performances observed during neurological examination of these children (Dare and Gordon, 1970; Ingram, 1973; Wolff and Hurwitz, 1966). This is a name with important neurological connotations. In neurological terms, a 'hard sign' such as a positive Babinski response, has power to help localize, lateralize or determine a specific lesion within the central nervous system. Sometimes a 'hard sign' connotes a specific disease. 'Soft signs' have no such specificity, a fact repeatedly emphasized in the sixties and seventies (Gomez, 1967; Kennard, 1960). Indeed at that time there was no evidence that 'soft signs' could reliably indicate damage or dysfunction in any part of the nervous system.

In the 1970s and 1980s, the controversy about the significance of 'soft signs' was elaborated by multiple contributors, who pointed out that special examinations, direct observations of performance and *measurement* of motor performance parameters were required (Gilberg and Rasmussen, 1982; Gubbay, 1978; Holden et al., 1982; Peters, Romine and Dykman, 1975; Spreen and Gaddes, 1969; Wolff, Gunnoe and Cohen, 1983). When so ascertained, 'soft signs' became much less equivocal and ephemeral. Finger and foot tapping speed and wrist turning were easily quantified and reproducible (Denckla, 1972), as were mirror movements (Stokman, Schafer and Shaffer, 1986), although of course not all authors agreed (Rutter, 1982). By the 1990s the psychiatric literature (rather than the neurologic) had become an arena where dysmorphologic physical findings and even historical allusions were dubbed 'soft signs'. 'Soft signs' were correlated with various psychiatric diagnoses, from schizophrenia to obsessive–compulsive disorder to social phobia (Cohen, Hollander, DeCaria et al., 1996; Hollander et al., 1996; Schaffer, Schonfeld, O'Connor et al., 1985).

So far, however, only motor soft signs, which are quite reproducible when properly measured in their dynamic setting, seem to have neurophysiological

information to yield. Because of the well-tried observation batteries for motor soft signs, for instance the PANESS (Guy, 1976; Tupper, 1987), the Neurologic Examination of the School-Age Child (Deuel, 1998), the Peabody Motor Development Survey (Boucher et al., 1993), the Bayley Scales of Infant Development (Bayley, 1969; Black, Dubowitz and Hutcheson, 1995) and because of some developmental norms (Denckla, 1974; Todor and Lazarus, 1986), soft signs have become reliably reproducible (Stokman et al., 1986). As reliable and reproducible, they are useful in the diagnosis and differential diagnosis of higher-order motor function deficits in children, while at the same time, new information concerning motor system subdivisions and neurotransmitter domains has allowed the motor soft signs to be more closely linked to known neuroanatomical sites and neurophysiological mechanisms. In regard to this linkage, they are likely to be heuristic in the study of normal development of higher-order motor function.

Developmental motor soft signs are readily ascertained within the context of a hands-on physical and neurological examination (Deuel, 1998). However, at the present time, the 'diagnosis' of an attention and learning disorder is seldom the province of the neurologist or pediatrician, but is often left in the hands of the local school district. This shift from medical to educational 'diagnosis' has divorced the term 'soft sign' completely from its roots in the neurological literature and its original meaning and purpose. It originally was used as a shorthand to narrow the differential diagnosis of the cause of the child's difficulty (Kennard, 1960), a process that is omitted for any child who is given an educational, rather than a medical, diagnosis. The differential diagnostic thought process, however, still should be carried out by examiners of children who have developmental motor 'soft' signs for reasons to be discussed in the description of each individual soft sign.

In the neurological literature, the word 'sign' is understood to mean an observable or elicitable finding during the neurological part of the physical examination. 'Signs' are conceptually very separate from 'symptoms'. 'Signs' are not part of the history, nor can they be derived from checklists or comments of the child's family or school teachers. The most well-known signs, such as Babinski's upgoing toe, clearly tip the neurological examiner off to an abnormal or damaged portion of the nervous system. Babinski's sign, for instance, indicates (usually) damage to the 'upper motor neuron' related to the toe that displays it. 'Soft signs', however, traditionally do not indicate an abnormality of a specific region or level of the nervous system, nor indicate any specific disease process (Barlow, 1974; Gomez, 1967). This traditional definition notwithstanding, 'soft signs', we now know, may indeed indicate specific nervous system damage or disease. Generally, 'soft signs' as hints of specific damage or disease are likely to be found with slight damage or very early in the course of a disease. For this reason, it is important that neurological physical examiners be aware of the differential diagnosis of each motor soft sign (i.e. know which soft sign might indicate what disease).

A further, seemingly contradictory, facet of motor 'soft signs' is that even when they are definitely present on focused examination, they may play no role at all in the functional disability of the child who presents with them, so the examiner is again required to make a judgment as to the significance of the sign for this particular child; i.e. answer the question "does this sign play any role at all in the functional disability of the child who presents with it?" Thus, evaluating motor soft signs and any related functional disabilities, in the context of the entire burden of the child's handicap, is a very important exercise for the examining professional. It appears that for some children, subnormal motor performance does not alter school performance or overall adjustment. For others, a quantitatively similar motor performance abnormality may have major effects on adjustment to the environment, both at home and at school. At times, the specific difficulty with motor performance is not apparent to caregivers, parents, and schoolteachers. Developmental dyspraxia, in particular, frequently goes unnoticed as an underlying cause of performance impairment.

The most commonly considered motor soft signs include clumsiness, dyspraxia, adventitious movements such as choreaform movements and synkinesis, and anomalies of manual dominance (Deuel and Robinson, 1987), as shown in Table 1. These four are in different categories of motor performance, each with its own developmental trajectory. When 'soft signs' are cited, they are most often developmental delays in one or several of these categories. However,

the fact that slow individual joint movements or lack of manual dominance was appropriate at some earlier age, does not imply that when it persists beyond that age, that the child will eventually 'grow out' of the soft sign or any related functional disability (Gilberg and Gilberg, 1989). The word 'sign' is not fully appropriate as the ascertainment of this type of motor delay or aberration requires the context of the entire pediatric and neurological exam, while a true neurological sign (e.g. the Babinski sign) is significant in and of itself. Slow and inaccurate finger tapping (as seen in clumsiness) could occur on the basis of spasticity, profound distal weakness or arthritis. It is only the *absence* of other, 'hard', physical findings that slow finger tapping is admissible as a 'soft sign', and after informed dismissal of the possibilities of remediable diseases and genetic disorders, as these all require medical measures beyond 'appropriate education placement'.

The examiner must, of course, observe the specific performances that allow ascertainment of the various 'soft signs'. This is especially important as the *outcome or product* of a motor performance may not be affected by mild or infrequently appearing abnormal motor behaviors. It is observation of the timing, direction and sequence of the movements as they are performed that allows the determination of normality or abnormality. Thus, the motor 'soft' signs might more appropriately be called 'dynamic' signs, since for their determination relevant actions must be observed, timed and localized.

The very most common motor soft sign is slowed speed (below expectation for age and verbal intelligence) of single joint movement. This slowing of the most rudimentary motions (e.g. index finger flexion and extension) is called *clumsiness*. The slowing may affect primarily distal joints or primarily proximal joints or face movements, or axial movements, or all combined. The slowing at individual joints is generally different at different joints, so that overall incoordination of compound movements is observed in fairly simple actions (spooning food to the mouth, manipulating clothing, implements, and sports objects). If 'extra time' is allowed for completion of complex multistage acts, the purely clumsy child may be successful. One clinical test frequently used is finger tapping speed, that has been measured and given normal values under many circumstances

TABLE 1

Motor Soft Signs

| Soft sign | Altered movement parameter | Outcome of intended action | Clinical test for soft sign | Differential diagnosis |
|---|---|---|---|---|
| *Clumsiness* | *Timing* slow single joint movements | Normal with 'extra timed' | Age-normed finger tapping, wrist turning, toe tapping (Denckla, 1974) | Upper motor neuron damage with spasticity and weakness, lower motor neuron, muscle or joint disease, cerebellar disease |
| | Slow and asynchronous multiple joint movements | | | |
| *Dyspraxia* | | | | |
| Ideational | *Sequence of individual acts* — rapid dexterous single joint movements | Abnormal with 'extra time' or repetition | Age-normed gestures, pantomime and use of objects (Deuel, 1992) | Static and progressive encephalopathies, stroke, metachromatic leukodystrophy, head trauma, cerebral palsy |
| Ideomotor | | | | |
| Mixed | | | | |
| Material-specific | | | | |
| Dysgraphia | *Sequence* of writing motions (all other motions normal) | | Age-normed writing, spell words presented orally, copy printed text (Deuel, 1995) | Cerebral cortex lesions |
| Dyspraxia of speech | *Sequence* of oral and pharyngeal motions | | Age-normed articulation tasks | Galactosemia, Fragile X (LeMay, 1992; Sommer, Gathof, Podskarbi et al., 1995) |
| *Involuntary movements* | | | | |
| Chorea | *Timing, direction, sequence* — abrupt rapid motions of body parts that often interrupt ongoing purposeful movements | Normal (depends on severity) | Observation of child during motor exam, have child stand, eyes closed, arms forward and pronated, wrists and fingers extended (Wolff and Hurwitz, 1966) | Sydenham chorea, collagen vascular disease, Wilson's disease, other basal ganglia diseases |
| Tics | *Timing, sequence* — rapid, repetitive, appear voluntary, briefly suppressible | Unintended (may appear intentional) | Observation or surreptitious observation (video tapes) | Encephalitis, cocaine, anticonvulsants, basal ganglia diseases with specific etiologies |
| Tremor | *Direction* — body part oscillates (does not maintain constant direction); may oscillate at rest and/or during voluntary movement | Abnormal with 'extra time' | Observation during motor exam, fine motor testing, finger–nose–finger test | Cerebellar disease, drug toxicity, hyperthyroidism, inherited disorders, weakness |
| Synkinesis | *None* — (for the body part in voluntary motion) | *Normal* (depends on severity and activity) | Command action of one body part (e.g. wrist turning, finger against thumb pressure) while observing actions of hand not engaged in voluntary actions | Agenesis of the corpus callosum, Klippel–Feil syndrome, weakness with excessive effort required of trivial acts (see text) |
| *Anomalies of manual dominance* | *None* | *Normal* | Handedness questionnaires, manual performance batteries | Stroke, cerebral dysgenesis, vascular malformation, porencephaly |

(Denckla, 1974; Knights and Norwood, 1980; Reitan and Wolfsun, 1985; Spreen and Gaddes, 1969). Slow and inaccurate finger tapping for age as seen in clumsiness could also occur on the basis of remediable disorders and genetic diseases that require further medical diagnosis and treatment as indicated in Table 1.

When clumsiness is present, it often affects the entire life-style of the child. Other children, parents, and teachers justifiably consider the child 'slow'. However, they often do not realize that this is a mechanical, rather than an oppositional, slowness. Authorities may even believe the child is deliberately avoiding completion of chores and punish the child accordingly. Such a reception by caregivers may cause secondary psychological ill effects. These are capable of being reversed with rational explanations of the mechanical difficulties.

On the other hand, isolated slow finger tapping or facial movements may cause the child very little trouble. Whether or not the clumsiness found in an exam actually has significance in terms of the child's ability to successfully compete in her environment must be judged on an individual basis. In fact, it might be said that there are only two reasons to evaluate soft signs. The first is when the soft sign is not a 'soft' sign, but really does indicate disease (for example, clumsiness due to spasticity caused by white matter disease), and the second is when the soft sign affects the child's daily living adversely (for example, she can never go out to recess because she has to finish writing out each spelling word fifteen times because she is so slow at writing that she cannot keep up during spelling class time).

The next most common soft sign is *dyspraxia* or the inability to learn or perform serial voluntary, age-appropriate movements. (David et al., 1981) This difficulty with completing skilled acts at an age-appropriate level persists no matter how much 'extra time' is allowed. In order to fulfill the definition of dyspraxia, there must be no loss of motor power, coordination, or sensory ability that could explain the performance deficit. The motor performance must be below expectation, not only for age but also for verbal IQ. There are several dyspraxia batteries (Bruiniks, 1978; Deuel and Doar, 1992; Gubbay, 1975) available that allow evaluation of age-appropriate motor sequences following the guidelines of Liep-

mann (Liepmann, 1908), who first described and categorized apraxia in adults. Dyspraxia, like clumsiness, can lead to ineffectual motions, but unlike clumsiness, individual motions themselves are not slowed, but are made generally in the wrong order. A common example is found in incorrect performance of the finger–nose–finger test. The child, despite repeated commands to put one forefinger on his nose and use the same forefinger to touch the examiner's finger, uses the other forefinger to touch the examiner's forefinger. This is, in fact, a normal response below the age of five. Gross motor acts may also be disrupted with dyspraxia. Despite repeated demonstrations, the child cannot skip, for instance. Children with dyspraxic motor deficits take no longer than their age mates to perform an act; however, its outcome is usually abnormal. The allowance of a 'long' time to perform does not help the outcome. Because of the normal motor speed this deficit is often unrecognized as a motoric problem by parents and teachers who report that "he can't learn to tie his shoes" and who may feel there is an intellectual deficit in the child, or a deliberate oppositional behavior. Secondary psychological effects due to misunderstandings of the deficit are at least as common with dyspraxia as with clumsiness. It is important to note that sometimes clumsiness accompanies dyspraxia.

The differential diagnosis of dyspraxia is fairly broad. Dyspraxia may be the first symptom of several childhood degenerative disorders, including subacute sclerosing panencephalitis, juvenile onset metachromatic leukodystrophy, or ceroid neuronal lipofucinosis. It is commonly seen in cerebral palsy.

There are objectively definable subtypes of dyspraxia in children. For example, some children have great difficulty in manipulating objects (opening locks, folding paper) but little difficulty in performing intransitive movements. These children may be classified as having ideational dyspraxia. Others encounter more trouble when the act involves intransitive motions of the limbs or body (for example, jumping jacks) and may be classified as ideomotor dyspraxia (Deuel and Doar, 1992) to follow Liepmann's scheme (Liepmann, 1908). There seems to be no evidence as yet that the differential diagnosis for these two types of dyspraxia is different in children. Most commonly, these two types of dyspraxia are both present in the same child (Deuel and Doar, 1992).

More limited dyspraxias, called material-specific dyspraxias, are well-recognized. They are called material-specific because the motor disability is only apparent when a particular type of cognitive material is necessary to prompt the motor execution phase of the task. Material-specific dyspraxias include dyspraxia of speech (Ferry et al., 1975; Rapin and Allen, 1988; Yoss and Darley, 1974), linguistic dysgraphia, and spatial dysgraphia (Deuel, 1995). Each has its own differential diagnosis (as shown in Table 1) and current modes of remediation. It is possible that new methods for diagnosis through functional brain imaging may result in less need for 'bypass remediation' in the future. At present, while these motor deficits are limited (a linguistic dysgraphic may be a talented flutist, for instance), they often severely impair the social and academic development of the afflicted, normally intelligent and normally dexterous child. This is particularly true of dyspraxia of speech (Ferry et al., 1975).

*Involuntary movements* are of two major types, one in which an unwanted movement appears irrespective of whether the afflicted child is attempting a voluntary movement. Choreas, some tremors, and tics (tics are considered hard rather than soft motor signs and are not considered further here) are of this type. The others are synkineses, or movements that occur during a willed motion but are present as unwilled, unintended activity of voluntary musculature.

There is ample evidence from the literature that choreaform movements are more common in populations of children with learning, language, attention and motor execution deficits than in children not so affected. However, the relationship of the choreaform movements to true chorea, and to the learning, language, and motor execution deficits is not clear. Stimulants in attention-enhancing doses do not change motor performance deficits such as clumsiness or synkinesis (Lerer and Lerer, 1976). Classically, true chorea manifests itself in sudden fast contractions of voluntary muscles. Although the movement may be complex, such as an arm-and-hand fling that resembles a voluntary wave goodbye, it is unwilled and purposeless. Such movements occur whether the limb is in voluntary play or not. At times, the afflicted individual seems to be weaving

the involuntary movements into a voluntary pattern. Most of such movements that are not due to a definable etiology are not severe enough to limit motor execution appreciably and are better termed 'choreaform' than 'chorea'. On the other hand, severity should not be a criterion for etiology. Whenever chorea is encountered or the slower chorea-athetosis, a differential diagnosis should be considered. It includes, of course, Sydenham's chorea, a part of the post-streptococcal rheumatic disease spectrum, juvenile lupus erythematosus, and several heritable degenerative diseases of the nervous system including Wilson's disease. Many of these conditions respond to specific medical treatments. Tics may very closely resemble chorea, and etiologies of chorea should at least be mentally considered when the clinical setting of a tic disorder warrants. The 'PANDAS' spectrum of tics and obsessive–compulsive behaviors is a case in point (Garvey et al., 1998).

Tremor is observed as involuntary oscillations of a body part, or even the whole trunk. These may occur when the affected body part is supported against gravity (resting tremor). Intention tremor is so called because as the body part (tested usually with the finger–nose–finger test) in voluntary play reaches its intended destination, the oscillations markedly increase, and may prevent the finger from coming to rest on the nose. Tremor may be of both types, for instance existing at rest and becoming much more severe with voluntary movement. The outcome of movements is often affected by tremor. Oscillations may often be seen in the graphic productions of children affected by essential tremor, for instance. Tremor has its own set of differential diagnostic considerations, including cerebellar disorders, juvenile Huntington's disease, other hereditary disorders, and benign familial tremor. Management of handicapping tremors is often feasible with specific medication.

Synkineses are involuntary movements in muscles not required to move to produce the willed effect. The synkinetic movement is induced by the intended voluntary effort. The synkineses are also called 'overflow' movements, and may occur in muscle groups homologous to the ones in voluntary play (mirror movements) or in quite distant musculature. In general, synkineses do not produce handicaps, although there is a hereditary form of mirror movements that is handicapping called Conrad's syndrome (Conrad et al., 1978). In the case of mirror movements, there should be suspicion of underlying joint, skeletal, muscle, nerve or brain pathology, although the movements themselves (as opposed to their possible underlying etiologies) are generally benign.

*Anomalies of manual dominance* are difficult to establish in the individual child. To establish 'pathological left-handedness' solidly by clinical criteria one needs to know that the child was originally right handed, in a manner comparable to adult hand preference change, or one needs both a comprehensive family history with no primary left-handed blood relatives, and additional evidence of left-hemisphere damage in the brain if the suspected condition is congenital. In any case the differential diagnostic suspicions should include joint, skeletal, muscle, nerve or brain pathology. The concept of pathological left-handedness, while hard to establish in individuals, is effectively applied to populations rather than to individuals. In an autistic population, for example Soper, Satz and Orsini (1986) reported left-handers and ambidextrous individuals in very high proportion compared to a general population of the same age, that exhibits no more than 15% of left-handed and ambidextrous people individuals. While pathological left-handedness can be positively established in some individuals, ambidexterity and other anomalous hand use remain of uncertain significance.

In summary, motor execution that is affected by the dynamic deficits we are discussing is one of two means (the other being speech) the child has for influencing its environment. Thus, motor soft signs, even when not significant of major nervous system lesions or diseases, may prove highly significant in the course of the development of an individual child. Speech, the other major means of influencing the environment, may help to compensate for motor deficits, or may itself be involved, as in the case of dyspraxia of speech.

## Motor development

In this section motor development and the motor milestones traditionally evaluated will be discussed, followed by an introduction to new concepts in the neurophysiological literature concerning types of memory and learning and how the recently defined skill and declarative memory systems may interact with the development of motor skills. How the motor system is currently conceptualized and how its anatomical sites might interact during motor development and motor skill learning will also be discussed.

It may be useful to preface this section with a discussion of the term 'development'. Initially, the term motor development was used, in the neurological literature at least, to denote changing and ever-improving parameters of motor skill during the growth of the child. The pattern of motor development has been well-documented and linked to many factors such as skeletal growth and development, physical size, practice, environmental demands, age, gender, and genetic disposition. A review of theoretical and observational articles concerning normal motor development and developmental soft signs is found in Deuel and Robinson (1987). One feature of the many observational works reviewed at that time was the importance of subject population selection. Anywhere from 100% of the subjects to approximately 15% of the subjects (depending clearly upon the selection criteria used for the study) demonstrated developmentally abnormal performances in their 'abnormal' populations, whereas up to 35% of their normal populations also demonstrated some sort of developmentally abnormal performance. This is merely a cautionary note to the reader of 'developmental' literature when evaluating studies of the developmental motor soft signs based on a-priori subject versus control, selection. Deuel and Doar (1992) tried another method when they studied 164 schoolchildren for praxis abilities using a standardized test. They found high correlations among age, I.Q. and praxis scores for the entire group. However, in the subgroup of children with praxis scores one standard deviation or more below the mean for age, there was no correlation among these factors: for example, the individual with a mean praxis score $-2.2$ SD below mean, and a F.S. I.Q. of 120. The 24-member subgroup, called apraxic because of their mild ($-1$ SD below mean) to severe ($-2.5$ SD below the mean) ideomotor and/or ideational apraxia clearly demonstrated a dissociation between I.Q. and praxis.

The timetable for normal development of motor activity is solidly established for humans and includes the well-known walking independently at 10–15 months of age, holding objects in the hand at 6–8 months, and transferring objects from one hand to the other at only a slightly later time (Frankenberg, Dodds, Archer et al., 1992). Beyond these activities that occur with a minimum of encouragement and without formal 'teaching' lies the bulk of human motor skills. The normal potential to exercise most motor skills comes from a combination of heritable and environmental factors. The latter includes observation of such activities by the learner, and deliberate tutelage to the learner by other people. What may appear to be rudimentary motor acts may actually be 'culturally determined' or 'acquired' skills. For example, before the age of two many toddlers can turn on the family television set. The toddler, however, does not spontaneously push any old button. Rather, initially he observes the act of older people, and notes that pushing one particular button leads to a gratifying burst of sound and color. After often observing this act and its result, the child tries to push the specific effective button and may rapidly succeed in producing sound and color.

Throughout infancy, toddlerhood, latency, and early adolescence it is clear that motor development is fed by a constant interplay of cognitive, motivational, perceptual and deliberate heuristic factors. The complexities of the interplay among these factors is just beginning to be appreciated and dealt with in the developmental literature and is being augmented by explorations of plasticity in the adult nervous system. Recently a plethora of visual recognition and discrimination capabilities have been found in human newborns, that seems to corroborate that visual perception is well developed far earlier than any but ocular mobility (Norcia et al., 1990). Reports concerning disease states, primate studies and functional imaging studies are beginning to sketch a theory of motor skill acquisition and maintenance quite different from those available earlier (Hadders-Algra, 2000).

In the 1950s and 1960s, neurologic teaching cited the 'poor vision' of newborns as an example of the fact that genetically programmed myelinization of certain central tracts was a prerequisite for specific sensory and motor developments. It was thought that the optic tracts and radiations do not myelinate until after 9 months gestation (Yakovlev and Lecours, 1967). However, these notions have radically changed starting with the information that in preterm births, early myelinization in visual pathways was found (Gilles et al., 1983). It is now known, for example, that before myelinization is discernable to sensitive imagery, diffusion tensor weighted imaging shows orientation of vectors in directions expected for myelin pathways (Vajapeyam et al., 2001). Put together, such findings suggest that perception, as well as age from conception, may be involved in systems maturation.

For motor systems, walking alone was said to come in association with full (assumption of 'pre-programmed') myelination of the cerebrospinal tracts at 1 year of age (Yakovlev and Lecours, 1967). There is now good evidence that prenatal myelination does take place in humans in long spinal tracts (Eyre, Miller, Clowry et al., 2000) and that a large number of factors including endogenous electrical activities (Ben-Ari, 2001) that may also induce and modulate spinal myelinization and cerebral competency, cerebral and cerebellar neuronal migration, synapse formation and eliminations. As well, environmental influences continuously interact to produce motor development from very early prenatal to young adult periods of human development (Penn and Schatz, 1999). If multiple intrinsic and environmental factors are involved, there may be opportunities for intervention to promote motor activities and development through manipulation of any one or several of the factors (other than gestational age) controlling motor system maturity.

One of the primary characteristics of motor development in childhood is that all motor competence seems to appear in association with repetitive practices. This is true in adulthood, but to a far lesser degree. After attempts and coaching, the young child practices and is able to master motorically complex skills such as tying shoelaces. Many gross motor skills may be learned quite early. Fine manual motor skills are also learned by practice but less early than gross motor skills.

These normal behavioral developments are taking place during the same time frame that neuroanatomical postnatal brain maturation is occurring, mainly development of synaptic relations (Rakic, Bourgeois and Goldman-Rakic, 1994) and myelinization (Gilles, 1976; Gilles et al., 1983) that lead to the formation of functional cognitive modules (Levy and Goldman-Rakic, 2000). It is now thought that interactions between structural and functional factors are continually reciprocally molding neuroanatomical and behavioral developments, and these changes continue well into adolescence (see Gilmore, 2003, this volume), and probably beyond. Evidence for these new generalizations continues to accrue. Methods such as magnetoencephalography, (Muller, Rothermel, Behen et al., 1998), various types of functional imaging (Jacobs, Chugani, Allada et al., 1995; Van Mier, Ojemann, Gopalan et al., 1998), continuum mechanical tensor maps (Thompson, Giedd, Woods et al., 2000) and diffusion tensor weighted imaging (Vajapeyam et al., 2001) are demonstrating detailed structural and connectional information. Construction of a timetable of integrative cognitive motor behaviors is, of course, hampered by the great difficulty of obtaining reliable functional images in the waking (therefore moving excessively) very young child.

Motor learning undoubtedly engages motor structures, sensory (especially kinesthetic) structures, and structures concerned with memory and executive (or decision-making) function. Memory, upon which motor and all other types of learning depend, used to be considered a fairly unitary function. It was divided up into time-related categories such as 'long'-term, 'short'-term and 'immediate' memory. It has become clear that there are other, qualitatively different domains of memory. At present, using the broad definition of memory as "the influence of prior experience upon current behaviors", memory can be divided into at least two or possibly three qualitatively separate categories, called skill or procedural memory (Mishkin et al., 1984), declarative or event memory (Hirsh, 1980; Squire and Cohen, 1984), and working memory (Goldman-Rakic, 1987). In addition to those major domains, there is material-specific memory (for instance, verbal as opposed to spatial memory) and modality-specific memory (for instance, visual versus auditory memory).

Several lines of evidence seem to substantiate the independence of all these types of memory. As well, the brain structures now known to support the different types of memory include the cerebellum and the striatum as well as neo- and archipallium.

In regard to the declarative versus skill memory dichotomy, the seminal work was in a human (Milner et al., 1968) who at first, after a bilateral hippocampectomy, appeared completely unable to lay down recent memories. It was found that this patient could learn new motor skills; however, he could not discuss or describe these new skills ('remember them') but only perform them. Later, in primates, it was demonstrated that the anatomic substrate of the skill memory differed from that for declarative memory (Mishkin and Petri, 1984); lesions of the hippocampal–amygdala region destroyed a monkey-equivalent of declarative memory (associative memory of a single experience), but skill-learning capacity remained intact. These investigators concluded that a form of conditioning (memory after repeated experiences, without effectual change until the experiences were complete) was taking place over pathways that did not involve the amygdala (well-known for its involvement in affective learning) and hippocampus. This finding allowed them to suggest that normally the declarative or fast-learning system (that is present only in higher vertebrates) confers the advantage of versatility in behavioral responses to current conditions, while the 'slow-learning' or skill learning provides reliability of responses to recurrent stimuli and depends upon a group of non-hippocampal structures (Mishkin and Petri, 1984; see DeLong, 2003, this volume).

In regard to acquisition of complex motor skills, evidence suggests that only the second type of memory (skill learning or slow or conditioning type of memory) is active in infant monkeys. Infant monkeys' power of skill retention, however, is as good as that of adult monkeys (Mishkin and Delacouer, 1975). In reviewing the brief (because it omits so many skills and it only goes up to the early latency period of human development, rather than through the end of adolescence when most motor skills are at their asymptote) motor milestones table (Table 2), it appears that all of the listed items could be supported by the slow-learning system. Although it has not been directly shown in humans, it seems likely that cortical/striatal/cerebellar structures, the most likely substrate of the skill or slow-learning memory, are the anatomical substrate of much very early motor development in human children. Depending on the individual child, often by 3 years, and certainly by 5

TABLE 2

Motor milestones

| Age of child | Typical motor achievements |
| --- | --- |
| Term birth | Regards faces; follows with eyes; flexes and extends all four extremities |
| 2 months | Smiles to a smile; pushes head up from prone with hands; turns head to either direction |
| 4 months | Rolls over from prone to supine; sits momentarily when placed in a sitting position; maintains head erect; claps hands together; arm waving toward objects; takes turns vocalizing with others |
| 6 months | Sits firmly when sat; reaches smoothly for object; grasps and maintains object in either hand; transfers it from hand to hand; feeds self finger foods |
| 8 months | Achieves sitting position; crawls; stands holding on; uses whole hand grasp; plays peek-a-boo by pulling a cloth off the head |
| 10 months | May get to standing; has a pincher grasp (separate control of thumb and forefinger); waves good-bye; gestures sooo-big |
| 12 months | Walks alone; holds a cup in both hands and can drink from it; points; says meaningful single words |
| 14 months | Runs; climbs; crosses midline with reaching; starts hand preference; holds a spoon using cross-palmar grasp |
| 16 months | Initiates self-help skills; undresses in part; imitates actions of adults; climbs stairs holding a railing |
| 18 months | Manipulates fine objects; plays imaginatively with toy cars and/or dolls; uses a fork and a toothbrush |
| 24 months | Jumps; throws; points to body parts; puts on some clothes; demonstrates hand preference; says two-word (or more) meaningful phrases |
| 3 years | Uses fork and spoon dexterously; pulls on clothes, copies circle; rides a three-wheeled toy; climbs stairs without holding onto a rail |
| 4 years | Stands on one foot; throws overhand; copies square; builds with Legos; manipulates puzzle pieces; tripod pencil grasp |
| 5 years | Walks a balance beam; hops on one foot; rides a two-wheeler; dresses completely; ties shoes; has a dynamic tripod pencil grasp; copies triangle |

years, evidence for fast declarative memory is clear in the normal child.

'Working' memory has been well described and tested in primates, and is highly pertinent to all motor performance. Goldman-Rakic and colleagues (1987) described mechanisms whereby a series of acts is represented or remembered 'on line' in the dorsal lateral prefrontal cortex and the related lateral medial dorsal thalamus. This type of representation allows serially appropriate deployment of individual motor acts within a given goal-directed behavior. It has been well characterized behaviorally and developmentally and has also been demonstrated by recordings at the single cell level. Without prefrontal cortex, internally cued and ordered acts, that lead to a completed skilled motor act are not possible. On the other hand, if sensory cues are presented serially, to induce each single motor act in an appropriate sequence, the entire behavior can be accomplished without prefrontal cortex (Deuel and Anderson, 1991; Deuel and Dunlap, 1979). Thus prefrontal damage to the primate makes sensory stimuli preeminent in eliciting motor behaviors (i.e. creates the state of being 'stimulus-bound').

MRI findings in head-injured human children poor at a working memory task (Levin et al., 1994) also point to a dissociation between verbal memory and delayed alternation changes, suggesting that there are two different neural substrates involved, at least between working and declarative types of memory in children. Since the 19th century, psychologists and neurologists have looked upon the motor system as a slave of the sensory systems. In simplest terms, it was considered the second and third 'response' parts of a three-part open loop system (see Fig. 1). There was a pyramidal motor system centered in primary motor cortex of the frontal lobe, that responded to messages from sensations by issuing commands to effector (lower motor) neurons via the direct and rapidly transmitting corticospinal tract. This hierarchical, unidirectional system operated independently of the extrapyramidal motor system centered in the basal ganglia and brainstem. That other, extrapyramidal system, operated by filtering its messages to lower centers via multisynaptic networks and was concerned with postural adjustments. It too was considered a serial unidirectional hierarchical system, but a less efficient one than the pyramidal system.

## MODEL OF MOTOR CONTROL

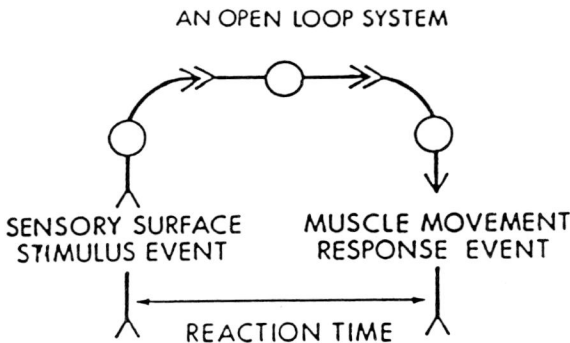

### AN OPEN LOOP SYSTEM

Fig. 1. The motor system as a unidirectional, three-element, open-loop device.

At this time, however, such old models appear invalid. The evidence is now quite clear that the 'two' motor systems generally act in concert. Now it appears that there is a single widely distributed multidirectional, multifunctional, motor system that processes in parallel as well as serially (Bonda et al., 1996; Gitelman et al., 1996; Kalaska and Crammond, 1992; Logan and Grafton, 1995). It is diagramed in Fig. 2. The anatomical components include at least cingulate cortex, supplementary motor areas, premotor areas, primary motor and sensory areas, anterior and parts of posterior parietal cortex, ventral and lateral thalamus, the basal ganglia, brainstem nuclei, tectum and cerebellum (Bucher et al., 1995; Ellerman et al., 1994; Grafton et al., 1992; Nicolelis et al., 1995).

Most recently, Rizzolatti and colleagues (Iacoboni et al., 1999; Rizzolatti et al., 1999) and others (Hasegawa et al., 2000) have documented by cellular recording areas of frontal cortex in adult monkeys that appear to be specialized, in the first instance for imitation of extremity and facial movements, and in the second for remembering and predicting movements. Neurons in the former region, that is analogous to Brodmann area 44 (part of Broca's area in the human) are active when the animal actually performs a hand movement, as well as when the animal is allowed to watch a similar movement by the appropriate hand of another monkey, even when the observing monkey's own hand and arm demonstrate no EMG activity. Rizzolatti's group have termed neurons active during viewing of movement 'mirror' neurons. Buccino carried out an fMRI study in adult humans showing essentially the same phenomenon, but extending the previous observations implicating frontal premotor and Broca's areas by demonstrating somatotopically situated regions within the previously implicated frontal and parietal regions (Buccino et al., 2001). Given that a preverbal animal such as the macaque has neurons specialized for imitation of motor acts, it is very tempting to speculate that the essentially preverbal normal 12-months-old human employs similar neural circuitry in elaborating pointing, waving bye-bye, and in facial expressive behaviors. Given the anatomical locations of the activations in the adult humans, it is quite likely that the implicated areas also play a role in the development of expressive speech, as noted by Miklosi (1999).

Considering these new models of normal development, the question "How do developmental soft signs fit into normal motor development?" may be reposed as "Are developmental motor soft signs simply developmental lags, or are they qualitatively different from any stage in normal motor development?" The answer, in most instances, is likely to be the latter. The good news is that the new concept of the motor system seems better able to explain 'motor soft signs' than the old hierarchical reflex models, that demanded 'damage' in the afferent, central, or efferent limb of one of the two separate systems before dysfunction could be conceptually accommodated. Now, more subtle interactive and quantitative explanations appear to be allowed by the new concepts of motor system physiology. With this new understanding of mechanisms, new preventative or restorative therapies may be found (Butters et al., 1994; Kinsbourne and Cook, 1971; Pellizer, Sargent and Georgopoulos, 1995; Thach, Goodkin and Keating, 1992; Tyszka, Grafton, Chew et al., 1994). The bad news is that a great deal of work will need to be done before the changes during normal development are understood, let alone their abnormalities as manifest in motor soft signs. With this rich complexity of interaction among neuroanatomical structures, even in the fully formed motor system, that seems to vary with the specific task being executed at the moment (Thach et al., 1992; Thach, Perry, Kane and Goodkin, 1993), and with the stage

## MODEL OF MOTOR CONTROL

### A MULTIPLE REDUNDANT & UNIQUE OPEN & CLOSED LOOP SYSTEM

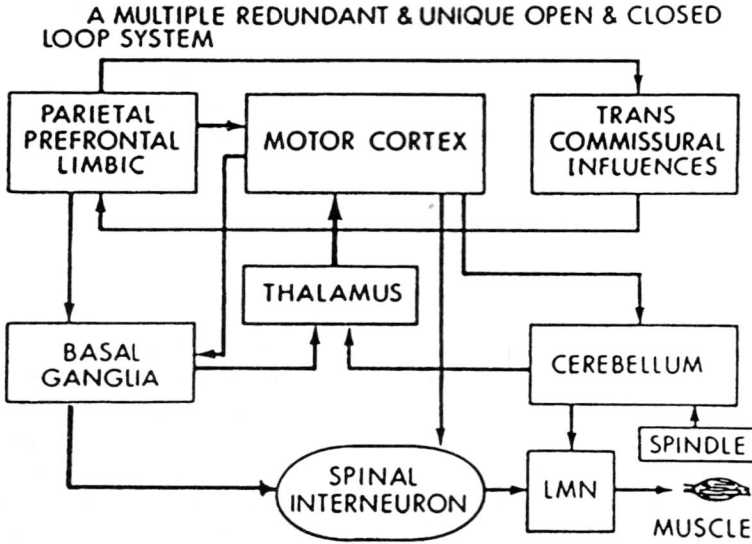

Fig. 2. The motor system as an as yet poorly understood multifunctional processing device that is distributed among all the levels of the nervous system.

of learning of the task (Pascual-Leone et al., 1994), it is certainly not yet possible to lay out a neat table of the neuroanatomical structures involved in each motor soft sign or higher-order motor execution deficit. Nonetheless, the generalization that they result from failures of interactions among subsystems of the three major neuroanatomic foci of the greater motor system seems warranted, pending further direct experimental evidence. It seems likely that basal ganglia (Mink and Thach, 1993) and possibly the thalamus (Bastian and Thach, 1995) will be found to be functionally different from normal in the child with adventitious movements, that the dyspraxic child will show primarily cerebral cortical changes both left and right (Graff-Radford and Biller, 1992), possibly dorsolateral prefrontally emphasized (Goldman-Rakic, 1987). The clumsy child may have functional differences from normal that are distributed between the cerebellum and the basal ganglia (Mink and Thach, 1993; Thach et al., 1993), with bilateral diffuse cortical changes (Habib et al., 1995) possible.

In the meantime, it seems wise to maintain differentiation of the different types of soft signs from one another. This is usually readily accomplished, based

on the clinical neurological examination as discussed earlier. The clinical differentiation anticipates confirmation by use of new neurophysiological techniques such as functional imaging.

### Nosology of motor soft signs

On the basis of all the foregoing considerations, it seems that a revision of the clinical nosology for motor soft signs is in order. Lumping all of the diverse motor abnormalities we have discussed here under the rubric motor soft signs is a current nosological trend. However, this lumping trend is somewhat regressive at this point. For one thing, it is confusing to the sensitive clinician and to the informed researcher (Missiuna and Polatajko, 1995) who cannot help but observe differentiated syndromes, components of the nervous system, remediations, and differential diagnoses for the different motor soft signs. For another, it is reducing the motor system back to its 19th century 'sensorimotor slave state' as depicted in Fig. 1.

Clinical nosologies and diagnostic and statistical manuals are meant to allow *principled* classification and subclassification of diseases, findings and pathologies. Therefore, such schemata generally have inclusion and exclusion criteria for allowing the 'diagnosis' of a given entity. Different conceptual grounds for inclusion and exclusion in decision-making may be assumed by different nosologies. Indeed, the two currently most used clinical nosologies of motor execution deficits or motor soft signs include the DSMIV (American Psychiatric Association, 1994) and the ICD-9 or the International Classification of Diseases, 9th edition (U.S. Department of Health and Human Services, 1991). These two nosologies have somewhat different conceptual methods of arriving at their suggested diagnoses. For DSMIV, there is explicit agreement that the disease or entity criteria are those of consensus among clinical psychiatrists (American Psychiatric Association, 1994, p. xxvii). DSMIV thus does not employ quantitative biological criteria, which, so far, are in general unavailable for psychiatric entities. On the other hand, the ICD-9 relies on biological criteria whenever possible. With that in mind, it may be of interest to look at the DSMIV diagnosis 'developmental coordination disorder', Code 315.4 (American Psychiatric Association, 1994, p. 53). It is presented as a unitary entity if certain broad neurological categories of disease are excluded (e.g. cerebral palsy, hemiplegia, or muscular dystrophy). The ICD-9, on the other hand, breaks Code 315.4 down into two subentities, clumsiness and dyspraxia (American Academy of Neurology, 1990, p. 38) as outlined in Table 1. The difference between the two is the subcategories of the ICD-9-DM diagnosis. Since it now seems clear that different motor activities engage different subsets of neuroanatomical substrates, it follows that, when considering motor developmental abnormalities (manifest in the four categories of motor soft signs discussed earlier) it becomes important to try to subdivide DSMIV's 315.4 along biologically distinct lines that faithfully reflect the differing underlying neuropathophysiologies of each sign, and medically provide as specific a differential diagnosis as possible for each.

While 'soft signs' may be appreciated in and of themselves, one diagnostic context in which they occur deserves special mention, namely, the autistic spectrum disorders. One of the primary 'diagnostic' findings in the 18-months-old autistic toddler is lack of pointing, or looking in the direction that others point or gaze (Baron-Cohen, Allen and Gill-

TABLE 3

Management of developmental motor disorders

| | |
|---|---|
| A | Recognition and evaluation of significance to 'burden of malfunction' |
| B | Elucidation (counsel RE: specific cognitive-motor *strengths* and weaknesses) to parents and teachers |
| C | Bypass methods (word-processing, tape-recording, cognitive mental rehearsal) |
| D | Remedial methods (OT, PT, adaptive PE) |
| E | Medication |
| F | In the future: sophisticated individualized evaluative methods (TCMS, FMR) leading to C, D, and E |

berg, 1992). These same children can be conditioned, using a technique called Applied Behavioral Analysis (Lovass, 1993) to perform pointing, in a sense demonstrating the 'apraxic' nature of this specific motor deficit in the autistic child. Individual motor movements are available but are not produced spontaneously unless the child is specifically conditioned to carry out the appropriate sequence (as in Applied Behavioral Analysis).

Finally, using these considerations about the neurophysiological underpinnings of the motor soft signs, and their developmental contexts, one may face the task of managing (or ignoring) the specific soft sign presented by the specific child within the context of that child's specific needs (Table 3).

If new methods of study and new models of motor system complexity are to serve the community of the disabled child, it will be through the community's acceptance of the challenge to subsume new facts into clinical practice, and by promoting, rather than burying, use of the newly available information. The reliability of ascertainment of different motor soft signs during development has increased in recent decades, due in part to the application of age-normed tests of motor performance in standard broad assessments of children, such as the Kaufman Assessment Battery for Children (Donders, 1982), the Peabody Motor Development Survey, (Boucher et al., 1993), the Bayley Scales of Infant Development (Black et al., 1995), the Halstead Reitan Neuropsychological Test Battery for Children (Reitan and Wolfsun, 1985), the PANESS (Tupper, 1987; see Molfese and Price, 2002, this volume). This has made possible increasingly detailed and specific diagnoses of the different soft signs and their cognitive contexts.

Purely mental processing deficits, such as the inability to focus attention, may be reliably ascertained. Limited and specific mental processing deficits (for example, dyslexia with dysgraphia) are now readily separable from motor or movement disorders on the one hand and from deficits in general cognitive power, such as mental retardation, on the other, using appropriate measures and normed test batteries. Tests, likewise, are now capable of separating purely sensory from more complex perceptual deficits, and primary from higher-order motor execution deficits. Given our current capabilities and knowledge, the diagnostic coding system might do best to reflect at least the subcategories of developmental disorders of motor execution that are readily separable by a trained clinician. Thus at the present time, at least three subcategories, clumsiness, dyspraxia and adventitious movements, seem relevant. A fourth subcategory, altered hand preference (common in Autistic Spectrum Disorders), is more problematical and less easily ascertained. Further, within each of these subcategories there are now specific differential diagnostic, prognostic, and management implications. Some unfortunate children may demonstrate all four subcatagories (Deuel, 1992) of motor soft signs.

## Conclusion

The last 10 years' study of brain functional organization has proceeded rapidly. In regard to motor soft signs in children, most recent research can now conceptually accommodate their presence in the absence of structural damage, or progressive disease. Functional imaging studies of awake behaving children, although very difficult to perform at young ages, are beginning to suggest that delay of integration between neural systems may play a major role in motor soft signs. Such on-line functional anatomical information may soon become diagnostically useful in terms of the clinical significance of motor soft signs. At present, a major responsibility of the examiner who finds motor soft signs is making a judgment on their significance, a significance that ranges from 'no contribution to the patient's clinical situation', to 'indication of underlying progressive disease'. For those motor soft signs that are clinically significant in terms of development, there are some fairly effective therapies at the present time, and as the mechanisms

of development become increasingly better understood, methods for actually preventing disability in individual children may become available.

## References

American Academy of Neurology: ICD-9-CM for Neurologists. Washington, DC: American Academy of Neurology, 1990.

American Psychiatric Association: Diagnostic and Statistical Manual of Mental Disorders (4th ed.). Washington, DC: American Psychiatric Association, 1994.

Armand J, Kably B: Critical timing of sensorimotor lesions for the recovery of motor skills in the developing cat. Experimental Brain Research: 93; 73–88, 1993.

Barlow C: 'Soft signs' in children with learning disorders. American Journal of Diseases of Children: 128; 605–606, 1974.

Baron-Cohen S, Allen J, Gillberg C: Can autism be detected at 18 months? The needle, the haystack, and the CHAT. British Journal of Psychiatry: 161; 839–843, 1992.

Bastian A, Thach WT: Cerebellar outflow lesions: a comparison of movement deficits resulting from lesions at the levels of the cerebellum and the thalamus. Annals of Neurology: 38; 881–892, 1995.

Bayley N: Manual for the Bayley Scales of Infant Development. New York, NY: The Psychological Corporation, 1969.

Ben-Ari Y: Developing networks play a similar tone. Trends in Neurosciences: 24; 354–360, 2001.

Black M, Dubowitz H, Hutcheson J, Bereson-Howard J, Starr R: A randomized clinical trial of home intervention for children with failure to thrive. Pediatrics: 95; 807–814, 1995.

Bonda E, Petrides M, Ostry D, Evans A: Specific involvement of human parietal systems and the amygdala in the perception of biological motion. Journal of Neuroscience: 16; 3737–3744, 1996.

Boucher E, Doescher S, Sugawara A: Preschool children's motor development and self-concept. Perceptual and Motor Skills: 76; 11–17, 1993.

Bruiniks R: Bruiniks-Oseretsky Test of Motor Proficiency. Minnesota: American Guidance Service, 1978.

Buccino G, Binkofski F, Fink GR, Fadiga L, Fogassi L, Gallese V, Seitz RG, Zilles K, Rizzolatti G, Freund H-J: Action observation activates premotor and parietal areas in a somatopic manner: and fMRI study. European Journal of Neuroscience: 13; 400–404, 2001.

Bucher S, Seelos K, Stehling M, Oertel W, Paulus W, Reiser M: High-resolution activation mapping of basal ganglia with functional magnetic resonance imaging. Neurology: 45; 180–182, 1995.

Butters N, Salmon D, Heindel W: Specificity of the memory deficits associated with basal ganglia dysfunction. Revue Neurologique: 150; 580–587, 1994.

Clements S: Minimal Brain Dysfunction in Children. (USPHS Publication #141) Washington, DC: U.S. Government Printing Office, 1966.

Cohen L, Hollander E, DeCaria C et al.: Specificity of neuropsychological impairment in obsessive–compulsive disorder: a comparison with social phobic and normal controls. Journal of Neuropsychiatry and Clinical Neuroscience: 8; 82–85, 1996.

Conrad B, Kriebel J, Hetzel W: Hereditary bimanual synkinesis combined with hypogonadotropic, hypogonadism and anosmia in four brothers. Journal of Neurology: 318; 263–274, 1978.

Dare M, Gordon N: Clumsy children: A disorder of perception and motor organization. Developmental Medicine and Child Neurology: 12; 178–185, 1970.

David R et al.: Report of the Task Force on Nosology of Higher Cerebral Function: A Proposed Nosology of Disorders of Higher Cerebral Function in Children. Minneapolis: Child Neurology Society, 1981.

DeLong GR: Disorders of memory in childhood with a focus on temporal lobe disease and autism. In Segalowitz SJ, Rapin I (Eds), Child Neuropsychology, Handbook of Neuropsychology, 2nd Edition, vol. 8, part II. Amsterdam: Elsevier, chapter 27, 2003.

Denckla M: Development of speed in repetitive and successive finger movements in normal children. Developmental Medicine and Child Neurology: 15; 635–645, 1972.

Denckla M: Development of motor coordination in normal children. Developmental Medicine and Child Neurology: 16; 729–741, 1974.

Deuel R: Motor skill disorders. In Hooper S, Hynd G, Mattison R (Eds), Developmental Disorders: Diagnostic Criteria and Clinical Assessment. Hillsdale, NJ: Earlbaum, pp. 239–281, 1992.

Deuel R: Developmental dysgraphia and motor skills disorders. Journal of Child Neurology: 10(Suppl. 6–8); 1995.

Deuel R: The neurological examination of the school aged and adolescent child. In David R (Ed), Pediatric Neurology for the Clinician. St. Louis, MO: Mosby, pp. 71–86, 1998.

Deuel R, Anderson T: Procedural and symbolic learning after large unilateral thalamic lesions in monkeys. In Vallar G, Wallesch C, Cappa S (Eds), Neuropsychological Disorders Associated with Subcortical Lesions. Oxford: Oxford University, pp. 98–125, 1991.

Deuel R, Doar B: Developmental dyspraxia: A lesson in mind and brain. Journal of Child Neurology: 7; 99–103, 1992.

Deuel R, Dunlap N: Role of frontal polysensory cortex in guidance of limb movements. Brain Research: 169; 183–188, 1979.

Deuel R, Robinson D: Developmental motor signs. In Tupper D (Ed), Soft Neurological Signs. New York, NY: Grune and Stratton, pp. 95–129, 1987.

Donders J: Validity of the Kaufman Assessment Battery for children when employed with children with traumatic brain injury. Journal of Clinical Psychology: 48; 225–230, 1982.

Ellerman J, Flament D, Kim S, Fu Q, Merkle H, Ebner T, Ugurbil K: Spatial patterns of functional activation of the cerebellum investigated using high field (4 T) MRI. NMR in Biomedicine: 7; 63–68, 1994.

Eyre J, Miller S, Clowry G, Conway E, Watts C: Functional cortico-spinal projections are established prenatally in the human fetus permitting involvement in the development of spinal centers. Brain: 123; 51–64, 2000.

Ferry P, Hall S, Hicks J: Dilapidated speech: Developmental verbal dyspraxia. Developmental Medicine and Child Neurology: 17; 749–756, 1975.

Frankenberg W, Dodds J, Archer P, Shaprio H, Bresnick B: The Denver II: A major revision and restandardization of the Denver Developmental Screening Test. Pediatrics: 89; 91–97, 1992.

Garvey M, Giedd J, Swedo S: PANDAS: The search for environmental triggers of pediatric neuropsychiatric disorders. Journal of Child Neurology: 13(9); 413–423, 1998.

Gesell A, Amatruda C: Developmental Diagnosis. New York, NY: Hoeber, 1947.

Gilberg I, Gilberg C: Children with preschool minor neurodevelopmental disorders, IV: Behavior and school achievement at age 13. Developmental Medicine and Child Neurology: 31; 3–13, 1989.

Gilberg C, Rasmussen P: Perceptual, motor and attentional deficits in seven-year-old children: Background factors. Developmental Medicine and Child Neurology: 24; 752–770, 1982.

Gilles F: Myelination in the neonatal brain. Human Pathology: 7; 244–248, 1976.

Gilles F, Leviton A, Dooling E: The Developing Human Brain: Growth and Epidemiologic Neuropathology. Boston, MA: John Wright, 1983.

Gilmore RO: Toward a neuropsychology of visual development. In Segalowitz SJ, Rapin I (Eds), Child Neuropsychology, Handbook of Neuropsychology, 2nd Edition, vol. 8, part II. Amsterdam: Elsevier, chapter 17, 2003.

Gitelman D, Alpert N, Kosslyn S, Daffner K, Scinto L, Thompson W, Mesulam M: Functional imaging of human right hemispheric activation for exploratory movements. Annals of Neurology: 39; 174–179, 1996.

Goldman PS: Functional development of the prefrontal cortex in early life and the problem of neuronal plasticity. Experimental Neurology: 32; 366–387, 1971.

Goldman-Rakic PS: Development of cortical circuitry and cognitive function. Child Development: 58; 601–622, 1987.

Gomez M: Minimal cerebral dysfunction (maximal neurologic confusion). Clinical Pediatrics: 6; 589–591, 1967.

Graff-Radford N, Biller J: Behavioral neurology and stroke. Psychiatric Clinics of North America: 15; 415–425, 1992.

Grafton S, Mazziotta J, Woods R, Phelps M: Human functional anatomy of visually guided finger movements. Brain: 115; 565–587, 1992.

Grattan L, Eslinger P: Long-term psychological consequences of childhood frontal lobe lesion in patient DT. Brain and Cognition: 20; 185–195, 1993.

Gubbay S: The Clumsy Child: A Study of Developmental Apraxic and Agnostic Ataxia. London: Saunders, 1975.

Gubbay S: The management of developmental apraxia. Developmental Medicine and Child Neurology: 20; 643–646, 1978.

Guy W (Ed): ECDEU Manual for Psychopharmacology. Rockville, MD, NIMH, pp. 383–406, 1976.

Habib M, Alicherif A, Balzamo M, Milandre L, Donnet A, Khalil R: Caracterisation du trouble gestuel dans l'apraxie progressive primaire: apport diagnostique et nosographique. Revue Neurologique: 151; 541–551, 1995.

Hadders-Algra M: The Neuronal Group Selection Theory: A framework to explain variation in normal motor development. Developmental Medicine and Child Neurology: 42; 566–572, 2000.

Hasegawa RP, Blitz AM, Geller NL, Goldberg ME: Neurons in monkey prefrontal cortex that track past or predict future performance. Science: 290; 1787–1789, 2000.

Hirsh R: The hippocampus, conditional operations, and cognition. Physiological Psychology: 8; 175–182, 1980.

Holden W et al.: Reliability of neurological soft signs in children: Reevaluation of the PANESS. Journal of Abnormal Child Psychology: 10; 163–172, 1982.

Hollander E, DeCaria C, Aronowitz B et al.: A pilot follow-up study of childhood soft signs and the development of adult psychopathology. Journal of Neuropsychiatry and Clinical Neuroscience: 3; 186–189, 1991.

Hollander E, Weiller F, Cohen L, Kwon J, Decaria C, Liebowitz M, Stein D: Neurological soft signs in social phobia. Neuropsychiatry, Neuropsychology, and Behavioral Neurology: 9; 182–185, 1996.

Iacoboni M, Woods RP, Brass M, Bekkiering H, Mazziota JC, Rizzolatti G: Cortical mechanisms of human imitation. Science: 286; 2526–2528, 1999.

Ingram T: Soft signs. Developmental Medicine and Child Neurology: 15; 527–530, 1973.

Jacobs B, Chugani HT, Allada V et al.: Developmental changes in brain metabolism in sedated rhesus macaques and vervet monkeys revealed by positron emission tomography. Cerebral Cortex: 5; 222–233, 1995.

Kalaska J, Crammond D: Cerebral cortical mechanisms of reaching movements. Science: 255; 1517–1523, 1992.

Kennard M: Value of equivocal signs in neurologic diagnosis. Neurology: 10; 753–764, 1960.

Kinsbourne M, Cook J: Generalized and lateralized effects of concurrent verbalization on a unimanual skill. Journal of Experimental Psychology: 23; 341–345, 1971.

Knights R, Norwood J: Revised normative data on the neuropsychological test battery for children. Ottawa, ON: Knights Psychological Consultants, 1980.

LeMay M: Left–right dissymmetry, handedness. American Journal of Neuroradiology: 13; 493–504, 1992.

Lerer R, Lerer M: The effects of methylphenidate on the soft neurological signs of hyperactive children. Pediatrics: 57; 521–525, 1976.

Levin H, Culhane K, Fletcher J, Mendelsohn D, Lilly M, Harward H, Chapman S, Bruce D, Bertolino-Kusnerik L, Eisenberg H: Dissociation between delayed alternation and memory after pediatric head injury: Relationship to MRI findings. Journal of Child Neurology: 9; 81–89, 1994.

Levy R, Goldman-Rakic P: Segregation of working memory functions within the dorsolateral prefrontal cortex. Experimental Brain Research: 133; 23–32, 2000.

Liepmann H: Drei Aufsätze aus dem Apraxiegebiet (Three essays on apraxia). Berlin: Karger, 1908.

Logan C, Grafton S: Functional anatomy of human eyeblink conditioning determined with regional cerebral glucose metabolism and position-emission tomography. Proceedings of the National Academy of Sciences of the United States of America: 92; 7500–7504, 1995.

Lovass O: The development of a treatment-research project for developmentally delayed and autistic children. Journal of Applied Behavioral Analysis: 26; 617–629, 1993.

Miklosi A: From grasping to speech: imitation might provide a missing link. Trends in Neuroscience: 44; 152–153, 1999.

Milner B et al.: Further analysis of the hippocampal amnesic syndrome: 14-year follow-up study of H.M. Neuropsychologia: 6; 215–234, 1968.

Mink J, Thach WT: Basal ganglia intrinsic circuits and their role in behavior. Current Opinion in Neurobiology: 3; 950–957, 1993.

Mishkin M, Delacouer J: An analysis of short-term visual memory in the monkey. Journal of Experimental Psychology (Animal Behavior): 1; 326–334, 1975.

Mishkin M, Malamut B, Bachevalier J: Memories and habits: Two neural systems. In Lynch G et al. (Eds), Neurobiology of Learning and Memory. New York, NY: Guilford Press, Chapter 2, 1984.

Mishkin M, Petri H: Memories and habits: Some implications for the analysis of learning and retention. In Squire L, Butters N (Eds), Neuropsychology of Memory. New York, NY: Guilford Press, 1984.

Missiuna C, Polatajko H: Developmental dyspraxia by any other name: Are they all just clumsy children? American Journal of Occupational Therapy: 49; 619–627, 1995.

Molfese V, Price B: Neuropsychological assessment in infancy. In Segalowitz SJ, Rapin I (Eds), Child Neuropsychology, Handbook of Neuropsychology, 2nd Edition, vol. 8, part I. Amsterdam: Elsevier, pp. 229–247, 2002.

Muller K, Ebner S, Homberg V: Maturation of fastest afferent and efferent central and peripheral pathways: No evidence for a constancy of central conduction delays. Neuroscience Letters: 166; 9–12, 1994.

Muller R-A, Rothermel R, Behen M, Muzik O, Magner T, Chugani H: Developmental changes in cortical and cerebellar motor control: A clinical and position emission study with children and adults. Journal of Child Neurology: 13; 550–556, 1998.

Nicolelis M, Baccala L, Lin R, Chapin J: Sensorimotor encoding by synchronous neural ensemble activity at multiple levels of the somatosensory system. Science: 268; 1353–1358, 1995.

Norcia A, Tyler C, Hamer R: Development of contrast sensitivity in the human infant. Vision Research: 30; 1475–1476, 1990.

Orten S: Word-blindness: In school children. Archives of Neurology: 14; 582–615, 1925.

Pascual-Leone A, Grafman J, Hallett M: Modulation of cortical motor output maps during development of implicit and explicit knowledge. Science: 263; 1267–1289, 1994.

Pellizer G, Sargent P, Georgopoulos A: Motor cortical activity in a context-recall task. Science: 269; 702–705, 1995.

Penn A, Schatz P: Brain waves and brain wiring: The role of endogenous and sensory driven neural activity in development. Pediatric Research: 45; 477–458, 1999.

Peters J, Romine J, Dykman R: A special neurological examination of children with learning disabilities. Developmental Medicine and Child Neurology: 17; 63–78, 1975.

Rakic P, Bourgeois J, Goldman-Rakic P: Synaptic development of the cerebral cortex: implications for learning memory and mental illness. Progress in Brain Research: 102; 227–243, 1994.

Rapin I, Allen D: Syndromes in developmental dyphasia and adult aphasia. Research Publications: Association for Research in Nervous and Mental Disease: 66; 57–75, 1988.

Reitan R, Wolfsun D: The Halstead–Reitan neuropsychological test battery: Theory and clinical interpretation. Tucson, AZ: Neuropsychology Press, 1985.

Rizzolatti G, Fadiga L, Gallese V: Resonance behaviors and mirror neurons. Archives Italiennes de Biologie: 137; 85–100, 1999.

Rutter M: Syndromes attributed to 'minimal brain dysfunction' in children. American Journal of Psychiatry: 139; 21–33, 1982.

Schaffer D, Schonfeld I, O'Connor P, Stokman C, Trautman P, Shafer S, Ng S: Neurological soft signs: Their relationship to psychiatric disorder and intelligence in childhood and adolescence. Archives of General Psychiatry: 42; 342–352, 1985.

Shaw L, Levine M, Belfer M: Developmental double jeopardy: A study of clumsiness and self-esteem in children with learning problems. Journal of Developmental Behavior Pediatrics: 3; 191–196, 1992.

Sommer M, Gathof B, Podskarbi T, Giugliani R, Kleinlein B, Shin Y: Mutations in the galactose-1-phosphate uridyltransferase gene of two families with mild galactosaemia variants. Journal of Inherited Metabolic Disease: 18; 567–576, 1995.

Soper L, Satz P, Orsini D: Handedness patterns in autism suggest subtypes. Journal of Autism and Developmental Disorders: 16; 155–167, 1986.

Spreen O, Gaddes W: Developmental norms for 15 neuropsychological tests age 6–15. Cortex: 5; 170–181, 1969.

Squire L, Cohen N: Human memory and amnesia. In Lynch G, McGaugh J, Weinberger N (Eds), Neurobiology of Learning and Memory. New York, NY: Guilford Press, pp. 3–64, 1984.

Stokman C, Schafer S, Shaffer D: Assessment of neurological 'soft signs' in adolescents. Reliability studies. Developmental Medicine and Child Neurology: 28; 428–439, 1986.

Thach WT, Goodkin H, Keating J: The cerebellum and the adaptive coordination of movement. Annual Review of Neuroscience: 15; 403–442, 1992.

Thach WT, Perry J, Kane S, Goodkin H: Cerebellar nuclei: Rapid alternating movement, motor somatotopy, and a mechanism for the control of muscle synergy. Revue Neurologique: 149; 607–628, 1993.

Thompson PM, Giedd JN, Woods RP, Evans AC, Toga AW: Growth patterns in the developing brain detected by using continuum mechanical tensor-maps. Nature: 404(6774); 190–193, 2000.

Todor J, Lazarus C: Exertion level and the intensity of associated movements. Developmental Medicine and Child Neurology: 28; 278–281, 1986.

Tupper D (Ed): NIMH Physical and Neurological Examination for Soft Signs, Appendix A. New York, NY: Grune and Stratton, pp. 339–353, 1987.

Tyszka J, Grafton S, Chew W, Woods R, Colletti P: Parceling of mesial frontal motor areas during ideation and movement using functional magnetic resonance imaging at 1.5 tesla. Annals of Neurology: 35; 746–749, 1994.

U.S. Department of Health and Human Services: ICO-9-CM (3rd ed). Washington, DC: DHHS Publication No. HS 89-160, 1991.

Vajapeyam S et al.: Use of diffusion tensor imaging to study discrete white matter fiber tract maturation after birth. Annals of Neurology: S98; 2001.

Van Mier H, Ojemann J, Gopalan B, Deuel R, Petersen S: Practice related changes during maze learning in children measured by FMRI. Neuroscience Abstracts: 26; 124, 1998.

Wolff P, Gunnoe C, Cohen C: Associated movements as a measure of developmental age. Developmental Medicine and Child Neurology: 25; 417–429, 1983.

Wolff P, Hurwitz I: The choreiform syndrome. Developmental Medicine and Child Neurology: 4; 160–165, 1966.

Yakovlev P, Lecours A: The myelogenetic cycles of regional maturation of the brain. In Minkowski A (Ed), Regional Development of the Brain in Early Life. Philadelphia: F.A. Davis, 1967.

Yoss D, Darley F: Developmental apraxia of speech in children with defective articulation. Journal of Speech and Hearing Research: 17; 399–416, 1974.

CHAPTER 16

# Somatosensory perception in children

Joseph E. Casey [a,*] and Byron P. Rourke [b]

[a,*] *Department of Psychology, University of Windsor, Windsor, ON N9B 3P4, Canada*
[b] *Yale University, New Haven, CT, USA*

***Nihil in intellectu quod non prius in sensu.***
*(Nothing in the intellect that was not previously in the senses.)*

A Scholastic version of an Aristotelian principle.

## Introduction

It has been some 10 years since the first edition of this chapter was published. It comprised a comprehensive review of matters related to the normal development and abnormal manifestations of somatosensory functions in children. The neuroanatomical pathways important to somatosensory perception were summarized. The developmental course for each of the major neuropsychological modalities typically assessed in children was described, as were the procedures by which these modalities are assessed. The literature addressing the reliability and validity of assessment procedures was reviewed. The nature and implications of somatosensory disorders in children were discussed, as were areas wherein future research might extend our understanding of brain–behaviour relationships. The emphasis for the chapter was decidedly on applied rather than basic research. Consequently, much of the literature reviewed involved the tests and procedures that have become associated with the Halstead–Reitan neuropsychological assessment batteries.

The vast majority of the literature relevant to the first edition of the chapter was published prior to 1985, with well over half the references predating 1980. This apparent trend toward less research activity focussing specifically on somatosensory functions in children was clearly evident from our current review of the literature. Incredibly few studies were published in the last 10 years that extended our first review of the literature. Those that have been published have been largely consistent with the results of earlier studies. Some recent studies have demonstrated tactile-perceptual impairments in certain clinical conditions, such as very low birth weight (DeMaio-Feldman, 1994) and attention deficit hyperactivity disorder (ADHD; Parush, Sohmer, Steinberg and Kaitz, 1997), thus providing further support for the notion that performance deficits on tactile-perceptual measures can occur in disorders that affect the brain diffusely or in conditions that are not ordinarily associated with damage to the neuroanatomical substrates specific to somatosensory perception (e.g., ADHD). Recent studies have also demonstrated that tactile-perceptual deficits are less sensitive to pathology or less predictive of outcome than deficits in other neuropsychological functions, again consistent with the earlier literature. Consider, for example, the study by Thompson, Francis, Stuebing et al., 1994. In their longitudinal study examining recovery following closed head injury, they compared 49 children and adolescents on motor, visual–spatial, and somatosensory measures. They found that tactile–spatial perception, at least as measured by the Tactile Form Perception Test (Benton, Hamsher, Varney and Spreen, 1983), was not sensitive to outcome, whereas measures of psychomotor skills were much more sensitive.

* Corresponding author. E-mail: jecasey@uwindsor.ca

Although supporting the findings of previous research, the few clinically oriented studies published since the first edition of this chapter have added disappointingly little to our neuropsychological understanding of somatosensory perception in children. Nonetheless, encouraging signs of progress, however meagre, are evident. The creative work of Eilers and her colleagues, discussed later in this chapter, introduces researchers and clinicians to a whole new direction for conceptualizing and studying tactile perception in children. Especially exciting in this regard is the further delineation of the tactile-perceptual system's potential role in the development of cognitive processes and of its potential as a modality for the treatment of certain developmental conditions, in this case hearing impairment.

In the interest of consistency with the other chapters of the *Handbook*, the comprehensive scope and depth of this chapter was retained. Unfortunately, this means that much of the literature pertinent to the current edition still derives from the 1970s and 1980s. However, reducing each of the sections to a summary would deprive the reader of the richness that characterizes this literature. The history of our knowledge of somatosensory perception and its disordered presentation in children would be neglected and the encyclopedic nature of the *Handbook* would be forsaken.

## Foundations

It has been suggested that "the basic aim of every neuropsychological assessment — be it with adults, adolescents, or children — is to produce a reliable and valid 'picture' of the relationships between the brain and behaviour" (Rourke, Bakker, Fisk and Strang, 1983, p. 112). Obviously, to accomplish such a goal, the assessment process must include a sufficiently broad and thorough sampling of behaviours so as to reflect principal areas of human functioning considered to be directly relevant to the status of the central nervous system. As such, the content of a comprehensive neuropsychological assessment usually includes an examination of visual, auditory, and tactile sensory-perceptual abilities, motor and psychomotor abilities, verbal and psycholinguistic skills, mnestic abilities, and 'higher-order' cognitive

functions such as concept-formation and problem-solving abilities (Rourke et al., 1983).

The psychological literature relevant to some of these ability areas is extensive, providing much information necessary to conduct a competent neuropsychological evaluation. For example, much has been written about the development of language abilities in children, and the features, both clinical and psychometric, of its pathological forms. In contrast, there has been relatively little study of the normal and abnormal development of somatosensory abilities and the clinical significance of its pathological manifestations. This is especially difficult to understand in view of the now classic investigations of both Piaget and Harlow which suggest that this sensory modality plays an important role in the cognitive and socioemotional development of the child (e.g., Harlow and Zimmerman, 1958; Piaget, 1952).

Despite this state of affairs, the examination of tactile-perceptual abilities is routinely incorporated into most neuropsychological assessments of children. To a large extent, the specific tests and procedures employed have been adopted, often without modification, from those that have been traditionally utilized in the evaluation of adult persons. In this chapter we focus on dimensions of tactile sensitivity in the developing child, summarizing the current literature. No attempt is made to deal with such dimensions at subsequent levels of development.

This chapter is organized into three sections. The introduction presents a brief history related to the assessment of tactile-perceptual skills and abilities in child neuropsychology, and provides a review of the functional neuroanatomy of the somatosensory system. The second section discusses the modalities of somatosensory perception that are typically evaluated in the course of a comprehensive neuropsychological assessment. For each of the tactile-perceptual modalities, developmental considerations and issues relating to the reliability and validity of the measurement techniques are addressed. The final section presents a summary of the major findings to emerge from this review. Also discussed are issues related to the interpretation of impaired performance on somatosensory measures, including the significance of early (i.e., developmental rather than acquired) somatosensory impairments. Finally, areas wherein future research might extend our understanding of brain–behaviour relationships in children are suggested.

## The Reitan–Kløve Sensory-Perceptual Examination

Since the seminal work of Ralph M. Reitan in the early 1950s, the systematic examination of the somatosensory system has been firmly ensconced in the major traditions of assessment within the field of child clinical neuropsychology. Reitan's collaboration with Halgrim Kløve produced the now standard battery referred to as the Reitan–Kløve Sensory-Perceptual Examination. This examination forms a part of what are considered to be the 'allied procedures' that ordinarily accompany the administration of the Halstead–Reitan Neuropsychological Test Batteries for Children. Although the examination also involves tests for auditory and visual imperception, its primary focus is on measures of tactile–haptic sensitivity. These procedures were designed to detect impairments of (1) simple tactile sensitivity under conditions of single and bilateral simultaneous stimulation, (2) finger recognition (localization), (3) finger graphaesthesia, and (4) stereognosis for forms (younger children) and coins (older children).

Reitan and Kløve did not carry out any reliability studies of this battery, but they did conduct several studies in which the validity of this examination was evaluated, either directly or indirectly. These are discussed in the appropriate sections of this chapter. More recently, Brown, Rourke and Cicchetti (1989) have reported some data relating to the test–retest reliability of the tactile imperception–suppression and finger agnosia subtests of the Reitan–Kløve examination; these are also discussed in the appropriate sections. However, before considering the neuropsychological tests and procedures designed to measure tactile-perceptual functioning, it would be well to review briefly the anatomical substrates relevant to the somatosensory system.

## Neuroanatomical substrates

Lesions can occur at any level within the fibre pathways that course from the peripherally located sensory receptors to the cerebral cortex. The pattern of the sensory loss as seen in conjunction with other neurological and/or neuropsychological findings is invaluable in determining the site of damage and the possible pathological process. Thus, a proper understanding of these anatomical systems, their course, and their functional correlates is necessary before one can render competent interpretations of neuropsychological findings. The information summarized below is based on the following sources: Barr and Kiernan (1983); Brodal (1981); Nieuwenhuys, Voogd and van Huijzen (1981).

There are five types (modalities) of cutaneous sensation for which the neuroanatomical substrates are well known. These include fine (discriminative) touch, vibration, light touch, temperature, and pain. The general sensory systems, which are distinguished from special sensory systems (i.e., visual, auditory, olfactory, vestibular), are usually divided into two main types based on neuroanatomical and functional considerations. The spinothalamic system, considered to be the more primitive of the two, is responsible primarily for the perception of pain and temperature. It is also referred to as the protopathic system. Since the functions of this system are routinely investigated as part of a neurological examination and are rarely, if ever, tested within the context of a neuropsychological assessment, this system will not be considered further. The interested reader can consult any of the sources listed above for more information about this system.

The second system, known variously as the medial lemniscus, dorsal column (or dorsal funiculus), or epicritic system, is concerned primarily with fine touch and the mediation of kinaesthetic information. This includes the tactile recognition of shapes or objects (stereognosis) and textures, and the ability to appreciate the position and movement of the limbs and body (proprioception). The discriminative quality of the information mediated by this system is obviously important for early learning and development. For example, the primary source of feedback necessary for the development of skills germane to Piaget's sensorimotor period (Piaget, 1954) is provided by this system. As a child exercises his/her elementary motor schemes, tactile and kinaesthetic feedback serve to direct and eventually refine these motor patterns, thus rendering them increasingly more complex and adaptive.

The receptor organs that transduce physical stimuli into the neural impulses and that ultimately give rise to the cutaneous modalities mediated by the epicritic system are fairly well understood. Unique to primates is the presence of Meissner's corpuscles; these are found most abundantly in the skin of the fingertips and to a lesser degree in the palmar surfaces of the hands. These receptors are particularly important for discriminative touch. Indeed, it is within these areas of glabrous (hairless) skin that two-point discrimination is the most acute. Pacinian corpuscles, found in both hairy and glabrous skin, mediate the sense of vibration. The principal receptors responsible for proprioceptive functions are the neuromuscular spindles, Golgi tendon organs, and endings innervating the capsules and ligaments of joints. In comparison to the axons that constitute the pathways of the protopathic system, those of the epicritic system are heavily myelinated. This enables the rapid transmission of information that is necessary for the execution of highly complex motor acts.

The cell bodies of the primary (i.e., first order) neurons are situated within the dorsal root ganglia. The end organs of their peripheral processes form the receptors that innervate the skin, joints, and tendons. Their central processes enter the spinal cord via the dorsal root, with the majority of the fibres ascending ipsilaterally in the dorsal funiculus (Fig. 1). The fibres that originate in the sacral, lumbar, and lower thoracic roots take a more medial position within the dorsal funiculus and comprise the fasciculus gracilis; those from the upper thoracic and cervical roots form the more lateral funiculus cuneatus. At the lower level of the medulla oblongata, these fibres terminate in the nucleus gracilis and cuneatus, respectively. The axons of the secondary neurons arising from these nuclei form the internal arcuate fibres as they cross the midline of the medulla. This pathway continues to ascend the brainstem, now contralateral to the nuclei from which it originated, as the medial lemniscus and ultimately terminates in the ventral posterior nucleus of the thalamus (VPL). The tertiary neurons of VPL send projections via the posterior limb of the internal capsule and the medullary centre (cerebral white matter) to the somaesthetic cortex located in the postcentral gyrus. It is only at this point that conscious awareness of the sensation is attained.

Of course, the pathways serving the epicritic modalities of the head do not ascend the spinal cord. Rather, these fibres enter the brainstem at the level of the mid pons and terminate ipsilaterally within their appropriate nuclei situated in the brainstem. Axons emerging from these nuclei cross the midline and join the contralateral medial lemniscus system. These axons terminate in the medial aspect of the ventral posterior nucleus of the thalamus which, in turn, sends the majority of its fibres to the lateral portion of the postcentral gyrus.

Another exception to the general organization of the epicritic system as described above involves those pathways for conscious proprioception from the lower limbs. The central processes of the dorsal root neurons enter the spinal cord and terminate at their segmental levels in the nucleus dorsalis. Axons from this nucleus ascend ipsilaterally as the dorsal spinocerebellar tract and enter the inferior cerebellar peduncle, with collaterals proceeding to the area rostral to the nucleus gracilis where they terminate. It is this latter pathway that is responsible for conscious proprioception from the lower limbs. Fibres emanating from this area join the medial lemniscus and continue as part of this system. An important feature of the epicritic system is its topographic arrangement of fibres which is maintained throughout its course. This gives rise to the precision with which somatosensory information is represented in the central nervous system (CNS).

The cortical areas representing the pharyngeal region, tongue, jaw, face, hand, arm, and thigh are found on the contralateral surface of the cerebral hemisphere as one moves from the most ventral to the most dorsal aspects of the somaesthetic strip. The cortical area for the remainder of the leg and the perineum is situated contiguously on the medial surface of the hemisphere. Reflecting their functional importance, the areas for the face (especially the lips) and the hands (especially the thumb and index finger) are disproportionately large relative to their actual physical size. The face has some ipsilateral representation as well as contralateral; however, the latter is predominant.

Posterior to the somaesthetic strip, in the superior parietal lobule, is the somaesthetic association cortex. It receives fibres from the postcentral gyrus and has reciprocal connections with certain nuclei of the thalamus. This association area is considered to be important for the recognition of objects or patterns presented tactually. This is accomplished through

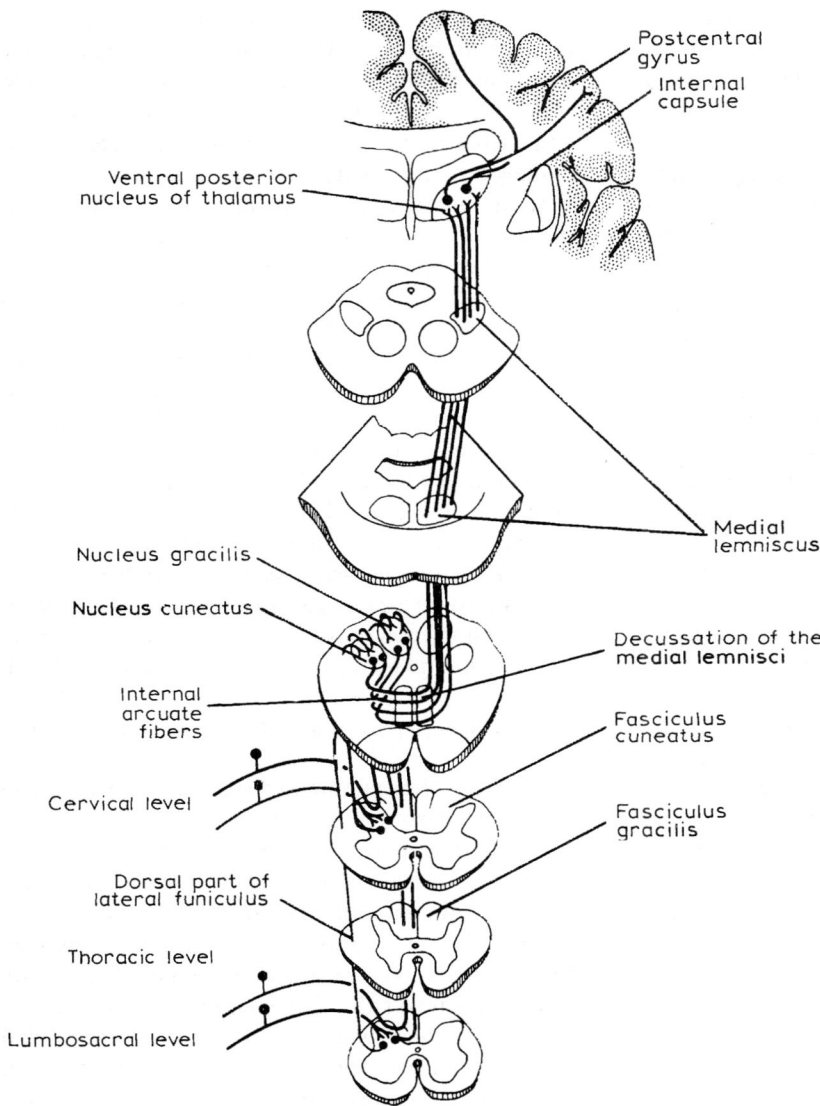

Fig. 1. The epicritic system for discriminative tactile sensation. (Adapted from Barr and Kiernan, 1983.)

the synthesis of tactile information regarding texture, shape, size, and weight of an object with the individual's past experiences. Destructive lesions involving the somaesthetic strip tend to disturb all aspects of epicritic sensation to the same degree, whereas lesions limited to the somaesthetic association cortex tend to disturb the more complex sensations (e.g., stereognosis) to a greater extent than the more elemental sensations (e.g., two-point discrimination, position sense). Unfortunately, this distinction in

the higher-order representation of tactile-perceptual functions has only been studied systematically in adults (e.g., Pause, Kunesch, Binkofski and Freund, 1989). Similar studies involving children have yet to appear in the literature.

Although all of the structures that constitute the epicritic system are present at birth, a considerable degree of myelination remains to occur. The course of postnatal myelination of the central nervous system has been discussed by Dekaban (1970). Those aspects that pertain to the epicritic system are summarized below.

At birth, the peripheral nerves supplying the segmental structures of the spinal cord are well myelinated, while the myelination of the posterior columns is at least well under way. Although there is indication that some myelination of the medial lemniscus is present throughout the brainstem, with some fibres being traceable to VPL, the myelination is not as extensive as that seen in the posterior columns. The only myelinated fibres found in the cerebral hemispheres are those few that, for the most part, are restricted to the primary projection afferents, a proportion of which course from VPL to the sensorimotor cortex.

The myelination of the epicritic system continues at a rapid pace during the first 18 months of life and occurs in a caudal to rostral direction. Whereas during the early period of infancy the myelination of the posterior columns clearly supersedes that of the corticospinal tracts, by 9 months of age the latter appear to be as well myelinated as the former. By 12 months of age, all spinal cord and brainstem tracts are well myelinated, as are the primary projection fibres of the cerebral hemispheres. In contrast, the long association fibres are less well developed, and the short association fibres, particularly those of the temporal and frontal lobes, even less so. By 18–24 months of age, the epicritic system is completely myelinated. In order to accommodate the physical development of the nervous system after this time, the sheaths continue to grow in a proportional manner, both in thickness and along the length of the nerve fibres.

This simplified account of the organization and postnatal development of the epicritic system is meant to introduce the reader to the main anatomical pathways relevant to the neuropsychological material covered in the remainder of this review.

## Neuropsychological modalities of somatosensory perception

### Simple tactile perception and suppression

Within the context of a neuropsychological assessment, the evaluation of simple tactile-perceptual functioning involves measuring the child's ability to localize tactile stimuli applied under conditions of single and double simultaneous stimulation, always without the aid of vision. Initially, the child is required to identify which of either hand or side of the face has been touched. If the child's performance is considered to be essentially intact (i.e., there is no evidence of imperception), then unilateral stimulations are interspersed with trials in which either both hands or one hand and the contralateral side of the face are touched simultaneously. Evidence of a suppression (also known as 'extinction') is represented by impaired performance on the bilateral simultaneous trials of the examination. Specific instructions for administering the most commonly used version of these procedures are available in Reitan (1984).

Evidence of tactile imperception and/or suppression on one side of the body is usually interpreted as being indicative of dysfunction within the area of, or adjacent to, the contralateral postcentral gyrus, the so-called somaesthetic strip (Rourke et al., 1983). Some consider unilateral suppression as a fairly common phenomenon of parietal lobe lesions, as in many cases of spastic hemiparesis (Paine and Oppé, 1966).

### Developmental considerations

The findings from normative studies suggest that the ability to detect tactile stimuli under conditions of single and double simultaneous stimulation is already well developed by the age of 5 years. Mairuro, Townes, Vitaliano and Trupin (1984) reported that there was no significant age effect on measures of imperception and suppression across the age groups that they studied (5- to 8-year-olds); they also reported that there was no significant difference between left- and right-hand performance. Although no statistical comparisons were provided, a visual inspection of the normative data of Knights and Norwood (1980) also suggests that little improvement in performance occurs for children aged 5 to 8 years. Data from Knights and Norwood (1980) for children 9 to 14 years of age indicate that, as a group, they make fewer errors as compared to the younger children. However, the difference is relatively small ($M = 0.42$ and 1.06, respectively) and is unlikely to be clinically meaningful.

Roeltgen and Roeltgen (1990) examined children 2 to 6 years of age and found a significant age effect on a test of double simultaneous stimulation of the hands. Children with known neurological disorders were excluded, as were left-handed children. Although multiple comparisons were not reported, an inspection of the means obtained for each of the four age groups suggests that children obtained ceiling performance at 3 to 4 years of age. Moreover, the results of error analyses revealed that more allaesthetic and suppression errors occurred following left-sided as compared to right-sided stimulation. An allaesthetic error was defined as one made by a child who, when touched on one hand, localized the stimulus to the contralateral hand.

Fink and Bender (1953) identified developmental patterns on tactile-perceptual measures by analysing separately the results of symmetrically (hand–hand; face–face) and asymmetrically (face–hand) applied bilateral touch stimuli in a sample of 300 normal 3- to 15-year-olds. It was found that the ability to localize symmetrical stimuli was well developed in 3-year-old children whereas the ability to localize asymmetrically applied stimuli developed more gradually, being present in 80% of the sample only by the age of 8 years. It was also found that all age groups demonstrated a face dominance on asymmetric stimulation that was manifested most often by a suppression of the stimulus applied to the hand.

Taken together, the results of these developmental studies suggest that (a) the ability to identify single and symmetrically placed double simultaneous tactile stimuli is well developed by approximately 3 years of age, (b) the ability to identify heterologous tactile stimuli does not develop fully until about age 8 years, and (c) regardless of age, under conditions of bilateral heterologous stimulation children are more likely to identify accurately the stimulus delivered to the face than the one delivered to the hand or some other area of the body. Developmentalists will recognize this last point as reflecting the proximodistal pattern of ontogenetic development.

*Reliability and validity*

Very few studies have evaluated the reliability of tactile-perceptual measures. One exception is a recently reported investigation of 248 children, aged 5 to 14 years, who had undergone neuropsychological assessment at least twice over an average of 2.6 years (Brown et al., 1989). The children were selected from a heterogeneous population of 3600 clinic-referred children, most of whom had been assessed for the purpose of evaluating a possible learning disability and/or perceptual problem to which it was thought that brain impairment might be a contributing factor. Test–retest reliabilities for all of the measures employed in the neuropsychological battery were determined by both Pearson product–moment correlations and intraclass correlations.

It was found that tactile-perceptual measures, in general, were less reliable than were measures reflecting other functional domains (e.g., psychometric intelligence, language and psycholinguistic abilities, motor abilities). Among the tactile-perceptual measures studied, the test of imperception and suppression tended to be the least reliable. Pearson product–moment correlations for both left- and right-hand dominant children ranged from 0.33 to 0.45; the corresponding intraclass correlations ranged from 0.19 to 0.38. However, the authors noted that the correlation coefficients for the tactile-perceptual tests might have been limited by the small range of scores typically obtained for such measures. In their sample, the number of errors with the right hand and left hand at first assessment were 1.6 (SD = 2.0) and 1.0 (SD = 1.6), respectively. At the second assessment, the number of errors were 0.76 (SD = 1.4) with the right hand and 0.61 (SD = 1.4) with the left hand.

Several case studies of children have reported the effects that lateralized brain lesions can have on simple tactile perception, particularly if the damage encroaches on the parietal lobe (for example, see Reitan, 1984, case no. 10; Rourke et al., 1983, case no. 1). While illustrative, such case studies do not address the clinical utility of simple tactile-perceptual measures. Given that errors rarely occur on these measures in normal children, the presence of impaired performance, in the absence of peripheral nervous system abnormality, would strongly suggest CNS dysfunction. However, as with most measures that rely on the pathognomonic sign approach, those of simple tactile-perceptual functioning would be expected to yield a high false-negative rate. Unfortunately of the many studies that have evaluated the sensitivity of various neuropsychological tests and measures to brain damage in children (e.g., Boll, 1974; Klonoff, Robinson and Thompson, 1969; Reed, Reitan and Kløve, 1965; Reitan, 1974;

Spreen and Benton, 1965), none has included in the data analyses tests of imperception and suppression. Thus, questions regarding the concurrent and predictive validity of these measures remain largely unanswered.

### Stereognosis

Impaired performance in the ability to identify objects by tactile perception only is referred to as 'astereognosis'. The examination procedure typically requires the child to identify various geometric shapes (e.g., cross, square, triangle, circle), placed singularly in the hand, by pointing to its match that is displayed along with the other stimulus figures. For older children, stereognosis for coins is also evaluated. The studies reviewed here are based on the tactile form recognition measures from the Reitan–Kløve Sensory-Perceptual Examination (Reitan, 1984).

The interpretive significance of lateralized impairment on stereognosis testing is similar to that for tactile suppressions. Thus, poor performance with the right hand would support a hypothesis of left parietal lobe dysfunction, and poor left-hand performance, right parietal lobe dysfunction (Rourke et al., 1983).

### Developmental considerations

Mairuro et al. (1984) found a significant main effect for age in their normative sample of 5- to 8-year-old children on the Tactile Form Recognition Test. Although the number of errors was small for all four age groups studied, the errors were considered somewhat more unusual for 7- and 8-year-olds. These results are consistent with the normative data of Knights and Norwood (1980), which also reveal that children performed virtually without error after the age of 8 years. Mairuro et al. (1984) also found that there was no significant difference between left- and right-hand performance for the younger (5- to 8-year-old) children.

In summary, the results of normative studies suggest that (a) the ability to recognize simple geometric shapes through touch is well developed in early childhood, (b) children make virtually no errors on such a task after the age of 8 years, and (c) left-

and right-hand performance in normal children is essentially the same.

### Reliability and validity

As of yet, no published study has examined the reliability of the Tactile Form Recognition Test. However, several studies have compared the performance of brain-damaged and normal children on many of the measures typically employed in the neuropsychological evaluation of children, including measures of tactile form recognition, finger-tip writing (symbol and number perception), and tactile finger localization from the Halstead–Reitan batteries for children. An early study by Boll (1972) found that a heterogeneous sample of children with brain damage (mean age of 12 years) performed significantly worse than an age- and sex-matched control group of normal children on the Tactile Form Recognition Test. However, of the five measures utilized in this study (Category Test, WISC Block Design subtest, Seashore Rhythm Test, Tactile Form Recognition Test, and Finger Oscillation Test), the Tactile Form Recognition Test yielded the smallest group difference. Boll and Reitan (1972) found no significant difference between a heterogeneous group of brain-damaged children and matched controls (overall age approximately 11 to 12 years) on the Tactile Form Recognition Test. In addition, there were no significant group differences in terms of discrepancies in performance between the two hands.

In contrast to these findings with older children, a significant difference, favouring normals, was obtained when a group of younger (5- to 8-year-old) brain-damaged children was compared with a group of normal children matched for age, race, and sex (Reitan, 1971). In addition, the left- and right-hand discrepancy score was significantly larger in the brain-damaged group. Employing the same sample, Reitan (1974) rank-ordered the neuropsychological tests based on the magnitude of the group differences. When both left- and right-hand rankings are combined, tactile form recognition emerges as the most sensitive of the tactile-perceptual measures. The single most sensitive tactile-perceptual measure was tactile form recognition with the left hand.

Reitan and Boll (1973) compared the performance of four groups of young children (average age approximately 7.4 years) on several neuropsychological measures, including tactile form recognition. The four groups studied were as follows: (1) a heterogeneous group of brain-damaged children; (2) a group of children classified as exhibiting minimal brain dysfunction (MBD), whose primary difficulties were academic in nature; (3) another group of children classified as having MBD and whose primary difficulties were behavioural in nature; and (4) a normal control group. It was found that the brain-damaged children performed significantly inferior to each of the other three groups. The control, MBD-academic, and MBD-behavioural groups did not differ from each other.

Tsushima and Towne (1977) compared a group of 'questionably' brain-damaged children with learning difficulties and a group of 6- to 8-year-olds who were experiencing learning difficulties but had no history of serious illness or trauma suspected of causing brain injury (e.g., prematurity, acute convulsive disorders, head trauma). They found that the groups did not differ in tactile form recognition ability with either hand.

The results of these studies suggest that (a) the ability to identify simple geometric forms is developed at an early age, (b) very few errors in performance can be expected in children aged 7 to 8 years, (c) poor performance in tactile form recognition is only likely to occur in children with frank brain damage, especially in younger (5 to 8 years) as compared to older (9 to 14 years) children, and (d) in a heterogeneous population of brain-damaged children, performance with the left hand appears to be more adversely affected than is that with the right hand. Presently, the sensitivity and specificity with which astereognosis would be expected to occur in children with unilateral lesions remains empirically undetermined.

## Graphaesthesia

A deficiency in the ability to identify symbols drawn on a part of the body is referred to as 'dysgraphaesthesia'. Ordinarily, for children 5 to 8 years of age, the task requires the child to identify without the aid of vision, elementary symbols (e.g., 'X', 'O') drawn on the fingertips. For older children, a restricted range of single-digit numbers is employed (e.g., 3

to 6). Several trials are administered to each finger of each hand in a counterbalanced fashion. The only standardized test of graphaesthesia is that included in the Reitan–Kløve Sensory-Perceptual Examination (Reitan, 1984).

The interpretive significance of dysgraphaesthesia errors (discussed in Rourke et al., 1983, and summarized below) is somewhat different than that of the other tactile-perceptual measures considered thus far. Whereas the presence of unilateral dysgraphaesthesia would suggest involvement of the contralateral parietal lobe, bilateral dysgraphaesthesia may arise from impaired functioning of the left cerebral hemisphere. The latter is due to the symbolic requirements of the task. Bilateral dysgraphaesthesia may also arise because of right cerebral hemisphere dysfunction; the putative bases for this hypothesis are the spatial aspects of the task. Thus, evidence of dysgraphaesthesia must be interpreted within the context of the entire neuropsychological examination.

### Developmental considerations

Mairuro et al. (1984) reported a significant age-effect on the Finger-tip Symbol Writing Test in their normative investigation of 5- to 8-year-old children for performance with both the left and right hands. Rather than being gradual, the improvement in performance appears most abrupt between the ages of 6 and 7 years. However, this trend is not evident in the Knights and Norwood (1980) data. Furthermore, the latter normative data also reflect what appears to be a gradual decrease in error rate for children 9 to 14 years of age for the Finger-tip Number Writing Test. Although no statistical comparisons are reported in either normative study, the data from each suggest that normal children demonstrate similar levels of performance with each hand.

### Reliability and validity

As with stereognosis measures, no study has reported the reliability of the graphaesthesia measures discussed herein. Many of the studies that have examined the validity of the finger-tip writing procedures (usually with the view to establishing their sensitivity to brain damage) have done so in conjunction with the other tactile-perceptual measures; these have been cited in previous sections of this chapter, particularly in that dealing with stereognosis.

Overall, the results of studies evaluating the effects of brain damage in older children on graphaesthesia are equivocal. Boll and Reitan (1972) found that a heterogeneous group of brain-damaged children performed significantly worse than did a normal control group on the Finger-tip Number Writing Test. However, there was no group difference in terms of the discrepancy in performance between the left and right hands.

Conversely, in a similar study, Boll (1974) found no difference between brain-damaged and control children for left- and right-hand performances analysed separately. In part, the discrepancy between the results of these two studies may have been due to the pooling of left- and right-hand scores in the Boll and Reitan (1972) study, thus giving rise to a more robust measure of graphaesthesia.

In younger children, the relationship between brain damage and dysgraphaesthesia is not quite as ambiguous. For example, it was demonstrated that 5- to 8-year-old brain-damaged children, as a group, exhibited significantly more dysgraphaesthesia errors relative to (a) age-matched groups of normal children (Reitan, 1971; Reitan and Boll, 1973), and (b) children diagnosed as MBD when compared on the left hand (Reitan and Boll, 1973). However, in groups of subjects for whom brain dysfunction is only suspected, such as in the MBD groups included in the Reitan and Boll (1973) study and the 'questionable brain disorder' group of Tsushima and Towne (1977), performance does not appear to be compromised. The results of a study by Nolan, Hammeke and Barkley (1983) of 7- to 13-year-olds are consistent with this notion. They found no significant difference among groups of control (non-brain-damaged), reading/spelling disabled, and math disabled children on Finger-tip Number Writing.

In summary, the findings from these studies, albeit tentative, suggest that dysgraphaesthesia (1) is not a sensitive measure of brain damage, especially when compared to other neuropsychological measures such as psychomotor tests, (2) is more likely to be observed in younger as compared to older children who have sustained brain damage, and (3) when present, is likely to be more pronounced with the left as compared to the right hand.

*Finger recognition*

Undoubtedly, the most extensively researched tactile-perceptual measure in the child neuropsychological literature concerns finger recognition. In essence, the child's task is to identify by any one of several methods (e.g., pointing, naming) the finger or fingers touched, usually while hidden. Several procedures for examining finger recognition ability have been employed, both clinically and experimentally. Although the results reported in the literature are based on these different procedures, there is sufficient consistency among the findings to render tentative conclusions regarding the reliability and validity of the finger recognition construct, and the methods for its evaluation.

Two particular procedures for testing finger recognition ability have been utilized more commonly than others. In its current form, the standardized procedure developed by Benton et al. (1983) comprises three parts, each consisting of 20 items (10 per hand). In the first part, with the hand in full view, the child must indicate the finger touched by the examiner. In part B, the child is required to localize the finger that has been touched, this time while it was hidden from view. In part C, again with the hand hidden from view, the child is required to identify pairs of fingers touched simultaneously. For all components of the test, the child's hand rests on the table with the palm up. Touches are made in the fingertips with the pointed end of a pencil. Acceptable responses include naming the finger touched (e.g., ring finger), pointing to the appropriate finger on a drawn outline of the hand, or calling out the number of the finger indicated on the drawing.

The version of this test included in the Halstead–Reitan batteries, referred to as Tactile Finger Recognition, is similar to part B of Benton's test in that it requires the child to identify fingers touched singularly while hidden from view. However, unlike Benton's test, the hand is placed palm down on the table and the fingers are touched by the examiner's own finger just proximal to the nail bed. Younger children (5 to 8 years of age) are required to point to the appropriate finger whereas older children (9 to 14 years of age) indicate which finger was touched by reporting its designated number (thumb = 1, index = 2, etc.). Four trials are administered to each finger of each hand (thus, a total of 20 trials per hand).

Ordinarily, evidence of unilateral finger agnosia implicates involvement of the contralateral parietal region. In contrast, evidence of bilateral deficiencies in finger recognition is often found in children who have a lesion confined to the right parietal region (Rourke et al., 1983).

*Developmental considerations*

Interest in the development of finger recognition ability, as well as in the clinical significance of finger agnosia in children, was sparked by the early observations of Gerstmann (1924) that finger agnosia in adults was a symptom of brain dysfunction. Furthermore, he considered the combination of finger agnosia, right–left disorientation, agraphia, and acalculia as a result of a focal lesion of the left parieto-occipital region (Benton, 1979). These findings led investigators to examine the relationship in children between finger recognition ability and arithmetic achievement (e.g., Benton, Hutcheon and Seymour, 1951; Strauss and Werner, 1938). However, as Benton (1955) pointed out, before the clinical significance of finger agnosia could be assessed, normative data documenting the development of finger recognition in children was necessary.

With this aim in mind, Benton (1955) studied 158 grade-school children within the age range of 5.5 to 9.5 years on a finger recognition task that was very similar to the one currently in use (i.e., Benton et al., 1983). It was found that there was a progressive increase in performance through the ages studied and that localizing the fingers with the aid of vision (part A) was the easiest task to perform, whereas localizing pairs of fingers without the aid of vision (part C) was the most difficult. The performance of boys and girls was not significantly different. Based on the children's level of performance, it was suggested that finger-localizing skills are already in the process of development before the age of 6 years and are not yet completely developed in the 9-year-old, as their performance was below that of the average adult.

Using the same task, Wake (Wake, 1956, 1957; summarized in Benton, 1979) extended these normative data to include 9- to 12-year-old children.

Whereas increases in overall performance were observed, these were less dramatic than those exhibited by the younger children, and were primarily attributable to skill development in the localization of pairs of fingers (part C).

Given that a disturbance in finger recognition had come to be associated with deficiencies in reading, writing, and arithmetic, Lefford, Birch and Green (1974) reasoned that the early indication of normal or pathological development of finger recognition ability might be of value in identifying children at risk for developing a learning disability. Thus, Lefford et al. (1974) studied the development of finger recognition in preschool children aged 3 to 6 years. Twelve experimental tasks that varied according to the method of stimulus presentation (e.g., visual, visual–tactile, tactile only) and the mode of response (e.g., finger–thumb opposition, pointing to the stimulated fingers, pointing to a pictorial representation of the stimulated fingers) were administered to all 167 children. On those tasks relevant to the present review, the thumb was always stimulated with one of the other fingers.

On the task in which the child received both visual and tactile information, a steady increase in performance was observed until approximately age 4 years, after which a plateau was reached. By age 5, 99% of the children were able to complete this task successfully. Localization ability based on touch alone increased steadily across the age groups, attaining a 91% accuracy rate in the oldest group of children. Performance also steadily improved on a task in which the child was required to identify on a drawing the fingers touched by the examiner. However, this ability to identify fingers represented pictorially was not considered to be fully developed even in the oldest group studied. These children, aged 5 years, 6 months to 5 years, 11 months, only achieved a 71% accuracy rate. In addition, it was reported that finger recognition ability did not develop uniformly for all fingers; rather, the index and little fingers differentiated first, followed by the middle and ring fingers.

Lefford et al. (1974) concluded that the data supported the notion that three cognitive processes, each with its own timetable, contributed to the development of finger recognition. The first process, labelled intrasensory differentiation, was represented by the child's ability to point to the finger that was touched while in full view. The second process to emerge was that of intersensory integration. The task representing this process required that the child point to the finger that was touched while hidden from view. Here, the child must integrate tactile and visual information in order to be successful. The third process to emerge included representational thinking, as in identifying the stimulated fingers on an outline drawing of the hand. The findings of Lefford et al. (1974) suggest that tests of finger recognition are not purely sensory measures, but that they also include a substantial cognitive component.

A significant age effect in the development of finger recognition was also demonstrated by Mairuro et al. (1984) in their normative study of 5- to 8-year-old children utilizing the Reitan–Kløve version of the finger recognition test. Although no statistical analyses were reported, an age effect is also apparent in the normative data of Knights and Norwood (1980). This is particularly evident among the years of 5 to 10, with virtually no difference being observed in the performance of 10- to 14-year-olds. Visual inspection of the data from both of these studies suggests that right- and left-hand performance is similar at each age level.

Based on the developmental and normative studies described above, several tentative conclusions appear warranted. First, the findings are consistent with the hypothesis that several cognitive processes underlie neuropsychological tests designed to measure finger recognition ability, with each achieving a developmental plateau at a different age. The data suggest that the earliest process to emerge, that of finger differentiation, is probably fully developed by the age of 5 years. Scores on finger recognition measures, representing the process of intersensory integration, do not attain a plateau until children reach an age of 9 or 10 years. Performance on finger recognition tasks requiring the additional process of representational thinking appears to improve continually beyond age 9 or 10. However, determining the upper limit is difficult because the measures employed in the study of older children are not sufficiently precise and comprehensive as, for example, those incorporated by Lefford et al. (1974). It will be recalled that acceptable modes of response in the Finger Localization Test of Benton et al. (1983)

include naming the fingers, calling out their numbers, or pointing to their counterparts depicted on a model. Whereas each of these involves representational thinking, they vary in their cognitive nature (e.g., verbal vs. visual–spatial) and, therefore, may exhibit a different chronological ascendancy. Nevertheless, the data suggest that the representational aspects of finger recognition, in general, develop after the process of intersensory integration, probably sometime between 12 years of age and adulthood.

Second, gender and handedness do not appear to be related to finger recognition ability. However, there is some evidence to suggest that psychometric intelligence is a mediating factor in children, with bright children performing better than children of average intelligence (Benton et al., 1983).

*Reliability*

In his normative study, Benton (1955) provided information regarding the homogeneity and retest reliability of the early version (50-item) of the Finger Localization Test. Based on a corrected odd–even correlation coefficient, the internal consistency of the total test was found to be 0.91 for the entire sample of 158 cases. Coefficients of internal consistency for parts A (20 items), B (20 items), and C (10 items) were 0.91, 0.86, and 0.72, respectively. Using equivalent forms, retest reliability for a 20-minute interval was found to be 0.70 in a sample of 46 cases, and for a 10-week interval, 0.75 in a different sample of 25 cases.

Brown et al. (1989) examined the long-term ($M = 2.6$ years) stability of the Tactile Finger Recognition Test (Reitan, 1984) in both right- and left-handed children aged 5 to 14 years. For right-handed children, coefficients derived from the Pearson product–moment correlation and the intraclass correlation were 0.33 and 0.31, respectively, for the right (dominant) hand and 0.39 and 0.38, respectively, for the left hand. Pearson product–moment correlation and intraclass correlation coefficients for left-handed children were as follows: 0.62 for both procedures for the right (nondominant) hand and 0.69 for both for the left hand.

Overall, the findings from these two studies suggest that the reliability of finger recognition tests is good to excellent over the short-term and somewhat less adequate over the long-term. Of course, the co-efficients of short- and long-term reliability are not directly comparable because they are based on different procedures. Estimates of short-term reliability are based on Benton's (1955) test, which incorporates items reflecting a wider range of difficulty than do those found in the Reitan–Kløve procedure, the latter upon which the long-term estimates of reliability (stability) are based. Therefore, a relatively more restricted range of scores would be expected to result from the latter procedure which, in turn, would attenuate the correlation coefficient. In addition, reliability (stability) coefficients are more likely to be confounded by factors that are operative when retesting follows a longer interval (e.g., significant developmental change, the implementation of an intervention programme).

*Validity*

Many studies have examined the validity of finger recognition measures. Those addressing the relationship of finger recognition to brain damage will be considered first, followed by those that seek to determine its concurrent and predictive validity in regard to disorders of reading and arithmetic.

A number of investigations have examined the sensitivity of finger recognition measures to brain damage. Reitan (1971) found that a heterogeneous group of 5- to 8-year-old children with brain damage performed more poorly than did a normal control group on the Tactile Finger Recognition Test. Although the performances of both the dominant and nondominant hands were impaired, that of the nondominant hand was worse, a finding that also obtained for the tactile-perceptual measures of stereognosis and graphaesthesia. Reitan and Boll (1973) also found that younger ($M = 7.4$ years) brain-damaged children performed significantly worse than did normal children, thus replicating the results of Reitan (1971). In addition, the performance of the brain-damaged group was poorer than that of a group of academically deficient children and a group of children exhibiting behavioural problems. The control, academically deficient, and problem-behaviour groups did not differ from each other on this test.

Boll and Reitan (1972) reported that older (average age approximately 12 years) brain-damaged

children as compared to normal children also demonstrated a significant impairment on the Tactile Finger Recognition Test. Moreover, the brain-damaged group exhibited a significantly greater discrepancy between right- and left-hand performance as compared to the control group. Boll (1974) found that a group of older (9- to 14-year-old) brain-damaged children performed more poorly than did normal children with the right hand, but not the left hand.

Research concerning the neuropsychological correlates of learning disabilities has fostered a renewed interest in finger agnosia that began with the seminal work of Strauss and Werner (1938). Drawing on the studies of Gerstmann (1924) and their own clinical experiences as impetus for their study, Strauss and Werner (1938) examined the relationship between deficiencies in 'finger schema' and problems in arithmetic. They investigated two groups of boys: one considered by teachers to demonstrate 'excellent achievement in arithmetic', the other, 'a special arithmetic disability'. Although it was concluded that an 'intimate' relationship existed between finger schema and arithmetic ability, the methodological and statistical shortcomings of this study render their conclusions questionable (Benton, 1979). A further attempt to elucidate the relationship between finger recognition ability and arithmetic achievement offered no support for such an association, either in normal children or in adolescents with mild retardation (Benton et al., 1951).

More recently, studies conducted by Rourke and his associates have demonstrated a relationship between tactile-perceptual abilities and arithmetic achievement. Subtyping 9- to 14-year-old children according to their patterns of reading, spelling, and arithmetic achievement, Rourke and Strang (1978) found that a group of children with outstanding deficiencies in mechanical arithmetic and average to above-average reading and spelling performed significantly worse on a composite measure of tactile-perceptual abilities (including finger recognition) than did the group with reading–spelling or the group with reading–spelling–arithmetic disabilities. These results, in conjunction with the findings of other studies (e.g., Rourke and Finlayson, 1978; Strang and Rourke, 1983) have led to the formulation of the nonverbal learning disabilities (NLD) syndrome of which deficiencies in arithmetic achievement and bilateral tactile-perceptual abilities are an integral part (Rourke, 1989). Moreover, it has been found that children classified as exhibiting the NLD syndrome demonstrate age-related decrements in performance in these areas and in areas of psychomotor, visual, perceptual, organizational, and nonverbal concept-formation and problem-solving abilities (Casey, Rourke and Picard, 1991). The results of these studies support the notion that (a) a relationship between finger recognition ability and arithmetic achievement exists, and (b) the nature of the relationship is not a simple or direct one. Rather, the deficiencies in either of these abilities are probably the result of some other factor or set of factors that are more cognitive in nature.

Several studies have examined the relationship between finger recognition and reading achievement. The findings of those studies evaluating the concurrent relationship have been mixed. For example, Croxen and Lytton (1971) found that a group of 9- to 10-year-old children with reading disabilities encountered significantly greater difficulty on a finger recognition task similar to that of Benton's (1955) than did a group of normal readers. A significant correlation between finger recognition and reading ability was reported by Hutchinson (1983), who examined three groups of children: those with normal language, dysphasic children, and children with language impairments other than dysphasia.

Reed (1967) investigated the relationship between lateralized deficiencies in finger recognition and reading achievement in children at two age levels. No relationship emerged between lateralized finger agnosia and reading achievement in children 6 years of age. However, in the 10-year-old children, the group that exhibited finger agnosia lateralized to the right side of the body read at a significantly lower level than did those who demonstrated finger agnosia lateralized to the left side.

In contrast to the above findings, Nolan et al. (1983) did not find evidence of differential performance on finger recognition among groups of 7- to 13-year-old children classified as normal, reading–spelling disabled, and arithmetic disabled. Other studies have also failed to demonstrate a relationship (e.g., Clements and Peters, 1962; Lyle, 1969).

A series of studies based on the Florida Longitudinal Project have addressed, among other things, the concurrent and predictive validity of finger recognition ability with respect to reading achievement (see Fletcher and Satz, 1984, for a review of the project and its results). A battery of neuropsychological and cognitive tests assembled for the purpose of predicting Kindergarten (KG) children at risk for subsequent academic learning problems was administered to a group of children at the beginning of KG and at the end of Grade 2 and Grade 5. Teacher-based measures of reading achievement were collected yearly from Grade 1 through Grade 6, and test-based measures of academic achievement were obtained at the end of Grades 2 and 5. It was found that finger recognition ability (assessed in KG) had the highest predictive value for Grade 2 reading performance among the measures employed (Satz, Taylor, Friel and Fletcher, 1978). Subsequent studies demonstrated that the predictive power of finger recognition tasks, based an KG performance, decreased with advancing grade levels, and that concurrent measures of verbal-conceptual abilities correlated better with reading in later grades (Fletcher and Satz, 1980; Fletcher, Taylor, Morris and Satz, 1982).

Lindgren (1978) also investigated the predictive validity of finger recognition for future reading disability. Several finger recognition tasks along with the Peabody Picture Vocabulary Test, Beery Developmental Test of Visual–Motor Integration, and a task of letter naming were administered to 100 kindergarten pupils. Achievement measures administered at the end of Grade 1 included teacher ratings of reading and arithmetic ability, and the Vocabulary and Comprehension subtests of the Gates–McGinitie Reading Test. It was found that poor readers scored significantly lower than adequate readers on all measures, with group differences being largest for letter naming, followed by finger recognition. Finger recognition performance alone correctly classified 75% of the children as either poor or adequate readers. Interestingly, finger recognition was also found to predict poor arithmetic achievement.

The results of studies examining the validity of finger recognition suggest that (a) it is a sensitive measure of brain damage in children, (b) in heterogeneous groups of brain-damaged children, finger agnosia is likely to be more evident, either in frequency or severity, with the left hand as compared to the right hand, (c) it is associated with academic deficiencies in both reading and arithmetic, but that the relationship is a complex one and is likely related to other aspects of cognitive functioning, and therefore, (d) the results of such measures are best interpreted within the context of a comprehensive neuropsychological examination.

## Discussion and implications for future research

When compared to other functional domains typically evaluated in the course of a neuropsychological assessment, the literature relevant to tactile-perceptual measures is relatively sparse. Nevertheless, our review suggests that some tentative conclusions are warranted regarding the contributions of tactile-perceptual measures to the understanding of brain–behaviour relationships in children.

It is clear that tactile-perceptual functions are usually compromised in children with frank brain injury. In general, age appears to be a mediating factor in the expression of these deficiencies: younger children (5- to 8-year-olds) tend to demonstrate greater impairments than do older children (9- to 14-year-olds). For measures of stereognosis, graphaesthesia, and finger recognition, the research findings demonstrate relatively consistently that impairments exhibited by brain-damaged children tend to be more evident for the left hand than for the right hand, regardless of age. In addition, it is suggested, based on the results of studies examining the sensitivity of neuropsychological measures to brain damage in children, that tactile-perceptual measures do not discriminate groups of children so afflicted from comparison groups as well as do measures reflecting most other functional domains (e.g., motor and psychomotor, problem-solving, and concept-formation). This view is supported by the study by Nici and Reitan (1986), which compared the relative degree of impairment among four categories of brain-related abilities (i.e., motor, somatosensory, general neuropsychological, and verbal/academic). In addition, the findings of Thompson et al. (1994) suggest that somatosensory measures are less sensitive than other measures to neuropsychological changes (recovery and maturation) that follow acquired brain injuries (in their study, closed head injury).

It is important to note that the aforementioned generalizations are based on studies that, for the most part, have employed heterogeneous groups of brain-damaged children. The neuropathological diseases represented in these groups, such as closed head injury, perinatal trauma, encephalitis, and infantile hemiplegia, are typical of the neurological conditions found in children. It is well recognized that the majority of these affect the parenchyma of the brain diffusely, rather than in a focal manner. Thus, the extent to which the above generalizations would follow from studies of children with lateralized or focal abnormalities remains speculative. Clearly, investigative studies employing groups of children with neurologically homogeneous and focal conditions, as is now common in the adult literature, are necessary to further our understanding of brain–behaviour relationships in children. Given that focal neuropathological disorders are uncommon in children as compared to adults, it appears that much of this research will need to rely on detailed case studies as well as long-term projects wherein a sufficiently large number of cases could accumulate to permit the appropriate utilization of statistical procedures.

It is reasonable to expect that the pathognomonic nature of tactile-perceptual impairments might make it difficult to discriminate target groups from comparison groups. That group differences do emerge despite this limitation inherent in tactile-perceptual measures suggests that, on an individual basis, evidence of impaired performance carries considerable diagnostic information. This view is supported by clinical experience and case-study data. Moreover, it is suggested that the presence of tactile-perceptual deficits in children suffering from brain injury may convey important prognostic information.

For example, during the acute phases of a significant insult to the brain (e.g., a severe traumatic brain injury), it is often the case that children exhibit bilateral deficits in somatosensory perception. With the passing of time — and, presumably, some recovery of brain function — a pattern of unilateral somatosensory imperception, suppression, or other tactile deficiency may emerge. That one side of the body remains affected while the other has 'recovered' is usually thought to mirror (a) 'general brain recovery' (e.g., the subsiding of brain edema), and (b) the probability of some degree of relatively permanent dysfunction in those skills and abilities subserved by some systems in the area of the brain contralateral to the affected side. Thus, the persistence of deficits in unilateral somatosensory perception is thought to hold some prognostic significance for neuropsychological skills and abilities. For example, right-sided somatosensory deficits that persist in the face of greatly diminished or absent left-sided deficits may suggest a very negative prognostic outcome for any aphasia that emerged at the time of the brain insult.

However, there is another dimension of the prognostic significance of somatosensory deficits that should be emphasized. This can be illustrated by continuing with our example of recovery following traumatic brain injury. It is usually the case that unilateral somatosensory deficits (that persist after an initial stage of bilateral impairment) decline in severity as a function of time since injury. However, this decline in the severity of somatosensory deficits may not be accompanied by a correlative decline in other skill and ability deficits. For example, it is common to observe a decline in right-sided somatosensory deficits that is not accompanied by a decline in aphasic signs. Thus, although the persistence of right-sided somatosensory deficits may be predictive of a poor outcome for any existing aphasic deficits, the decline of these right-sided somatosensory deficits may not be — and, usually, is not — necessarily linked to a decline in the linguistic disturbances that were exhibited following the brain insult.

*Significance of early somatosensory experiences and impairments*

In the developmental presentation of the NLD syndrome, basic and early emergent deficits in tactile-perceptual skills are thought to play a very significant role in the eventual manifestations of impaired problem-solving, concept-formation, and related cognitive abilities (Rourke, 1989, 1995b). One of the conceptual bases for this linkage is the position of Piaget (1954) regarding the importance of intact sensorimotor functioning as one of the early developmental pillars upon which formal operational thought is based.

It is clear that the 'world' of the young child is, in the main, one that could be characterized as searching, locating, encountering, and exploring objects in the physical world. The manipulations of the elements of this world are generally through the contact senses of touch and taste. Of course, one would not want to suggest a diminished role for vision in this process. Indeed, the processes of searching, locating, and exploring are greatly enhanced thereby. However, the young child's encounters with the physical world are largely haptic in nature. It is clear that smooth affectional encounters between persons, regardless of age or stage of development, are greatly enhanced by the presence of intact somatosensory capacities. Indeed, one would be inclined to maintain that intimate exchanges between persons would be all but impossible without such capacities. Clearly, the early bonding between parent and child that is thought to be so important for subsequent psychosocial development is largely a function of exchanges through the somatosensory systems.

With growth and maturity, the child comes to depend more on the distance senses for knowledge of the world. The encounters with this world are largely representational in nature rather than characterized by immediate physical contact, haptic or otherwise. Nevertheless, the knowledge gained through immediate haptic contact, especially during the early phases of development, is thought by many to be essential for normal intellectual growth.

Of interest in this regard is the case of S.B., a 52-year-old man whose vision was partially restored after what was until that point a lifetime of blindness (Gregory, 1972). S.B. demonstrated that he could, without any special training, recognize by sight, or represent by drawings, objects that he had experienced tactually at some time during his life. For example, after his vision was restored, he was able to read immediately by sight numbers and upper case letters, symbols that were presented to him as raised forms on wooden blocks when he was a youngster in the school for the blind. Not only could he not recognize lower case letters, symbols for which he had no previous tactile experience, he also exhibited considerable difficulty in learning them. These findings are consistent with the notion that information acquired through the tactile modality is important for intellectual development.

Also of interest is the work of Eilers and her colleagues who have demonstrated the influence of early tactile experiences on cognitive development. For example, one study evaluated the effects of tactile stimulation on phonological development of young hearing-impaired children. Two groups of children from classrooms for the profoundly hearing-impaired were followed over a 3-year period (Eilers, Fishman, Oller and Steffens, 1993). Children in the experimental group were provided with tactile vocoders that converted acoustic information into tactile stimuli. A set of solenoid vibrators enables the user to experience a real-time spectral display of sound as a dynamically moving pattern of sensation on the skin. At baseline, all children produced little intelligible speech and did not differ significantly in phonological production abilities. By Year 3, the tactilely aided group showed significantly greater gains in production than did the comparison group, a difference that was largely due to improvements in consonant production. These findings illustrate the influence of tactile perception and intersensory integration on cognitive development (in this case, phonological production) and suggest that incorporating early tactile stimulation as part of an intervention programme may have significant remedial benefits for some neuropsychological disorders.

Another line of research has demonstrated the prognostic implications of early tactile-perceptual impairments. Although the findings have been mixed, recent studies have provided evidence supporting the association between delays in the development of finger recognition and reading disabilities. Research based on the Florida Longitudinal Project has demonstrated convincingly that evidence of finger agnosia in preschoolers is predictive of subsequent problems in learning to read. However, it has also been shown that the strength of this association is decreased in older children with reading disabilities. Thus, it appears that the relationship between these two variables is not a direct one, but rather that both are dependent upon other, and possibly related, developmental processes.

It may be that the cognitive processes thought to be fundamental to the development of finger recognition (viz., intrasensory differentiation, intersensory integration, and representational/symbolic thinking) play an important role in the development of reading skills. Indeed, a model proposed by Goldberg and Costa (1981), which was later adapted by Rourke (1982, 1989) to embody neurodevelopmental dimen-

sions, is consistent with this notion. It is thought that systems within the right cerebral hemisphere are especially critical for the acquisition of new skills. Important elements to this process involve the capacity for intermodal integration and the ability to deal with novel, or otherwise complex, information for which there is no preexisting neural code. In contrast, systems within the left cerebral hemisphere are thought to be crucial for the stereotypic application of codes that have been previously learned. From a rational perspective, one can conceive of the learning-to-read process, by definition a novel task initially, as involving intrasensory differentiation (e.g., visual discrimination of letters), intersensory integration (e.g., association of graphemes and phonemes), and representational/symbolic thinking (e.g., appreciating the semantic content of words and phrases). As the child becomes more proficient in each of these skills, they are expected to be increasingly under the control of left hemisphere systems. Empirically, evidence exists that supports this hypothesized progression (e.g., Bakker, 1979). Whereas this likely represents a simplified account of the learning-to-read process, it serves to illustrate how deficiencies in one or more of these processes might influence performance on tasks of both finger recognition and reading.

Finally, it has become clear that tactile-perceptual deficits, hypothesized to be among the primary deficits in NLD (Rourke, 1989, 1995a), are outstandingly poor in children with NLD (Casey et al., 1991; Harnadek and Rourke, 1994). This is also the case in many forms of paediatric neurological disease wherein the NLD phenotype is manifest (Rourke, 1995b).

Although the contributions that measurements of somatosensory skills have made to our understanding of brain–behaviour relationships in children are clearly evident from this review, considerable progress remains to be realized. The outstanding issues of 10 years ago remain. These focus on the lack of information regarding the reliability of somatosensory measures and the virtual absence of studies examining groups of children with focal neuropathological conditions for which specific hypotheses concerning brain–behaviour relationships could be tested. That early tactile interventions based on sound neuropsychological theory and scientific procedures might provide new avenues for the treatment of cognitive disorders in children also deserves our research attention.

# References

Bakker DJ: Hemispheric differences and reading strategies: Two dyslexias? Bulletin of the Orton Society: 23; 15–27, 1979.

Barr ML, Kiernan JA: The Human Nervous System: An Anatomical Viewpoint. New York: Harper and Row, 1983.

Benton AL: Development of finger-localization capacity in school children. Child Development: 26; 225–230, 1955.

Benton AL: The neuropsychological significance of finger recognition. In Bortner M (Ed), Cognitive Growth and Development: Essays in Memory of Herbert G. Birch. New York: Brunner/Mazel, pp. 85–104, 1979.

Benton AL, Hamsher K DeS, Varney NR, Spreen O: Contributions to neuropsychological assessment. New York: Oxford University Press, 1983.

Benton AL, Hutcheon JF, Seymour E: Arithmetic ability, finger-localization capacity and right–left discrimination in normal and defective children. American Journal of Orthopsychiatry: 21; 756–766, 1951.

Boll TJ: Conceptual vs. perceptual vs. motor deficits in brain-damaged children. Journal of Clinical Psychology: 28; 157–159, 1972.

Boll TJ: Behavioural correlates of cerebral damage in children aged 9 through 14. In Reitan RM, Davison LA (Eds), Clinical Neuropsychology: Current Status and Applications. Washington, DC: V.H. Winston and Sons Inc., pp. 91–120, 1974.

Boll TJ, Reitan RM: Motor and tactile-perceptual deficits in brain-damaged and normal children. Perceptual and Motor Skills: 34; 343–350, 1972.

Brodal A: Neurological Anatomy in Relation to Clinical Medicine. New York: Oxford, 1981.

Brown SJ, Rourke BP, Cicchetti DV: Reliability of tests and measures used in the neuropsychological assessment of children. Clinical Neuropsychology: 3; 353–368, 1989.

Casey JE, Rourke BP, Picard EM: Syndrome of nonverbal learning disabilities: Age differences in neuropsychological, academic, and socioemotional functioning. Developmental Psychopathology: 3; 329–345, 1991.

Clements SD, Peters JE: Minimal brain dysfunctions in the school-age child. Archives of General Psychiatry: 6; 195–197, 1962.

Croxen ME, Lytton H: Reading disability and difficulties in finger localization and right–left discrimination. Developmental Psychology: 5; 256–262, 1971.

Dekaban A: Neurology of Early Childhood. Baltimore, MD: William and Wilkins, 1970.

DeMaio-Feldman D: Somatosensory processing abilities of very low-birth weight infants at school age. The American Journal of Occupational Therapy: 48; 639–645, 1994.

Eilers RE, Fishman LM, Oller DK, Steffens ML: Tactile vocoders as aids to speech production in young hearing-impaired children. The Volta Review: 95; 265–293, 1993.

Fink MD, Bender MB: Perception of simultaneous tactile stimuli in normal children. Neurology: 3; 27–34, 1953.

Fletcher JM, Satz P: Developmental changes in the neuropsychological correlates of reading achievement: a six-year longitudinal followup. Journal of Clinical Psychology: 2; 23–37, 1980.

Fletcher JM, Satz P: Preschool prediction of reading failure. In Levine MD, Satz P (Eds), Middle Childhood: Development and Dysfunction. Baltimore, MD: University Park Press, pp. 153–182, 1984.

Fletcher JM, Taylor HG, Morris R, Satz P: Finger recognition skills and reading achievement: A developmental neuropsychological analysis. Developmental Psychology: 18; 124–132, 1982.

Gerstmann J: Fingeragnosie: Eine umschriebene Störung der Orientierung am eigenen Körper. Wiener klinische Wochenschrift: 37; 1010–1012, 1924.

Goldberg E, Costa LD: Hemisphere differences in the acquisition and use of descriptive systems. Brain and Language: 14; 144–173, 1981.

Gregory RL: Eye and Brain: The Psychology of Seeing. New York: World University Press, 1972.

Harlow HF, Zimmerman RR: The development of affectional responses in infant monkeys. Proceedings of the American Philosophical Society: 102; 501–509, 1958.

Harnadek MCS, Rourke BP: Principal identifying features of the syndrome of nonverbal learning disabilities in children. Journal of Learning Disabilities: 27; 144–154, 1994.

Hutchinson BB: Finger localization and reading ability in three groups of children ages three through twelve. Brain and Language: 20; 143–154, 1983.

Klonoff H, Robinson GC, Thompson G: Acute and chronic brain syndromes in children. Developmental Medicine and Child Neurology: 11; 198–213, 1969.

Knights RM, Norwood JA: Revised Smoothed Normative Data of the Neuropsychological Test Battery for Children. Ottawa, ON: Author, 1980.

Lefford A, Birch HG, Green G: The perceptual and cognitive basis for finger localization and selective finger movement in preschool children. Child Development: 45; 335–343, 1974.

Lindgren SD: Finger localization and the prediction of reading disability. Cortex: 14; 87–101, 1978.

Lyle JG: Reading retardation and reversal tendency. Child Development: 40; 833–843, 1969.

Mairuro RD, Townes BD, Vitaliano PP, Trupin EW: Age norms for the Reitan–Indiana Neuropsychological Test Battery for children. In Glow RA (Ed), Advances in the Behavioral Measurement of Children: A Research Annual. Greenwich, CT: Jai Press Inc., pp. 159–173, 1984.

Nici J, Reitan RM: Patterns of neuropsychological ability in brain-disordered versus normal children. Journal of Consulting and Clinical Psychology: 54; 542–545, 1986.

Nieuwenhuys R, Voogd J, van Huijzen C: The Human Central Nervous System: A Synopsis and Atlas. Berlin: Springer, 1981.

Nolan DR, Hammeke TA, Barkley RA: A comparison of the patterns of the neuropsychological performance in two groups of learning disabled children. Journal of Clinical Child Psychology: 12; 22–27, 1983.

Paine RS, Oppé TE: Neurological Examination of Children. London: Heinemann Medical Books Ltd., 1966.

Parush S, Sohmer H, Steinberg A, Kaitz M: Somatosensory functioning in children with attention deficit hyperactivity disorder. Developmental Medicine and Child Neurology: 39; 464–468, 1997.

Pause M, Kunesch E, Binkofski F, Freund H-J: Sensorimotor disturbances in patients with lesions of the parietal cortex. Brain: 112; 1599–1625, 1989.

Piaget J: The Origins of Intelligence in Children. New York: International Universities Press, 1952.

Piaget J: Construction of Reality in the Child. New York: Basic Books, 1954.

Reed JC: Lateralized finger agnosia and reading achievement at ages 6 and 10. Child Development: 38; 213–220, 1967.

Reed HBC Jr, Reitan RM, Kløve H: Influence of cerebral lesions on psychological test performances of older children. Journal of Consulting Psychology: 29; 247–251, 1965.

Reitan RM: Sensorimotor functions in brain-damaged and normal children of early school age. Perceptual and Motor Skills: 33; 655–664, 1971.

Reitan RM: Psychological effects of cerebral lesions in children of early school age. In Reitan RM, Davison LA (Eds), Clinical Neuropsychology: Current Status and Applications. Washington, DC: Winston and Sons, pp. 53–89, 1974.

Reitan RM: Aphasia and Sensory-Perceptual Deficits in Children. Tucson, AZ: Neuropsychology Press, 1984.

Reitan RM, Boll TJ: Neuropsychological correlates of minimal brain dysfunction. Annals of the New York Academy of Sciences: 205; 65–88, 1973.

Roeltgen MG, Roeltgen DP: Asymmetrical lateralized attention in children. Developmental Neuropsychology: 6; 25–37, 1990.

Rourke BP: Central processing deficiencies in children: Toward a developmental neuropsychological model. Journal of Clinical Neuropsychology: 4; 1–18, 1982.

Rourke BP: Nonverbal Learning Disabilities: The Syndrome and the Model. New York: Guilford Press, 1989.

Rourke BP: Introduction and overview: The NLD/white matter model. In Rourke BP (Ed), Syndrome of Nonverbal Learning Disabilities: Neurodevelopmental Manifestations. New York: Guilford Press, pp. 1–26, 1995a.

Rourke BP: Syndrome of Nonverbal Learning Disabilities: Neurodevelopmental Manifestations. New York: Guilford Press, 1995b.

Rourke BP, Bakker DJ, Fisk JL, Strang JD: Child Neuropsychology: An Introduction to Theory, Research, and Clinical Practice. New York: Guilford Press, 1983.

Rourke BP, Finlayson MAJ: Neuropsychological significance of variations in patterns of academic performance: Verbal and visual–spatial abilities. Journal of Abnormal Child Psychology Psychology: 6; 121–133, 1978.

Rourke BP, Fisk JL, Strang JD: Neuropsychological Assessment of Children: A Treatment-oriented Approach. New York: Guilford Press, 1986.

Rourke BP, Strang JD: Neuropsychological significance of variations in patterns of academic performance: motor, psychomotor, and tactile-perceptual abilities. Journal of Pediatric Psychology: 3; 62–66, 1978.

Satz P, Taylor GH, Friel J, Fletcher JM: Some developmental and predictive precursors of reading disabilities: a six-year follow-up. In Benton AL, Pearl D (Eds), Dyslexia: An Appraisal of Current Knowledge. New York: Oxford University Press, pp. 315–347, 1978.

Spreen O, Benton AL: comparative studies of some psychological tests for cerebral damage. Journal of Nervous and Mental Disease: 140; 323–333, 1965.

Strang JD, Rourke BP: Concept-formation/non-verbal reasoning abilities of children who exhibit specific academic problems with arithmetic. Journal of Clinical Child Psychology: 12; 33–39, 1983.

Strauss A, Werner H: Deficiency in the finger schema in relation to arithmetic disability. American Journal of Orthopsychiatry: 8; 719–725, 1938.

Thompson NM, Francis DJ, Stuebing KK, Fletcher JM, Ewing-Cobbs L, Miner ME, Levin HS, Eisenberg HM: Motor, visual–spatial, and somatosensory skills after closed head injury in children and adolescents: A study of change. Neuropsychology: 8; 333–342, 1994.

Tsushima WT, Towne WS: Neuropsychological abilities of young children with questionable brain disorders. Journal of Consulting and Clinical Psychology: 45; 757–762, 1977.

Wake FR: Finger localization in Canadian school children. Paper presented at the meeting of the Canadian Psychological Association, Ottawa, Ontario, June 1956.

Wake FR: Finger localization scores in defective children. Paper presented at the meeting of the Canadian Psychological Association, Toronto, Ontario, June 1957.

# Subject Index *

---

\* Underlined page numbers indicate in-depth treatment.